OXFORD MEDICAL PUBLICATIONS

A new system of anatomy

A new system of anatomy
A dissector's guide and atlas

Lord Zuckerman

Professor Emeritus, University of Birmingham
Professor Emeritus, University of East Anglia

Second edition

revised in collaboration with
Dr Deryk Darlington
Department of Anatomy, University of Birmingham, and
Professor F. Peter Lisowski
Department of Anatomy, University of Hong Kong

Oxford New York Toronto Melbourne
OXFORD UNIVERSITY PRESS
1981

Oxford University Press, Walton Street, Oxford OX2 6DP

OXFORD LONDON GLASGOW
NEW YORK TORONTO MELBOURNE WELLINGTON
IBADAN NAIROBI DAR ES SALAAM LUSAKA CAPE TOWN
KUALA LUMPUR SINGAPORE JAKARTA HONG KONG TOKYO
DELHI BOMBAY CALCUTTA MADRAS KARACHI

First edition 1961
Second edition 1981

British Library Cataloguing in Publication Data

Zuckerman, Solly, *Baron Zuckerman*
A new system of anatomy.—2nd ed.
—(Oxford medical publications).
1. Human dissection   2. Anatomy, Human
—Laboratory manuals
I. Title   II. Darlington, Deryk
III. Lisowski, Peter   IV. Series
611'.0028   QM34   79–41193
ISBN 0-19-263137-3
ISBN 0-19-263136-5 (*paperback*)

*Printed in Great Britain by
Butler & Tanner Ltd, Frome and London*

Preface to second edition

The term 'anatomy' is used in the title of the *New System* in its strict sense of dissection by 'cutting asunder', and not more generally to signify the body of knowledge which comprehends all that is known about the structure and relations of the parts of the human frame. To make the purpose and design of the book absolutely clear, I have now subtitled it '*A Dissector's Guide and Atlas*'.

In essence, the book provides a series of instructions which the average medical student should be able to follow on his or her own in the dissecting room, without calling unduly for help from demonstrators. To this end, the text was repeatedly revised before it was originally published, and also furnished with a comprehensive series of realistic illustrations, as opposed to idealized pictures of what a student was supposed to see when he dissected.

Needless to say, the structure of the body has not changed in the twenty years since the book has been in use. Experience has, however, shown where some further changes can be made both to simplify even more the task of the student and to allow for the fact that the never-ending expansion of the medical curriculum as a whole has meant that the hours that medical students are expected to spend in the dissecting room have, in some schools, had to be reduced. The same principle which governed the design and writing of the first edition has therefore been used to delete, where possible, instructional detail whose omission it is felt will not be prejudicial to the amount of anatomical knowledge which is indispensable to the medical student both in his further studies and in his subsequent professional career. Experience has also indicated the advisability of rearranging the suggested order of dissection of a few parts of the body, particularly of the upper part of the neck. The instructions for the dissection of the heart have been simplified, and a new section added to deal with the practical problems of dissecting the brain when shortage of material does not allow of each group of students being given two specimens to study. The sections on the limbs and the abdomen have been least changed. New paragraphs of instructions on surface anatomy have been added to help the student study the actions of muscles and movements of joints.

A few illustrations have been omitted as being unnecessary when text has been reduced, for example in the description of the thoracolumbar fascia, and a limited number of new ones added. At the same time, the opportunity has been taken to reverse some figures so as to make their left to right orientation constant. Others have been reduced in size when doing so has not affected clarity.

Obviously, the more time a student devotes to his dissection the better will be his knowledge of the structure of the body. The custom in the Birmingham Medical School when I launched the book was to devote some 300 hours to the dissection of the whole body. I am assured that the present text could be satisfactorily mastered in about 200.

A further simplification has been introduced by changing the nomenclature used in the book. In the original edition I mainly followed the international system known as the Paris *Nomina Anatomica*, or PNA, and, as far as possible, the English versions of the Latin terms. But with the continuing decline in the teaching of Latin in schools, and with the failure of the international *Nomina Anatomica* to come into general use, it has been thought sensible to make no reference at all in the text to Latin terms except where they are in common use. In those exceptional cases where no PNA Latin form was ever available, the book continues to employ whatever English term for a structure is in commonest use in English-speaking countries.

The original double-entry index has been retained, and Latin entries are now followed by the English terms. The Index can thus serve as an English–Latin, Latin–English dictionary for those anatomical terms used in the text; but it cannot be regarded as either an exhaustive or as a necessarily accurate guide to the latest, the fourth, edition of the *Nomina Anatomica*. The aim has been to maintain as great a degree of compatibility with the current international terminology as English usage allows.

I am grateful to several colleagues in schools other than Birmingham who were kind enough to write to me after the book first appeared, pointing out minor textual errors which inevitably seem to creep in regardless of the care that is taken to avoid them. The necessary corrections were made in the second and later impressions of the First Edition, Dr Peter Dallas Ross, who had given unstintingly of his help in the preparation of the book, undertaking their collation.

The close examination of the text which has resulted in such changes as have been introduced in this Edition was mainly the work of Dr Deryk Darlington and Professor Peter Lisowski. Dr Darlington was also responsible for the new instructions for the dissection of the brain (pp. 6.30 to 6.35) and Professor Lisowski for those dealing with the dissection of the heart (pp. 3.29 to 3.38). I am grateful to Professor Charles Oxnard, at whose suggestion some paragraphs on surface anatomy have been added and the lists of contents of the separate parts of the body modified.

The untimely death of Mr W. J. Pardoe, with whom I had worked so closely in devising the illustrations of the book, deprived me of his help in producing the new figures required for this edition. For these I owe thanks to Mr John Petty, and also to Mr Norman Fahy, who was responsible for Figures 5.23 and 5.108.

Lord Zuckerman
May 1979

Preface to first edition

Teachers of medical students have long agreed that some traditional parts of the curriculum must be streamlined if the student of today is to have time to learn about the many new fields of knowledge which now affect the practice of medicine. Indeed, with the accelerating growth of scientific knowledge, pruning would be necessary even if one were to contemplate an increase in the duration of a medical student's university life from its present span of six years to, say, seven or even eight. These considerations led me, some fifteen years ago, to reorganize the course of topographical anatomy in my own Department, and later, after experimenting with such texts as were available, to design a new practical book from the sequence of dissections which we adopted. My aim was to provide a guide to the course of instruction in regional anatomy which precedes clinical studies, and which, in the United Kingdom, leads to the Second Professional Examination in Medicine (the 'Second MB'). A first draft of such a dissecting manual was issued for use in typescript form eight years ago. Minor modifications were subsequently made in the text and then, starting some four years ago, the entire book was re-written in the light of the experience we had gained, and on the basis of an extensive series of new dissections specially made for the purpose.

Topographical anatomy is essentially a visual discipline, and my text accordingly deals only with the kind of anatomy that can be demonstrated and learnt in the dissecting room. All matters irrelevant to this purpose have, as far as possible, been excluded. The principle I have followed is to give directions for dissection and examination from which the student should be able to make his own observations and discoveries. As now published, the text has been rigorously and extensively tested in the dissecting room on numerous cadavers and by hundreds of dissectors. The sequence of dissections that is described covers the entire body, and can be adapted to practical courses of any desired duration, provided that a total of at least 300 hours is devoted to work in the dissecting room.

Knowing that the average student soon forgets the mass of anatomical detail he is sometimes enjoined to learn, and with the object of encouraging the kind of study which provides a three-dimensional idea of the structure of the body, I have tried to eliminate detail which has no apparent scientific or educational value, or which, to the best of my knowledge, has little obvious clinical significance.

No two anatomists are likely to agree precisely about what constitutes unnecessary detail in the dissecting room. On the principle that a student should be asked to dissect only what can be dissected adequately, we hold that he should be discouraged from spending precious time trying to reveal features which can be demonstrated only on special preparations (for example, preparations which display the lymphatic system), and which can be conveniently learnt from a textbook. On the other hand, structures which can be easily demonstrated on the cadaver may not necessarily be important either scientifically or clinically, whereas something important may be difficult to display. How one draws a line between these two extremes is a matter of personal judgement. No one would deny that the student should have a clear idea of the course of the vagus nerve, or of the ureter, or of the ulnar nerve. These are all important structures. Correspondingly, it is generally agreed that the veins can usually be disregarded in a dissection. But if this latter principle were carried too far, it would mean that the student left his anatomical studies without knowing the disposition of the external jugular veins, or without knowing that the right suprarenal vein is so short that the right suprarenal gland is very closely applied to the inferior vena cava. The emphasis of a dissection might also be influenced by the ease with which some particular and relatively 'unimportant' dissecting room feature can be displayed. If, to give a specific example, the posterior superior alveolar branches of the superior alveolar nerves were difficult to display, I should not suggest to the medical student that he tries to dissect them, in spite of their clinical interest. In fact, however, they are easily dissected, and for that reason we suggest that our students do so.

In my view it is not the function of a pre-clinical department to teach the applied anatomy which is the concern of the surgeon or physician. When he moves from the Department of Anatomy to his clinical studies, the student should certainly be expected to appreciate what is involved anatomically in, say, the surgical approach to the heart or in the conditions of foot-drop or ulnar paralysis, after he has been told what these things mean from the point of view of medical practice. But I should not expect him to make a clinical diagnosis of foot-drop or ulnar paralysis merely on the basis of his work in the dissecting room. The primary purpose of a medical student's studies in the dissecting room, during his first or first and second pre-clinical years, can only be to provide an adequate knowledge of structure with which to articulate what is learnt in other parts of the medical curriculum. I am talking, of course, of the student who proposes following a career in some branch of medical practice, and not of the small number who are likely to make anatomy itself their field of specialist study.

I have introduced into the text no more and no less osteology than the student needs to understand how the soft parts of the body relate to its bony structure. The educational value of such osteological matters with which I have not dealt is extraneous to the understanding of dissecting room anatomy.

After experimenting with several methods of illustration, from simple line drawings to untouched photographs, I finally decided to rely mainly on touched-up photographs of actual dissections which display what a student should see when he follows the text. So far as possible figures have been placed either on the page opposite to the relevant text, or on the same page. A few have been repeated.

The nomenclature used is, wherever possible, an English equivalent of the Paris *Nomina Anatomica* (PNA) as agreed at the Sixth International Congress of Anatomists held in Paris in 1955, and as revised at the Seventh Congress in New York in 1960. The international convention about the omission of hyphens between vowels has also been followed, but with regret and, at times, even with dismay. Further details about nomenclature are given on pages 0.6 to 0.11.

In most British dissecting rooms four students are concerned in a single dissection of the head and neck, which early on entails the removal of the skull-cap (calvaria) and, later, of other parts of the specimen, the remains of which finally have to be bisected. The method described in my own text is to bisect the head and neck at an early stage, as this makes it easier for pairs of students to dissect simultaneously without getting in each other's way. This technique, which was suggested to me by Dr F. P. Reagan, a former member of my staff, is very easy for the student to follow, and also makes it possible to examine cranial features from both their medial and lateral aspects. As indicated in the text, however, the stage where the bisection is performed can be deferred, if that is desired. Another technique that is advocated is decalcification of the temporal bone, in order to simplify the dissection of the middle and internal ear.

In the Department of Anatomy in the University of Birmingham the 300 hours of dissection my text entails are easily fitted into a student's first year in the Medical School. This obviates the need for lecturers and demonstrators to deal at one and the same time with overlapping years of students in the dissecting room—otherwise an inevitable consequence of the more conventional five-term course of most British schools. In order to help the student a certain amount of repetition and summarization has been deliberately introduced into the text of this dissecting manual (particularly in the section on the head and neck, whose dissection does not follow as flowing a course as that of other parts of the body). For convenience, a brief statement of the layout of the lymphatic system has been included as an appendix to this book. Under the Birmingham system the student also has an opportunity to consolidate what he learns in the dissecting room through separate classes in Surface and Radiological Anatomy. Courses on Neurology, in which Neuro-anatomy and Neuro-physiology are combined, and on Growth, are given when the student has completed his studies in the dissecting room.

The average total time devoted to the study of the different parts of the body in my own dissecting room is as follows:

Upper Limb	44 hours
Lower Limb	44 hours
Thorax	23 hours
Abdomen	75 hours
Head and Neck	117 hours

While the form, content and style of this book are my responsibility, it could never have been written without the loyal co-operation of many who have served on the staff of my Department over the past eight years. I wish especially to acknowledge my debt to Professor C. F. V. Smout, who willingly accepted a large part of the practical burden of introducing our shortened practical course and of preparing the first duplicated text we issued. In this work Dr D. Darlington and Dr W. P. Dallas Ross also gave considerable help, as they later did in seeing that my final text was as consistent as possible in the use of the PNA terminology and in arranging the index. To both of them, as also to Dr P. Beavon, Dr S. H. Green, Dr R. W. Heslop, Dr J. T. Hobbs, Dr F. P. Lisowski, Dr G. D. Officer, Dr J. B. Pearson, and Dr W. L.

Whitehouse, I owe a great deal for the care with which they carried out dissection after dissection in order to provide the material for the illustrations, and to help check the text which is now published; as well as for their help with the proofs, an arduous task in which other lecturers on the staff of the Department also assisted. To Mr W. J. Pardoe I am as grateful for the tolerance he showed over my exigent demands as I am appreciative of his skill in elaborating a system of illustration which provides a more realistic representation than a line drawing of what the medical student actually sees in the dissecting room. Here I owe thanks, too, to Mr T. F. Spence, for his assistance both in photography and dissection. To my secretary, Miss E. R. Lawton, I am greatly indebted for her care in typing successive drafts of the text. I am grateful, too, to Mr E. A. Sims for providing an inordinate amount of material for special dissection, and to the hundreds of students who were the unwitting 'guinea-pigs' in an experiment of producing a new book on anatomy.

My indebtedness extends beyond the confines of my own Department. Professor A. L. d'Abreu, Dean of the Medical School in the University of Birmingham and Professor of Cardiac Surgery, Professor W. Melville Arnott, William Withering Professor of Medicine in the University of Birmingham, Professor F. A. R. Stammers, Professor of Surgery in the University of Birmingham, Professor J. Dixon Boyd, Professor of Anatomy in the University of Cambridge, Professor A. J. E. Cave, Professor of Anatomy in the Medical College of St Bartholomew's Hospital in the University of London, have all read my text and been generous in encouragement and constructive comment.

S. Zuckerman
University of Birmingham, 1961

Contents

2.2   The front and medial side of the thigh   2.17
   Osteology   2.17
   Surface anatomy   2.19
   Reflection of the skin   2.19
   Dissection of the front and medial side of
     the thigh   2.20

2.3   The back of the thigh and the popliteal fossa   2.32
   Osteology   2.32
   Surface anatomy   2.32
   Reflection of the skin   2.33
   Dissection of the back of the thigh and the
     popliteal fossa   2.33

2.4   The hip joint   2.39
   Osteology   2.39
   Dissection of the hip joint   2.40

2.5   The leg and the foot   2.42
   Osteology   2.42
   Surface anatomy   2.48
   Reflection of the skin   2.48
   Dissection of the front of the leg and
     dorsum of the foot   2.49
   Dissection of the back of the leg   2.57
   Dissection of the sole of the foot   2.61

2.6   Joints of the lower limb   2.67
   The knee joint   2.67
   The interosseous membrane of the leg   2.72
   The ankle joint   2.73
   The tibiofibular joints   2.75
   The joints of the foot   2.76
   The arches of the foot   2.78

Part 3: The thorax

3.1   The chest wall   3.2
   Osteology   3.2
   Surface anatomy   3.7
   Dissection of the chest wall   3.7

3.2   The pleura and mediastinum   3.12
   The removal of the anterior chest wall   3.12
   The removal of the lungs   3.15
   The mediastinum   3.17
   The right side of the mediastinum   3.19
   The left side of the mediastinum   3.22

3.3   The heart   3.24
   The examination of the heart *in situ*   3.24
   The removal of the heart   3.27

   The surface of the heart   3.28
   The interior of the heart   3.31

3.4   The lungs   3.39
   The surfaces of the lungs   3.39
   Dissection of the lungs   3.42

3.5   The posterior and the superior mediastinum   3.43
   The cardiac plexus   3.43
   The thoracic duct   3.45
   The trachea   3.46
   The oesophagus   3.47
   The descending thoracic aorta   3.48

3.6   The joints of the thorax   3.49
   The costovertebral joints   3.49
   The sternocostal joints   3.50
   The action of the muscles of respiration   3.51

Part 4: The abdomen

4.1   The pelvis   4.3
   Osteology   4.3
   Surface anatomy   4.4

4.2   The perineum   4.5
   Surface anatomy   4.5
   Superficial dissection of the male perineum   4.5
   Superficial dissection of the female
     perineum   4.7
   The disposition of the pelvic viscera   4.7
   The ischiorectal fossa   4.8
   Deep dissection of the male perineum   4.11
   Deep dissection of the female perineum   4.14

4.3   The anterior abdominal wall   4.17
   Surface anatomy   4.17
   Reflection of the skin and superficial fascia   4.18
   The oblique and transverse muscles of the
     abdominal wall   4.20
   The inguinal canal   4.23
   The scrotum and its contents   4.27
   The rectus abdominis muscle and the rectus
     sheath   4.29
   The thoracolumbar fascia   4.30
   The blood supply of the anterior abdominal
     wall   4.32
   The nerve supply of the anterior abdominal
     wall   4.33
   The functions of the abdominal muscles   4.34

4.4   The peritoneal cavity   4.35
   The ligaments attached to the umbilicus   4.36

Part 6: The brain

Introduction

The dead body which you will study was injected shortly after death with a solution which usually consists of a mixture of industrial alcohol, formalin, carbolic acid, and glycerin. The injection is generally made into the femoral artery at the upper end of the right thigh, and the fluid perfuses the whole body. The tissues are, therefore, both sterilized and preserved, at the same time as the glycerin prevents them from becoming too hardened. Every effort has been made to ensure that when you dissect you will not run any hazard of being infected by bacteria or viruses that may have been in the body at the time of death.

Different medical schools have different ideas about the proportions of the ingredients used to make up the injection liquid. Most of these differences are arbitrary, but some are made necessary by climatic conditions, preservation usually being more difficult in hot than in temperate zones. Once preservation of the cadaver has been achieved, it is customary in some schools to render the arteries of the body more conspicuous with a coloured injection mass. This is done in various ways, one of the commoner being to inject a mixture of starch and carmine into the arterial system through the same opening in the femoral artery through which the preserving fluid was introduced.

Do not be surprised if it turns out that someone has a better-preserved body to dissect than you have (or vice versa). A large number of factors influence the way injection fluid flows through the body.

It is convenient to dissect in pairs, except in the case of the thorax, abdomen, and head and neck, where dissections are usually made by groups of four. Your main concern will necessarily be the cadaver which you are dissecting, but always allow colleagues who are working on other bodies to see what you are doing, and, whenever possible, check your own findings on their dissections.

Section 0.1

How to dissect

Instruments

Scalpels and forceps are the main instruments you will use. Your scalpels should be sharp, and furnished with blades of at least two different sizes. Scalpels with expendable blades are the most convenient, and blades with a sharply-curved cutting edge will be found the most useful. These should be changed frequently. To avoid accidents, be careful how you carry your scalpels when not in use. Note that the term 'heel' is applied to that part of the blade closest to the shaft.

You should have at least two pairs of forceps, one with broad, the other with fine serrated jaws. A stout pair of toothed forceps is useful when you reflect skin, and you will find those with a weak spring less tiring to use.

Scissors are also necessary, and again you will find it useful to have more than one pair.

Because they do not rust, it is a better investment to buy instruments made of stainless steel, or of good quality plated steel.

It is well to equip yourself, too, with a metal probe or seeker, and a magnifying glass. You may find it useful to have both a blunt and a sharp-pointed seeker. Other instruments which you will occasionally need, such as bone forceps, an amputation-saw (or tenon-saw), a frame-saw and a double-edged skull-saw, and a long-bladed knife, will be provided as part of the equipment of the dissecting room [Fig. 0.1].

The cadaver

The institutional arrangements for disposing of the dead vary from country to country, and except in very primitive parts of the world every death has to be officially notified to the authorities. Bodies are made available for dissection only under strictly controlled regulations, and, apart from bodies of people who have expressly asked that their remains be used for medical science, those that become available to medical schools are usually those of the indigent whose remains have not been claimed by relatives for ritual burial or cremation. Anatomy schools in countries where the expectation of life is high, that is to say about seventy years or more, will as a rule receive only senile cadavers. In the years from 1950 to 1960 the average age of male and female subjects in the dissecting room of the Birmingham School of Anatomy was 72. The senile body not only differs from the body of a young person in lacking teeth (i.e. in being edentulous) and having atrophied masticatory muscles and thinned jaw bones, but also in the relative proportions of various other structures. Some bodies may be emaciated, others may have a lot of subcutaneous and other fat. Not surprisingly, many of the bodies which come to the dissecting room reveal the marks of previous disease. You may even find that the cadaver you are dissecting is that of a person who died of cancer. In that case you may have to study the affected parts on some other body.

While the general arrangement of the muscles, vessels, and nerves which make up the body follows the same pattern you will discover during the course of your dissection that anatomical details vary considerably from one individual to another. So do not be surprised, for example, if in the cadaver you are dissecting, an artery arises from some main trunk differently from the way described. Indications are given in the text about those structures which are most variable in their disposition.

Another point worth noting from the start is that the appearance of the tissues in the cadaver is very unlike that of the same tissues in the living body. For example, arteries are differentiated more easily from veins in the living body than in the dead; different planes of fascia are separable more readily on the operating-table than you will find possible in the cadaver you are dissecting; and organs and muscles are more fixed in position in the cadaver. Their colour, texture, and surface-markings are also different in the living as compared with the body prepared for dissection by the injection of fixatives. Note, too, that the degree of distension of different parts of the alimentary canal are bound to differ in the cadaver you dissect from what would be expected in a healthy person. It is unlikely that someone whose body would be referred to a dissecting room would have eaten much solid food before death. At the same time mortuary attendants sometimes distend the terminal part of an otherwise empty alimentary tract, that is to say, the rectum, with tow, so making its appearance different from what it would normally be during life. All the figures used to illustrate this book are realistic representations of what your dissection will expose.

The techniques of dissection

Before you begin to dissect, it is *essential* that you read these instructions.

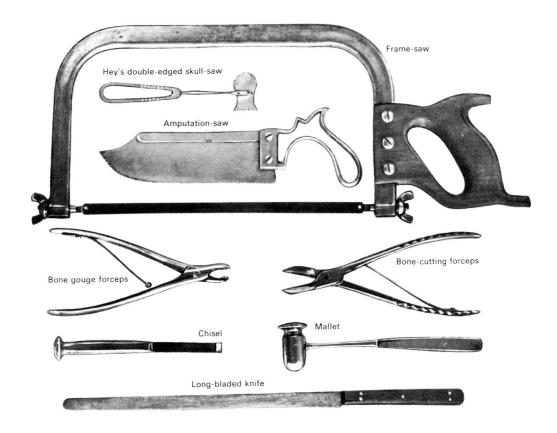

Hey's double-edged skull-saw

Frame-saw

Amputation-saw

Bone gouge forceps

Bone-cutting forceps

Chisel

Mallet

Long-bladed knife

Fig. 0.1 Dissecting instruments.

Reflection of skin

You will be told the exact position of every skin incision you have to make. Cut through the skin, remembering that it is rarely more than 2 mm thick. A decrease in resistance as you cut will tell you when you reach the subcutaneous tissue.

To detach the skin from the subcutaneous tissue, use stout forceps to grip the angle where two incisions meet, and cut with your scalpel between the skin and the underlying subcutaneous tissue or fascia. As you lift the skin away (this is called 'reflecting the skin') pull on it, and continue cutting close to, and parallel with its under-surface, keeping the flap tense as you reflect it away. Most of your reflections will be made so that the flap you lift is left attached by one edge. The skin can then be replaced, between periods of dissection, over the part you are studying.

Reflection of fascia

The subcutaneous tissue between the skin and whatever structure it overlies (usually muscle) consists of fatty connective tissue known as superficial fascia, and a deeper layer of non-fatty membranous fascia called the deep fascia. The cutaneous nerves and vessels ramify in the superficial fascia, having pierced the deep fascia. Using a scalpel and forceps, the superficial fascia is then reflected from one of the edges of the area laid open by the reflection of skin. As it is turned

back, care must be taken lest you inadvertently cut some of the cutaneous nerves or arteries which you may be asked to study.

Cleaning muscles, nerves, and arteries

By 'cleaning' a muscle, a nerve or a vessel, one means completely removing the connective tissue and fat or fascia by which it is ensheathed. This is done with forceps and scalpel, where necessary piecemeal. When you dissect do not hesitate to remove small veins, or for that matter, large veins, unless specifically told not to do so.

When you are asked to 'define' a nerve or artery, or a muscle, you are meant to carry on with the process of cleaning until the whole structure concerned is clearly and cleanly exposed. The same meaning attaches to the word 'following' a nerve or artery.

Any tissue that is removed from the body should be put into a receptacle so that it can eventually be buried.

Most of your dissection will be made with a sharp scalpel and forceps.

By 'blunt dissection' is meant the process of isolating a structure without using the blade of a knife. Blunt dissection often involves pulling a nerve or artery to one side, so must be carried out with care. One can, for example, separate a vessel which is bound by connective tissue to a nerve by pushing the points of closed forceps, or scissors, between them, and then gently opening the blades. Or one can separate them by pushing gently with the handle of a scalpel.

Do not be rough, but never be afraid to use your fingers to feel the structures which you have to clean and isolate. If, for example, it is necessary to cut through a muscle, be quite certain that you can define its edges, and if possible first insinuate a finger between it and the structures on which it is lying. As a preliminary to inserting your finger, it may be necessary to push gently with the handle of a scalpel.

There is almost no limit to the amount of dissection that can be done on a particular part. Most of the figures by which this book is illustrated necessitated finer dissection than you will be expected to undertake in the time you have available. This does not, however, justify hasty or inadequate dissection. Never regard your examination of a particular part or region as completed until you really have exposed the structures described in the text.

You may sometimes find that some of the muscles you are dissecting are unexpectedly friable and that they tear. All you can do to overcome this shortcoming is to examine the muscle or part concerned on somebody else's dissection.

The skeleton

Bones form the framework of the body, and dissecting rooms are usually furnished with one or more articulated skeletons to which you can refer when dissecting. You will find it even more useful to have at hand the bones of the particular part on which you are working. The bones of the limbs help you to understand the action of the muscles that rise from and become inserted into them, while those of the pelvis and the skull help you to understand the position of different soft structures, and the points of emergence of vessels and nerves.

Preservation of the dissection

After each period of study it is essential that the whole body, or any individual part that is being dissected, should be wrapped up in order to prevent loss of moisture and hardening of the specimen. Moisten the parts that you are dissecting from time to time. Preserving fluid containing glycerin is most useful for this purpose. You should not allow any lamps that you may have above your table to come too close to the cadaver, as this will increase the rate of evaporation.

Structures that cannot be adequately dissected

You will have no difficulty in dissecting the muscles, the visceral organs, and the main vessels and nerves of the body. Some anatomical structures that are important functionally cannot, however, be studied adequately by the straightforward methods of dissection which you will be using. The main one is the lymphatic system. This consists of a network of minute channels and associated nodes that are found in

most parts of the body. All you will see, and then only in some of your dissections, are well-defined solid lumps of matted tissue of varying shape, usually embedded in fascia. These are lymph nodes. When you dissect the thorax you will also come across the main collecting duct of the whole lymphatic tree. But this is about all you will see of the system. Since you cannot construct a coherent picture of the anatomical distribution and connection of the lymph ducts and nodes from your dissection, a general account of the whole system is given as an Appendix.

Your dissection will also fail to reveal some of the more detailed parts of the nervous system of the body. The brain and the spinal medulla comprise the central nervous system, from which motor nerves pass to all parts of the body, and towards which nerve fibres transmitting sensory impulses from peripheral structures (such as the retina of the eye or the skin) pass. But another major part of the nervous system of the body is the autonomic nervous system. This consists of so-called sympathetic and parasympathetic fibres which pass to the viscera (e.g. the heart, lungs, and alimentary tract) and which are associated with visceral sensory fibres. The action of the parasympathetic nerves is often the reverse of that of the sympathetic fibres. For example, while sympathetic nerve impulses to the iris of the eye make the pupil dilate, those transmitted down the associated parasympathetic fibres cause it to constrict.

The cell bodies of the motor fibres which innervate the viscera lie outside and not within the central nervous system, as is the case for motor fibres which innervate striated ('voluntary') muscles. The autonomic nerve cells are aggregated into ganglia which lie either along the course of the nerves themselves or within the organs which they supply. The peripheral autonomic cells are controlled by other nerve cells that lie within the central nervous system. The general arrangement of the fibres that constitute what is called the sympathetic outflow, and their organization into the sympathetic trunk, is explained on page 0.9. Parasympathetic fibres emerge from the central nervous system as part of the nerves which spring from the brain itself and from those that arise from the terminal or sacral part of the spinal cord. Autonomic nerve fibres pass from the sympathetic ganglia to the smooth muscles of the blood vessels and the viscera and various glands. The abdominal organs receive their autonomic fibres mainly from additional ganglia placed in an intermediate position between the sympathetic trunk and the viscera themselves. The sympathetic fibres which pass to the blood vessels of the limbs and to those of the musculature and the skin of the rest of the body run in the ordinary nerves which you will be exposing.

Some of the peripheral plexuses formed by sympathetic nerve fibres cannot be adequately dissected. Except in a few regions of the body, you will not be able to display parasympathetic fibres as a separate entity.

Section 0.2

The sequence of dissection

The dissecting instructions set out in this book are designed for the study of the parts of the body in the following order: Upper Limb, Lower Limb, Thorax, Abdomen, Head and Neck, and Brain. If required, the order of dissection can, however, be varied as follows:

1. The Upper Limb can be dissected before the Thorax; the Thorax before the Head and Neck and Abdomen, and the Lower Limb before the Abdomen (e.g. Lower Limb, Upper Limb, Thorax, Head and Neck, Abdomen). For such sequences no modification of the dissection instructions is required.

2. The trunk or the Head and Neck can be dissected before either of the limbs. If this is desired the instructions should be modified as follows:

   a. If the Head and Neck are to be dissected first, you must start on the shoulder region, following the instructions for the dissection of the Upper Limb up to the point where the limb is about to be detached [pp. 1.2–1.23]. Both upper limbs should be left attached to the body and the instructions followed from the start of the Head and Neck [p. 5.2] as far as the Bisection of the Head [p. 5.23]. Then instead of removing the right half of the head from the cadaver according to instruction 8 of page 5.24 you should remove the half which seems to be the less firmly attached to the trunk. The horizontal section for this removal should then be made higher up, just below the cricoid cartilage [pp. 5.16 and 5.20], rather than at the level of the first rib as directed in the text. From then on dissection of the head and neck can proceed according to the sequence as given.

   b. When it is intended to start with the Thorax, you must first dissect the shoulder region by following the in-

structions for the Upper Limb from page 1.2 to page 1.23. Although one of the upper limbs must be detached before you can proceed to the dissection of the thorax, it is desirable not to do this on both sides. Despite some consequent inconvenience, keeping one limb attached will facilitate your study of the junctional zone between the thorax, neck, and upper limb.

   c. If the Abdomen has to be studied before the Lower Limb, the dissection of the pelvis and perineum must be delayed and a start made on the anterior abdominal wall [p. 4.17]. The text can then be followed to the end of the chapter on the posterior abdominal wall [p. 4.81]. The student must then dissect the gluteal region, thigh and hip joint, and detach both lower limbs [pp. 2.2–2.41] before returning to the Abdomen and completing the study of the pelvis, perineum [pp. 4.3–4.16], and pelvic cavity [pp. 4.82–4.102].

The eventual completion of the dissection of the limbs can be deferred as long as is desired provided precautions are taken to prevent the parts becoming too dry.

3. The dissection of the Abdomen is not recommended before that of the Thorax.

In addition to changing the order in which the parts of the body are studied, the sequence of dissection of the Head and Neck can also be varied with regard to the stage at which the head is bisected and the stage at which the deep muscles of the back and the spinal medulla are examined. These variations are dealt with on pages 5.23–5.24 in the instructions for bisecting the head.

The Brain will be studied by dissecting separate specimens that have been specially fixed soon after death.

Section 0.3
Terminology

General terms of position

For the purpose of description the body is considered as being in what is called the **anatomical position**. In this position the subject is assumed to be standing, the feet together, the arms to the side, and with the head and eyes and the palms of the hands facing forwards. To ensure consistency of description it is important to keep the anatomical position constantly in mind.

The position of structures relative to each other in the body is defined in relation to the following planes [Fig. 0.2]:

The **Median Plane.** This is the back-to-front vertical plane which cuts through the body in the midline. This plane bisects the body into symmetrical right and left halves.

A **Sagittal Plane.** This is any vertical plane parallel to the median plane.

A **Frontal Plane.** This is any vertical plane at right angles to the median plane. It is often called a **coronal plane.**

A **Transverse Plane.** This is any **horizontal plane** through the body at right angles to both the sagittal and frontal planes.

Any structure lying closer than another to the midline of the body is said to be **medial** to it, and any further from the midline **lateral**. Every structure automatically has a medial and a lateral aspect. A point or plane in space closer than another to the head-end of the body is said to be **superior** to it, and, conversely, the point or plane further away is **inferior**. The terms **cranial** and **caudal** replace the terms 'superior' and 'inferior' in descriptions of the embryo, and they are also sometimes replaced by the terms **rostral** and **caudal** in descriptions of the brain. The terms **proximal** and **distal** are used in describing parts of the limbs which are closer to or further from the attachment of the limbs to the trunk.

The front surface of the body, or of any structure in the body, is called its **anterior** surface, and conversely the back of any structure is denoted by the term **posterior**. The terms **ventral** and **dorsal** are synonymous with 'anterior' and 'posterior'. The term **supine** refers to the body lying on its back, i.e. dorsal surface. The term **prone** refers to the body lying on its face, i.e. ventral surface. The hand is said to be supinated when the **palmar** surface faces forwards as in the anatomical position. When the hand is rotated so that the palmar surface faces posteriorly it is said to be pronated. The sole of the foot is known as the **plantar** surface. When the plantar surface is turned medially, the foot is **inverted**; when laterally, **everted**.

Structures which lie near to the surface of the body are described as **superficial** to others which lie on a **deep** plane. The term **external** describes structures outside an area, space, or structure, and the term **internal** describes those within. Sometimes, however, these terms are used in a completely different sense, as synonymous with the terms 'lateral' and 'medial'. This practice should be avoided.

When referring to structures of the wrist and hand, the terms **radial** and **ulnar** are often used instead of 'lateral' and 'medial'. This avoids any confusion due to the fact that when the hand is pronated its lateral border (i.e. the side of the thumb) lies 'medial' to the side of the little finger, which in the supinated position is medial.

Descriptive terms of general application

Aditus. An aditus is an entrance or opening.

Ala. An ala is a wing-like process.

Alveolus. An alveolus is a deep narrow pit, such as a tooth-socket.

Ampulla. The term 'ampulla' is used to describe the dilated part of a duct. The Roman ampulla was a narrow-necked flask.

Ansa. An ansa is a loop, usually the loop of a nerve.

Antrum. An antrum is a cavity.

Aponeurosis. An aponeurosis is a glistening sheet of fibrous connective tissue from which muscle fibres arise, or into which they run.

Arteries. Arteries are blood vessels which conduct blood from the **heart**. The largest artery of the body, the **aorta,** leaves the heart and is nearly 3 cm in diameter. The division of this and subsequent major branches leads to a continuous increase in their number and spread, with a concomitant progressive decrease in size. The smallest arteries, or **arterioles,** end in the capillary bed.

Bone. Bone is a special form of connective tissue in which calcium salts are deposited and which provides a framework, or skeleton, for the other tissues of the body. Most muscles arise from and become attached to bone.

Bursa. A bursa is a membranous sac containing a little viscous fluid. Bursae are usually found in the tissues where friction develops, such as where a tendon crosses a bony prominence. The lining of a bursa resembles that of a synovial joint (see **Joints),** and bursae may form

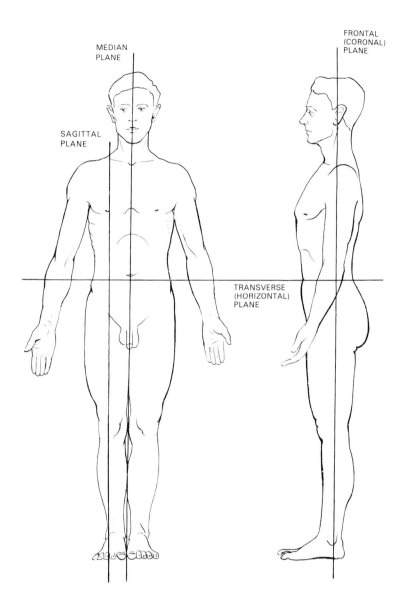

MEDIAN
PLANE

SAGITTAL
PLANE

FRONTAL
(CORONAL)
PLANE

TRANSVERSE
(HORIZONTAL)
PLANE

Fig. 0.2 The planes of the body.

synovial sheaths to surround tendons as they cross other tendons or bone.

Canal. A canal is a tubular and relatively narrow channel, or tunnel, often through a bone. A **canaliculus** is a small canal.

Capsule. A capsule is a fibrous or membranous envelope surrounding an organ. An **articular capsule** surrounds each synovial joint, being attached to the bones just beyond the limits of the joint cavity.

Cartilage. Cartilage is a firm white tissue, from which most parts of the bony skeleton are formed and which persists to protect the surfaces of bones and joints.

Caruncle. A caruncle is a small fleshy eminence.

Cauda. The term 'cauda' means 'tail'.

Cavity. Hollow spaces (or potential spaces) within the body or its organs are often called cavities.

Cervix. The term 'cervix' (=neck) is applied to the neck-like portion of an organ.

Chiasma. A chiasma is a crossing of fibres in the form of an X. The term is used particularly to describe nerve fibres which cross each other in the median plane of the body.

Commissure. A commissure is a band of fibres which join corresponding right and left parts of an organ across the median plane. It is most often applied to bundles of nerve fibres in the brain or spinal medulla.

Corpus. The term 'corpus' means 'body'.

Cortex. The outer part, or rind, of some organs is called the cortex, as distinguished from their inner part, or core, called the **medulla.**

Crest. A crest is a projecting ridge, especially one which surmounts a bone.

0.7

Crus. The term 'crus' means a 'leg' and is sometimes applied to a structure that resembles a leg or stalk.

Decussation. A decussation is the same thing as a chiasma.

Digitation. A digitation is a finger-like process of muscle.

Disc. A disc is a flat round structure. The term is applied to plates of cartilage in joints.

Duct. A duct is a tube for the passage of fluid, especially the secretions of the **glands.** A **ductule** is a narrow duct.

Epithelium. Epithelium is the layer of cells which forms the external surface of the skin, or which lines the cavities of the digestive, respiratory, and urogenital organs, the serous cavities, the inner coats of the blood and lymphatic vessels, the glands and the cavities (ventricles) within the brain. The epithelium of the skin forms the **epidermis.** The epithelium of the digestive, respiratory, and urogenital organs is moistened by a film of mucus and is known as the **mucous coat.** The microscopic structure of epithelium varies according to its situation. Blood vessels are lined with an epithelium consisting of flattened cells, a pavement epithelium or **endothelium.** The serous cavities are lined by a similar pavement epithelium called **mesothelium.**

Fascia. The tissue which lies immediately deep to the skin is known as the subcutaneous tissue. It usually consists of a layer of connective tissue which contains fat, and of a deeper and more fibrous layer which adheres to the surface of the underlying muscle and vessels. These layers are known as the **superficial** and **deep fascia** respectively. They vary in consistency from one part of the body to another. Fascia also surrounds every muscle, organ, vessel, and nerve in the body.

Fasciculus. A fasciculus is a small bundle, and the term is usually applied to collections of nerve fibres.

Filum. Literally a thread, 'filum' is the name given to several thread-like structures such as the **filum terminale,** the thread-like lower end of the pia mater of the spinal medulla.

Fold. The term 'fold' is used to describe a ridge formed where a membrane doubles back on itself.

Folium. The term 'folium' means a 'leaf'. The plural 'folia' is applied to the folds of the cortex of the cerebellum.

Foramen. A foramen is a hole, often in a bone or between adjacent bones.

Fossa. Literally a 'ditch', the term usually refers to a shallow depression or cavity.

Fovea. A fovea is a small pit or fossa.

Frenulum. A frenulum is a small fold of the mucous coat which limits the movement of the structure to which it is attached.

Fundus. The term 'fundus' is sometimes used to denote the widest part of a hollow organ.

Ganglion. A ganglion is a swelling on the course of a nerve, and usually corresponds to a collection of nerve cells.

Genu. The terms 'genu', literally a 'knee', and **geniculum** (a little knee) are sometimes applied to a bent part of a structure.

Gyrus. A gyrus is a fold or convolution of the cerebral cortex.

Hilum. A hilum is a depression or notch where blood vessels enter or leave an organ.

Humour. The term 'humour' is applied to the fluids of the eye.

Infundibulum. An infundibulum is a funnel-shaped passage.

Interdigitate. Interdigitation is the interlocking of structures by finger-like processes, as when the fingers of the two hands are interposed.

Invaginate. A membrane, such as the peritoneum, is invaginated when a part of its wall is pushed inwards, so that the structure which invaginates the membrane becomes partly ensheathed by it.

Isthmus. An isthmus is the narrow part of a duct or other passage, or a narrow strip of tissue connecting two wider parts of an organ.

Joints. Bones meet each other (articulate) at joints. Where the bones are connected by fibrous tissue, the joint is known as a **fibrous joint** (e.g. a suture between two bones of the skull). Where they are united by cartilaginous tissue, the joint is known as a **cartilaginous joint** (e.g. the **pubic symphysis**). Where a space intervenes between the articulating ends of bones, so that the joint is movable, the joint is called a **synovial joint.** In such cases an **articular capsule** of fibrous tissue connects the ends of the bones, and the capsule is lined by a **synovial membrane,** which secretes a lubricating fluid (e.g. the shoulder or hip joints).

Labium. A labium is a lip.

Lamina. A thin plate of bone or cartilage or a thin layer of the softer tissues may be referred to as a 'lamina' (plural, 'laminae'). **Stratum** is also used (in Latin) to denote 'layer'.

Ligament. A ligament is a band of fibrous connective tissue by which bones are connected to each other. In the thorax and abdomen, bands of connective tissue which support the viscera are also known as ligaments.

Lobe. A lobe is part of an organ, often separated from the rest by fissures. A **lobule** is a small lobe.

Meatus. A meatus is a passage or opening.

Muscle. Muscles vary in shape and size, but always consist of masses of special contractile cells which are under nervous control. It is usual to describe a muscle as possessing an **origin** and an **insertion,** in the sense that when the muscle contracts, the insertion moves towards the origin. It is perhaps more useful to regard a muscle as possessing attachments which are approximated when the whole muscle contracts. The origin of a muscle is sometimes called the **head,** and the contractile part the **belly.** The actions or functions of muscles cannot be inferred simply from their bony attachments; nor is it safe to analyse the muscles involved in a particular movement merely on the basis of their relations. Accurate statements on matters such as these need to be based on electrophysiological studies of the living body. In the text which follows, you will find the following terms applied to muscles:

A **fusiform muscle** is a spindle-shaped muscle in which the bundles of muscle-fibres are arranged in a longitudinal manner throughout its length.

A **bipennate muscle** is a muscle in which the fibres are arranged in bundles at each side of a central tendon.

A **multipennate muscle** is a muscle in which the bundles of muscle-fibres run into one of several tendinous prolongations which extend into the substance of the muscle.

Nerves. The nerves of the body are divided into twelve pairs of **cranial nerves,** which emerge from the brain, and thirty-one pairs of **spinal nerves,** which arise from the spinal medulla in segmental series (eight cervical, twelve thoracic, five lumbar, five sacral, and one coccygeal). The spinal nerves emerge from the intervertebral foramina which lie on each side between adjacent vertebrae. They pass laterally into the trunk or neck.

A typical spinal nerve [Fig. 0.3] is formed by the union of a **dorsal root,** which springs from the posterior aspect of the spinal medulla, and a **ventral root,** which springs from the anterior aspect. The dorsal root consists of sensory (afferent) fibres, and is characterized by a swelling called the **spinal ganglion,** which contains the cell bodies of the sensory nerve fibres. The ventral root consists of motor (efferent) nerve fibres. The nerve trunk formed by the union of the two roots splits almost immediately into a **dorsal ramus,** which supplies the deeper muscles of the back and the overlying skin, and a **ventral ramus.** The latter is usually by far the bigger, and supplies the muscles and skin on the lateral and ventral aspects of the body. The nerve supply of the limbs is derived entirely from the ventral rami of the spinal nerves.

Just after the trunks of the twelve thoracic and upper two lumbar spinal nerves split into ventral and dorsal rami, the ventral ramus gives off a small branch which passes laterally into a vertically-disposed beaded nerve, called the **sympathetic trunk,** which lies on either side of the vertebral column [Fig. 0.3]. Each of these branches is called a **white ramus communicans,** and passes to one of the nodes or **ganglia** on the sympathetic trunk. The ganglia of the sympathetic trunk contain nerve cells on which

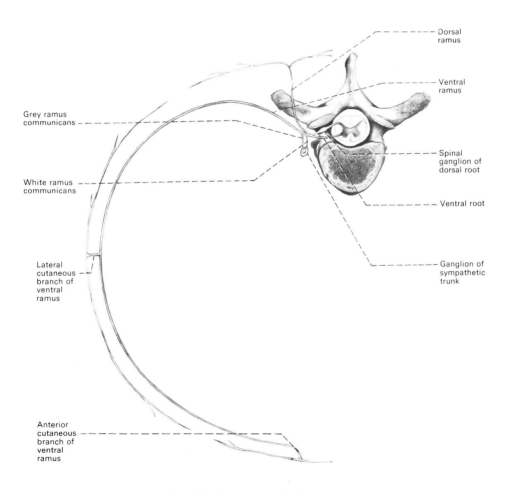

Fig. 0.3 A typical spinal nerve.

the fibres of the white ramus communicans end (= 'synapses'). Nerve processes from the cells then pass out of the ganglion and rejoin the trunk of the spinal nerve as the **grey ramus communicans.** The fibres in the white ramus communicans are medullated and are known as preganglionic fibres. Those which originate from the cell bodies within the ganglion and pass out in the grey ramus communicans are non-medullated and are known as post-ganglionic fibres.

Neuron. Neurons or nerve cells are the functional units of the nervous system. Each is composed of a **cell body,** or perikaryon, where the nucleus of the cell is situated, and one or more processes. One of the processes, called the **axon,** is structurally different from the others, which are called **dendrites.** The axon is a slender process, which is usually longer than the dendrites, and is often of considerable length.

Some axons possess a sheath of lipid material called myelin, and are called myelinated or **medullated nerve fibres.** (The paleness of the white matter of the brain and spinal medulla is due to the presence of these fibres.) Axons which do not have a medullary sheath are called **non-medullated nerve fibres** (unmyelinated fibres).

Node. A node is a swelling or protuberance. A **nodule** is a small node.

Notch. A notch is an indentation or depression, chiefly on the border of a bone.

Nucleus. The Latin word 'nucleus' means a 'kernel' or 'nut'. As an anatomical term the word 'nucleus' is most frequently used to describe an aggregation or cluster of nerve cells.

Papilla. A papilla is a small nipple-shaped elevation.

Periosteum. The periosteum is the fibrous membrane which surrounds a bone.

Plexus. A plexus is a network of nerves or vessels.

Pouch. The term 'pouch' is applied to pockets of peritoneum in the abdomen.

Process. A process is an appendage or projection from the main part of a bone or organ.

Punctum. Literally a 'point', the term 'punctum' refers to a minute opening.

Ramus. A ramus is a branch, and when translated is the term used to describe the smaller arteries, veins, and nerves. It is specifically used untranslated to describe the ventral and dorsal branches of the spinal nerves.

Raphe. A raphe is a seam, sometimes raised, where two similar sheets of tissue (e.g. skin or muscle) unite, usually in the midline of the body.

Rete. 'Rete', literally a 'network', is used to describe elaborate plexuses of small canals or vessels.

Retinaculum. A retinaculum is a band of connective tissue, usually connected at both ends to bone, which retains tendons or other structures in place.

Rima. 'Rima' can be translated 'cleft' or 'fissure', and refers to a narrow oval or oblong opening.

Root. The root of a nerve or organ is the part by which it is attached to another structure.

Sac. A sac is a bag-like cavity, or pouch.

Septum. A septum is a dividing wall or partition. A **septulum** is a small septum.

Sheath. A sheath is a tubular structure, often surrounding a tendon.

Sinus. A sinus may be a recess, a cavity or hollow space, a dilated channel for venous blood, or a small tunnel.

Space. Some clearly demarcated segments of the tissues, or potential cavities, are called 'spaces'.

Spine. A spine is usually a small, often sharp-pointed, projection from a bone.

Stria. A stria is a streak or stripe, often slightly elevated.

Stroma. This term denotes the supporting fibrous framework of a tissue.

Substantia. The term 'substantia' means 'substance' or 'matter' and is sometimes translated as such.

Surface. The surfaces of the bones and viscera are separated from each other by **borders.**

Sulcus. A sulcus is a groove, but is used untranslated to describe the fissures between the gyri of the cerebrum.

Taenia. Literally a flat 'band' or 'tape', the term 'taenia' may be applied to a narrow strip of muscle.

Tegmen. A tegmen is a cover or roof.

Tela. The word 'tela' means a 'web', and is used to describe thin web-like membranes. It is usually translated 'tissue'.

Tendon. A tendon is a cord of connective tissue in which muscle-fibres end, so that the pull of the muscle becomes concentrated into a small area, and by which muscle becomes attached to bone or other structures.

Trabecula. The word 'trabecula' means a 'beam' or 'bar'. A trabeculated structure comprises a network of strands or bundles.

Tract. A tract is a collection or bundle of fibres, often nerve fibres, having similar origins and terminations.

Trigonum. A trigonum is a triangular space or area.

Trochlea. A trochlea is a pulley.

Tuber. A tuber is an enlargement or swelling.

Tubercle. A tubercle is an eminence on a bone, usually less rough than a tuberosity.

Tuberosity. A tuberosity is a rough eminence on a bone.

Tunica. A tunica is a coat and is often translated as such. The muscle coat and the mucous coat are parts of the wall of many hollow viscera.

Uvula. Literally a 'little grape', the term, when used without qualification, usually refers to the small fleshy appendage that hangs from the soft palate in the midline.

Vallecula. A vallecula is a wide depression or furrow.

Valve. A valve is a fold in an artery, vein, or duct which prevents the reflux of its contents. **Valvula** is a small valve.

Vas. Vas (= vessel) is used untranslated to denote a tubular structure.

Veins. Veins return the blood from the capillaries to the heart. Generally their walls are thinner than those of their corresponding arteries.

Velum. The Latin word 'velum' means a 'veil' or 'curtain', and is occasionally used to name a sheet-like structure.

Viscus. A viscus is any organ of the digestive, respiratory, or urogenital systems, or any ductless gland. 'Viscera' is the plural of 'viscus', and is commonly applied to the contents of the abdominal and thoracic cavities.

Charts of contents

The introduction to the dissection of each part of the body is prefaced by a Chart of Contents in which there is set out, in a tabular form, the main features of that part of the body. The charts are an organized checklist of the main anatomical structures that will be encountered during dissection.

Chart of contents of the upper limb

COMPONENTS	REGIONS			
	Shoulder Axilla	**Arm**	**Forearm**	**Hand**
Bones	scapula clavicle	humerus	radius ulna	carpals metacarpals phalanges

Joints	acromioclavicular
	     shoulder
	sternoclavicular
		elbow	proximal radio-ulnar
			     wrist
			distal radio-ulnar
				hand

Muscles	extensors and
	     abductors
	flexors and
	     adductors
		extensors
		
		flexors
			extensors and
			     supinators
			flexors and
			     pronators
				intrinsic

Nerves	brachial plexus	radial musculocutaneous median ulnar	posterior interosseous radial median ulnar	terminal branches
Arteries	axillary	brachial	radial ulnar	palmar arches digital
Veins *superficial* *deep*	cephalic axillary	cephalic brachial	cephalic basilic radial ulnar	dorsal digital palmar
Lymph nodes *superficial* *deep*	axillary	cubital		

Part 1

The upper limb

The upper limb consists of the shoulder, arm, forearm, and hand, these four anatomical regions being separated from each other by the shoulder joint, elbow joint, and wrist joint. By moving your own limb, note the movements that occur at these joints. Movement is free and extensive at the shoulder joint, and includes flexion (when the arm is moved forwards in front of the body), extension (when it is moved backwards behind the body), abduction (when it is raised from the side away from the body), and adduction (when the arm is moved towards the side of the body from the position of abduction). The movements that are made when swinging or rotating the arm at the shoulder, as occur when you serve at tennis or bowl a ball, are called circumduction.

Movement at the elbow joint is restricted to flexion, when the hand is raised to touch the shoulder, and extension, when the arm is straightened. Similarly, the wrist can be bent backwards and forwards, that is, extended and flexed, as well as abducted and adducted. Movements of supination and pronation of the forearm occur at two small joints at the upper and lower ends of the two forearm bones. With the arm beside the trunk the forearm is supinated when the position of the palm is such that the thumb is lateral. Pronation occurs when the palm is turned so that the thumb becomes medial.

The main movements of the thumb and fingers are those of flexion, extension, abduction, and adduction, with the thumb having a rather wider range of movement. Flexion of the fingers produces a clenched fist, and extension an open hand. Separating the fingers from one another is called abduction, and bringing them together adduction. Functionally the thumb can be said to represent half of the hand. Its range and power of movement is unique, and is not paralleled anywhere in the animal world.

The anatomy of the hand is important since it is involved in nearly half of all industrial accidents.

Because they act on the shoulder and arm, you start your dissection by examining the superficial muscles of the back. You then dissect the muscles of the anterior surface of the chest wall, since they, too, move the arm. When these have been studied you dissect the axilla (the arm pit) through which all the blood vessels and nerves from the neck pass into the arm. After this you remove the upper limb from the rest of the body, and continue with its dissection separately.

The shoulder region

The only bone of the upper extremity which articulates directly with the trunk is the clavicle. Its medial end forms a joint with the upper part of the sternum. Its lateral end is joined to a flat triangular bone called the scapula, which is situated on the upper part of the back, and which does not articulate directly with any bone of the trunk. The position of the scapula at any moment is determined by the pull of muscles which connect it with the vertebral column and ribs on the one hand, and the humerus, the bone of the arm, on the other, the head of the humerus articulating with the scapula at the shoulder joint. The upper limb is thus held to the trunk by muscles which pass to the shoulder girdle (the clavicle in front and the scapula behind), and from the shoulder girdle to the humerus.

Osteology

The clavicle

The clavicle [Fig. 1.1] is subcutaneous throughout its whole length. Examine the bone as it lies *in situ* on the skeleton. Note that it braces back the shoulder, thus allowing the upper limb to swing clear of the trunk. In its medial two-thirds the clavicle is round and convex forwards; its lateral third is flat and concave forwards; its inferior surface is grooved and ridged.

Now examine a disarticulated clavicle, and from the information already given, determine the side of the body to which it belongs. This is an exercise which it is useful to repeat when any bone is studied.

The **sternal articular surface** of the clavicle is oval and may extend for a short distance on to the inferior aspect of the bone. Return to the skeleton and note that the bone articulates medially not only with the sternum but also with the first costal cartilage.

Also notice the oval facet at the extremity of the flattened lateral end of the clavicle which articulates with the acromion of the scapula.

Turn again to a skeleton and at the same time also examine a disarticulated scapula.

The scapula [Fig. 1.2]

The scapula is a flat triangular bone from which a large **spine** projects posteriorly, and a small coracoid process supero-

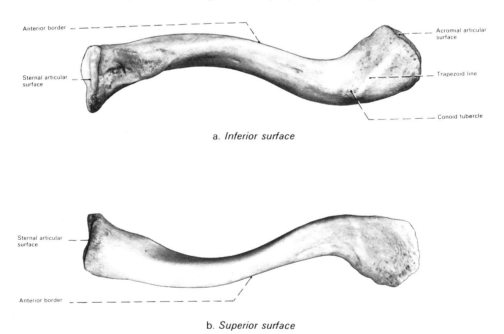

a. *Inferior surface*

b. *Superior surface*

Fig. 1.1 The left clavicle. The trapezoid line and conoid tubercle give attachment to the coracoclavicular ligament. They are not referred to in the text.

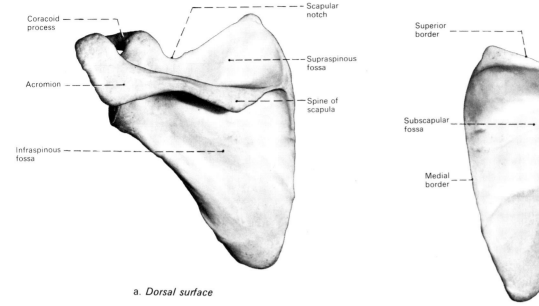

a. *Dorsal surface*

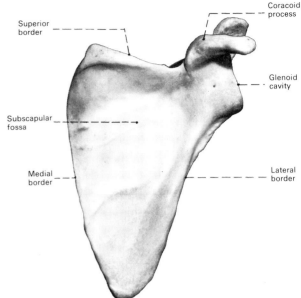

b. *Costal surface*

Fig. 1.2 The left scapula.

laterally. The spine ends in the flattened **acromion** which overhangs the shoulder joint. Because it is so easily felt, the tip of the acromion is a landmark in the living body.

Examine the **coracoid process.** Infero-laterally to it is the shallow, pear-shaped, **glenoid cavity.** This is where the head of the humerus articulates with the scapula to form the shoulder joint. To the infero-medial side of the coracoid process is the **scapular notch.** The base or body of the coracoid process is disposed vertically, but the tip is directed forwards and slightly laterally. As you will see, the tip of the coracoid process can be palpated in the living body.

Study the flat triangular body of the scapula. It has three borders, superior, lateral, and medial; three angles called lateral, superior, and inferior; two surfaces, a costal in relation to the ribs, and a dorsal which faces backwards. The costal surface constitutes the **subscapular fossa** and the dorsal surface is subdivided by the spine into a **supraspinous fossa** and an **infraspinous fossa.**

The sternum

Next examine the sternum on a skeleton [Fig. 1.3]. It lies in the midline of the front of the chest, and the upper seven ribs articulate with it through the intermediary of costal cartilages. A concave **jugular notch** forms its upper border, and about 4 cm below this is a projection called the **sternal angle,** where the upper and smaller part of the sternum, called the **manubrium of the sternum,** joins the body of the bone. A horizontal plane drawn through the sternal angle marks the level of the second costal cartilage in front, and the intervertebral disc between the fourth and fifth thoracic

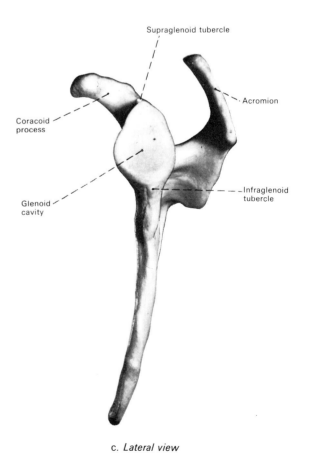

c. *Lateral view*

1.3

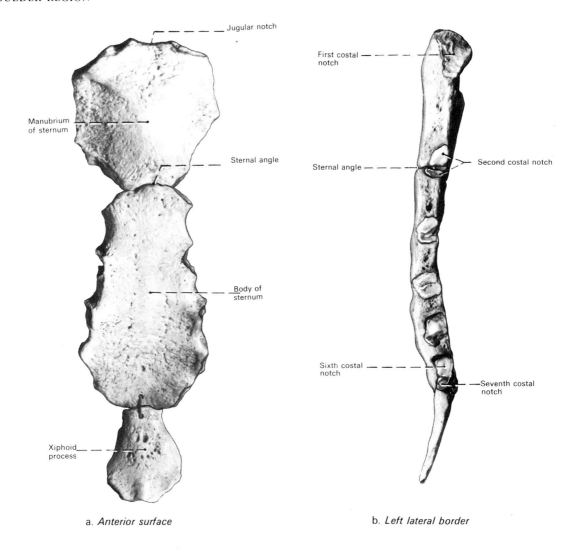

a. *Anterior surface*   b. *Left lateral border*

Fig. 1.3 The sternum.

vertebrae behind. The sternal angle is used as a landmark when counting the ribs.

You will see that the **body of the sternum** ends at the level of the seventh costal cartilage by merging with the **xiphoid process** of the bone, which up to adolescence is cartilaginous. The junction of the xiphoid process and the body of the sternum lies in the plane of the ninth thoracic vertebra.

The humerus

Now examine the humerus, both separately and as part of a skeleton [Fig. 1.4].

The humerus is one of the long bones of the body, and consists of a shaft, an upper, and a lower end. At this stage of your dissection, you will be concerned only with the upper half of the bone.

First look at the hemispherical **head** which articulates

with the glenoid cavity of the scapula. At the periphery of the head there is a constriction called the **anatomical neck,** and below this are the **greater tubercle** and the **lesser tubercle.** Immediately below these tubercles the bone is constricted again at the **surgical neck,** a name which signifies the fact that it is here that the bone not uncommonly fractures.

Between the two tubercles is the **intertubercular groove.** Laterally, just below the groove, and about halfway down the shaft, is the well-marked **deltoid tuberosity** into which the deltoid muscle is inserted.

Surface anatomy

The shoulder

Begin by examining the surface anatomy of the shoulder region [Fig. 1.5]. This is very much easier to do on a living

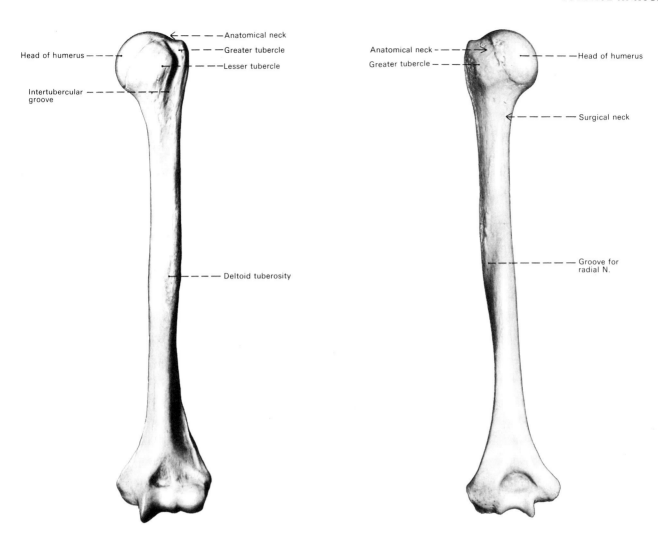

Anatomical neck
Greater tubercle
Head of humerus
Lesser tubercle
Intertubercular groove
Deltoid tuberosity

Anatomical neck
Greater tubercle
Head of humerus
Surgical neck
Groove for radial N.

Fig. 1.4 The left humerus.

person than on a cadaver, on which you will be able to confirm only a few of the more obvious points.

First look at and feel the horizontal bony ridge that separates the front of the chest from the neck. It is formed by the clavicle. Below it, the front of the chest is covered by a large triangular muscle called the pectoralis major, whose lateral edge can be seen and felt in the anterior wall of the axilla. On the living body you can also see and feel below the clavicle a depression called the **infraclavicular fossa.** Above the clavicle you can see the lower part of the **posterior triangle of the neck.** This triangle is bounded medially by the sternocleidomastoid muscle, which will stand out if the face is turned towards the opposite shoulder, and laterally by the cervical part of the trapezius muscle, which becomes prominent when the shoulders are raised against resistance. The sternocleidomastoid is a large strap-like muscle which extends between the medial third of the clavicle below and

the mastoid process above. The latter is the boss of bone which stands out on the skull immediately behind the ear.

Feel deeply in the lateral part of your own infraclavicular fossa. The bone you press on is the tip of the coracoid process of the scapula [Fig. 1.2]. The process is partly covered by the medial edge of the clavicular part of the deltoid muscle. Lateral to this you can feel the head of the humerus covered by the deltoid muscle. The position of the head will become clearer if the arm is rotated. The bone which overhangs the shoulder joint is the acromion of the scapula. The deltoid muscle forms the rounded contour of the shoulder. Its fibres arise in part from the clavicle and in part from the scapula, and converge on to a tuberosity, called the deltoid tuberosity, in the middle of the shaft of the humerus. With the arm at the side of the body, feel on the back for the inferior angle of the scapula and note that it lies at about the level of the seventh rib.

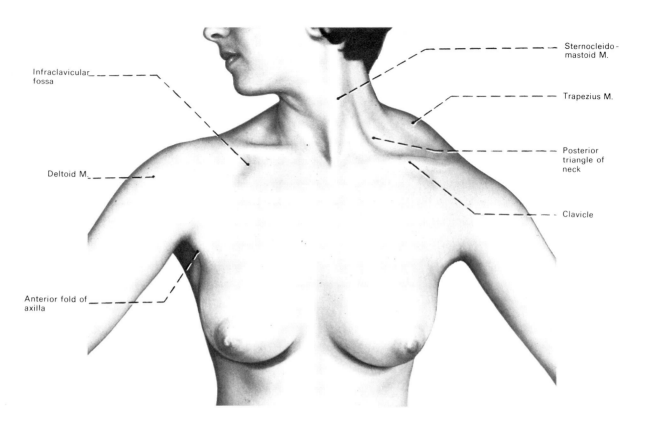

The infraclavicular fossa is sometimes called the delto-pectoral triangle because it corresponds to a gap between the attachment of the pectoralis major to the medial part of the clavicle and the attachment of the deltoid muscle to the lateral part. The boundaries of the triangle can be made to stand out by pressing the hands together in front of the chest.

The axilla

Return to the cadaver and examine the boundaries of the axilla. You will be able to feel with your thumb and finger that the anterior and posterior walls of the axilla are muscular. The medial wall is formed by the muscles which lie directly on the chest wall. Later you will see that the lateral wall is a very restricted area on the medial side of the upper part of the arm.

The back

When you have noted these points turn the cadaver over so that it lies face downwards. Locate the external occipital protuberance, which is a prominence at the back of the skull immediately above the nape of the neck. The nape is the uppermost part of the neck in the midline behind. From here run your fingers down the vertebral column, so as to feel the spinous processes. At the lower end of the vertebral column feel the sacrum between the two hip-bones, and run your fingers along either iliac crest laterally and forwards

until they stop at the anterior superior iliac spine. The latter is a prominent landmark which can be felt with great ease.

Reflection of the skin of the back

The object of the first part of your dissection is to expose and study the muscles which connect the scapula and humerus with the trunk.

Make the following incisions through the skin, carrying your scalpel just into the subcutaneous tissue [Fig. 1.6]:

1. A midline vertical incision from the external occipital protuberance to the upper end of the **natal cleft** between the buttocks.

2. Four transverse incisions across the body:
   i. At the level of the upper border of the iliac crest, extending to the **axillary line** of the body. This is a line which passes downwards from the middle of the axilla along the side of the body.
   ii. At the level of the spinous process of the seventh cervical vertebra (this is the most prominent spinous process you can feel at the nape of the neck), and extending to the tip of the acromion of the scapula.
   iii. A transverse incision across the back, midway between the upper and lower transverse incisions you have already made, and extending to the axillary line.

This incision will be approximately at the level of the inferior angle of the scapula.

iv. From the external occipital protuberance, and extending laterally halfway towards the base of the mastoid process.

Beginning in the midline, carefully reflect the skin from the subcutaneous fat, pulling laterally as you increase the size of your flap. In the neck take care that you do not reflect the skin beyond the lateral border of the trapezius muscle; if you go beyond this line you may damage structures in the posterior triangle. As you separate the skin from the underlying fat, do not be concerned as you cut through small cutaneous nerves. These are usually associated with small blood vessels.

The cutaneous nerves

The cutaneous nerves which you cut near the midline of the body emerge in series and are branches of the **dorsal rami of the spinal nerves.** You will see and divide other small nerves nearer the lateral margin of the body. These are the **lateral cutaneous branches of the ventral rami of the spinal nerves.** They, too, emerge in series. All these are sensory nerves, which end in the skin itself, and are so distributed that no surface area is without a sensory nerve supply.

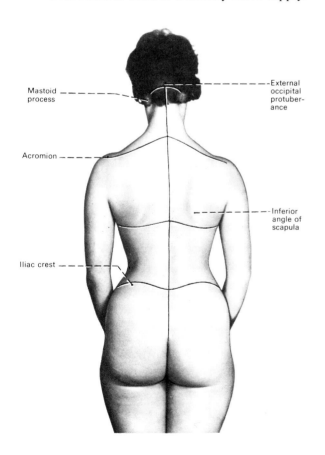

Mastoid process

External occipital protuberance

Acromion

Inferior angle of scapula

Iliac crest

Fig. 1.6 Skin incisions of the back.

Superficial muscles of the back

Having isolated a few of these cutaneous nerves, remove the fat from the underlying muscles. You will find that the fat is enmeshed in dense but watery connective tissue, which is frequently stained brown. The staining, called 'hypostatic staining', is due to fluid which has gravitated through the body while it was lying on its back. Because of its colour and texture you may find it difficult to distinguish the fascia from the underlying muscle, and particularly from its more medial fibrous (aponeurotic) part. Proceed very carefully. Embedded in the tough fascia at the upper end of the neck is the stout dorsal ramus of the second cervical nerve. This, the **greater occipital nerve,** is the most prominent of the posterior cutaneous nerves of the back of the neck, and you should try to isolate it as you clean the underlying muscle, the trapezius, which it pierces. When the muscle is thoroughly cleaned you will see that practically the whole of the back is covered by two long, flat and broad muscles, the trapezius above and the latissimus dorsi below. If the dissectors on the opposite side have reached a similar stage in their dissection, note that the shape formed by two trapezius muscles is a trapezoid [Fig. 1.7].

Examine the attachment of these muscles carefully, referring to a skeleton when necessary, in order to identify the features of the bone that may be concerned. When studying the various muscles try to work out their actions on yourself. Muscles become more prominent and firmer when they contract, particularly against resistance.

The trapezius muscle [Fig. 1.7]

You will see that each trapezius takes origin from the external occipital protuberance and from the adjacent part of two ridges of bone which arch laterally from the protuberance over the back or occiput of the skull (the superior nuchal lines of the occipital bone); from a vertically-disposed fascial band in the midline of the neck called the **ligamentum nuchae;** from the spinous process of the seventh cervical vertebra; and from the spinous processes of all the thoracic vertebrae, including the supraspinous ligament which binds their tips together. The word 'nuchal' refers to the nape of the neck. The ligamentum nuchae is a septum of fibrous tissue which extends from the occipital bone to the seventh cervical vertebra, being attached to the tip of the spinous process of each cervical vertebra in turn. It separates the muscles on the two sides of the back of the neck. In animals with a long neck the ligament contains elastic tissue.

Having verified the extensive origin of the trapezius, trace the muscle to its insertion. You will see that its lower fibres are attached to the superior border of the crest of the spine of the scapula, while those fibres which take origin from the neck run without interruption to the adjacent posterior border of the lateral third of the clavicle.

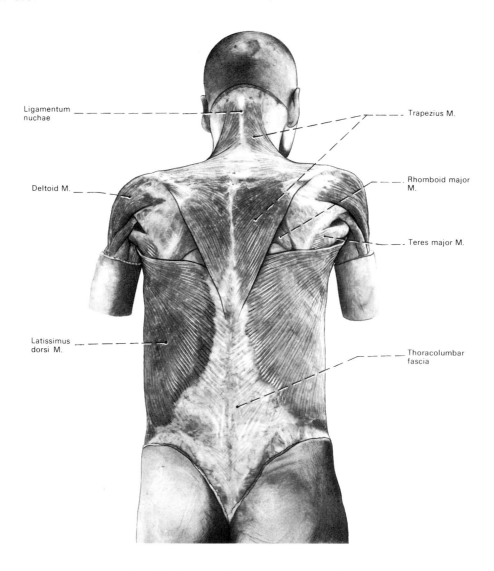

Fig. 1.7 The superficial muscles of the back.

When muscles contract they approximate the point or area of their insertion to that of their origin. Bearing this in mind, it will be clear that when the two trapezius muscles act together they brace back the shoulders and pull back (retract) the head. If one muscle works independently of the other, it draws the head to its own side. If the upper fibres of the muscle worked independently they would elevate the shoulder. Try out these movements on yourself. Pick up a weight with one hand, and with the other feel the sloping upper lateral border of the trapezius muscle of the side carrying the weight. Note that it is firmly contracted. At a later stage you will see that the middle and lower fibres of a muscle called the serratus anterior, which is inserted into the costal surfaces of the superior and inferior angles of the scapula and the intervening medial border, combine functionally with the trapezius to rotate the scapula when the arm is raised above the head.

The latissimus dorsi muscle [Fig. 1.7]

Now examine the latissimus dorsi muscle, the upper and medial part of which is overlapped by the trapezius. The origin of the latissimus dorsi muscle from the midline of the body will be seen to be aponeurotic (an aponeurosis is a flattened tendon).

Complete the isolation of the lower lateral border of the trapezius from underlying structures. In order to protect two flat, thin muscles, the rhomboid major and rhomboid minor, which lie deep to the trapezius, slide the handle of a scalpel under the lower part of the trapezius and then detach the origin of the lower 10 cm of the muscle from the spinous processes of the vertebrae.

Now turn the lower part of the muscle upwards in order to expose the origin of latissimus dorsi fully. You will see that the latissimus dorsi muscle arises from the spinous processes of the lower six thoracic vertebrae and from a dense **thoracolumbar fascia,** which attaches it to the lumbar and sacral vertebrae and the posterior part of the iliac crest.

The insertion of the latissimus dorsi muscle cannot be verified at this stage, but note that it sweeps round the lateral margin of the body as it passes to be inserted into the floor of the intertubercular groove of the humerus. You should be able to feel the muscle contract when you adduct your arm against resistance—for example, by pressing your hand against your thigh—by palpating your own latissimus dorsi muscle where it approaches the humerus.

Movements of the shoulder joint

The movements of the arm take place at the shoulder joint, and consist of extension, flexion, medial rotation, lateral rotation, adduction, and abduction [Fig. 1.8]. Note again that extending the arm means moving it directly backwards from the body. Flexing it is the opposite movement. Medial rotation is rotating the arm inwards, and lateral rotation the opposite. Adduction is drawing the arm towards the midline of the body, and abduction is the opposite movement. Circumduction is defined on page 1.1. You should try out all these movements on yourself.

If you now study the disposition of the latissimus dorsi from the point of view of its action, you will see that the muscle acts on the arm, in a variety of movements, with the body fixed, and on the body when the arms are fixed. For example, in exercises on a horizontal bar, the contraction of the muscle would raise the body.

The accessory nerve

The lower part of the trapezius has already been separated from its origin. Using scissors, separate the remainder as far superiorly as the spinous process of the seventh cervical vertebra by cutting upwards from below, about 1 cm lateral to the spinous processes and taking care not to damage the underlying muscles [Fig. 1.9]. Then turn the trapezius laterally to find a nerve and vessels on its deep surface. The nerve is called the accessory nerve. Clean and trace the nerve as far as possible. Then, taking care not to cut the nerve, incise the trapezius horizontally from the root of the neck until you reach the anterior free border of the muscle just above its insertion into the clavicle. Clean the accessory nerve and associated vessels so that they stand out as in Fig. 1.9, removing all the veins and also the small branches of the artery.

The thoracodorsal nerve

Now define the upper and lateral borders of the latissimus dorsi. Push your fingers downwards under the upper border and upwards under the upper part of the lateral border so as to free this part of the muscle from the chest wall. Search for and isolate a nerve and vessels running into the muscle. Now divide the muscle. Start the incision at the upper border at a point just medial to the inferior angle of the scapula. End the incision at a point on the lateral border of the muscle just above the attachment of the muscle to the ninth rib [Fig. 1.10].

If you now insinuate your fingers beneath the lower part of the latissimus dorsi, separating the muscle from underlying structures, you will get a convincing demonstration of its origin from the thoracolumbar fascia and the lower ribs. Having done so, detach the muscle from the ribs. Turn the upper part of latissimus dorsi upwards towards the arm and from the trunk, and find the nerve to the muscle entering its deep surface [Fig. 1.11]. This nerve is called the thoracodorsal nerve.

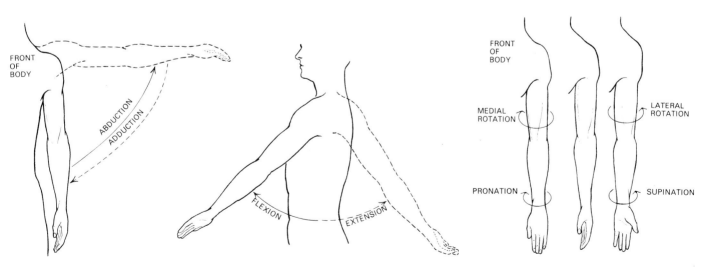

Fig. 1.8 The movements of the arm.

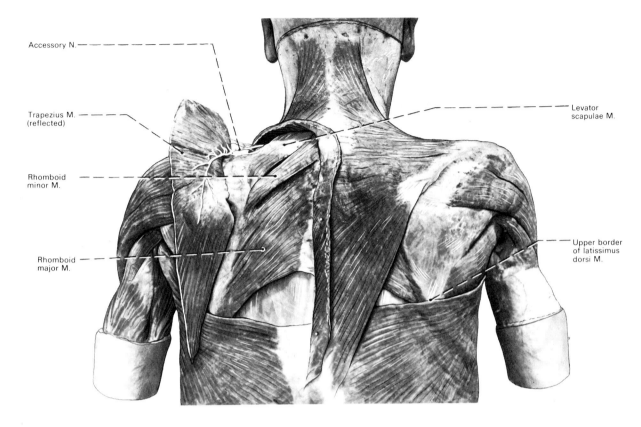

Accessory N.

Trapezius M.
(reflected)

Rhomboid
minor M.

Rhomboid
major M.

Levator
scapulae M.

Upper border
of latissimus
dorsi M.

Fig. 1.9 Reflection of the left trapezius muscle.

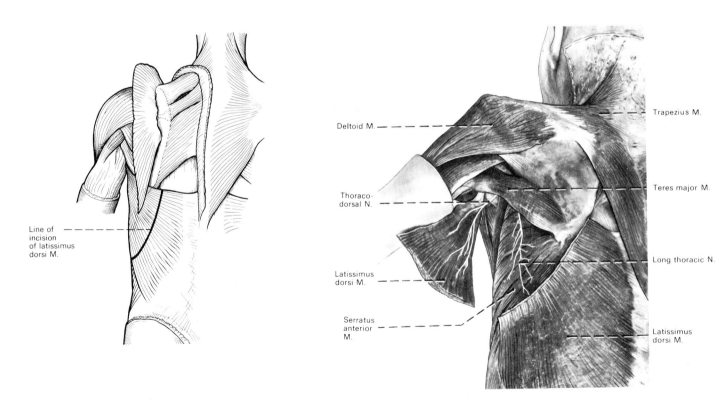

Line of
incision
of latissimus
dorsi M.

Fig. 1.10 Division of the left latissimus dorsi muscle.

Deltoid M.

Thoraco-
dorsal N.

Latissimus
dorsi M.

Serratus
anterior
M.

Trapezius M.

Teres major M.

Long thoracic N.

Latissimus
dorsi M.

Fig. 1.11 The left thoracodorsal nerve.

1.10

The levator scapulae and rhomboid muscles

When you turned the trapezius laterally, you exposed a sheet of muscle which consists of three separate muscles that pass between the midline of the back and the medial border of the scapula. They are, from above down, the levator scapulae, rhomboid minor, and rhomboid major [Fig. 1.9]. These should now be rapidly cleaned and traced from their origins towards their insertions.

The origin of **levator scapulae** from the transverse processes of the upper four cervical vertebrae cannot be confirmed at this stage, but trace the muscle to its insertion into the medial border of the scapula, from the superior angle to the root of the spine. The levator scapulae is concerned with elevating the shoulder.

Next examine the thin, strap-like **rhomboid minor muscle.** Note its origin from the spinous processes of the seventh cervical and first thoracic vertebrae, and trace it to its insertion into the medial border of the scapula at the root of the spine.

Then examine the **rhomboid major muscle.** It will be seen to arise from the spinous processes of the second, third, fourth, and fifth thoracic vertebrae and the intervening supraspinous ligaments. Trace it to its insertion into the medial border of the scapula, from the root of the spine to the inferior angle.

The rhomboids retract the scapula to the midline.

The levator scapulae and the rhomboids are supplied by branches of the fifth cervical nerve (C.5). The levator scapulae also receives fibres from the third and fourth cervical nerves (C.3 and C.4).

After using the handle of a scalpel to separate them from the underlying thin flat muscle called the **serratus posterior superior muscle,** cut through the rhomboid muscles near their origins from the spinous processes of the vertebrae. Do not spend unnecessary time in dissecting the serratus posterior superior. Then look for the **dorsal scapular nerve** from C.5 descending beneath the levator scapulae to enter the rhomboid muscles on their deep surfaces.

Reflection of the skin of the pectoral region

The cadaver should now be turned into the supine position (on its back). In the next part of the dissection you examine the pectoral muscles and the axilla. The contents of the axilla are the axillary vessels which carry blood to and from the upper limb, and the brachial plexus of nerves which innervate the muscles and skin of the limb. The axilla also contains a mass of fat and groups of intercommunicating lymph nodes which, in spite of their practical importance when cancer occurs in the breast, can rarely be satisfactorily identified in the cadaver. Before beginning to dissect the anterior chest wall, you should revise the surface anatomy of this region, and read an account of the mammary gland in a reference book on anatomy. The prepared cadavers of the dissecting room are usually old people, in whom it is practically impossible to make out the detailed structure of the mammary gland, which consists mainly of fat. No useful purpose will be served by spending any time on its dissection.

Make the following incisions through the skin [Fig. 1.12], taking care not to cut too deeply and thereby damaging cutaneous nerves and subcutaneous veins:

1. From the jugular notch along the whole length of the clavicle as far as the acromion of the scapula. This incision should be extended till it meets the lateral end of the horizontal incision you made in the skin of the back from the spinous process of the seventh cervical vertebra to the acromion.
2. Downwards on the lateral surface of the arm from the lateral end of the last incision to a point halfway down the arm.
3. From the end of the second incision transversely across the front of the arm as far as its medial surface.
4. A vertical incision from the jugular notch to the lower end of the sternum.
5. A horizontal incision from the lower end of the sternum, extending laterally to the axillary line, in the female cadaver cutting immediately below the attachment of the breast.

Reflect the flap of skin, including the areola and nipple, laterally from the midline, until it meets the flap of skin you previously isolated on the back. The skin must be completely detached from the chest and axillary region. Reflect the skin from the upper part of the arm, turning it medially so as to remove all the remaining skin from the axilla.

The mammary gland

In the female remove the mammary gland from above downwards by separating it from the underlying muscle, which is called the pectoralis major. As you remove it, you may find strands of fibrous tissue which anchor the gland to the deep fascia on the pectoralis major muscle. You may also sometimes note an important extension of the mammary gland into the axilla, called the axillary tail. If this is not obvious, do not search for it.

The supraclavicular nerves

See if you can find muscle fibres within the fascia anterior to and below the clavicle. These belong to the **platysma,** which is a quadrilateral subcutaneous sheet of muscle fibres which arise from the superficial fascia and skin of the shoulder and upper chest wall, and which extends upwards to the face. You will examine this muscle when you dissect the head and neck. Dissect the platysma fibres over and just below the clavicle, and as you do so try and pick up in their

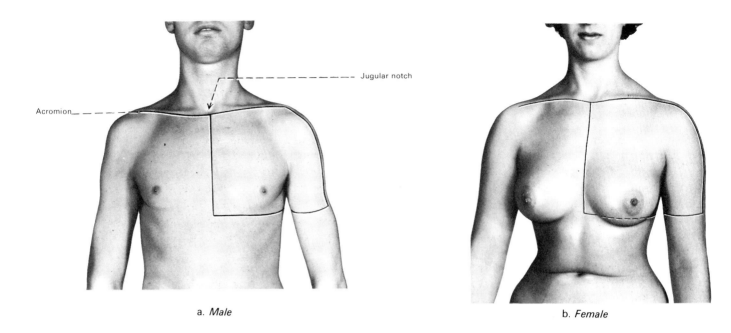

a. *Male* b. *Female*

Fig. 1.12 Skin incisions of the pectoral region.

substance the **medial, intermediate,** and **lateral supraclavicular nerves.** The lateral supraclavicular nerves will be found far laterally on the top of the shoulder, and the intermediate nerves below the middle of the clavicle. Most probably you will not find the medial nerves, which are very small. They lie below the medial end of the clavicle. All these nerves are cutaneous branches of the ventral rami of the third and fourth cervical nerves, which help to form the cervical plexus which is studied when you come to dissect the head and neck. They pass over the clavicle and are distributed as far down as the second intercostal space. If they are not readily apparent pass on to the next stage of your dissection.

The intercostal nerves and vessels

Now dissect the superficial and deep fascia from the pectoralis major muscle, noting as you do so that at the medial end of each intercostal space (space between ribs), the deep fascia is pierced by a small artery which is called the **perforating branch of the internal thoracic artery** and by an **anterior cutaneous branch of the intercostal nerve.** The two internal thoracic arteries run vertically on either side of the deep aspect of the sternum. Their perforating branches supply the mammary gland.

The intercostal nerves are branches of the thoracic nerves and encircle the chest wall between the intercostal muscles which fill the spaces between the ribs. As you proceed laterally, note that the deep fascia is also perforated in the more lateral part of each intercostal space by **lateral cutaneous branches of the intercostal nerves.** Carry your separation of the deep fascia as far as the lateral (lower) border of the

pectoralis major, where it becomes continuous with the fascia of the floor of the axilla.

Branches of the axillary nerve

Remove the deep fascia from the deltoid muscle over the shoulder. As you do so you may find cutaneous nerves perforating the muscle. They are cutaneous branches of the axillary nerve, which is also the motor nerve of the deltoid muscle. These cutaneous branches appear from behind the posterior border of the deltoid and run forwards in the fascia covering the muscle. You will see the trunk of the axillary nerve itself at a later stage in your dissection, lying between the upper end of the humerus and the deep surface of the muscle.

In the space between the deltoid muscle and the pectoralis major muscle, you will see the **cephalic vein.** This vein drains superficial structures on the lateral aspect of the upper limb.

The pectoral muscles

The pectoralis major muscle

You can now see [Fig. 1.13] that the pectoralis major muscle arises by three heads:

1. A **clavicular part** from the anterior aspect of the medial half of the clavicle.
2. A large **sternocostal part** from the anterior surface of the sternum and the adjacent upper six costal cartilages.
3. A small slip of variable size, called the **abdominal part,** from an aponeurosis on the upper part of the abdominal

wall. This is the aponeurosis of the external oblique muscle of the abdomen, which is the most superficial muscle of the abdominal wall. The exact situation of the lowest horizontal skin incision you made will determine how much of this lower part of pectoralis major is exposed.

Follow the fibres of the clavicular part of the pectoralis major laterally. You will see that they pass anterior to the upper fibres of the sternocostal part, under cover of which the lower fibres of the muscle curl to form part of a tri-laminar band. This, as you will see later, becomes inserted on the crest of the greater tubercle, the lateral lip of the inter-tubercular groove of the humerus, under the anterior border of the deltoid muscle.

At a convenient moment examine your own pectoralis major muscles. Push the palms of your hands against each other in front of your body (adduction). You will see these muscles standing out. Next grasp the anterior fold of the axilla which is formed mainly by the pectoralis major muscle and note which parts of it act when the arm is moved against resistance. During flexion, the clavicular part is most active; during adduction and extension the sternocostal part, and both parts when the arm is rotated medially.

The pectoral nerves

Now cut through the clavicular part of the pectoralis major as close as possible to its origin from the clavicle, and turn it downwards from the clavicle. You will see that blood vessels and a nerve or nerves enter the deep surface of the upper part of the muscle. The nerve is the **lateral pectoral nerve.** Cut away and reflect the sternocostal and abdominal parts of the muscle from its origin, and turn it laterally from the sternum and costal cartilages, taking care not to disturb the layer of fascia which lies deep to it. When the whole muscle is reflected laterally you will see a small triangular muscle, the pectoralis minor, which is pierced by the **medial pectoral nerve** and vessels as they pass to the overlying pectoralis major, which this nerve also supplies [Fig. 1.13].

The clavipectoral fascia

You have already seen that the deep fascia which you reflected from the surface of the pectoralis major muscle blended with the **axillary fascia.** The clavipectoral fascia on the under-surface of the pectoralis major, and covering the pectoralis minor, continues superiorly above the upper border of the latter and is attached to the undersurface of the clavicle, where it ensheathes a small muscle called the **subclavius,** which is closely applied to the bone. The name

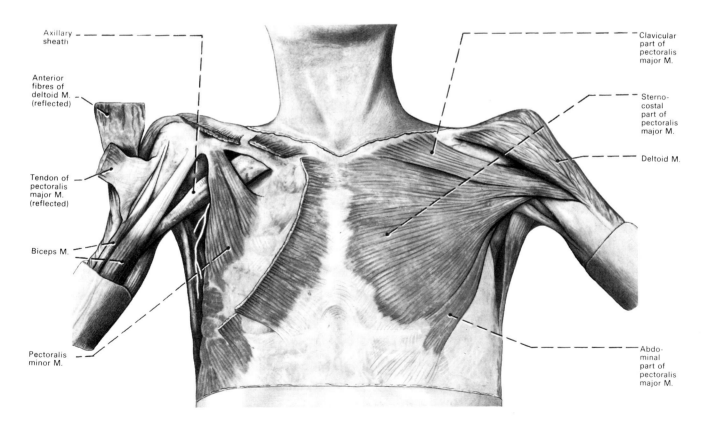

Fig. 1.13 The pectoral muscles.

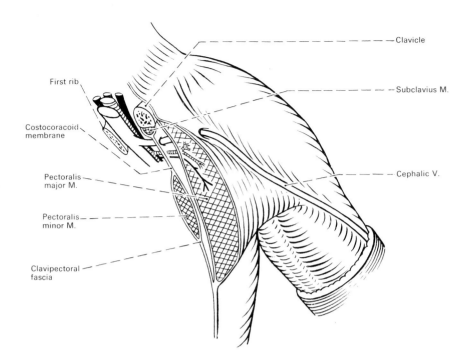

Clavicle

Subclavius M.

First rib

Costocoracoid
membrane

Cephalic V.

Pectoralis
major M.

Pectoralis
minor M.

Clavipectoral
fascia

Fig. 1.14 Schematic view of the anterior wall of the left axilla.

'costocoracoid membrane' is often given to that part of the clavipectoral fascia which intervenes between the upper border of the pectoralis minor and the clavicle [Fig. 1.14]. This membrane is pierced by the prominent cephalic vein and by the thoracoacromial artery, a branch of the axillary artery which supplies the pectoralis major muscle. It is also pierced by the lateral pectoral nerve. If your specimen does not show the costocoracoid membrane clearly, do not spend valuable time trying to clean these structures, which, deep to the membrane are associated with the apical axillary lymph nodes.

The cephalic vein [Fig. 1.14]

The cephalic vein begins on the dorsum of the hand and drains the lateral part of the upper limb. It ascends in the arm between the deltoid and pectoralis major muscles, and having pierced the costocoracoid membrane, it enters the axillary vein, which is the main venous trunk from the arm. The cephalic vein is not a large vessel, but is important because when the axillary vein is obstructed from any cause, distal to the opening of the cephalic, the cephalic vein becomes the main vessel carrying away the venous blood from the upper limb.

The pectoralis minor muscle

Now remove the clavipectoral fascia from the surface of the pectoralis minor muscle [Fig. 1.13] which will be seen to be small and triangular in shape. It arises by three slips from the second, third, fourth, or the third, fourth, and fifth ribs near the costal cartilages, and passes upwards and laterally

to be inserted, as will be seen later in the dissection, into the coracoid process of the scapula. It is innervated by the medial and lateral pectoral nerves, the same two nerves which supply the pectoralis major. Its action is to draw the shoulder downwards.

Using the handle of the scalpel, carefully separate the upper margin of the pectoralis minor from the fascia and structures which lie deep to it. Carefully cut through and dissect away the clavipectoral fascia at the lower border of the subclavius muscle, taking care not to injure the muscle itself. As you clear the fascia the axillary vessels will come into view, ensheathed in their own fascia, in the space between the clavicle and the upper border of the pectoralis minor. They are passing over the first rib under cover of the clavicle.

Now cut through the pectoralis minor near its origin from the ribs and turn it aside. This will at once open up the axilla.

The axilla

When dissecting the axilla you must proceed with the greatest care, in order to avoid cutting important structures accidentally. Before you start, it is therefore useful to get a general idea of the nerve and blood supply of the upper limb.

With the exception of some cutaneous branches to the medial side of the arm from the second, third, and sometimes fourth intercostal nerves, the motor and sensory nerves of the upper limb are branches of a plexus of nerves called the brachial plexus [Fig. 1.15].

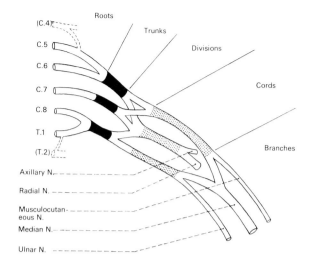

(C.4)
Roots
C.5
C.6
C.7
C.8
T.1
(T.2)
Trunks
Divisions
Cords
Branches
Axillary N.
Radial N.
Musculocutan-
eous N.
Median N.
Ulnar N.

Fig. 1.15 Schema of the left brachial plexus.

The brachial plexus

This plexus begins in the neck as **roots** formed by the ventral rami of the fifth, sixth, seventh, and eighth cervical, and the first thoracic spinal nerves (referred to for convenience as C.5, 6, 7, 8, and T.1), often augmented by small branches from C.4 and T.2. The plexus descends into the upper limb in the triangular gap between the clavicle, the first rib, and the superior border of the scapula. The roots of C.5 and C.6 unite to form a **superior trunk** of the plexus. The root of C.7 is continued as a **middle trunk**, and the roots of C.8 and T.1 unite to form an **inferior trunk.** Each trunk then divides into **anterior** and **posterior divisions** [Fig. 1.15]. The anterior division of the superior and middle trunks unite to form the **lateral cord** of the plexus, the anterior division of the inferior trunk is continued as the **medial cord,** and the posterior divisions of all three trunks unite to form the **posterior cord.** Each cord gives off collateral and terminal branches which become the nerves of the limb.

The lateral cord gives off the **musculocutaneous nerve** which supplies three muscles of the arm, the coracobrachialis, the biceps, and part of the brachialis. The lateral cord then joins a large branch of the medial cord to form the **median nerve,** which is a main nerve of the muscles and skin of the anterior part of the forearm and hand. The other terminal and main branch of the medial cord is the **ulnar nerve,** which supplies the muscles and skin of the medial side of the anterior part of the forearm and hand.

The posterior cord of the plexus gives off the **axillary nerve,** which supplies the deltoid muscle, and then continues as the **radial nerve,** which is the source of most of the nerves which innervate the skin and muscles of the back of the arm, forearm, and hand. In addition to these terminal branches, smaller nerves are given off to various structures from the roots, trunks, divisions, and cords of the plexus. Those which come off from the roots and trunks are sometimes referred to as supraclavicular branches of the plexus, to differentiate them from the infraclavicular branches given off by the divisions and cords.

The axillary artery

The arterial trunk of the upper limb is the axillary artery [Fig. 1.16]. It begins at the lateral border of the first rib, continuous with the **subclavian artery,** and ends at the lower border of the axilla, where it continues as the **brachial artery.**

The axillary artery also enters the axilla in the space between the clavicle, the first rib, and the superior border of the scapula. It is soon crossed by the pectoralis minor, so that for purposes of description the artery can be divided into three parts, a part above, a part behind, and a part below that muscle. The artery first lies on the first intercostal space and the first digitation of a muscle called the serratus anterior, and then on the posterior axillary wall. The cords of the brachial plexus lie above and behind the first part of the artery, but as they descend in the axilla they move medially, so that their relation to the second part of the artery is connoted by their names, the lateral cord lying lateral, the posterior cord posterior, and the medial cord medial to the artery. By the time the third part of the artery is reached, the cords have broken up into their terminal branches, and the median and musculocutaneous nerves lie lateral to the artery, between it and the coracobrachialis muscle. The axillary nerve lies between the artery and the subscapularis muscle, which lies posterior to the artery; the radial nerve lies between the artery and the muscles of the posterior axillary wall, and the ulnar nerve and the medial cutaneous nerve of the forearm lie on the medial side of the artery.

The axillary vein

All the venous blood of the upper limb is drained by the axillary vein [Fig. 1.16], which begins at the lower border of the axilla as a continuation of the **basilic vein** and which is soon joined by the companion veins of the brachial artery. The axillary vein receives tributaries corresponding to the branches of the axillary artery (except the thoracoacromial vein, which usually enters the cephalic vein), and at the lateral border of the first rib it becomes the **subclavian vein.** Throughout its course the axillary vein lies on the medial aspect of the axillary artery and is closely related to the lateral axillary lymph nodes. It is, therefore, liable to become obstructed if these nodes are enlarged as a result of, say, cancer of the breast.

Dissection of the axilla

When dissecting the axilla and, indeed, most parts of the body, small veins are likely to get in the way. Do not hesitate to divide and trim away any except the main veins (for example, the axillary vein itself). Smaller veins are very vari-

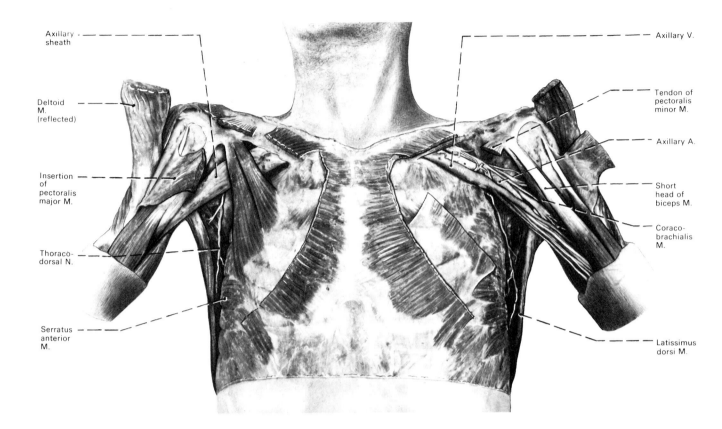

Axillary sheath

Deltoid M. (reflected)

Insertion of pectoralis major M.

Thoraco-dorsal N.

Serratus anterior M.

Axillary V.

Tendon of pectoralis minor M.

Axillary A.

Short head of biceps M.

Coraco-brachialis M.

Latissimus dorsi M.

Fig. 1.16 The axillary sheath and its contents. Most of the left pectoralis minor muscle has been excised and the left axillary sheath opened.

able in their anatomical distribution, and the extent to which they stand out differs from cadaver to cadaver. Their appearance in the dead body is little indication of what they look like normally.

With this general idea of the arrangement of the axillary vessels and nerves in mind, incise the anterior edge of the fascia which forms the floor of the axilla (the axillary fascia). Reflect it as far posteriorly as possible, but again be careful not to divide two and sometimes three fairly prominent cutaneous nerves which emerge from the upper intercostal spaces and pass laterally to the medial side of the arm.

Then divide the remains of the fascia, below the pectoralis minor, as close as possible to the chest wall, and reflect this fascia laterally, taking with it all the fat and lymph nodes which occupy the axilla, still being careful not to cut cutaneous nerves. Detach the fascia when the deltoid muscle is reached, and so remove the fat and lymph nodes. In this way the structures on the lateral wall of the axilla will be brought into view.

The lymph nodes usually appear as dense grey matted lumps and vary in prominence, definition, and number from cadaver to cadaver. They are very important both physiologically and clinically, and it is unfortunate that neither they nor the lymphatic vessels which enter and leave them can be properly dissected in the usual injected and preserved

dissecting-room body. It is for that reason that a general account of the whole lymphatic system is given as an Appendix. To display them adequately necessitates special preparations.

The axillary sheath

First identify the fascial sheath containing the axillary vessels and brachial plexus [Fig. 1.16]. When you have found them, clean the cutaneous nerves that run transversely across the lower part of the axilla to the arm from the upper intercostal spaces. They are the lateral cutaneous branches of the second, third, or fourth intercostal nerves, and since they pass into the arm they are called the **intercostobrachial nerves.** Having followed them across the axilla, divide them.

Now open the axillary sheath and clean the axillary vessels. To get a clear exposure, remove any tributaries of the axillary vein, but take care not to injure the accompanying nerves. Look for a vertically-disposed nerve lying on the large muscle which is closely applied to the side of the chest wall. The muscle is the **serratus anterior,** and the nerve which supplies it one of the supraclavicular branches of the brachial plexus, called the **long thoracic nerve.** Clean the serratus anterior muscle as far as possible and deal similarly with two vertically-disposed strap-like muscles that bound

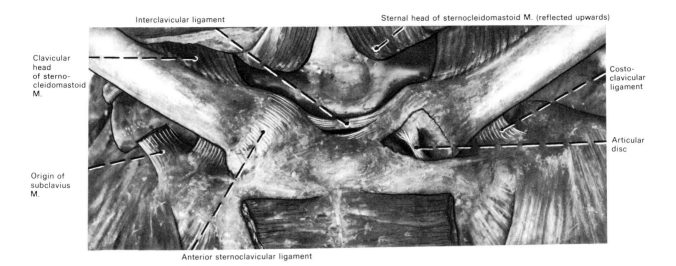

Interclavicular ligament

Sternal head of sternocleidomastoid M. (reflected upwards)

Clavicular head of sterno-cleidomastoid M.

Costo-clavicular ligament

Articular disc

Origin of subclavius M.

Anterior sternoclavicular ligament

Fig. 1.17 The sternoclavicular joint. Most of the left anterior sternoclavicular ligament has been excised.

the lateral wall of the axilla, and which are called the **short head of the biceps** and the **coracobrachialis muscles.** The coracobrachialis lies on the medial side of, and is smaller than, the biceps [Fig. 1.16]. The three muscles that form the posterior axillary wall (the subscapularis, latissimus dorsi, and teres major muscles) will be exposed later.

In order to get the clearest possible view of the axillary vessels and the branches of the brachial plexus, the clavicle will have to be displaced laterally by opening the sterno-clavicular joint and removing the structures which tie the clavicle to the first rib and first costal cartilage.

The sternoclavicular joint

Since you will destroy the joint when it is opened, it must be studied at this stage.

The sternoclavicular joint is a synovial joint which allows the medial or sternal end of the clavicle to glide on the manubrium of the sternum and the first costal cartilage, with both of which it articulates. Even though it is covered by the sternal head of the sternocleidomastoid muscle, the joint is easily palpable in the living body. Later, when the thorax is dissected, you will have the opportunity of verifying the important structures which are related to its posterior surface.

First detach the tendon by which the sternal head of the sternocleidomastoid muscle arises from the anterior surface of the manubrium of the sternum, and clean the anterior surface of the sternoclavicular joint [Fig. 1.17]. The **articular capsule** will readily come into view, and a weak **interclavicular ligament** connecting the sternal ends of the two clavicles may be seen. The capsule is reinforced in front and behind by strong ligaments. In the interior of the joint there is a strong **articular disc.** Open the joint near the sternal edge

and identify this disc. Note that it is attached to the capsule in front and behind, to the clavicle above, and to the first costal cartilage below. Lying on the medial aspect of the subclavius muscle is a short but powerful accessory ligament of the joint called the **costoclavicular ligament.** Define this ligament. Sever the attachments of both the subclavius muscle and the costoclavicular ligament from the first rib and costal cartilage, directing the blade of your scalpel from the lateral to the medial side. As you do this be careful not to injure the underlying subclavian vein. Then separate the articular disc from the clavicle without disturbing its attachments to the remainder of the joint.

Incise the part of the sternocleidomastoid muscle that arises from the medial third of the clavicle (the clavicular head of the muscle), and leaving the disc *in situ,* carefully lever the clavicle from its bed and turn it laterally [Fig. 1.18]. As you do so look for two narrow and thin strap-like muscles which ascend into the neck, the sternohyoid and sternothyroid. The first arises from the clavicle and the adjacent part of the manubrium of the sternum (and will, therefore, be partly separated from its origin), and the second from the manubrium of the sternum and the first costal cartilage. More laterally search for a vertically-disposed delicate nerve which passes into the subclavius muscle. It springs from the roots of C.5 and 6. This nerve, as well as the medial supraclavicular nerve, which you may have already seen, innervates the joint.

The axillary vessels

With the clavicle turned aside, the axillary vessels and the infraclavicular branches of the brachial plexus are fully displayed in the space which lies between the clavicle in front and the first rib behind and slightly below.

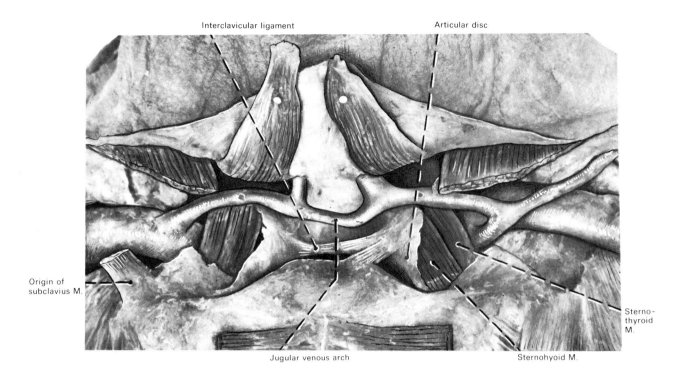

Fig. 1.18 The posterior relations of the sternoclavicular joint. The sternal heads of the sternocleidomastoid muscles are reflected upwards.

In order to expose the nerves of the axilla fully, an effort should first be made to identify the main branches which arise from the three parts of the axillary artery and to note their distribution [Fig. 1.19]. As you do so, remove their associated veins, as usual. It should be emphasized now that the arterial branches are very variable in their origin, and that you should not be surprised if they are not disposed in accordance with the following description. When the branches have been identified they can be severed from the main artery.

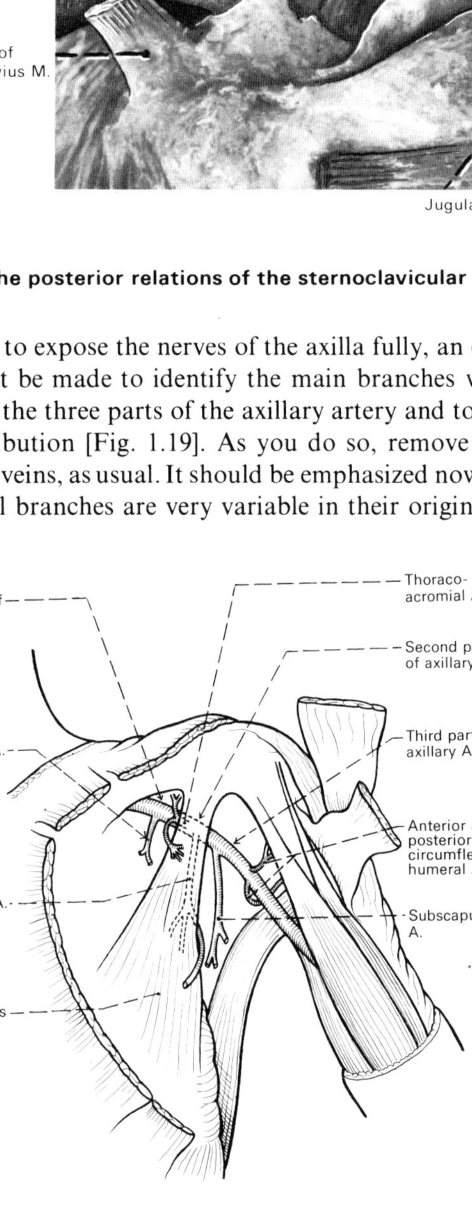

The branches of the axillary artery

From the first part of the axillary artery above the level of the pectoralis minor there usually springs the **highest thoracic artery,** which is a small branch to the chest wall. From the second part, under cover of the muscle, arise first the **thoracoacromial artery,** which is a more prominent vessel that pierces the clavipectoral fascia. It normally gives branches which diverge laterally, medially, and inferiorly to supply the chest wall. A second branch of the second part of the axillary artery is the **lateral thoracic artery,** which descends on the lower border of the pectoralis minor muscle. It sends branches to the chest wall and to the lateral aspect of the mammary gland. From the third part of the axillary artery springs the **subscapular artery,** which is the largest branch of the axillary artery. It runs along the lower border of the subscapularis muscle to supply it throughout its extent. It gives off a large branch called the **circumflex scapular artery,** and this vessel, together with its parent trunk, is mainly responsible for an important arterial anastomosis around the scapula. Two other branches of the third part are the **anterior** and **posterior circumflex humeral arteries,** which form an arterial circle around the surgical neck of the humerus, supplying the shoulder joint and adjacent muscles.

Fig. 1.19 The branches of the axillary artery.

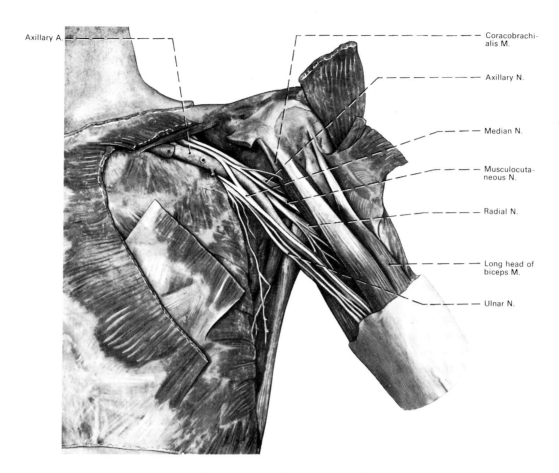

Fig. 1.20 The branches of the left brachial plexus.

What has been described is the more usual arrangement of the branches of the axillary artery. Note again that they may be very differently disposed in the cadaver you are dissecting. For example, the thoracoacromial artery may arise not from the second, but from the first part of the axillary artery, and all the branches of the third part may arise by a common stem. Occasionally, the axillary artery divides into two main trunks called the **radial artery** and the **ulnar artery.** These normally begin at the termination of the brachial artery (the continuation of the axillary artery) in front of the elbow joint.

When the relationship of the main axillary vein to its artery and to the adjacent nerves has been studied, remove a section of the main vein. This done, you will be able to examine the small flap-like valves in its interior. These prevent the backflow of blood.

The brachial plexus

Branches of the lateral cord

By this time you will have exposed several large nerves [Fig. 1.20]. Crossing in front of the lower part of the axillary artery is the main termination of the medial cord of the

brachial plexus. It will be seen to join the termination of the lateral cord in a V-shaped formation to form the median nerve. Use this nerve as your point of reference in the dissection of the branches of the plexus.

Trace the **median nerve** distally for a short distance as it descends on the lateral aspect of the artery. Having identified the terminal branch of the lateral cord which contributes to the median nerve, begin from below to find the branches of the lateral cord, and as the nerves come into view clean them carefully and trace them as far as possible to their destination. Pull the coracobrachialis muscle aside. The branch of the lateral cord which you will see piercing the muscle is the **musculocutaneous nerve.** A careful dissection of this nerve will reveal a branch it sends to supply the coracobrachialis muscle before the main trunk disappears into the substance of the muscle.

Tracing the lateral cord further upwards you will come to the **lateral pectoral nerve** on its way to the pectoralis major. You should have seen this nerve when you dissected that muscle [p. 1.13].

Branches of the medial cord

Now retrace your steps and follow the medial cord upwards from the point at which it sends its contribution to the

1.19

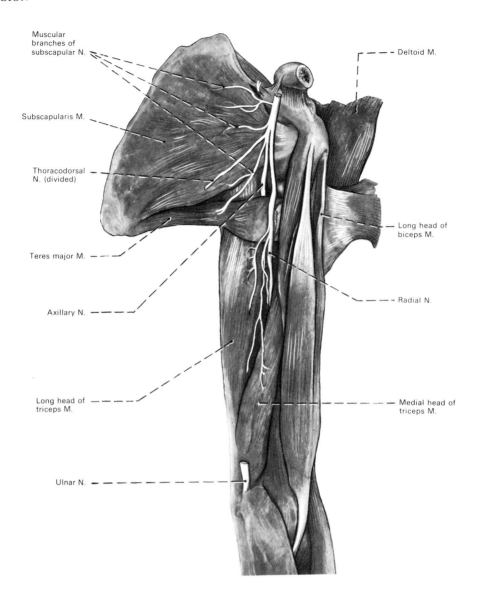

Muscular branches of subscapular N.

Subscapularis M.

Thoracodorsal N. (divided)

Teres major M.

Axillary N.

Long head of triceps M.

Ulnar N.

Deltoid M.

Long head of biceps M.

Radial N.

Medial head of triceps M.

Fig. 1.21 The posterior cord of the left brachial plexus.

median nerve. The next big branch you will then encounter is the **ulnar nerve,** descending on the medial aspect of the axillary artery and between it and the axillary vein, which lies on the medial side of the artery. The more delicate branch of the medial cord alongside it is the **medial cutaneous nerve of the forearm,** also between the axillary artery and vein. Following the medial cord a little further upwards, you will find a branch called the **medial cutaneous nerve of the arm.** This nerve descends on the medial aspect of the axillary vein. Much further up in the axilla identify the **medial pectoral nerve** as it pierces the pectoralis minor, which it supplies before it passes into the deep surface of the pectoralis major. You have already seen this nerve [p. 1.13].

Branches of the posterior cord

If the axillary artery is turned aside a large nerve lying underneath it will be exposed. This is the **radial nerve.** It is the main terminal branch of the posterior cord of the brachial plexus.

Before it leaves the axilla the radial nerve will be seen to send a cutaneous branch to the posterior aspect of the arm, and a muscular branch to a muscle which lies behind the coracobrachialis. This muscle is the long head of triceps [Fig. 1.21]. The triceps is the main muscle of the back of the arm.

As you continue to trace the posterior cord upwards, the **axillary nerve** will come into view as it turns backwards

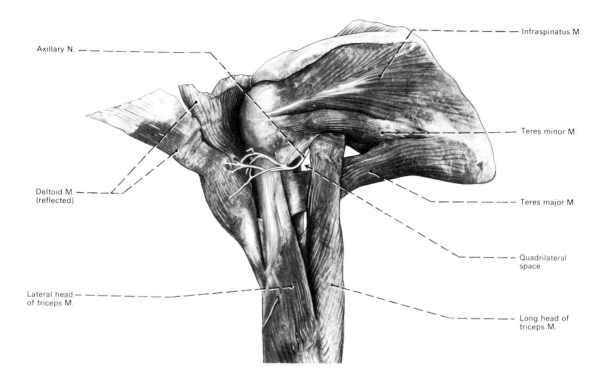

Axillary N.

Infraspinatus M.

Teres minor M.

Deltoid M.
(reflected)

Teres major M.

Quadrilateral
space

Lateral head
of triceps M.

Long head of
triceps M.

Fig. 1.22 The axillary nerve. The quadrilateral space is not referred to in the text.

below the lower border of a muscle, the **subscapularis muscle** [Fig. 1.21], which occupies the costal surface of the scapula. Immediately below the point where the nerve turns is a muscle called the teres major. To the lateral side of the nerve as it passes between these two muscles is one of the heads of the triceps muscle—the lateral head—and to its medial side the long head of the same muscle, which you will dissect at a later stage.

After it has reached the back of the arm the axillary nerve winds round the neck of the humerus [Fig. 1.22] and supplies the deltoid and teres minor muscles and an area of skin on the lateral aspect of the arm.

Now complete the cleaning of the muscles on the posterior wall of the axilla. Trace the posterior cord further upwards, and as you clean it, find the upper and lower branches of the **subscapular nerve** and the **thoracodorsal nerve** to the latissimus dorsi which spring from it [Figs 1.21 and 1.23]. The upper branch (or branches) of the subscapular nerve supplies the subscapularis muscle, and also gives a branch to the shoulder joint. The lower branch (or branches) of the subscapular nerve passes to the lower part of the subscapularis and to the teres major muscles. The thoracodorsal nerve will be seen to enter the deep surface of the latissimus dorsi near its upper border.

The serratus anterior muscle

Now examine the origin of the serratus anterior muscle [Fig. 1.23]. First complete the cleaning of the muscle, which is closely applied to the chest wall. It arises by eight fingerlike processes or digitations from the upper eight ribs. If the lower four digitations are traced medially, they will be seen to interdigitate with a muscle on the superficial aspect of the abdominal wall called the external oblique muscle of the abdomen. Do not carry your dissection further into the abdominal region.

Now look at the first digitation of the serratus anterior muscle. It will be seen to arise from the second as well as from the first rib. Follow the muscle to its insertion on to the costal surface of the medial border of the scapula. It will then be seen that the first digitation passes to the superior angle, the second and third (possibly also the fourth) digitations spread along the costal aspect of the medial border, while the remaining digitations converge on the costal surface of the inferior angle of the bone.

It will be obvious that since most of the muscle is inserted into the inferior angle, its main function is to rotate the scapula so that the arm can be raised above the head, an action in which the serratus anterior is associated with the trapezius. Another function of the serratus anterior is to draw the scapula forwards, a movement called protraction, thus extending the reach of the outstretched limb. Try these movements on yourself. If the origin and insertion of the muscle are further considered, it will be obvious that the serratus anterior plays an important part in maintaining the scapula in contact with the chest wall, so that if this muscle, for any reason, becomes paralysed, the scapula becomes

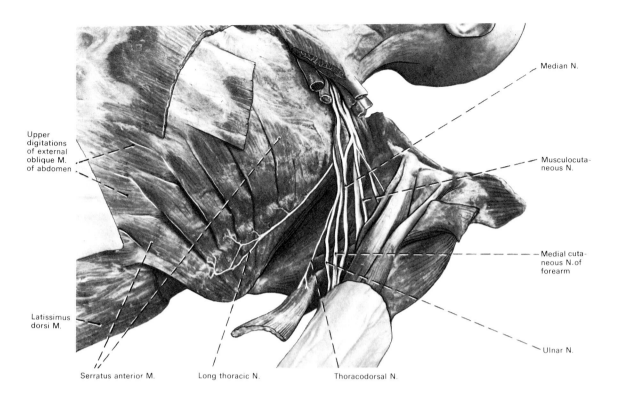

Median N.

Musculocuta-
neous N.

Upper
digitations
of external
oblique M.
of abdomen

Medial cuta-
neous N. of
forearm

Latissimus
dorsi M.

Ulnar N.

Serratus anterior M.   Long thoracic N.   Thoracodorsal N.

Fig. 1.23 The serratus anterior muscle and the brachial plexus.

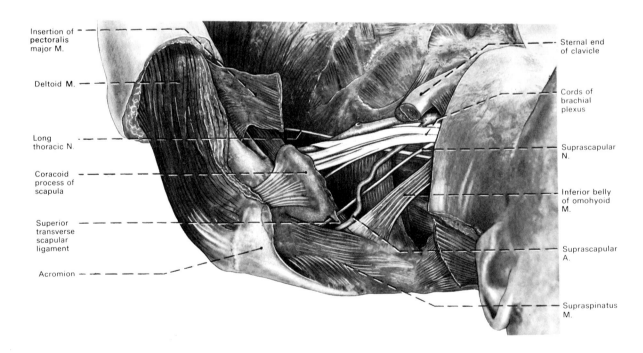

Insertion of
pectoralis
major M.

Sternal end
of clavicle

Deltoid M.

Cords of
brachial
plexus

Long
thoracic N.

Suprascapular
N.

Coracoid
process of
scapula

Inferior belly
of omohyoid
M.

Superior
transverse
scapular
ligament

Suprascapular
A.

Acromion

Supraspinatus
M.

Fig. 1.24 The omohyoid muscle and the suprascapular nerve (viewed from above). The lateral part of the left clavicle, the pectoral
muscles, the anterior fibres of the deltoid muscle, and most of the trapezius muscle have been excised.

'winged', that is to say, it stands out from the back of the body like a wing. Earlier in the dissection you saw the **long thoracic nerve** descending on the surface of the muscle to supply it. It is derived from the ventral rami of the fifth, sixth, and seventh cervical nerve roots.

Now turn the cadaver over on to its face, and examine the serratus anterior muscle from behind.

Having done so, divide the serratus anterior, starting from below, leaving the major part of the muscle and the nerve supplying it on the trunk. At this stage you can obtain a particularly good view of the contents of the axilla from the posterior aspect. Try to identify the structures you see.

Detachment of the limb

The next step in your dissection is to remove the upper limb from the trunk. Begin by completely separating the accessory nerve from the lower part of the trapezius muscle in which it is embedded. Then divide the levator scapulae near its insertion into the upper part of the medial border of the scapula, preserving the nerves supplying it. More laterally, on the superior border of the scapula, find the origin of a small strap-like muscle, called the **omohyoid** [Fig. 1.24]. The part you will see is the inferior belly. You should trace this muscle upwards as it passes into the neck. Divide the inferior belly and then look for the **scapular notch** on the superior border of the scapula just lateral to the attachment of the omohyoid. You will find that it is converted into a foramen by the **superior transverse scapular ligament.** If you dissect beneath the ligament you will find a nerve, the **suprascapular nerve,** running through the foramen to supply the scapular muscles on the dorsal surface of the scapula. The artery which usually runs above the ligament is the **suprascapular artery.** Divide both the nerve and the artery as close to the scapula as possible.

Turn the cadaver on to its back. Then pick up the axillary vessels and the brachial plexus and tie them with string. Divide them at the inferior border of the clavicle and tie them to that bone. Finally, sever all the remaining structures by which the limb is attached to the trunk. These will consist only of muscular branches of blood vessels and some folds of skin.

The limb will now be completely detached from the body.

Section 1.2
The arm

The next phase of your dissection deals with the front of the arm and a fossa (the cubital fossa) which lies in front of the elbow joint. It is a simple dissection, and the main structures which you will expose during its course are the biceps and brachialis muscles, which flex the elbow joint, and the origins of certain muscles of the forearm, and especially of the flexors and extensors of the wrist joint. The main extensor of the elbow joint, the triceps muscle, lies on the back of the arm and will be seen later. You will also be able to follow the large nerves and vessels you exposed in the axilla.

Osteology

The humerus

Begin by examining the humerus again [Fig. 1.25]. Identify the prominent **medial** and **lateral epicondyles** at the lower end of the bone, and the **medial** and **lateral supracondylar ridges** running into them from above. Note the lateral articular surface, called the **capitulum,** which articulates with the radius, and the medial articular surface, called the **trochlea,** which extends on to the posterior surface of the bone and articulates with the ulna. On the anterior surface

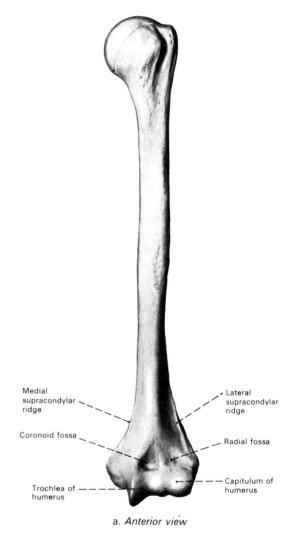

Medial supracondylar ridge

Lateral supracondylar ridge

Coronoid fossa

Radial fossa

Trochlea of humerus

Capitulum of humerus

a. *Anterior view*

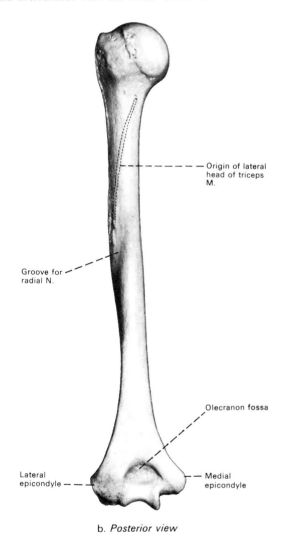

Origin of lateral head of triceps M.

Groove for radial N.

Olecranon fossa

Lateral epicondyle

Medial epicondyle

b. *Posterior view*

Fig. 1.25 The left humerus.

note the shallow **radial fossa** above the capitulum. This receives the head of the radius when the forearm is flexed. Note also the deeper **coronoid fossa** above the trochlea anteriorly, which in similar circumstances receives the coronoid process of the ulna. Now look at the posterior surface of the bone and note the **olecranon fossa** above the trochlea [Fig. 1.25]. It houses the olecranon of the ulna when the forearm is extended.

You have already noted the **deltoid tuberosity** into which the deltoid muscle is inserted. Opposite this the coracobrachialis muscle is inserted into the shaft. From this level distally the brachialis muscle takes a broad origin from the lower half of the front of the shaft. On the back of the bone the lateral head of the triceps takes a linear origin from the upper half of the shaft, and the medial head of triceps takes

a broad origin from the lower half of the shaft. Between these two heads identify a shallow and sometimes faint spiral groove in the bone. This is the **groove for the radial nerve.**

The radius and ulna

Before proceeding with your dissection, also examine the bones of the forearm [Fig. 1.26]. Articulate them. The radius lies on the lateral side of the forearm and the ulna on the medial side. The proximal end of the radius is a small circular head which articulates with a notch, called the **radial notch,** on the lateral side of the proximal part of the ulna. The superior surface of the **head of the radius** is slightly cupped. If you look at an articulated skeleton, you will see that this cupped surface articulates with the capitulum of the

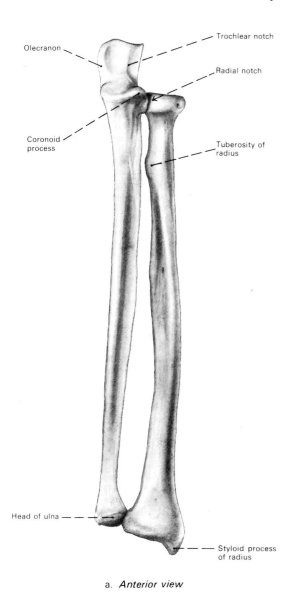

a. *Anterior view*

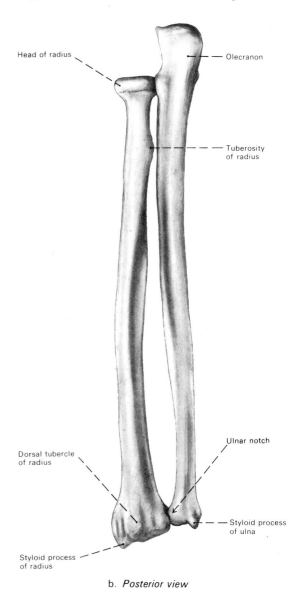

b. *Posterior view*

Fig. 1.26 The left radius and ulna.

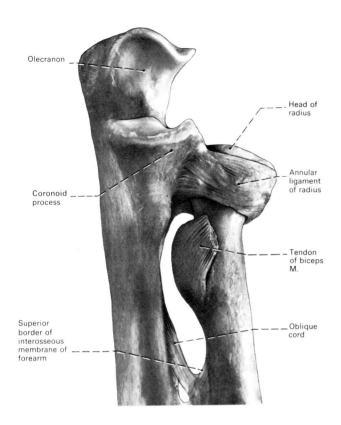

Olecranon

Head of radius

Annular ligament of radius

Coronoid process

Tendon of biceps M.

Superior border of interosseous membrane of forearm

Oblique cord

Fig. 1.27 The annular ligament of the left radius.

humerus. In the living body the head of the radius is held in position by the **annular ligament of the radius** [Fig. 1.27], which is attached to the anterior and posterior borders of the radial notch on the ulna.

The rough area of bone immediately distal to the head is called the **tuberosity of the radius.** The biceps muscle is inserted into the posterior aspect of this tuberosity. Identify the large **trochlear notch** at the proximal end of the ulna, bounded by the **olecranon** proximally, and the smaller **coronoid process** anteriorly. The triceps muscle is inserted into the superior surface of the olecranon, and the brachialis muscle is inserted into the coronoid process.

Examine the distal ends of the two bones. The **head of the ulna** is at the distal end (not the proximal end, as in the radius). Note that it terminates medially in a **styloid process,** and that it articulates laterally with an **ulnar notch** on the medial side of the distal end of the radius. The radius, in contradistinction to the ulna, widens from above down. The radius also ends distally in a styloid process. When the two bones are articulated, you will see that the styloid process of the radius extends for 2 cm below that of the ulna. This is a point of importance in fractures of the lower end of the radius, when the relative position of these two prominences may be altered.

Surface anatomy

The arm

Now study the surface anatomy of the arm and elbow joint. Place your left hand on your right shoulder, immediately below the acromion of the scapula. By rotating your right arm you should be able to recognize the head of the humerus, with the greater tubercle on its lateral aspect, and the lesser tubercle on its antero-medial aspect. The lesser tubercle can be felt only when the arm is laterally rotated at the shoulder joint as far as possible. The insertion of the deltoid into the middle of the shaft of the humerus is easily defined. On each side of the shaft, immediately below this level, you can feel a supracondylar ridge, which, when followed down, merges with an epicondyle. Both supracondylar ridges and both epicondyles can be felt, the medial epicondyle being the more prominent. The cord-like structure you can feel behind the medial epicondyle is the ulnar nerve. About 5 cm below the insertion of the deltoid, and immediately above the lateral supracondylar ridge, the radial nerve leaves its groove on the back of the humerus and passes to the anterior compartment of the arm.

You will easily locate the olecranon of the ulna. When the forearm is extended it lies in the same horizontal plane as the epicondyles of the humerus. With a finger on each of these three bony points flex the forearm [Fig. 1.28]. You will find that the points form the angles of an equilateral triangle. These details are of importance when a fracture in the region of the elbow joint is suspected.

Examine the prominent biceps muscle on the front of the arm [Fig. 1.29]. On either side of this muscle there are shallow grooves called the **medial** and **lateral bicipital grooves.** The vein in the lateral groove is the cephalic vein. Place your fingers into the medial groove, pressing them laterally and posteriorly. The artery that can be felt pulsating in this position is the brachial artery, and is continuous with the axillary artery. In the upper part of the arm the ulnar nerve, and in the lower part the median nerve, lie on the medial side of the artery.

The cubital fossa

Now examine the cubital fossa, at the bend of the elbow [Fig. 1.30]. Put a finger into the fossa and pronate the forearm, that is to say, turn your forearm so that the palm of your hand faces downwards. The muscles which form the boundaries will then be readily distinguished. The muscle on the medial side is the pronator teres; that on the lateral the brachioradialis. The prominent tendon in the middle of the fossa is the tendon of biceps, and passing from it you can feel a thick band of fascia called the bicipital aponeurosis, which sweeps medially to blend with the deep fascia of the forearm. In the fossa on the medial side of the biceps tendon you can feel an artery pulsating. This again is the brachial artery, covered by the bicipital aponeurosis. In the roof of

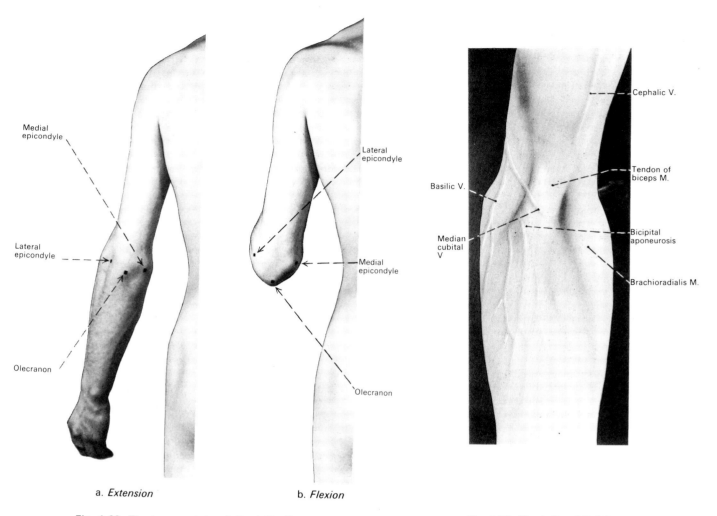

a. *Extension*

b. *Flexion*

Fig. 1.28 The bony points of the left elbow.

Fig. 1.30 The left cubital fossa.

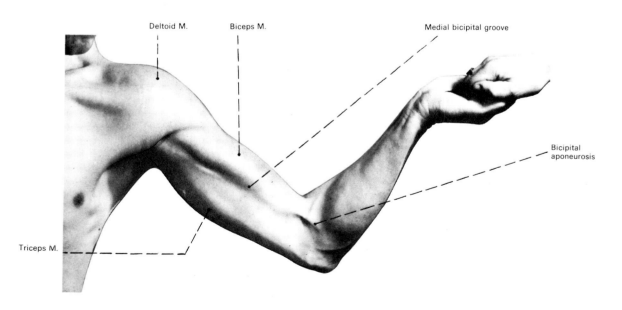

Fig. 1.29 Surface anatomy of the left arm.

the fossa one or two subcutaneous veins will be prominent. Their arrangement is variable, but often the median cubital vein may be seen connecting the cephalic and basilic veins.

Try to palpate the head of the radius with your thumb and finger. It lies immediately below the lateral epicondyle of the humerus on the medial side of the brachioradialis muscle. It is more easily felt from behind. If the forearm is pronated and supinated (the reverse movement of pronation) this bony prominence will be felt to rotate within the annular ligament of the radius.

Reflection of the skin

Begin the dissection of the detached limb. Incise the skin along the midline to 5 cm below the elbow. Then make an annular incision around the forearm at this level [Fig. 1.31].

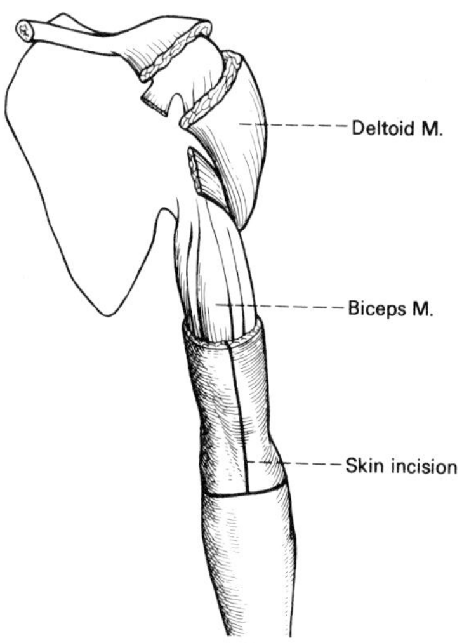

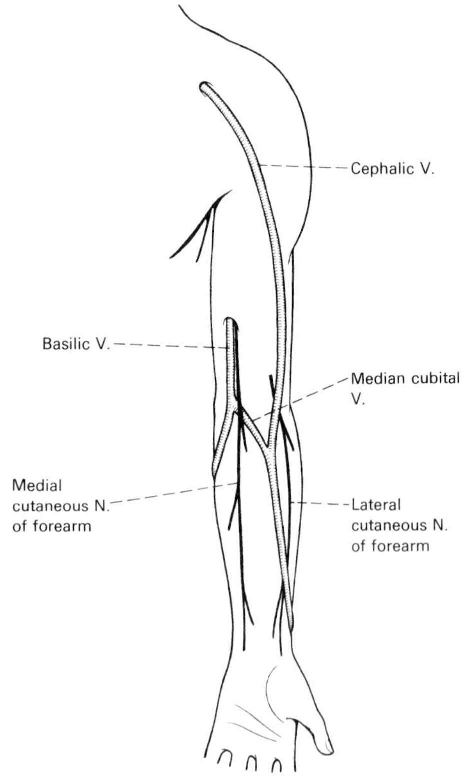

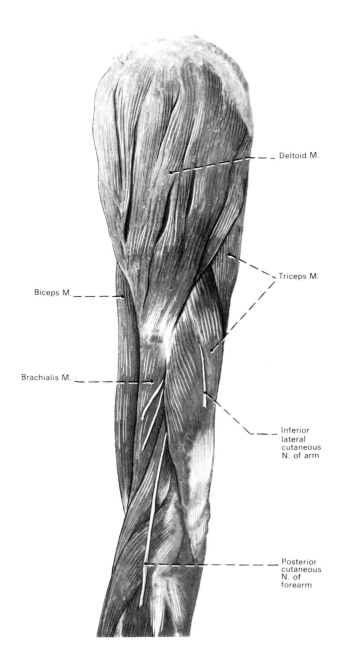

Fig. 1.32 The cutaneous nerves and superficial veins of the upper limb.

Fig. 1.33 The left deltoid muscle.

Remove the skin completely from the arm, and then remove the superficial fascia, looking out for the **medial and lateral cutaneous nerves of the forearm** as you do so [Fig. 1.32]. Note the position of the veins in the roof of the cubital fossa, since they are commonly used for intravenous injections. Trace the **cephalic** and **basilic veins** as they ascend on the lateral and medial sides of the biceps muscle respectively. Note that the basilic vein pierces the deep fascia about the middle of the arm. You will find the medial cutaneous nerve of the forearm lying close to it.

Now clean the deep fascia, but do not remove it. It is attached to the supracondylar ridges of the humerus, forming the medial and lateral intermuscular septa of the arm. This fact will be demonstrated more clearly later, when you incise the fascia. Below the elbow the fascia blends with the bicipital aponeurosis of the biceps tendon.

Structures around the shoulder joint

The deltoid muscle

Complete the cleaning of the deltoid muscle, dividing the deep fascia for this purpose [Fig. 1.33]. A feature of the deltoid muscle is that its central portion consists of a number of short tendons into which muscle fibres are inserted obliquely. This arrangement, called multipennate, makes the muscle extremely powerful. The origin of the deltoid from the clavicle and the scapula, and its insertion into the humerus, should be clearly defined on the cadaver and then on the skeleton.

Now make a transverse incision through the muscle close to its attachment to the borders of the clavicle, acromion, and spine of the scapula. The muscle should now be turned down to display the important structures which lie deep to it.

The axillary nerve [Fig. 1.34]

Pick up and clean the axillary nerve, and follow it round the neck of the humerus. It divides into an anterior branch, which winds round the humerus to the anterior border of the muscle, which it supplies by several branches, some of which pierce the muscle to become cutaneous nerves to the overlying skin; and a posterior branch which supplies not only the deltoid but also the teres minor muscle, and which ends as a cutaneous nerve, the **superior lateral cutaneous nerve of the arm,** which turns round the posterior border of the deltoid to become cutaneous.

Below and medial to the axillary nerve you may find the small **posterior cutaneous nerve of the arm,** a branch of the radial nerve. Do not spend time following this nerve.

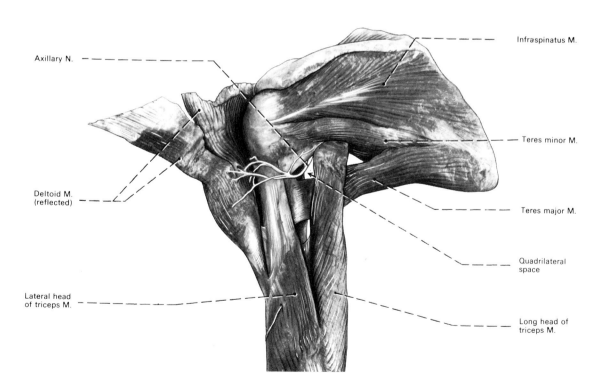

Fig. 1.34 The posterior aspect of the left shoulder joint. The quadrilateral space is not referred to in the text.

Axillary N.

Infraspinatus M.

Teres minor M.

Deltoid M. (reflected)

Teres major M.

Quadrilateral space

Lateral head of triceps M.

Long head of triceps M.

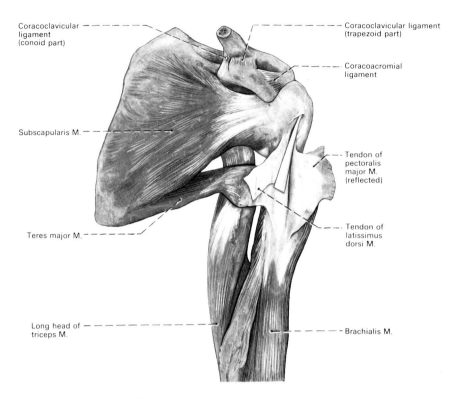

Coracoclavicular ligament (conoid part)

Coracoclavicular ligament (trapezoid part)

Coracoacromial ligament

Subscapularis M.

Tendon of pectoralis major M. (reflected)

Tendon of latissimus dorsi M.

Teres major M.

Long head of triceps M.

Brachialis M.

Fig. 1.35 The anterior aspect of the left shoulder joint.

The ligaments of the coracoid process

Now identify the coracoid process of the scapula and clean and define the ligaments attached to it [Fig. 1.35].

The **coracoclavicular ligament,** which ties the lateral end of the clavicle to the coracoid process, consists of a postero-medial **conoid ligament** and an antero-lateral **trapezoid ligament,** the former being a thick round ligament and the latter a thinner quadrilateral one.

The **coracoacromial ligament** is a triangular band whose base is attached to the lateral border of the coracoid process and whose apex is fixed to the acromion lateral to the clavicle. A **coracohumeral ligament** willl be seen later.

The muscles around the shoulder joint

Clean and define the tendon of the subscapularis, as it passes immediately in front of the shoulder joint to its insertion into the lesser tubercle of the humerus. Turn the limb, and on the greater tubercle identify the tendons of three muscles, the **supraspinatus, infraspinatus,** and **teres minor** muscles, in that order from above down [Fig. 13.4]. Clean these muscles, which arise from and cover the dorsal surface of the scapula. In order to expose the supraspinatus [Fig. 1.36], the clavicular insertion of trapezius must be divided close to the bone.

The subacromial bursa

A bag formed by loose connective tissue that will now come

into view between the acromion and the upper end of the humerus is the subacromial bursa, which should be removed as far as possible.

The deltoid muscle

With a scapula and humerus by your side, look again at the muscles which you have cleaned. The deltoid [Figs 1.33 and 1.34] will be seen to arise as a continuous sheet from the lateral third of the clavicle, the lateral border of the acromion, and the inferior border of the crest of the spine of the scapula. Follow it to its insertion into the deltoid tuberosity. It is obvious that this muscle is an abductor of the upper limb as you can see for yourself if you move your arm away from your body by pressing against a wall, when the muscle stands out very clearly. You can also see that its anterior fibres flex and medially rotate, and that the posterior fibres extend and laterally rotate the upper limb. You have already seen that the muscle is supplied by the axillary nerve.

The supraspinatus and infraspinatus muscles

Follow the supraspinatus muscle [Figs 1.36 and 1.43] to its origin from the supraspinous fossa on the scapula, and in so far as you can, to its insertion on the uppermost facet on the greater tubercle of the humerus. As you do so, clean away any remains of the subacromial bursa, but at this stage do not incise the coracoacromial ligament. The supraspinatus

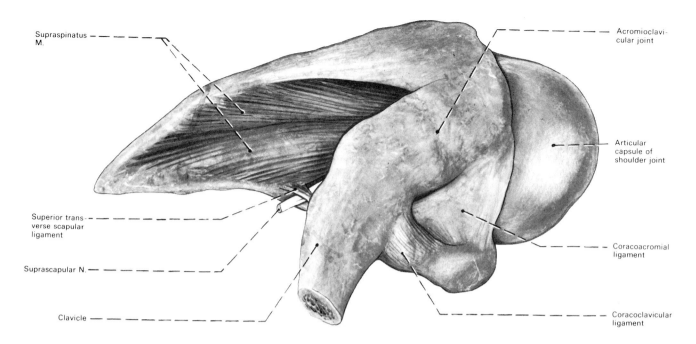

Supraspinatus M.

Superior transverse scapular ligament

Suprascapular N.

Clavicle

Acromioclavicular joint

Articular capsule of shoulder joint

Coracoacromial ligament

Coracoclavicular ligament

Fig. 1.36 The left supraspinatus muscle (viewed from above).

will be seen to blend with the articular capsule of the shoulder joint. The action of this muscle, which you will see in its entirety when the shoulder joint is dissected, is to stabilize the head of the humerus as the deltoid abducts the limb.

The infraspinatus muscle [Fig. 1.34] should be traced to its origin from the infraspinous fossa on the scapula, and then to its insertion into the middle facet on the greater tubercle of the humerus, where it also blends with the capsule of the shoulder joint. Both the supraspinatus and infraspinatus muscles are innervated by the suprascapular nerve. This nerve arises from the superior trunk of the brachial plexus, and as you have already seen, passes through the scapular notch.

The teres minor muscle [Fig. 1.34]

Now look at the teres minor muscle. It is a small round muscle which arises from the upper part of the dorsal surface of the lateral border of the scapula, below the origin of the long head of the triceps. Trace it to its insertion on the lowest facet of the greater tubercle of the humerus. Note that it, too, blends with the capsule of the shoulder joint. It is innervated by the posterior branch of the axillary nerve.

If you examine the attachments of the infraspinatus and teres minor muscles on the cadaver and verify them on the skeleton, you will see that they must be lateral rotators of the upper limb.

The subscapularis muscle

Now turn the arm over, and examine the muscle which fills

the subscapular fossa on the costal surface of the scapula [Fig. 1.35]. This is the subscapularis muscle. Follow it to its insertion on to the lesser tubercle of the humerus, and into the capsule of the shoulder joint. Note that it is a direct anterior relation of the joint. This large muscle is supplied by the subscapular nerves, which spring from the posterior cord of the brachial plexus. If you follow the muscle from its origin to its insertion, you will see that it must be a medial rotator of the upper limb.

It should be noted that all four short muscles of the shoulder joint (the supraspinatus, infraspinatus, teres minor, and subscapularis) are inserted into the articular capsule, forming a musculotendinous cuff around the joint which retains the head of the humerus in contact with the glenoid cavity of the scapula, and thus maintains the stability of the shoulder joint.

The teres major muscle

Now examine the muscle which lies immediately to the lateral side of subscapularis. This is the teres major [Figs 1.34 and 1.35]. Follow it to its origin from the lower part of the dorsal surface of the lateral border of the scapula. You will see that it arises below the teres minor and that it extends down as far as the inferior angle of the scapula. Clean its insertion into the crest of the lesser tubercle, which is the medial lip of the intertubercular groove on the humerus. Note that when it contracts it must medially rotate, adduct, and extend the upper limb. It is supplied by the lower branch of the subscapular nerve.

1.31

Structures on the front of the arm

You must now reflect the deep fascia from the front and back of the arm and from the elbow region. Make central vertical incisions through the fascia on the front and back of the arm, and a circular incision at the level of the elbow joint. Then reflect the fascial flaps medially and laterally from the vertical incisions. The **medial** and **lateral intermuscular septa** now come into view. They give origin to certain muscles and divide the arm into anterior and posterior compartments.

The biceps muscle

The biceps is the most superficial muscle of the anterior compartment, which is seems to fill. Behind it is the brachialis, closely applied to the front of the humerus. The posterior compartment on the back of the arm is filled by the triceps, which arises by three heads.

At this stage you can see that the biceps arises by two tendinous heads [Fig. 1.38]. Later, you will see that the **short head** is thick and flattened, and that it arises with the coracobrachialis from the tip of the coracoid process. The **long head** is a narrow tendon which starts inside the shoulder

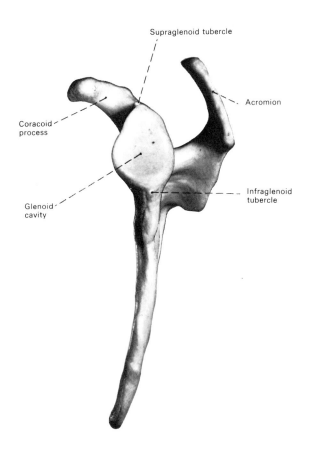

Fig. 1.37 The lateral aspect of the left scapula.

Supraglenoid tubercle

Acromion

Coracoid process

Infraglenoid tubercle

Glenoid cavity

joint from a tubercle, the supraglenoid tubercle, at the apex of the glenoid cavity [Fig. 1.37]. Examine this tubercle on the scapula. The course of the tendon of the long head within the joint, where it arches over the head of the humerus, will be seen later. It emerges from the articular capsule, sheathed in synovial membrane, and passes down the intertubercular groove, within which it is held by a transverse ligament of the shoulder joint.

Both tendinous heads pass into elongated fleshy bellies which fuse together in the lower part of the arm, where they become continuous with a flattened tendon which is inserted into the posterior part of the tuberosity of the radius [Fig. 1.38]. You will be able to study the insertion at a later stage of your dissection.

The brachialis muscle

The brachialis muscle [Fig. 1.35] arises as a fleshy mass from the front of the lower half of the humerus, and from the two intermuscular septa. Expose its upper part, and note that this embraces the insertion of the deltoid muscle. Below you can see that the muscle covers the front of the elbow joint before ending in a thick tendon which is inserted, as you will see later, into the tuberosity of the ulna on the front of the coronoid process.

The biceps and brachialis muscles are flexors of the elbow joint. If you bend your arm at the elbow against resistance, you will see the whole of this anterior muscle mass, in particular the biceps, standing out.

The vessels and nerves [Fig. 1.38]

Pick up the **brachial artery** with its companion veins, on the medial side of the biceps muscle. Clean the artery, and remove the veins. You will see that the brachial artery is relatively superficial, but that it is overlapped to a variable extent by the biceps. Note its oblique course. At its origin the artery lies on the medial aspect of the humerus, whereas at its termination, it is midway between the two epicondyles. Verify the fact that from above down the artery lies on the long head of triceps, then on the medial head, then on the insertion of coracobrachialis and finally on brachialis.

Then study the relationship of the nerves to the vessel [Fig. 1.38]. You will see that the **median nerve** is at first lateral to the artery. About the middle of the arm it crosses the vessel, usually anteriorly, and in the lower half of the arm the nerve is medial to the artery.

Observe that the **ulnar nerve** is medial to the artery in the upper half of its course, but that later it pierces the medial intermuscular septum and descends in the posterior compartment of the arm, where it comes to lie in the groove behind the medial epicondyle.

Now look for the **radial nerve** lying behind the beginning of the brachial artery, between it and the long head of triceps. The nerve is passing to the back of the arm.

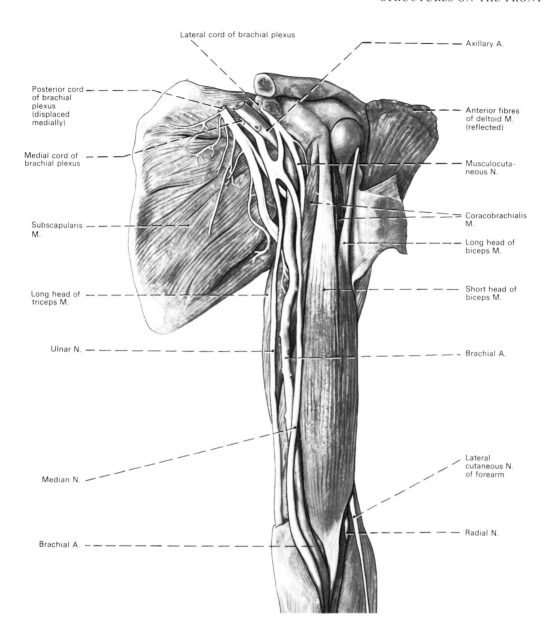

Lateral cord of brachial plexus

Axillary A.

Posterior cord of brachial plexus (displaced medially)

Anterior fibres of deltoid M. (reflected)

Medial cord of brachial plexus

Musculocutaneous N.

Coracobrachialis M.

Subscapularis M.

Long head of biceps M.

Short head of biceps M.

Long head of triceps M.

Brachial A.

Ulnar N.

Median N.

Lateral cutaneous N. of forearm

Radial N.

Brachial A.

Fig. 1.38 The front of the left arm.

You will have noticed three or four branches of the brachial artery. They supply adjacent muscles and take part in an anastomosis around the elbow joint. The one passing deeply with the radial nerve is called the **profunda brachii artery**; the one accompanying the ulnar nerve is called the **superior ulnar collateral artery.** Do not spend unnecessary time dissecting these vessels.

You can now study the **musculocutaneous nerve** throughout its course in the arm [Fig. 1.38]. Arising from the lateral cord of the brachial plexus, it will be seen to descend into the arm between the axillary artery and the coracobrachialis muscle. Here it gives off a small branch to the muscle, which you have already seen [p. 1.19]. At the lower border of the

axilla the nerve passes through the coracobrachialis muscle. Trace it as it descends under cover of the biceps on the brachialis muscle. It supplies both these muscles, and the nerve to the brachialis also supplies the elbow joint. Near the bend of the elbow the nerve emerges at the lateral side of the biceps and pierces the deep fascia to supply the skin. It is subsequently known as the lateral cutaneous nerve of the forearm.

The coracobrachialis muscle

The attachments of the coracobrachialis muscle [Fig. 1.38] should now be confirmed. Follow it from its origin from the tip of the coracoid process, by a tendon common to it and the short head of biceps, to its insertion into the medial border of the shaft of the humerus, opposite the deltoid tuberosity. The muscle is a flexor and a weak adductor of the upper limb.

Structures on the back of the arm

The radial nerve

Clean and trace the radial nerve in the arm, at the same time as you study the triceps muscle [Fig. 1.40]. Start where the nerve arises from the posterior cord of the brachial plexus. Here it will be found behind the axillary artery. If you turn the arm over you can see that the nerve then descends behind the upper part of the artery between the long head and medial head of the triceps. From this point it is accompanied by its companion artery, the profunda brachii, which, as you have seen, is a branch of the brachial artery. The nerve descends to the lateral border of the arm, deep to the triceps, running for a short time in the groove for the radial nerve on the back of the humerus.

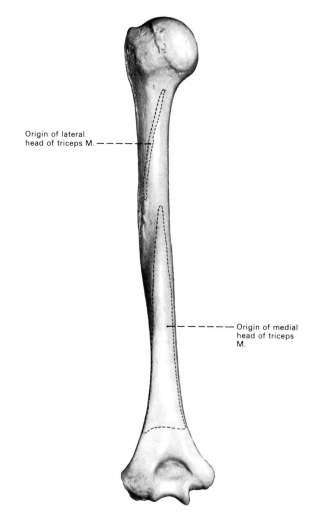

Origin of lateral head of triceps M. — — — —

— — — — — — — Origin of medial head of triceps M.

Fig. 1.39 The humeral origins of the left triceps muscle.

The triceps muscle [Fig. 1.40]

Now study the triceps muscle. One of its three heads, the **long head,** has a tendinous origin from the infraglenoid tubercle of the scapula. You will see that it lies medial to the lateral head and superficial to the medial head. These arise directly from the posterior surface of the humerus [Fig. 1.39]. The **lateral head** arises from the narrow oblique ridge on the humerus, which marks the upper part of the groove for the radial nerve, and from the lateral intermuscular septum. The **medial head,** which is covered by the other two parts of the muscle, has an extensive origin from the back of the humerus, starting below the groove for the radial nerve, and reaching almost to the trochlea. It also arises from the medial intermuscular septum.

You will be able to see that the fibres of the triceps become inserted into the superior surface of the olecranon of the ulna. The muscle is an extensor of the elbow joint. If you try to straighten your bended arm against resistance you will feel your triceps becoming prominent just below the posterior border of the deltoid muscle.

Separate the upper end of the long head of triceps from the upper part of the lateral head and find the radial nerve between them. It may help if you first find the nerve on the front of the arm. Now insert a pair of forceps along the course of the nerve beneath the lateral head, remembering that the nerve runs obliquely across the back of the arm [Fig. 1.40]. Gently cut down on to the forceps and so divide the lateral head of the muscle. Turn aside the two halves of the lateral head and display the radial nerve and the medial head of the triceps.

The branches of the radial nerve

As you clean the radial nerve you will inevitably see the branches it sends to the three heads of triceps. Try to identify two cutaneous branches which also spring from it in the arm. You may already have seen the origin of the first, the **posterior cutaneous nerve of the arm,** in the axilla; the nerve supplies an area of skin on the posterior aspect of the arm. The **inferior lateral cutaneous nerve of the arm** [Fig. 1.40] pierces the lateral head of the triceps muscle just below the insertion of the deltoid muscle. It supplies the skin of the lateral surface of the lower half of the arm. The **posterior cutaneous nerve of the forearm** also arises from the radial nerve as it lies on the back of the humerus. It pierces the deep fascia about the middle of the arm and supplies an area of skin in the lower part of the back of the arm and the middle of the back of the forearm.

The radial nerve should now be followed forwards as it pierces the lateral intermuscular septum. Turn the arm over and pick up the nerve in the anterior compartment of the arm, between the brachialis muscle on its medial side, and the origin of one of the muscles of the forearm, the brachioradialis, laterally [Fig. 1.41]. As you continue cleaning

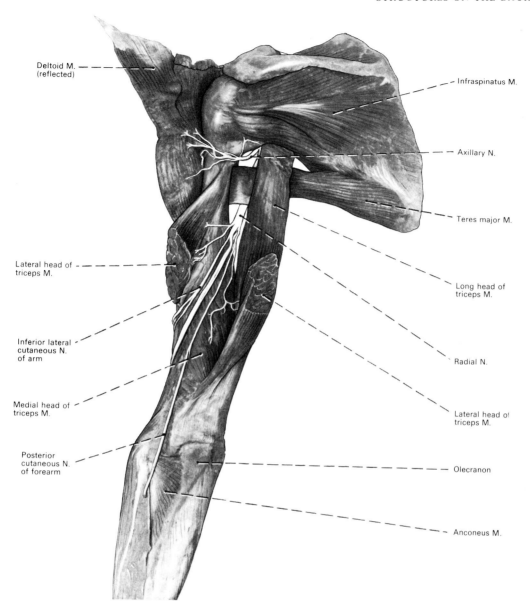

Deltoid M.
(reflected)

Infraspinatus M.

Axillary N.

Teres major M.

Lateral head of
triceps M.

Long head of
triceps M.

Inferior lateral
cutaneous N.
of arm

Radial N.

Medial head of
triceps M.

Lateral head of
triceps M.

Posterior
cutaneous N.
of forearm

Olecranon

Anconeus M.

Fig. 1.40 The back of the left arm. The lateral head of the triceps muscle has been divided and the two parts turned aside.

the nerve, try to find the branches it sends into these muscles, and also to another muscle of the forearm that arises close to the brachioradialis, the extensor carpi radialis longus. At the level of the lateral epicondyle you will see that the radial nerve gives off a **deep branch** called the **posterior interosseous nerve.** If you pull the brachioradialis and the extensor carpi radialis longus aside you may see that this nerve passes backwards and that it pierces a muscle called the supinator. The **superficial branch** (or main trunk of the radial nerve) continues into the forearm.

Joints of the shoulder girdle

Before proceeding with the dissection of the forearm, complete the examination of the joints of the shoulder region,

beginning with the acromioclavicular joint. Turn the deltoid muscle away from the joint and detach the trapezius muscle from its remaining attachment to the acromion and spine of the scapula, thereby removing the muscle completely.

The acromioclavicular joint

The acromioclavicular joint is an articulation between the clavicle and the acromion of the scapula. The joint, which is subcutaneous and easily palpated, is a synovial plane joint, allowing gliding movement between the two articulating surfaces. Clean the articular capsule and define its accessory ligaments [Fig. 1.42]. The most important is the **coracoclavicular ligament,** consisting of two powerful ligamentous bands, the **conoid** and **trapezoid ligaments** which you should have already seen. This ties the lateral end of

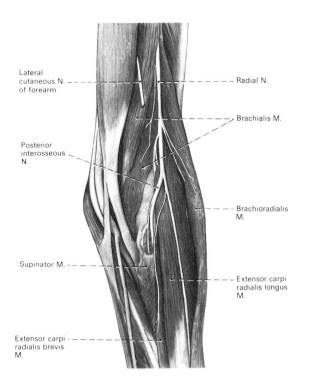

Lateral
cutaneous N.
of forearm

Radial N.

Brachialis M.

Posterior
interosseous
N.

Brachioradialis
M.

Supinator M.

Extensor carpi
radialis longus
M.

Extensor carpi
radialis brevis
M.

Fig. 1.41 The left brachioradialis muscle and radial nerve. The arm is viewed from the antero-lateral aspect and the brachioradialis muscle has been pulled aside.

the clavicle to the coracoid process of the scapula. Note its attachment to the inferior surface of the clavicle, and to the coracoid process of the scapula.

Now examine the strong **coracoacromial ligament** which, besides being an accessory ligament of the acromioclavicular joint, protects the shoulder joint and helps to prevent the upward displacement of the humerus. Note again the triangular shape of the ligament, and that it is attached by its apex to the tip of the acromion in front of the articular facet and by its base to the lateral border of the coracoid process.

The interior of the acromioclavicular joint

Now open the acromioclavicular joint. Do this by incising right through its capsule so that the clavicle is separated from the acromion. Hinge the clavicle forwards on the coracoclavicular ligament and examine the articular surfaces. You will usually find an incomplete **articular disc** which partially separates the articular surfaces.

Next, saw through the spine of the scapula at its junction with the acromion [Fig. 1.43] and hinge the detached acromion forwards on the coracoacromial ligament, which is still attached by its base to the coracoid process. Clear away that part of the subacromial bursa which was beneath the ligament, and complete the cleaning of the supraspinatus muscle, noting that its insertion blends with the upper part of the capsule of the shoulder joint.

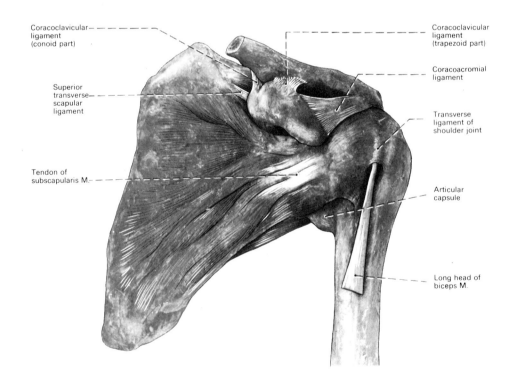

Coracoclavicular
ligament
(conoid part)

Coracoclavicular
ligament
(trapezoid part)

Coracoacromial
ligament

Superior
transverse
scapular
ligament

Transverse
ligament of
shoulder joint

Tendon of
subscapularis M.

Articular
capsule

Long head of
biceps M.

Fig. 1.42 The left shoulder and acromioclavicular joints.

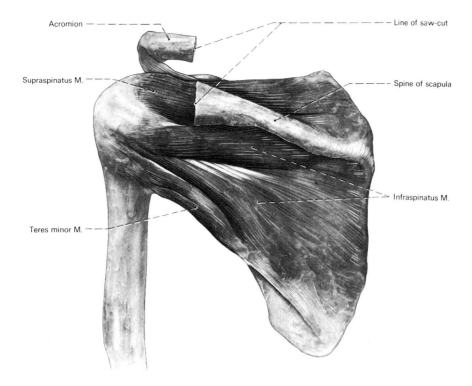

Acromion — — — — —

Supraspinatus M. — — —

Teres minor M. — — —

Line of saw-cut

Spine of scapula

Infraspinatus M.

Fig. 1.43 The removal of the left acromion. The acromion is elevated.

Movements of the shoulder girdle

The sternoclavicular joint and the acromioclavicular joint are joints of the shoulder girdle. All movements of the shoulder joint are associated with reciprocal movements of the shoulder girdle, and any movement of the scapula must result in some movement of the clavicle. In elevation and depression of the shoulder, movement at the sternoclavicular joint takes place between the clavicle and the articular disc. Elevation of the shoulder is produced by the upper fibres of the trapezius and the levator scapulae, and is limited by the costoclavicular ligament. Depression is produced chiefly by gravity, assisted by the lower fibres of the trapezius, pectoralis minor, and subclavius muscles, and is limited by the first rib and the sternoclavicular ligaments. In forward and backward movement of the shoulder, the clavicle and articular disc move on the manubrium of the sternum. Forward movement is produced by the serratus anterior, which pulls the medial border of the scapula forwards, backward movement by the trapezius, rhomboid major, and rhomboid minor muscles. The acromioclavicular joint allows the scapula to glide on the clavicle when the former rotates as the arm is thrust forward, or when it is elevated above the head. The acromioclavicular joint also comes into play in elevation and depression of the shoulder; it enables the scapula to maintain close contact with the chest wall as it moves.

Try to study these various movements on your own body and the muscle groups that produce them.

The shoulder joint

The shoulder joint must now be examined. It consists of an articulation between the globular head of the humerus and the shallow glenoid cavity of the scapula. It is a synovial joint of the ball and socket type. You can already see that the **articular capsule** covers the head of the humerus and is attached to the anatomical neck of the humerus. When the joint is opened you will have a better opportunity of confirming this attachment. Look at the front of the joint [Fig. 1.42] and note that the tendon of the long head of biceps emerges from inside the capsule. It is held in place in the intertubercular groove by a small band of fibrous tissue, called the **transverse ligament of the shoulder joint,** which acts as a retinaculum stretching across the groove.

Relations of the shoulder joint

Note that the subscapularis muscle, with the axillary vessels and infraclavicular branches of the brachial plexus, lie in front of the joint, whilst the infraspinatus and teres minor muscles lie behind the joint. The supraspinatus muscle lies above it [Figs 1.44 and 1.45].

Abduct the arm in order to see the inferior relations of the joint, and particularly the position of the axillary nerve. It appears to be almost adherent to the capsule [Fig. 1.40]. Medial to the axillary nerve is the long head of the triceps, and below the nerve is the teres major.

1.37

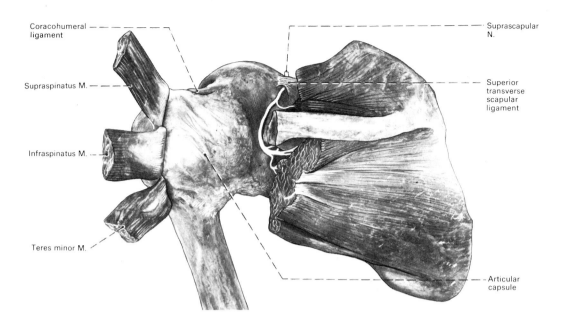

Coracohumeral
ligament

Supraspinatus M.

Infraspinatus M.

Teres minor M.

Suprascapular
N.

Superior
transverse
scapular
ligament

Articular
capsule

Fig. 1.44 The posterior aspect of the left shoulder joint.

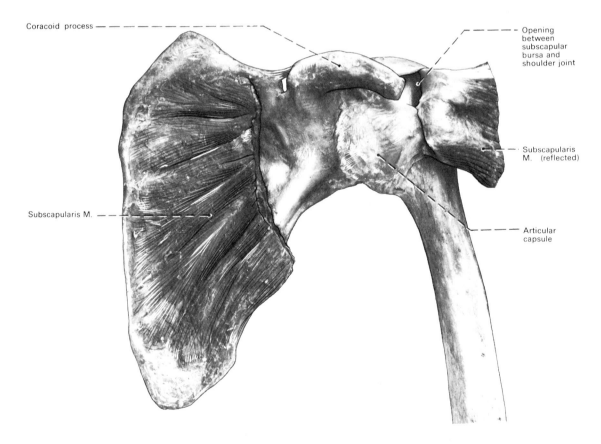

Coracoid process

Subscapularis M.

Opening
between
subscapular
bursa and
shoulder joint

Subscapularis
M. (reflected)

Articular
capsule

Fig. 1.45 The anterior aspect of the left shoulder joint.

The coracohumeral ligament

Now dissect on the upper aspect of the joint, in front of the tendon of the supraspinatus muscle, and define a broad band, called the coracohumeral ligament [Fig. 1.44], which strengthens the upper part of the articular capsule and passes from the base of the coracoid process to the front of the greater tubercle of the humerus. Note that its posterior border blends with the tendon of supraspinatus.

The articular capsule

In order to expose the articular capsule completely you must now divide several muscles. Cut the conjoint tendons of the biceps and coracobrachialis 2 cm from their origin, and turn the main parts of these muscles away from the joint. Divide the teres major transversely through its midpoint, and the long head of triceps 2 cm below its origin. Now divide the supraspinatus, infraspinatus, and teres minor muscles, in each case making a transverse cut about 5 cm from their insertions. If you then turn back the distal end of each muscle [Fig. 1.44], the posterior part of the capsule will be exposed, and you will be able to confirm that it is attached to the rim of the glenoid cavity. Note again that the tendons of these three muscles blend with the capsule of the joint. As you turn back the infraspinatus you may find a bursa between it and the capsule; this bursa may occasionally open into the joint. Find the cut end of the suprascapular nerve as it passes beneath the superior transverse scapular ligament [p. 1.23]. Then, reflecting as necessary the supraspinatus and infraspinatus, trace the nerve as it passes round the lateral border of the spine of the scapula into the infraspinous fossa, giving branches to both muscles [Fig. 1.44].

Turn the arm over, and divide the subscapularis muscle in a similar manner to the other three muscles. As you turn its distal end towards the humerus, look for a bursa which constantly lies between the upper part of its tendon and the articular capsule [Fig. 1.45]. This bursa, which is called the **subscapular bursa,** always communicates with the joint cavity. Note that the anterior part of the capsule, like the posterior part, is attached to the margin of the glenoid cavity.

Forcefully separate the humerus from the scapula, and note the wide gap you have made between the bones. In keeping with the wide range of movement of which the joint is capable, the articular capsule is very thin and lax. The joint is, in fact, the most unstable joint in the body, and is commonly dislocated.

It will be obvious to you that the muscles whose tendons blend with the capsule of the joint form a musculotendinous cuff in front, above, and behind the joint. These muscles maintain the head of the humerus in the glenoid cavity whichever way the humerus is moved relative to the scapula [Fig. 1.46]. The shoulder joint thus depends for its stability

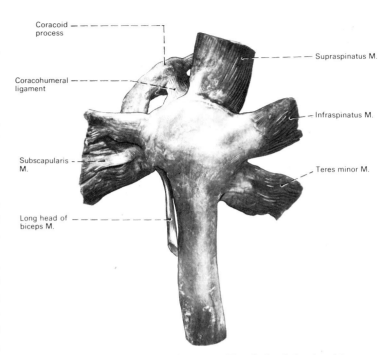

Fig. 1.46 The 'musculotendinous cuff' of the left shoulder joint (lateral view). The muscles inserted into the head of the humerus have been divided and reflected laterally.

on the tone of the muscles around it, and not on the strength of its capsule or on ligaments.

The interior of the shoulder joint

The joint should now be opened from behind by means of a vertical incision through the capsule, 1 cm from its scapular attachment. Then splay the joint like a hinge and study its interior [Fig. 1.47]. You will see that the capsule is attached above to the margins of the articular surface of the glenoid cavity of the scapula, outside a rim of cartilage, called the **labrum glenoidale,** which is attached to the edge of the cavity. You can now easily confirm that the capsule is attached below to the anatomical neck of the humerus, extending down to the shaft of the bone for a short distance medially.

The labrum deepens the shallow glenoid cavity, which, like the head of the humerus, is covered with shiny articular hyaline cartilage.

Synovial membrane provides on its inner surface a slimy lubricant for the joint. It lines the capsule and covers the outer surface of the labrum glenoidale. It also ensheathes the tendon of the long head of biceps and is prolonged on that tendon for a short distance outside the joint, extending down as far as the surgical neck of the humerus. The capsule is thus perforated by the long head of biceps. It is also deficient under the tendon of the subscapularis, and sometimes beneath the tendon of the infraspinatus, allowing the synovial membrane to herniate in the form of bursae. It should be noted that the tendon of the biceps, though within the capsule of the joint, lies outside the synovial cavity.

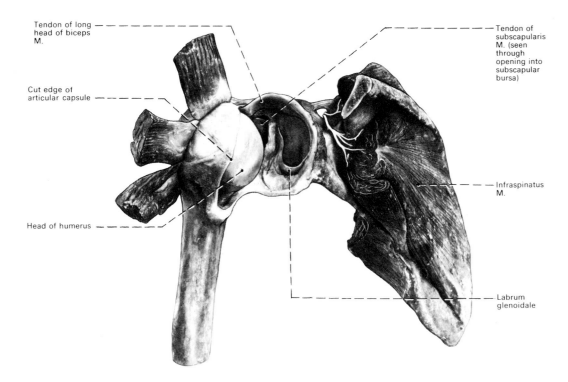

Tendon of long
head of biceps
M.

Cut edge of
articular capsule

Head of humerus

Tendon of
subscapularis
M. (seen
through
opening into
subscapular
bursa)

Infraspinatus
M.

Labrum
glenoidale

Fig. 1.47 The labrum glenoidale and the interior of the left shoulder joint (posterior view).

Now look at the long head of biceps above the head of the humerus, and note its attachment to the supraglenoid tubercle. Below it you will see the opening from the shoulder joint into the subscapular bursa and, through this opening, the tendon of the subscapularis muscle.

Pull the head of the humerus from the glenoid cavity so as to stretch the anterior part of the articular capsule. You may then see three thickenings in it called the **superior, middle,** and **inferior glenohumeral ligaments.** They are all attached to the anterior margin of the glenoid cavity.

Movements of the shoulder joint

Before beginning the dissection of the forearm, try to work out the actions of the muscles which control the shoulder joint. Note that the joint is innervated by the suprascapular, axillary, and lateral pectoral nerves, the three nerves which supply most of the muscles by which it is moved. This will help you to remember much of what you have dissected so far. Note again that the movements which occur at the joint are accompanied by compensatory movements of the joints of the shoulder girdle.

Flexion of the arm (forward movement) is performed by the coracobrachialis, biceps, and pectoralis major and the anterior fibres of the deltoid.

Extension (backward movement) is performed by the latissimus dorsi, teres major, and the posterior fibres of the deltoid.

Abduction is performed chiefly by the deltoid, assisted by the supraspinatus.

Adduction is performed chiefly by the pectoralis major, the latissimus dorsi, and the coracobrachialis, assisted by the teres major and teres minor.

Lateral rotation is performed by the teres minor and infaspinatus.

Medial rotation is performed by the pectoralis major, latissimus dorsi, subscapularis, and teres major.

Circumduction is a combination of these movements.

You should examine the movement of these various muscle groups on your own shoulder region.

Remember that the four short muscles which are inserted into the head of the humerus and into the articular capsule (supraspinatus, infraspinatus, teres minor, and subscapularis) maintain the head of the humerus in apposition with the glenoid cavity of the scapula, when the joint is moved by the larger and more powerful muscles which act on it.

Section 1.3
The front of the forearm

Like the arm, the forearm consists mostly of muscles, of which those on the anterior aspect are mainly flexors of the wrist joint and fingers, and those on the posterior aspect extensors. The flexors are in general more massive than the extensors, and the decreasing girth of the forearm as the wrist is approached mainly reflects the fact that the fleshy bellies of the forearm muscles, the origins of many of which extend upwards on to the lower part of the lateral and medial supracondylar ridges of the humerus and also on to the intermuscular septa attached to them, give way to tendons in the distal half of the forearm. Those muscles which extend on to the humerus are weak flexors and extensors of the elbow joint.

Osteology

The radius and ulna

Turn either to an articulated skeleton or to isolated specimens of the humerus, ulna, and radius which you can fit together. Note again how the two bones of the forearm articulate not only with the humerus but also with each other [Fig. 1.48]. As you have already seen, the proximal end or **head of the radius** articulates with the **radial notch** on the lateral surface of the ulna, to which it is held by the **annular ligament of the radius** [Fig. 1.27]. Similarly, the distal end or **head of the ulna** articulates with the **ulnar notch** on the medial side of the lower widened end of the radius. These articulations make it possible for the radius to rotate by rolling over the ulna.

Hold the radius and ulna together in the supinated position. You will see that the medial border of the shaft of the radius and the lateral border of the shaft of the ulna are sharp. These are the interosseous borders of the bones. They are joined by a thin ligamentous sheet called the **interosseous membrane of the forearm** [Fig. 1.49].

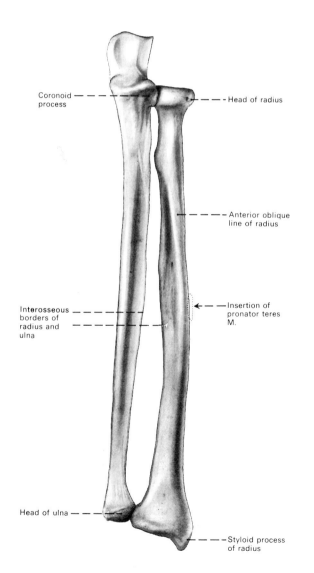

Coronoid process — Head of radius — Anterior oblique line of radius — Insertion of pronator teres M. — Interosseous borders of radius and ulna — Head of ulna — Styloid process of radius

Fig. 1.48 The left radius and ulna (anterior view).

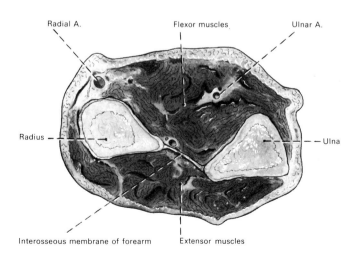

Radial A. — Flexor muscles — Ulnar A. — Radius — Ulna — Interosseous membrane of forearm — Extensor muscles

Fig. 1.49 Cross-section of the left forearm (viewed from above). The radius is slightly pronated.

In cross-section each bone has a roughly triangular shaft whose surfaces are demarcated by somewhat indistinct anterior and posterior borders as well as by the sharp interosseous border [Figs 1.48 and 1.49]. The anterior surfaces of both bones and the anterior surface of the interosseous membrane form a long shallow basin from which the flexor muscles of the wrist and fingers arise, their common head of origin extending upwards to the medial epicondyle of the humerus. The extensor muscles arise from a corresponding posterior basin, and extend upwards on to the lateral epicondyle and the lower part of the lateral supracondylar ridge of the humerus.

On the lateral surface of the shaft of the radius, at the point of maximum curvature of the bone, you will find a small, somewhat roughened ridge, into which the pronator teres muscle is inserted [Fig. 1.48]. The anterior border of the radius appears to pass just in front of this roughening, and upwards it follows an oblique course across the bone to the tuberosity into which the biceps is inserted. This upper extension of the anterior border is called the **anterior oblique line** of the radius.

The radius and ulna are held together at the wrist in such a way that a single articular surface is formed for the carpal bones of the wrist [Fig. 1.50], with which the five metacarpal bones articulate.

The carpal and metacarpal bones

On the skeleton note that there are eight carpal bones arranged in two rows of four [Fig. 1.51]. From the lateral

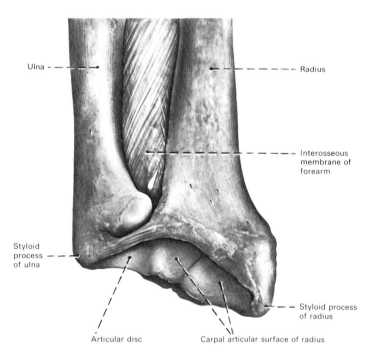

Ulna

Radius

Interosseous membrane of forearm

Styloid process of ulna

Articular disc

Carpal articular surface of radius

Styloid process of radius

Fig. 1.50   The distal ends of the left radius and ulna (anterior view).

to the medial side the proximal row comprises the **scaphoid, lunate, triquetral,** and **pisiform bones.** The distal row consists of the **trapezium, trapezoid, capitate,** and **hamate bones.** Note the shape, size, and position of the scaphoid bone, which is a common site of fracture, and the groove flanked by a prominent crest on the anterior surface of the trapezium, called the **tubercle of the trapezium.** As you will see later, the groove lodges the tendon of a muscle called the flexor carpi radialis. Also note the hook-shaped process on the hamate, which is called the **hook of the hamate,** and the small spherical pisiform , which you can see rides on the palmar aspect of the triquetral bone. Note the shape of the metacarpal bones, and particularly the rounded heads of the four medial metacarpal bones. These form the knuckles. Note that there are three phalanges for each of the fingers, but two only for the thumb.

Surface anatomy

Pronate your own left forearm at the same time as you press with the fingers of your right hand into the fossa below your elbow joint. You will feel the most lateral part of the mass of flexor muscles contracting. This is the pronator teres muscle. Look again at the skeleton. The muscle arises superficially from the medial epicondyle of the humerus, in common with other flexor muscles, and deeply from the front of the coronoid process of the ulna, medial to the bigger area into which the brachialis is inserted. You cannot feel the insertion of the muscle, which lies deep to a group of extensor muscles on the lateral side of the forearm.

With the forearm pronated you can easily feel the posterior border of the ulna intervening between the flexor and extensor groups of muscles, both of which are arranged, as you will see later, in superficial and deep layers.

You will have noticed that the distal end or head of the ulna is smaller than the proximal end, and that the reverse condition holds in the case of the radius [Fig. 1.48]. You can feel that both bones are somewhat superficial in the lower half of the forearm, and whatever the position of the forearm, you will have no difficulty in palpating the prominent styloid process of the radius. The more slender styloid process of the ulna is better felt with the forearm in a semipronated position. At a later stage you will find out the names of the ligaments which connect the styloid processes with the hand, as well as the prominent tendons which run in front of the wrist joint, and those which you can feel passing in bony grooves on the back of the distal ends of the ulna and radius.

Reflection of the skin

Now continue with the dissection of the front of the forearm.

The skin and superficial fascia should be removed separ-

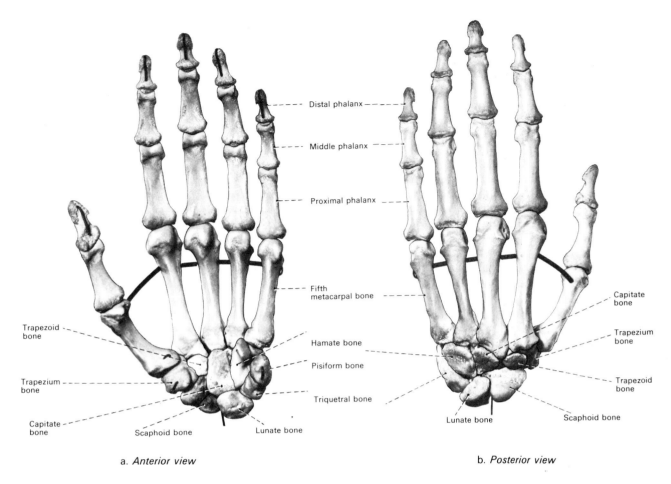

a. *Anterior view*   b. *Posterior view*

Fig. 1.51   The bones of the left hand.

ately, after making a midline vertical incision on the anterior surface, with transverse incisions at the level of the distal crease at the wrist. Reflect the skin flaps laterally and medially, and clear away the superficial fascia, noting any cutaneous nerves as you do so [Fig. 1.32].

If you examine the deep fascia in front of the elbow, you will be able to define the special thickening called the **bicipital aponeurosis** which, as you have already seen, springs from the upper part of the tendon of the biceps [Fig. 1.52]. The aponeurosis blends with the deep fascia on the medial side of the upper part of the forearm. Remove the deep fascia of the forearm, with the exception of the bicipital aponeurosis, and so display the superficial muscles on the front of the forearm. Clean these muscles.

The cubital fossa

The brachioradialis muscle

The most lateral muscle of the forearm is the brachioradialis [Fig. 1.52]. You can see that it arises from the upper two-thirds of the lateral supracondylar ridge of the humerus. It

becomes tendinous about midway down the forearm and is inserted into the lateral side of the distal end of the radius. It is essentially a flexor of the elbow joint. You can demonstrate this on yourself. With the forearm in the semi-pronated position, flex the elbow against resistance and observe that the brachioradialis stands out. Deep to it on the lateral margin of the forearm which you are dissecting identify two other muscles, the extensor carpi radialis longus and extensor carpi radialis brevis.

Clean the brachioradialis muscle, taking care not to damage the radial nerve which lies deep to it, and also clean the pronator teres [Figs 1.52 and 1.53]. These muscles form the inferior boundaries of the cubital fossa.

The contents of the fossa should now be explored. First identify the tendon of biceps. Clean and trace it as it passes to its insertion into the radial tuberosity. Now remove the bicipital aponeurosis to find the brachial artery, which lies on the medial side of the tendon of biceps. Separate the muscles to display the artery's two terminal branches; the radial artery passing laterally and superficially, and the ulnar artery passing medially and deeply.

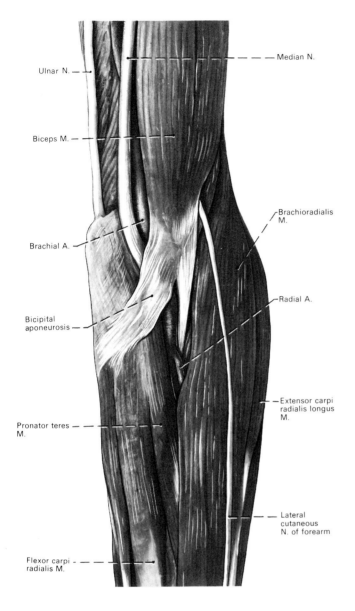

Fig. 1.52   Structures anterior to the left elbow joint.

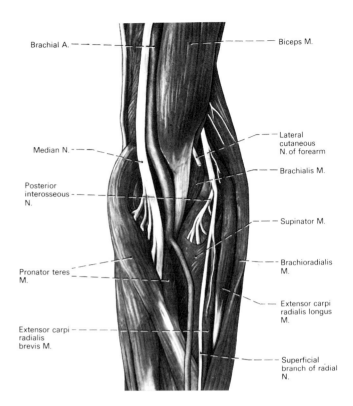

Fig. 1.53   The left cubital fossa.

can be seen closely applied to the neck of the radius. It forms a small part of the floor of the fossa.

The radial nerve

Pick up the radial nerve between the belly of the brachio-radialis and the distal part of the brachialis. As you clean the nerve, again note its deep branch, the posterior inter-osseous nerve, passing into the supinator muscle [Fig. 1.53]. You will study it at a later stage in the posterior compartment of the forearm. Trace the superficial branch of the radial nerve as it passes deep to the brachioradialis. Close to the wrist you will see that it passes dorsally behind the tendon of the muscle [Fig. 1.54].

Structures on the front of the forearm

The radial artery

Clean the radial artery and trace its course in the forearm, at the same time removing its companion veins. Start at its origin in the cubital fossa [Fig. 1.52], and then, pulling the brachioradialis aside, trace and clean it downwards, noting its relations to adjacent structures. It lies successively on the insertions of the biceps, supinator, and pronator teres muscles, and on the flexor digitorum superficialis, flexor pollicis longus, and pronator quadratus muscles, and finally on the radius itself. It turns back at the wrist, behind some slender tendons that pass to the thumb [Fig. 1.54].

The pronator teres muscle [Fig. 1.53]

Clean the median nerve, on the medial side of the brachial artery, and trace it down as it passes into the forearm through the pronator teres. Note the two heads of this muscle. The part superficial to the nerve is the **humeral head.** It arises from the medial epicondyle, and a variable amount of the humerus above the epicondyle; the part deep to the nerve is the **ulnar head,** which arises from the front of the coronoid process.

Now trace the insertion of the **brachialis** into the anterior aspect of the coronoid process. Note that it forms the major part of the floor of the cubital fossa. By pulling the brachio-radialis aside, part of another muscle, the supinator,

1.44

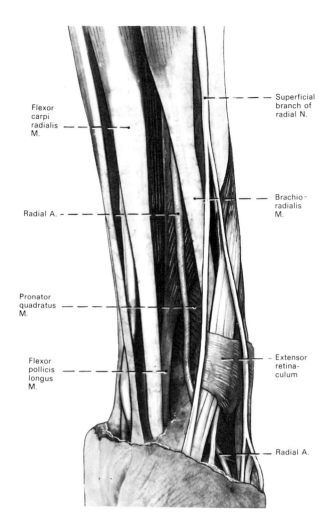

Flexor carpi radialis M.

Radial A.

Pronator quadratus M.

Flexor pollicis longus M.

Superficial branch of radial N.

Brachio-radialis M.

Extensor retina-culum

Radial A.

Fig. 1.54   The radial nerve and artery at the left wrist.

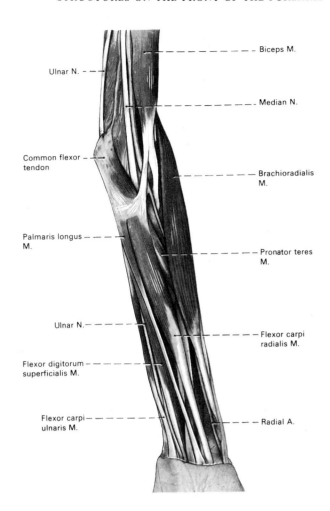

Ulnar N.

Common flexor tendon

Palmaris longus M.

Ulnar N.

Flexor digitorum superficialis M.

Flexor carpi ulnaris M.

Biceps M.

Median N.

Brachioradialis M.

Pronator teres M.

Flexor carpi radialis M.

Radial A.

Fig. 1.55   The superficial muscles of the front of the left forearm.

The superficial muscles of the forearm

Examine the muscles that arise from a common flexor tendon which is attached to the medial epicondyle of the humerus [Fig. 1.55]. You have already cleaned the **pronator teres.** The muscle immediately medial to it is the **flexor carpi radialis.** In the middle of the forearm the fleshy belly of this muscle gives way to a long tendon, which passes to the wrist. On its medial side is the **palmaris longus** (if present) and the **flexor carpi ulnaris,** whose tendon also passes to the wrist. Deep to these muscles is another muscle, the **flexor digitorum superficialis,** part of which springs from the common flexor tendon. Its tendons are inserted, as you will see later, into the fingers.

Define the insertion of the pronator teres into the radius halfway along the convex lateral surface of the bone, and then divide the muscle transversely just distal to the point at which the belly of the muscle becomes independent of the other muscles which arise from the common flexor tendon. Then separate the flexor carpi radialis and palmaris longus from the underlying flexor digitorum superficialis, and divide them transversely in the middle of the forearm. As you turn them aside, you may pick up the branches sent to them by the median nerve. The origin of the flexor digitorum superficialis can now be studied. Part of it arises from the common flexor tendon. A small slip of the muscle can also be seen rising from the upper part of the medial side of the coronoid process of the ulna, as can the more prominent and broader radial head which comes prominently into view at this stage, arising from the anterior oblique line of the radius. The muscle ends in four tendons which pass into the hand.

Detach the radial head of the flexor digitorum superficialis from the bone. Under cover of it you will find a muscle, the flexor pollicis longus, arising from the shaft of the radius and the interosseous membrane. Pull on this muscle, which requires practically no cleaning, and watch its single tendon move the thumb. Immediately to the medial side of the muscle is the belly of the deep flexor of the fingers, the flexor digitorum profundus.

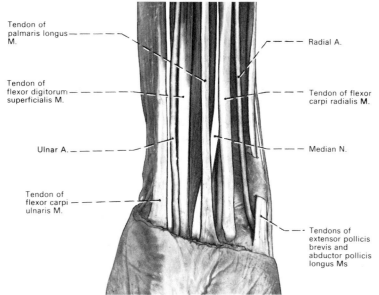

Tendon of palmaris longus M.

Tendon of flexor digitorum superficialis M.

Ulnar A.

Tendon of flexor carpi ulnaris M.

Radial A.

Tendon of flexor carpi radialis M.

Median N.

Tendons of extensor pollicis brevis and abductor pollicis longus Ms

Fig. 1.56   Structures anterior to the left wrist.

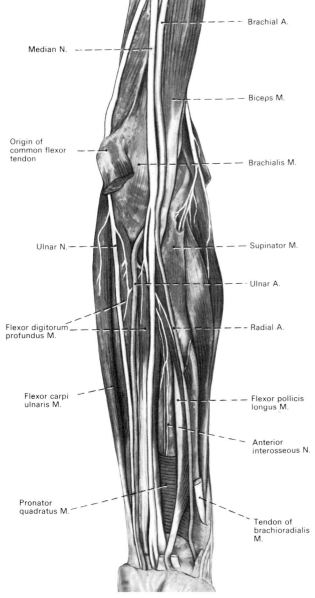

Median N.

Origin of common flexor tendon

Ulnar N.

Flexor digitorum profundus M.

Flexor carpi ulnaris M.

Pronator quadratus M.

Brachial A.

Biceps M.

Brachialis M.

Supinator M.

Ulnar A.

Radial A.

Flexor pollicis longus M.

Anterior interosseous N.

Tendon of brachioradialis M.

Fig. 1.57   The deep muscles of the front of the left forearm.

The median nerve [Fig. 1.57]

Now pick up the median nerve in the cubital fossa, between the two heads of the pronator teres [Fig. 1.53]. Note that the ulnar head of the muscle separates the median nerve from the ulnar artery, which lies posterior to the muscle. Follow the nerve from this point as it runs on the deep surface of the flexor digitorum superficialis, to which it will be found to be adhering. The muscle on which it lies is the flexor digitorum profundus, which also ends below in four flexor tendons to the fingers. Observe carefully that the nerve is very superficially disposed at the wrist, with the flexor digitorum superficialis on its medial and the flexor carpi radialis on its lateral aspect [Fig. 1.56].

The narrow palmaris longus tendon, when present, overlies the nerve. The tendon enters the palm by passing superficial to a transverse fibrous band called the flexor retinaculum. Do not follow the median nerve further at this stage, but quickly identify the branches it sends to the pronator teres, flexor carpi radialis, palmaris longus, and flexor digitorum superficialis muscles. Just distal to the cubital fossa, also find a deep branch of the median nerve. This, the **anterior interosseous nerve,** descends on the interosseous membrane, accompanied by vessels, between the flexor pollicis longus and the flexor digitorum profundus. It supplies the former and the radial half of the latter. Trace the anterior interosseous nerve until it disappears, near the wrist, under a small transversely-disposed rhomboidal muscle which passes from the anterior surface of the ulna to the radius [Fig. 1.57]. This muscle is the pronator quadratus, which the anterior interosseous nerve also

supplies. The anterior interosseous nerve ends at the wrist by supplying the wrist joint and intercarpal joints.

The ulnar artery

Return to the cubital fossa and pick up the ulnar artery at its origin from the brachial artery [Fig. 1.57]. Note that it passes deep to the ulnar head of the pronator teres [Fig. 1.53] as well as under the flexor digitorum superficialis. Trace the artery as it runs downwards and medially on the flexor digitorum profundus [Fig. 1.57]. Near its origin it will be seen to lie under cover of the muscles arising from the common flexor tendon, and lower down beneath the flexor carpi

1.46

ulnaris. The nerve on its medial side is the ulnar nerve, which supplies the medial half of the flexor digitorum profundus and the flexor carpi ulnaris. The artery is relatively superficial at the wrist where, with the ulnar nerve, it passes superficial to the flexor retinaculum [Fig. 1.62] to enter the palm. Note now that the median nerve passes under the retinaculum.

Near its origin the ulnar artery gives off an important, but very short, **common interosseous artery,** and this should be merely identified at this stage. This vessel divides at the upper border of the interosseous membrane into **anterior and posterior interosseous arteries** which, with the corresponding nerves, run down on the front and back of the membrane respectively.

The ulnar, radial, and interosseous arteries all give branches which help to form an anastomosis around the elbow joint, and similar branches which contribute to an anastomosis around the wrist joint. Do not spend any time searching for these small vessels.

The ulnar nerve

Look behind the medial epicondyle of the humerus and pick up the ulnar nerve [Fig. 1.57]. If you feel your own arm at this point you will easily identify the nerve. Follow the nerve on your specimen and note that it passes between a head of origin of the flexor carpi ulnaris muscle from the medial epicondyle, and another which the muscle obtains from the medial surface of the olecranon and from a fascial aponeurosis attached to the posterior border of the ulna. The nerve then lies on the flexor digitorum profundus. From this point the nerve should be traced distally under the flexor carpi ulnaris and on the flexor digitorum profundus. About the middle of the forearm it is joined by the ulnar artery and the two descend together as far as the hand.

The deep muscles of the forearm [Fig. 1.57]

Now re-examine the origins and insertions of the brachioradialis and the pronator teres. Note again the nerve supply to the first from the radial nerve, and to the second from the median nerve. Observe again that the brachioradialis is essentially a flexor of the elbow joint.

The superficial flexors should now be turned aside in order to study the attachments and nerve supply of the supinator and pronator quadratus muscles. At the same time look again at a disarticulated radius and ulna. Note the depression which lies immediately distal to the radial notch on the ulna. It lodges but gives no attachment to the tendon of the biceps muscle. This depression will be seen to be bounded posteriorly by the sharp **supinator crest** from which part of the supinator muscle takes origin.

Turn to your dissected specimen, and you will see that the **supinator muscle** consists of a superficial part which arises from the lateral epicondyle and a deep part which passes from the supinator crest of the ulna laterally to wrap itself round the upper part of the radius, reaching to the anterior oblique line [Figs 1.57 and 1.78]. It is obvious that the muscle must supinate the forearm from the pronated position.

Examine the **pronator quadratus muscle,** under the superior border of which you have already seen the anterior interosseous nerve disappearing. Note the attachment of the muscle to the front of the lower quarter of the ulna and radius.

Verify the origins of the **flexor pollicis longus** from the shaft of the radius, and the **flexor digitorum profundus** from the shaft of the ulna, and see how the two muscles appear to run into each other on the interosseous membrane.

Now examine in further detail the insertions of the two powerful flexors of the elbow joint, the biceps and brachialis muscles. If you follow the tendon of biceps distally you will find that it is inserted into the posterior part of the radial tuberosity. A bursa lies between the tendon and the smooth anterior part of the tuberosity. You can demonstrate its presence by opening it with a scalpel. The brachialis can be seen to be inserted into the anterior aspect of the coronoid process of the ulna.

Note that the brachialis is only a flexor of the elbow. The biceps, in addition to being a flexor of the elbow, is the most powerful supinator of the forearm, in which action it is reinforced by the supinator muscle. You can verify this by first pronating your own forearm, flexing the elbow and then observing that your biceps swells when you supinate against resistance.

Section 1.4
The palm of the hand

Surface anatomy

Examine the surface of your own wrist and hand [Fig. 1.58]. Look first at the transverse creases at the wrist. The distal crease indicates the proximal border of the flexor retinaculum, which forms the roof of a tunnel for the flexor tendons of the wrist and finger joints, as they pass into the palm. The proximal crease roughly indicates the level of the wrist joint.

The rounded muscle mass on the radial (lateral) aspect of the palm is known as the **thenar eminence.** It is formed by the short muscles of the thumb, and is bounded medially by the radial longitudinal crease of the palm. A similar mass on the ulnar (medial) aspect of the palm, known as the **hypothenar eminence,** is formed by the short muscles of the little finger. The proximal transverse crease at the base of each finger is distal to the position of the metacarpophalangeal joint, but the two distal transverse creases on each digit almost correspond to the two interphalangeal joints. Feel the thick web of muscle joining the thumb and the index finger. This is formed on the palmar aspect by the transverse

head of a muscle called the adductor pollicis, and on the dorsal aspect by another muscle called the first dorsal interosseous muscle.

The thumb, as you will realize, is set at an angle to the plane of the palm. Forward movement away from the palm is termed abduction, the converse movement adduction. Medial movement across the palm is called flexion, the converse extension. Opposition is the movement whereby the palmar aspect of the thumb touches the palmar aspect of another finger of the same hand. Try these movements on your own thumb.

Reflection of the skin

Start by reflecting the skin of the palm. To do this satisfactorily the fingers should be pinned to a board. Make the following incisions through the skin [Fig. 1.58]:

1. Along the ulnar border of the palm, as far as the base of the little finger.
2. A transverse incision across the bases of the fingers, extending to the radial border of the palm.
3. Central incisions along the thumb and one or more fingers.

Remove the skin from the palmar surface of the hand by turning the skin flap laterally before completely detaching it. Remove the skin from the fingers by turning the skin flaps aside. To do this without injury to the underlying structures will tax both your skill and patience, for while the superficial fat will protect deeper structures from your knife in some places, the fat is not evenly distributed, and at the palmar creases is wholly absent. Here the skin is adherent to an underlying **palmar aponeurosis** [Fig. 1.59] and great care will be needed if this and the palmar cutaneous nerves are not to be mutilated.

Structures in the palm and fingers

The pulp of the finger

Examine the pulp of the finger. This is the fleshy part of the front of the distal part of each finger. When the skin is removed from the finger, you may see that it is attached to the periosteum covering the underlying bone by a number of radially-arranged fibrous septa. In this way the pulp of the finger becomes divided into separate compartments.

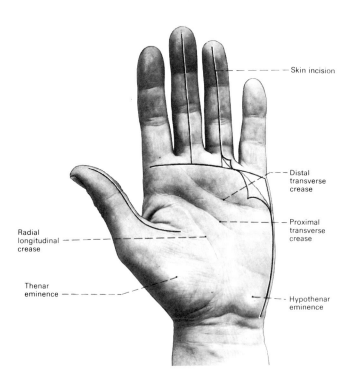

Fig. 1.58 The palmar surface of the left hand (showing skin incisions).

Skin incision

Distal transverse crease

Proximal transverse crease

Radial longitudinal crease

Thenar eminence

Hypothenar eminence

1.48

These are limited proximally by a septum at the level of the distal interphalangeal joint. This attaches the skin to the distal end of the **digital fibrous sheath** surrounding the flexor tendons [Fig. 1.60]. In this way a closed 'pulp space' is defined. These anatomical facts are important because of the way infections of the fingers are contained.

The palmar aponeurosis [Fig. 1.59]

Look out for some transversely-disposed muscle fibres in the subcutaneous tissue at the base of the hypothenar eminence. They constitute the **palmaris brevis muscle,** which is attached to the flexor retinaculum, the palmar aponeurosis, and the skin. If you divide the muscle, which is of little importance, you will see that it overlies the ulnar artery and nerve. At this point it will be possible to pick up the **palmar cutaneous branch of the ulnar nerve.**

When the palmar aponeurosis is cleaned it will be seen to be a dense triangular band of fibrous tissue, which is attached by its apex to the transversely-disposed flexor retinaculum adjacent to the palmaris longus tendon. This tendon becomes continuous with the aponeurosis, the base of which divides at the fingers into four slips, between which the digital vessels and nerves and some thin muscles called the lumbrical muscles will be seen passing distally [Fig. 1.60]. Note that each slip divides into two, and so forms

an arch for the flexor tendons of the fingers. Follow the slips as they pass distally to blend with the proximal ends of the digital fibrous sheaths in which the flexor tendons are held to the phalanges. The sheaths should now be exposed on those fingers from which you have removed the skin.

Pick up the **palmar digital nerves** and **palmar digital arteries** to one or two fingers at the base (i.e. the distal part) of the aponeurosis, and trace them distally; do not disturb those to the radial side of the index finger or those to the thumb.

The fascial spaces of the palm

From the palmar aponeurosis thin fascial septa pass deeply between the flexor tendons to merge with the fascia over the deep muscles of the palm. The septa which enclose the flexor tendons to the index finger and the first lumbrical muscle, sometimes collectively called the oblique septum [Fig. 1.61], form the boundary between the medial and lateral palmar fascial spaces, which lie deep to the tendons of the flexor digitorum profundus. The **lateral space** lies superficial to the transverse head of the adductor pollicis muscle, and the **medial space** anterior to the interosseous muscles between the third and fourth, and fourth and fifth metacarpal bones.

With these facts in mind, detach the apex of the palmar

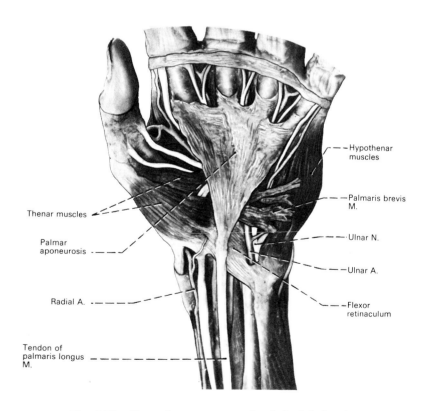

Fig. 1.59 The palmar aponeurosis of the left hand.

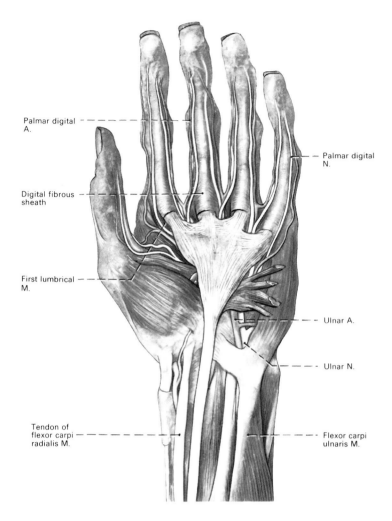

Palmar digital
A.

Palmar digital
N.

Digital fibrous
sheath

First lumbrical
M.

Ulnar A.

Ulnar N.

Tendon of
flexor carpi
radialis M.

Flexor carpi
ulnaris M.

Fig. 1.60   Superficial dissection of the left palm.

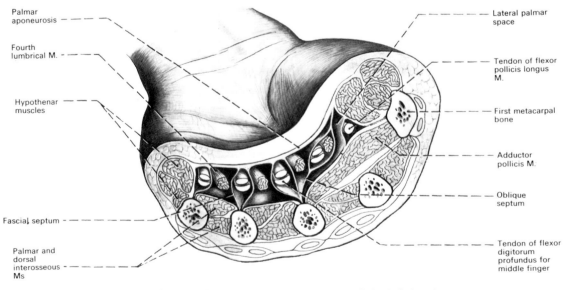

Palmar
aponeurosis

Fourth
lumbrical M.

Hypothenar
muscles

Fascial septum

Palmar and
dorsal
interosseous
Ms

Lateral palmar
space

Tendon of flexor
pollicis longus
M.

First metacarpal
bone

Adductor
pollicis M.

Oblique
septum

Tendon of flexor
digitorum
profundus for
middle finger

Fig. 1.61   A schematic transverse section of the left hand.

aponeurosis from the flexor retinaculum and reflect it towards the fingers, taking care not to injure the underlying structures. As you throw the palmar aponeurosis forward the fascial septa will come into view and should be divided.

The fascial spaces are of importance to the surgeon, since they confine pus which may collect when deep infections occur in the hand.

The flexor retinaculum

Now examine the flexor retinaculum [Fig. 1.62]. It is a tough band of fibrous tissue which measures about 2.5 cm transversely, and 2 cm proximo-distally, and which is attached on each side to the margins of the carpal bones. It converts the carpal arch into the **carpal tunnel,** through which the tendons of the flexor digitorum superficialis, flexor digitorum profundus, and the flexor pollicis longus, as well as the median nerve, pass into the palm [Fig. 1.63]. Clean the retinaculum and define the ulnar nerve and artery as they pass over it into the palm under cover of a small fibrous

band [Fig. 1.62]. Note again how the tendon of the palmaris longus passes over (or fuses with) the retinaculum.

Clean the median nerve and note that just distal to the flexor retinaculum it divides into medial and lateral terminal branches, and that the latter gives off a stout muscular branch which supplies the thenar muscles.

The thenar eminence and muscles

Now clean the muscles which make up the thenar eminence. Its surface consists of two muscles, the **abductor pollicis brevis** laterally and the **flexor pollicis brevis** medially [Fig. 1.64]. These two muscles should be separated from each other and divided transversely about their middles. By turning aside their cut ends you expose another thenar muscle. This is the small but important **opponens pollicis** [Fig. 1.62]. Trace the attachments of these short muscles of the thumb, noting that all three arise together from the flexor retinaculum and the tubercles of the scaphoid and trapezium bones. On the ulnar side of the opponens pollicis is the **oblique head**

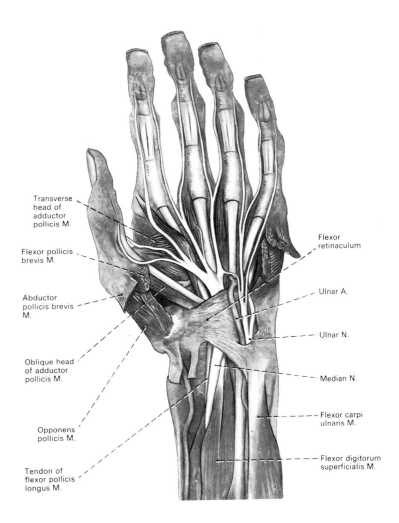

Transverse head of adductor pollicis M.

Flexor pollicis brevis M.

Abductor pollicis brevis M.

Oblique head of adductor pollicis M.

Opponens pollicis M.

Tendon of flexor pollicis longus M.

Flexor retinaculum

Ulnar A.

Ulnar N.

Median N.

Flexor carpi ulnaris M.

Flexor digitorum superficialis M.

Fig. 1.62 The flexor retinaculum of the left hand.

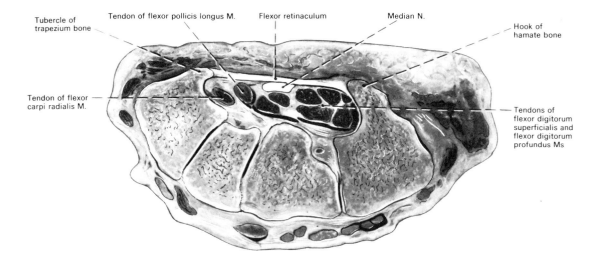

Tubercle of trapezium bone

Tendon of flexor pollicis longus M.

Flexor retinaculum

Median N.

Hook of hamate bone

Tendon of flexor carpi radialis M.

Tendons of flexor digitorum superficialis and flexor digitorum profundus Ms

Fig. 1.63   Cross-section through the left carpal bones to show the flexor retinaculum (viewed from above).

of the adductor pollicis muscle, which arises from the base of the second and third metacarpal bones and the capitate bone; the more prominent transverse head of the adductor arises from the palmar surface of the third metacarpal bone. You will now be able to see that both heads insert into the base of the proximal phalanx of the thumb.

The abductor and flexor will be found to be inserted together on the radial side of the base of the proximal phalanx of the thumb, a sesamoid bone (i.e. a small seed-like bone that develops in a tendon) usually being present in the tendon. The opponens pollicis will be found to be inserted into the radial border of the first metacarpal bone. These three muscles are supplied by the median nerve. Their functions will be studied later.

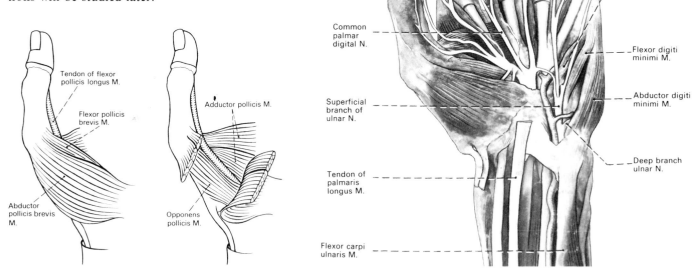

Tendon of flexor pollicis longus M.

Flexor pollicis brevis M.

Adductor pollicis M.

Abductor pollicis brevis M.

Opponens pollicis M.

Common palmar digital N.

Superficial branch of ulnar N.

Tendon of palmaris longus M.

Flexor carpi ulnaris M.

Opponens digiti minimi M.

Flexor digiti minimi M.

Abductor digiti minimi M.

Deep branch ulnar N.

Fig. 1.64   The left thenar muscles. In the right-hand figure the abductor pollicis brevis and flexor pollicis brevis muscles have been divided and reflected proximally.

Fig. 1.65   The palmar digital nerves of the left hand.

The ulnar nerve and artery

Return now to the ulnar nerve and artery at the base of the hypothenar eminence [Fig. 1.65]. Trace them back into the forearm and note that as they pass into the palm over the flexor retinaculum they lie lateral to the pisiform bone and medial to the projecting hook of the hamate. At the base of the hypothenar eminence you will see that the ulnar nerve divides into a **superficial branch** and a **deep branch,** and that the ulnar artery gives off a **deep palmar branch** which accompanies the deep branch of the nerve.

Follow the superficial branch of the nerve. You will see that it divides into a **palmar digital nerve,** which supplies the ulnar aspect of the palm and the ulnar side of the little finger, and a **common palmar digital nerve** which subdivides into two branches which supply the adjacent sides of the little finger and ring finger. You may notice that the latter nerve sends a **communicating branch** to join the most medial digital branch of the median nerve.

Examine the deep branch of the ulnar nerve, and note that it supplies all the muscles of the hypothenar eminence.

The hypothenar eminence and muscles.

Taking care not to damage the ulnar artery and nerve, clean and define the muscles of the hypothenar eminence [Fig. 1.65]. Medially on the surface lies the **abductor digiti minimi** and laterally on the same plane is the **flexor digiti minimi.** These two small muscles take origin from the flexor retinaculum, from the pisiform bone and from the hook of the hamate bone, and are inserted into the medial side of the base of the proximal phalanx of the little finger. Cut transversely through the middle of the abductor and flexor muscles. Deep to them you will see the minute **opponens digiti minimi** muscle, which has the same origin as the other two short muscles. It is pierced by the deep branch of the ulnar nerve and is inserted into the medial part of the shaft of the fifth metacarpal bone. The abductor and flexor have the actions indicated by their names. Palpate the ulnar border of your own hypothenar eminence and forcibly abduct your little finger. As you do so you can feel the abductor digiti minimi contracting.

The median nerve [Fig. 1.65]

Now return to the median nerve. You have seen that its lateral branch supplies the muscles of the thenar eminence. Trace the prominent cutaneous branches it gives to the sides of the thumb and the lateral side of the index finger. A fine branch from the latter passes to the first lumbrical muscle. This branch is easy to find, but also to snap.

Follow the distribution of the medial branch of the median nerve, and trace branches, **common palmar digital nerves,** to the adjacent sides of the index, middle, and ring fingers and also, if you can, to the second lumbrical muscle. These nerves divide into **palmar digital nerves** which pri-

marily supply the palmar surface of the fingers, but also give branches to the dorsum of the distal phalanx of the thumb and the dorsum of the middle and distal phalanges of the index, middle, and half the ring fingers [Fig. 1.75]. This arrangement is variable, so do not try to do more than find dorsal branches to one finger. You may already have found the thin nerve by which the most medial branch of the median nerve communicates with the most lateral branch of the ulnar nerve.

The superficial palmar arch

Next study the superficial palmar arch [Fig. 1.66]. This is formed almost entirely from the **ulnar artery,** but the arch is completed laterally by a branch from one of the terminal branches of the radial artery (either the **superficial palmar branch of the radial artery,** a small vessel which passes over the thenar muscles from the point where the radial artery turns backwards behind the tendons of the muscles of the thumb to the back of the wrist, or a branch from either the princeps pollicis artery or the radialis indicis artery, which

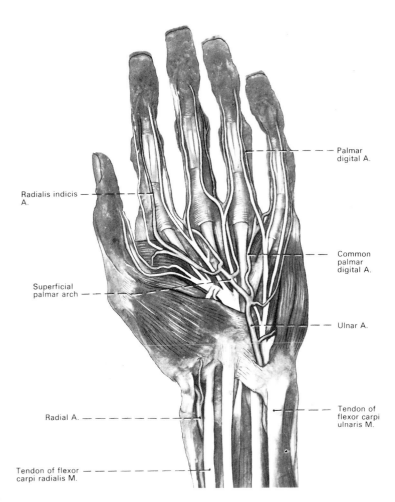

Radialis indicis A.

Superficial palmar arch

Radial A.

Tendon of flexor carpi radialis M.

Palmar digital A.

Common palmar digital A.

Ulnar A.

Tendon of flexor carpi ulnaris M.

Fig. 1.66 The superficial palmar arch. In this hand the radialis indicis artery completes the superficial palmar arch, and in fact appears to arise from it.

are branches of the main terminal part of the radial artery, when it returns to the deep aspect of the palm).

The arch is very superficial, lying immediately beneath the palmar aponeurosis, with the branches of the median nerve, flexor tendons, and lumbrical muscles deep to it. Note its position in the palm, where it is very vulnerable to deep cuts. It lies proximal to the proximal transverse palmar crease, and within the space enclosed by two vertical lines from the ulnar margin of the ring finger and the radial margin of the middle finger.

The three **common palmar digital arteries** given off from the convexity of the arch, as shown in Fig. 1.66, supply the fingers and should be traced distally.

The flexor tendons in the palm

Now clear away the superficial structures from the middle of the palm and so expose the flexor tendons and the lumbrical muscles. Cut through the flexor retinaculum and divide the median nerve at the wrist and turn it distally. Also divide the ulnar artery where it becomes the superficial palmar arch. As you turn the nerve back you expose the oblique head of the adductor pollicis muscle.

The tendons of the flexor digitorum superficialis and flexor digitorum profundus are surrounded beneath the flexor retinaculum by the **common flexor synovial sheath** [Fig. 1.67]. The tendon of the flexor pollicis longus is enclosed in a similar synovial sheath. Sometimes the sheaths are separate, but in most cases they communicate beneath the flexor retinaculum. They begin about 2.5 cm proximal to the flexor retinaculum.

The **sheath of the flexor pollicis longus tendon** extends as far as the insertion of the tendon into the base of the distal phalanx of the thumb. The common flexor synovial sheath

extends as far as the middle of the palm, except for that part which surrounds the flexor tendons of the little finger. This part extends as far as the insertion of the flexor digitorum profundus tendon into the base of the distal phalanx.

The flexor tendons in the fingers

Examine the arrangement of the flexor tendons on the index, middle, and ring fingers. The tendons are surrounded by **digital synovial sheaths** which are entirely separate from the common flexor sheath, which ended in the middle of the palm. They run in the **digital fibrous sheaths** which are attached to the margins of the phalanges [Fig. 1.68].

Open these fibrous sheaths. You will see that they are particularly thick over the shafts of the phalanges, the **annular part of the fibrous sheath,** and very thin over the joints, the **cruciform part of the fibrous sheath.** Tubular synovial sheaths, within the fibrous sheaths, surround the tendons. Next define the relationship of the tendons of the flexor digitorum superficialis and those of the flexor digitorum pro-

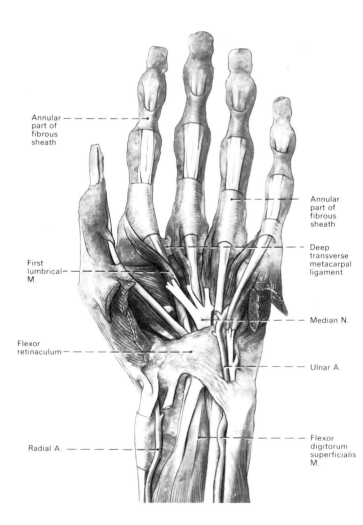

Fig. 1.68 The digital fibrous sheaths of the left hand.

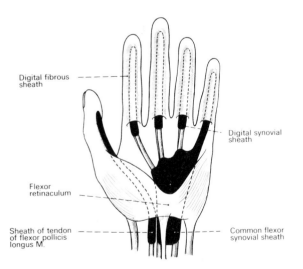

Fig. 1.67 The synovial sheaths of the flexor tendons of the left hand.

fundus. Note how the former split to enclose the latter [Fig. 1.69]. Follow the tendons to their insertions, the superficialis into the margins of the middle phalanx of each finger, and the profundus into the base of the distal phalanx. Note the fibrous bands called **vincula longa** and **vincula brevia** by which these tendons are attached to the phalanges [Fig. 1.70]. These vincula carry blood vessels to the tendons. Next trace the tendon of flexor pollicis longus to its insertion into the base of the distal phalanx of the thumb.

The lumbrical muscles

Clean the four lumbrical muscles between the deep flexor tendons in the palm. The first and second arise from the lateral aspects of the tendons of flexor digitorum profundus to the index and middle fingers respectively; the third and fourth will be found to arise by two heads from the adjacent sides of the tendons of flexor digitorum profundus to the middle and ring, and ring and little fingers respectively [Fig. 1.71]. Follow the tendon of each lumbrical muscle as it

passes to the radial side of the metacarpophalangeal joint. At a later stage you will see that it is inserted chiefly into the expansion of the tendons of the extensor muscles to the corresponding digit. A careful dissection will reveal a further slip of the tendon of the lumbrical muscle passing into the base of the proximal phalanx.

The lumbricals flex the metacarpophalangeal joints, and are essentially concerned with the fine movements of the hand. The two lateral lumbricals are innervated by the median nerve and the two medial ones by the ulnar nerve.

Clean away the synovial sheaths from the tendons of the flexor digitorum superficialis and the flexor digitorum profundus, and divide the tendons at the wrist. Turn them down in order to expose the deep muscles of the hand, the deep palmar arch, and the deep branch of the ulnar nerve. As this is done you may be able to see that the nerves supplying the two medial lumbrical muscles spring from the deep branch of the ulnar nerve. Divide these fine branches if you see them.

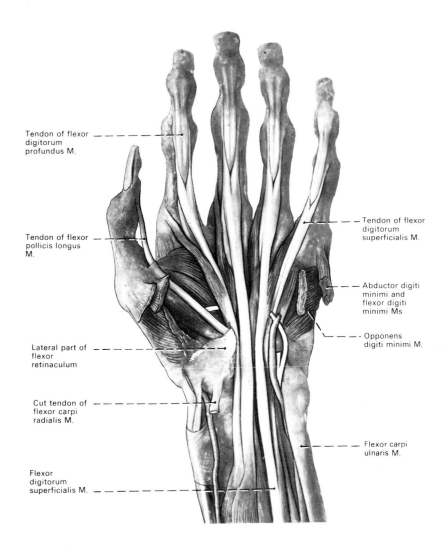

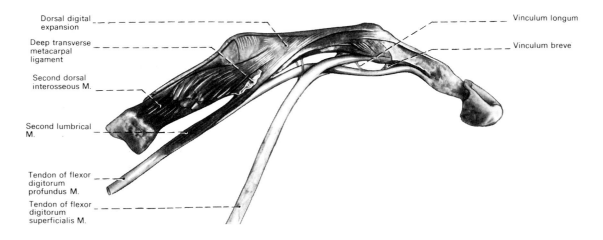

Dorsal digital expansion

Deep transverse metacarpal ligament

Second dorsal interosseous M.

Second lumbrical M.

Tendon of flexor digitorum profundus M.

Tendon of flexor digitorum superficialis M.

Vinculum longum

Vinculum breve

Fig. 1.70   The insertions of the long flexor tendons in the left middle finger.

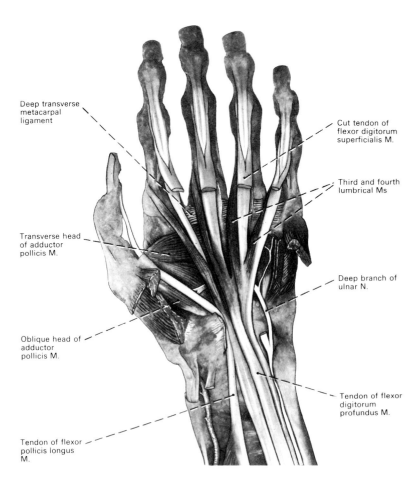

Deep transverse metacarpal ligament

Transverse head of adductor pollicis M.

Oblique head of adductor pollicis M.

Tendon of flexor pollicis longus M.

Cut tendon of flexor digitorum superficialis M.

Third and fourth lumbrical Ms

Deep branch of ulnar N.

Tendon of flexor digitorum profundus M.

Fig. 1.71   The lumbrical muscles of the left hand.

1.56

The adductor pollicis muscle

Now re-examine the adductor pollicis and study its two heads [Fig. 1.71]. The **oblique head,** as already noted, has a fairly extensive origin from the bases of the second and third (sometimes even the fourth) metacarpal bones, and from the adjacent carpal bones and their ligaments. The wide **transverse head** arises from the shaft of the third metacarpal bone. Trace the transverse head to its insertion into the ulnar side of the proximal phalanx of the thumb, and the oblique head into both sides of this phalanx. The muscle is innervated by the ulnar nerve and its function is to adduct the thumb, i.e. to draw it across the palm. Carefully divide both heads of the muscle near their insertions and turn them aside.

The interosseous muscles

Now find and clean the interosseous muscles [Fig. 1.72]. These are the deepest muscles of the palm, and as their name suggests, they lie between the bones of the hand. They are arranged in a ventral or palmar series of four **palmar interosseous muscles,** which are smaller than the four **dorsal inter-** **osseous muscles,** which can be seen easily from both sides of the hand.

The palmar interosseous muscles

The small first palmar interosseous muscle will be found deep to the oblique head of the adductor pollicis. Examine its origin from the base of the first metacarpal bone. The other three palmar interosseous muscles should now be found, one arising from the ulnar side of the second metacarpal bone, and the other two from the radial sides of the fourth and fifth metacarpal bones. The muscles are unipennate, that is, their fibres are directed to one side only of their tendon of insertion.

Trace the tendons of the second, third, and fourth palmar interosseous muscles as they pass deep to the **deep transverse metacarpal ligament** which connects adjacent metacarpophalangeal joints of the fingers. The first palmar interosseous muscle is inserted into the base of the proximal phalanx of the thumb. The second is inserted into the ulnar side of the dorsal digital expansion of the extensor tendon to the index finger. The third and fourth are inserted into the radial

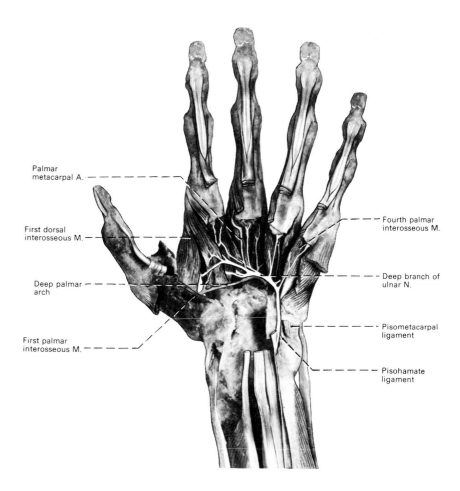

Palmar metacarpal A.

First dorsal interosseous M.

Deep palmar arch

First palmar interosseous M.

Fourth palmar interosseous M.

Deep branch of ulnar N.

Pisometacarpal ligament

Pisohamate ligament

Fig. 1.72 The interosseous muscles and the deep branch of the ulnar nerve.

sides of the dorsal digital expansions of the ring and little fingers respectively. You will see, therefore, that, with the exception of the first, the palmar interosseous muscles pass into the sides of the extensor tendon expansions on the dorsum of the digits. These are dissected and described later.

This arrangement allows the palmar interosseous muscles to adduct the thumb, index, ring, and little fingers towards the axis of the hand which runs through the third metacarpal bone and the middle finger.

The dorsal interosseous muscles

The four dorsal interosseous muscles lie between the metacarpal bones, deep to the unipennate palmar interosseous muscles [Fig. 1.73]. You will see that they are bipennate muscles—that is to say, the muscle fibres are directed to both sides of a central tendon; and that they arise from the adjacent sides of the first and second, the second and third, the third and fourth, and the fourth and fifth metacarpal bones. Clean them and trace them towards their insertions. You will obtain a better view of the insertion of an interosseous muscle if one of the deep transverse metacarpal ligaments is cut.

You will see that the first dorsal interosseous muscle is inserted into the radial side of the proximal phalanx of the index finger. The second and third dorsal interosseous muscles pass to the middle finger, the former being inserted into the radial side of the dorsal digital expansion and the base of the proximal phalanx, and the latter into the ulnar side of the dorsal digital expansion only. The fourth dorsal interosseous muscle is inserted into the ulnar side of the dorsal digital expansion of the ring finger and also sends a slip to be inserted into the base of the proximal phalanx of the same finger.

All the interosseous muscles are supplied by the deep branch of the ulnar nerve.

The actions of the interosseous muscles

The arrangement of the dorsal interosseous muscles permits them to abduct the index, middle, and ring fingers from the axis of the middle finger.

Remember that the thumb and little fingers possess their own abductors.

When the palmar and dorsal interosseous muscles act together, the adducting and abducting effects balance each

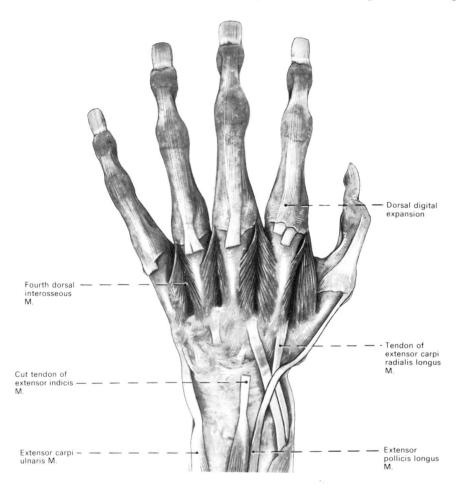

Fourth dorsal interosseous M.

Cut tendon of extensor indicis M.

Extensor carpi ulnaris M.

Dorsal digital expansion

Tendon of extensor carpi radialis longus M.

Extensor pollicis longus M.

Fig. 1.73   The dorsal interosseous muscles of the left hand (posterior view).

1.58

other, and they merely flex the metacarpophalangeal joints.

It should be obvious that the interosseous muscles, like the lumbricals, play an important part in all fine movements of the fingers.

You should now study these various movements in your own hand. In particular feel in the first intermetacarpal space when you either abduct or flex your index finger against resistance at the metacarpophalangeal joint. You will feel your first dorsal interosseous muscle hardening.

The deep branch of the ulnar nerve

Pick up the ulnar nerve at the wrist and find its deep branch, as it pierces the opponens digiti minimi muscle [Fig. 1.72]. Follow it as it crosses the palm. This important branch supplies no fewer than fourteen of the small muscles in the hand (the three muscles of the hypothenar eminence, the adductor pollicis, the two medial lumbrical muscles, the four palmar interossei and the four dorsal interossei). You need not try to pick up more than a few of these branches, but trace the main nerve to where it disappears into the adductor pollicis.

The deep palmar arch

The artery which you will find piercing the first dorsal interosseous muscle is the termination of the **radial artery.** Trace it from here across the palm as it runs medially on the bases of the metacarpal bones, and on the interossei, as far as the fifth metacarpal. Here it is joined by the **deep palmar branch of the ulnar artery,** to form the deep palmar arch [Figs 1.72 and 1.74]. This arch gives off three **palmar metacarpal arteries** which join the common palmar digital arteries which spring from the superficial arch. These vessels stand out only in a well-injected specimen, so do not waste time on their dissection. Merely note that the common palmar digital arteries from the superficial palmar arch, having been joined by the three palmar metacarpal arteries from the deep arch, divide into branches which supply the adjacent sides of the fingers and the ulnar side of the little finger. The deep

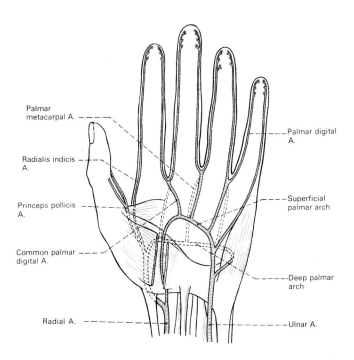

Fig. 1.74 The palmar arches.

arch is much smaller than the superficial arch. It is accompanied by the deep branch of the ulnar nerve and lies on the metacarpal bones and interossei, covered by the flexor tendons and lumbricals.

Earlier on you saw the radial artery turning back at the wrist behind some tendons passing to the thumb. It returns to the palm, as you have seen, by piercing the first dorsal interosseous muscle. Where it pierces the muscle, the radial artery, as already noted, gives off a vessel, the **princeps pollicis artery,** which divides into two branches which run along the sides of the thumb. A further branch, the **radialis indicis artery,** will be found running along the radial border of the index finger. Sometimes the princeps pollicis and radialis indicis arteries arise by a common stem.

Section 1.5

The back of the forearm and hand

Reflection of the skin

To begin this dissection first remove the skin from the back of the forearm and hand and also from the back of the thumb and from the back of at least two fingers.

Find the cutaneous nerves in the exposed superficial fascia, and get an idea of the areas in which they are distributed [Fig. 1.75]. In the forearm, you will find the **posterior cutaneous nerve of the forearm** (a branch of the radial nerve); the **medial cutaneous nerve of the forearm** (from the medial cord of the brachial plexus); and on the dorsum of the hand, the **dorsal digital nerves,** branches of the ulnar and radial nerves. The large and highly variable venous plexus on the back of the hand drains into the cephalic and basilic veins. Remove these veins.

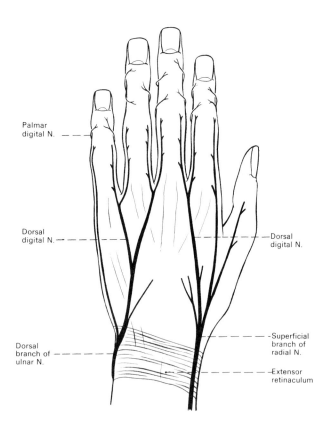

Palmar
digital N.

Dorsal
digital N.

Dorsal
digital N.

Superficial
branch of
radial N.

Dorsal
branch of
ulnar N.

Extensor
retinaculum

Fig. 1.75 The cutaneous nerves of the dorsum of the left hand.

Structures on the back of the forearm

The extensor retinaculum [Fig. 1.76]

Next clear away the superficial fascia and expose the deep fascia. Note that this forms an annular thickening on the back of the wrist called the extensor retinaculum (it corresponds to the flexor retinaculum on the opposite side of the wrist), which is attached medially to the triquetral bone and pisiform bone and laterally to the distal end of the radius. The extensor tendons of the hand pass beneath it, each in a tunnel of its own. Do not cut the retinaculum but remove the remainder of the deep fascia so as to expose the superficial muscles on the dorsum of the forearm [Fig. 1.76].

The superficial extensor muscles of the wrist and fingers [Fig. 1.76].

Look first in the elbow region, and you will see the **extensor carpi radialis longus** emerging just below the **brachioradialis.** Below the long extensor and on a slightly deeper plane, for it has a deeper origin, you will see the short extensor, called the **extensor carpi radialis brevis.** Medial to this is the **extensor digitorum,** and if you glance at its distribution in the hand you will see that it divides into tendons which pass to each of the four fingers. Next comes the **extensor digiti minimi** passing to the little finger, and then the **extensor carpi ulnaris,** which ends at the wrist.

In the interval between the short extensor of the wrist and the extensor of the fingers you will see emerging in the lower third of the forearm the tendons of the **abductor pollicis longus** and the **extensor pollicis brevis,** which are closely applied together, and medial to them the tendon of the **extensor pollicis longus** [Fig. 1.77].

Now look at the articulated radius and ulna and refer to Fig. 1.26b. You will see that these tendons lie in grooves at the distal ends of these bones. Note especially the **dorsal tubercle of the radius** and the deep groove on its medial side for the tendon of extensor pollicis longus. This muscle has an oblique pull. Now verify the dorsal tubercle on your own wrist. It is a landmark in locating the position of the extensor tendons.

The tendons of all these muscles are surrounded by short synovial sheaths as they pass beneath the extensor retinaculum, closely applied to the bone.

Now clean the superficial extensor muscles, and first examine their origins. The extensor carpi radialis longus will be found to arise from both the lateral supracondylar ridge on the humerus, and the adjacent lateral intermuscular septum below the brachioradialis. The extensor carpi radialis brevis, extensor digitorum, extensor digiti minimi, and extensor carpi ulnaris will be found to arise by a common tendon, called the common extensor tendon, which is attached to the lateral epicondyle of the humerus.

Between the proximal ends of the extensor carpi ulnaris and the flexor carpi ulnaris you will have seen a further short triangular muscle. This is the **anconeus** [Fig. 1.76], a weak extensor of the elbow joint. Clean it, and you will find that it arises at its apex from the lateral epicondyle of the humerus. It is inserted by its base into the lateral border of the olecranon and the roughly triangular depression at the upper end of the shaft of the ulna. As you define the short upper border of the muscle you may find a small nerve entering its deep surface. This branch of the radial nerve has descended through the triceps.

The extensor carpi radialis brevis also takes origin from the radial collateral ligament of the elbow joint. Examine the aponeurosis that is attached to the posterior border of the ulna. You will see that parts of both the flexor and extensor carpi ulnaris arise from it.

The insertions of the extensor tendons

Now trace the tendons of the extensor carpi radialis longus and of the extensor carpi radialis brevis to their insertions, and as you do this, open the appropriate compartment in the extensor retinaculum on the back of the wrist. You will see that the extensor carpi radialis longus becomes attached to the base of the second metacarpal bone, and the extensor carpi radialis brevis to the base of the third metacarpal bone [Fig. 1.82].

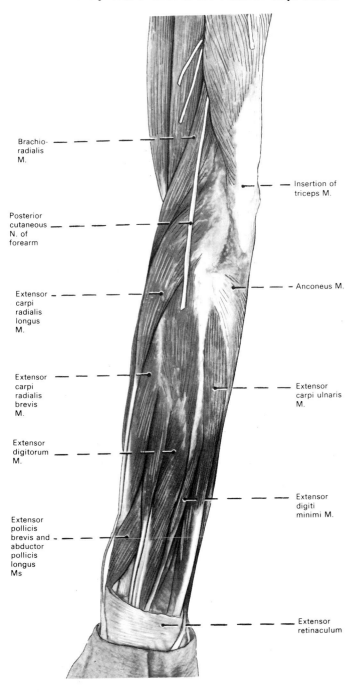

Brachio-radialis M.

Posterior cutaneous N. of forearm

Extensor carpi radialis longus M.

Extensor carpi radialis brevis M.

Extensor digitorum M.

Extensor pollicis brevis and abductor pollicis longus Ms

Insertion of triceps M.

Anconeus M.

Extensor carpi ulnaris M.

Extensor digiti minimi M.

Extensor retinaculum

Fig. 1.76 The superficial muscles of the back of the left forearm.

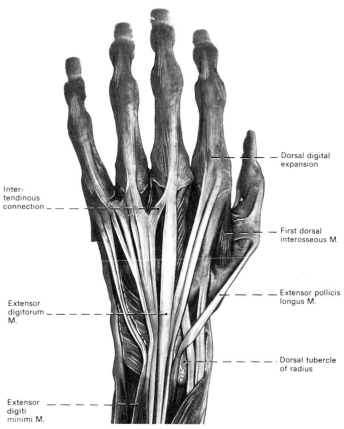

Inter-tendinous connection

Extensor digitorum M.

Extensor digiti minimi M.

Dorsal digital expansion

First dorsal interosseous M.

Extensor pollicis longus M.

Dorsal tubercle of radius

Fig. 1.77 The dorsum of the left hand and fingers.

1.61

The extensor digitorum will be seen to divide into four tendons on the dorsum of the hand. Follow each tendon as it passes to be inserted mainly into the bases of the middle and distal phalanges, again opening the appropriate compartment of the extensor retinaculum. Each tendon also sends a small slip into the base of the proximal phalanx. Over the dorsum of the metacarpophalangeal joint and the proximal phalanx of each finger there is a tendinous hood, called the **dorsal digital expansion.** If you clean this carefully you will be able to demonstrate its extent and attachments. You will find that the tendons of the extensor digitorum are incorporated into their appropriate expansions, into which the tendons of the lumbrical and interosseous muscles also pass. When confirming these points do not cut into the dorsal digital expansions.

At this stage you will not be able to see the slips sent by the extensor tendons to the proximal phalanges; you will have an opportunity of looking for them later on. It should be noted also that the tendons to the middle, ring, and little fingers are connected to each other on the back of the hand by **intertendinous connections** [Fig. 1.77]. These connections make it impossible, starting with a clenched fist, to extend any one of these fingers fully by itself. The index finger has the greatest freedom of movement. Confirm that the tendon to this finger is entirely independent.

Now trace the insertion of the tendon of the extensor digiti minimi into the dorsal digital expansion of the little finger, and that of the extensor carpi ulnaris into the base of the fifth metacarpal bone. As before, incise the extensor retinaculum.

The deep extensor muscles

Divide the extensor digitorum near its origin and, if necessary, the extensor carpi radialis brevis as well, in order to reveal the deep muscles in the back of the forearm [Fig. 1.78]. Clean these muscles. From above downwards, and proceeding in a medial direction, they are the **supinator,** the **abductor pollicis longus,** the **extensor pollicis brevis,** the **extensor pollicis longus,** and the **extensor indicis.**

The posterior interosseous nerve [Fig. 1.78]

You will recall that when you were dissecting the elbow region, you found that a branch of the radial nerve, the posterior interosseous nerve, passed backwards through the supinator muscle at the level of the lateral epicondyle. Pick up the posterior interosseous nerve as it emerges from the supinator on the dorsum of the forearm and trace it downwards, first on the abductor pollicis longus and then on the interosseous membrane of the forearm. You may see some of the branches it sends to the superficial and deep muscles on the back of the forearm. With the exception of the extensor carpi radialis longus and brachioradialis, which are supplied by the radial nerve itself, the posterior interosseous

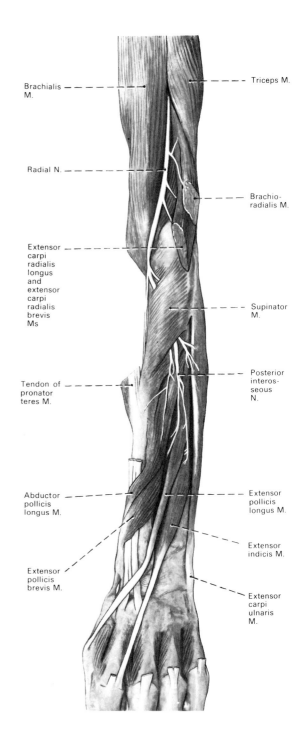

Fig. 1.78   The deep muscles of the back of the left forearm.

nerve supplies all these muscles. It also supplies the wrist joint and intercarpal joints.

Attachments of the deep extensor muscles

Re-examine the extensive origin of the supinator muscle from the lateral epicondyle of the humerus, from the radial collateral ligament of the elbow joint, from the annular ligament of the radius, and from the supinator crest on the ulna. Follow the muscle to its insertion. Note again that it completely surrounds the upper end of the neck and shaft of the radius, except medially, and that it extends down as far as the anterior oblique line.

Now study the attachments of the deep muscles of the back of the forearm [Fig. 1.78]. Look at the abductor pollicis longus. It arises from both bones of the forearm and from the intervening interosseous membrane. You will see that the extensor pollicis brevis arises from the radius, and the extensor pollicis longus and the extensor indicis from the ulna. Follow the tendons distally and open the remaining compartments in the extensor retinaculum. As you follow these muscles to their insertions, note again that the tendon of the extensor pollicis longus is hooked round the dorsal tubercle of the distal end of the radius.

Study the insertions of the tendons of these three muscles of the thumb; the abductor into the base of the first metacarpal bone; the extensor brevis into the base of the proximal phalanx; and the extensor longus into the base of the distal phalanx. Note that the extensor indicis is inserted into the dorsal digital expansion of the index finger.

Now observe on your own hand the actions of the abduc-

tor pollicis longus and of the extensors of the thumb. Move the thumb forcibly and note how the tendons stand out.

The arrangement of the extensor tendons at the wrist

The order in which the tendons of the extensor muscles lie at the wrist is of importance to the surgeon when he is dealing with cuts involving one or more of these tendons, for he must be able to identify them. On the dissected specimen, identify these tendons from the radial to the ulnar side as follows [Fig. 1.79]: abductor pollicis longus and extensor pollicis brevis (which run together), extensor carpi radialis longus, extensor carpi radialis brevis, extensor pollicis longus, extensor digitorum with the extensor indicis deep to it, extensor digiti minimi, and extensor carpi ulnaris.

Surface anatomy of the wrist

Before proceeding further, study the surface anatomy of your own wrist in order to help you fix in your mind some of the observations you have already made in your dissection. Start with the palmar surface facing upwards.

The conspicuous tendon lying immediately lateral to the midline, which stands out when you flex your wrist forcibly, is that of the flexor carpi radialis [Fig. 1.80]; on its ulnar side (when present) is the more prominent tendon of the

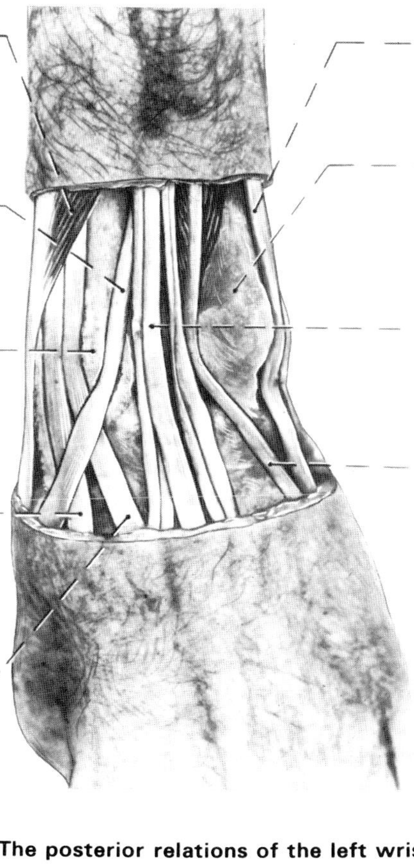

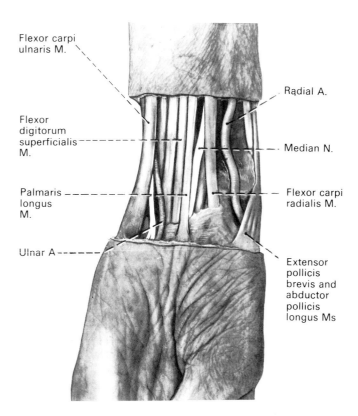

Fig. 1.79 The posterior relations of the left wrist joint.

Fig. 1.80 The anterior relations of the left wrist joint.

palmaris longus. The median nerve lies relatively superficial, immediately behind the tendon of palmaris longus, on the ulnar aspect of the tendon of the flexor carpi radialis. The radial artery lies both on the pronator quadratus and on the radius, on the radial aspect of the flexor carpi radialis. You can feel the artery pulsating at this point. The muscle mass on the medial aspect of the flexor carpi radialis is the flexor digitorum superficialis. Medial to this is the tendon of the flexor carpi ulnaris passing into the pisiform bone.

In the interval between the tendon of the flexor carpi radialis and the base of the thumb is the scaphoid bone. This extends into the floor of a depression at the base of the thumb called the 'anatomical snuff-box'. The triquetral bone forms a conspicuous prominence distal to the head of the ulna on the ulnar border of the dorsum of the hand. The pisiform bone rests on this bone and can be located on the front of the wrist, usually between the two creases in the skin of the wrist.

By extending the thumb the tendinous boundaries of the 'anatomical snuff-box' will become prominent [Fig. 1.81]. The anterior boundary of this landmark is formed by the conjoint tendons of the abductor pollicis longus and the extensor pollicis brevis, and the posterior boundary by the tendon of the extensor pollicis longus. The bony floor of the 'snuff-box' is formed chiefly by the scaphoid bone. Distal to the scaphoid is the trapezium articulating with the base of the first metacarpal bone to form the important carpometacarpal joint of the thumb. On the floor of the 'snuff-box' is the radial artery which has entered from the anterior surface of the wrist by passing under the tendons of the abductor pollicis longus and extensor pollicis brevis

muscles, and which is on its way to return to the palm through the first dorsal interosseous muscle.

In the superficial fascia forming the roof of the 'anatomical snuff-box' is the origin of the cephalic vein.

Again verify the relative positions of the styloid processes of the radius and ulna.

The radial artery

Now return to your dissected specimen, and pick up the radial artery at the wrist. Clean it and follow it beneath the tendons of the abductor pollicis longus and the extensor pollicis brevis; then through the 'anatomical snuff-box'; and then beneath the tendon of the extensor pollicis longus [Fig. 1.82]. It then passes between the two heads of the first dorsal interosseous muscle to enter the palm, where it has been found already. If the lateral head of the latter muscle is divided close to its origin, the complete course of the artery in this region will be seen more clearly.

The dorsal interosseous muscles [Fig. 1.82]

Clean all the dorsal interosseous muscles and trace their insertions into the dorsal digital expansions and the bases of the proximal phalanges. Study this arrangement carefully,

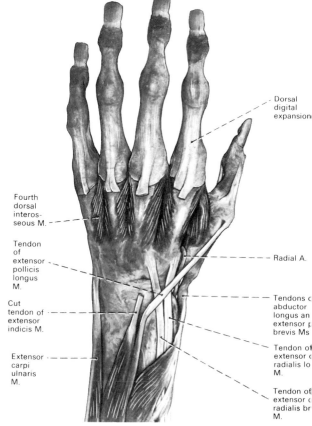

Fig. 1.82 The radial artery and the dorsal interosseous muscles of the left hand.

Labels on Fig. 1.82:
- Dorsal digital expansion
- Fourth dorsal interosseous M.
- Tendon of extensor pollicis longus M.
- Cut tendon of extensor indicis M.
- Extensor carpi ulnaris M.
- Radial A.
- Tendons of abductor pollicis longus and extensor pollicis brevis Ms
- Tendon of extensor carpi radialis longus M.
- Tendon of extensor carpi radialis brevis M.

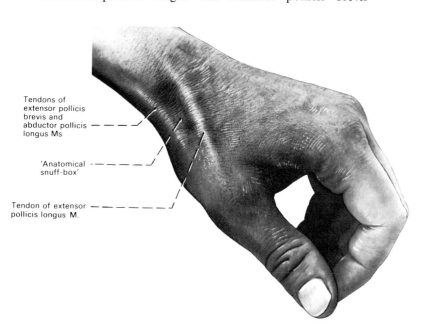

Labels on Fig. 1.81:
- Tendons of extensor pollicis brevis and abductor pollicis longus Ms
- 'Anatomical snuff-box'
- Tendon of extensor pollicis longus M.

Fig. 1.81 The 'anatomical snuff-box'.

otherwise the action of these important muscles as abductors of the fingers will not be understood.

The long flexor and extensor muscles of the forearm

Having examined the various long flexor and extensor muscles in your specimen, try and study their action on your own forearm and hand. Note that they help flex and extend the wrist, the first carpometacarpal, and metacarpophalangeal and interphalangeal joints. The long flexor and extensor muscles that are inserted into the carpal bones steady the wrist joint so as to allow those flexors and extensors that insert more distally to act on the distal joints.

The joints of the elbow, wrist, and hand

Except for the joints of the elbow, wrist, and hand, you have now completed the dissection of the upper limb.

The elbow joint and the proximal radio-ulnar joint

In order to dissect the elbow joint, carefully remove all the structures from the vicinity of its articular capsule and ligaments. This is your last opportunity to verify the attachments of the muscles in this region. Note again the common origins of the flexor and extensor muscles from the epicondyles of the humerus. At this stage you also get a particularly good view of the supinator muscle.

The **articular capsule** of the elbow joint surrounds the joint surface, and will be found to be thin anteriorly and posteriorly, but to be reinforced medially and laterally by ligaments which are merely thickenings of the capsule [Fig.

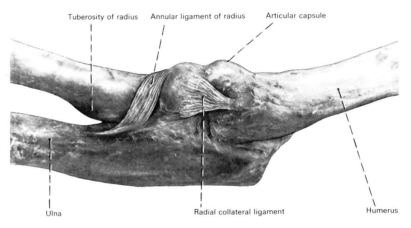

Tuberosity of radius   Annular ligament of radius   Articular capsule

Ulna   Radial collateral ligament   Humerus

a. *Lateral view (with forearm pronated)*

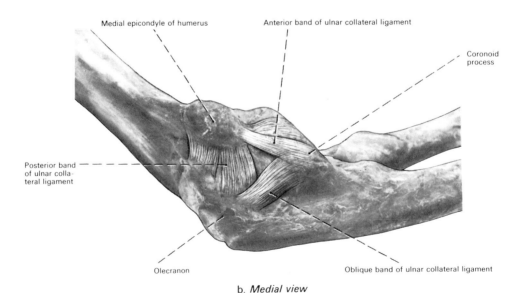

Medial epicondyle of humerus   Anterior band of ulnar collateral ligament

Coronoid process

Posterior band of ulnar collateral ligament

Olecranon   Oblique band of ulnar collateral ligament

b. *Medial view*

Fig. 1.83 The left elbow joint.

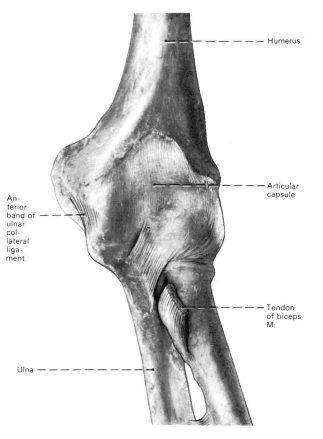

Fig. 1.83 c. *Anterior view* (*with forearm supinated*)

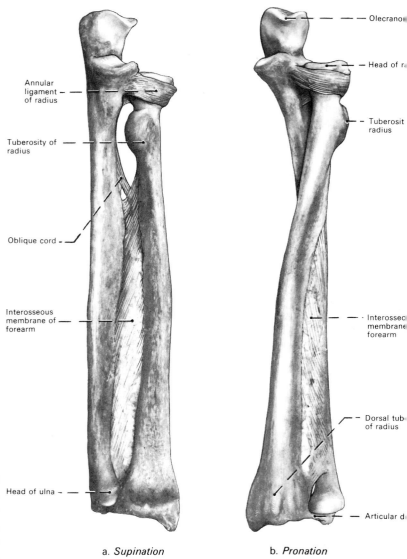

a. *Supination*   b. *Pronation*

Fig. 1.84   The left radio-ulnar joints.

1.83]. Scratch with the point of the scalpel and try to define the **ulnar collateral ligament.** It is triangular, with its apex attached to the medial epicondyle. From the apex two ligamentous bands should be traced downwards to the coronoid process and olecranon respectively. Some oblique ligamentous fibres form a third band which connects these two processes together and so completes the triangle.

Next trace the **radial collateral ligament** of the joint. It, too, is triangular. It extends from the lateral epicondyle above to the **annular ligament of the radius** below.

Then open the joint by incising the front of the capsule horizontally, and so expose the **synovial membrane.** Note that the membrane is continuous with that of the proximal radio-ulnar joint. Hyperextend the joint in order to display the fat between the synovial membrane and the articular capsule, and expose completely the annular ligament, which surrounds the head of the radius; and the **quadrate ligament,** which forms a floor for this ring.

The elbow joint, like all hinge joints, is capable of movement through a single transverse axis. Movement is confined to flexion (by brachialis chiefly, assisted by biceps, brachioradialis, and pronator teres) and extension (by triceps and anconeus).

Having confirmed the attachment of the muscles of the forearm from the radius and ulna and the intervening inter-

osseous membrane, remove them, and clean the membrane throughout its entire extent [Fig. 1.84]. Proximal to the membrane you will see the thin ligamentous **oblique cord** which passes from the medial side of the ulna above to the radius below, in a direction at right angles to the fibres of the interosseous membrane.

Rotate the forearm so as to perform the movements of pronation and supination. These involve the proximal and distal radio-ulnar articulations. It will be seen that the ulna remains stationary, while the head of the radius rotates within the annular ligament above, and the distal end rotates around the head of the ulna below. The axis of rotation is represented by a line which passes through the centre of the head of the radius, and extends obliquely downwards through the centre of the styloid process of the ulna.

1.67

The wrist joint and the distal radio-ulnar joint

Cut the anterior part of the capsule of the distal radio-ulnar joint. Free the head of the radius from the annular ligament of the proximal radio-ulnar joint. The quadrate ligament below the annular ligament can now be clearly seen. Divide it and the interosseous membrane, and separate the bones sufficiently to define the attachments of the **articular disc** of the wrist joint and the distal radio-ulnar joint.

The articular disc [Fig. 1.85] will be seen to be a triangular plate of fibrocartilage which is attached by its apex to the lateral surface of the base of the styloid process of the ulna, and by its base to the radius at the lower margin of the ulnar notch.

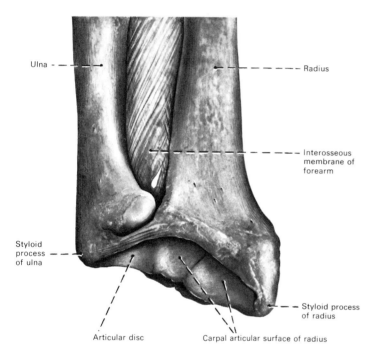

Fig. 1.85 The distal radio-ulnar joint.

At this stage verify the insertion of the flexor carpi radialis as it passes between the lateral attachments of the flexor retinaculum. The tunnel through which it passes should be opened on its medial aspect.

The lower end of the radius and the articular disc articulate with the scaphoid, lunate, and triquetral bones and constitute the wrist joint.

Define the **articular capsule** of the joint, noting that while thin anteriorly and posteriorly, it is reinforced on each side. Open the capsule from the front by a horizontal incision, leaving the **ulnar collateral ligament of the wrist** and the **radial collateral ligament of the wrist** intact. Hyperextend the joint, and examine the articular surfaces [Fig. 1.86]. Examine the thickened fibrous bands which constitute the radial and ulnar collateral ligaments of the joint. Try to make out the movements of which the joint is capable, by examining the movements of your own wrist. You will see that the joint can move on a transverse axis (anteroposterior movement) and on an axis at right-angles to it (abduction and adduction). Combinations of these movements can result in circumduction.

The joints of the hand

The intercarpal joints

The intercarpal joints and the **midcarpal joint** between the two rows of carpal bones should now be opened from behind by making a horizontal incision between the two rows of carpal bones. You can see that the carpal bones are bound together by **dorsal, palmar,** and **interosseous intercarpal ligaments,** with a common joint cavity between them. Only the cavity of the **pisiform joint** with the triquetral bone is separate. The pisiform bone is held in position by a **pisohamate ligament** and a **pisometacarpal ligament** [Fig. 1.72]. Functionally these are extensions of the flexor carpi ulnaris tendon from the pisiform bone. Gliding movements occur at the intercarpal joints.

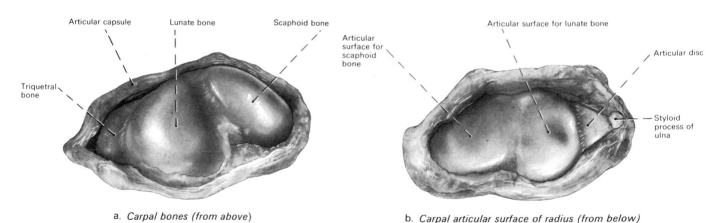

a. *Carpal bones (from above)*

b. *Carpal articular surface of radius (from below)*

Fig. 1.86 The left wrist joint.

The carpometacarpal joints

The carpometacarpal joints of the hand should be exposed from their posterior aspect, the **dorsal carpometacarpal ligaments** incised and the metacarpal bones flexed strongly. These joints are built on much the same plan as are the intercarpal joints, being reinforced by **palmar carpometacarpal ligaments** and dorsal carpometacarpal ligaments. They also allow gliding movements.

The carpometacarpal joint of the thumb

The carpometacarpal joint of the thumb is a very important joint and must be examined closely. Except for an articulation between the auditory ossicles of the ear, this is the only saddle joint in the body, and it allows a very free range of movement.

Test on your own thumb and on your dissected specimen the wide range of movement that occurs at the joint. Note that the movement of opposition combines flexion with medial rotation.

Open the capsule from the lateral aspect and separate the trapezium from the first metacarpal bone. Examine the saddle-shaped articular surfaces.

The metacarpophalangeal and interphalangeal joints

Each metacarpophalangeal joint and interphalangeal joint has a complete capsule, the sides of which are reinforced by strong **collateral ligaments.** On the anterior aspect of each joint is a thick fibrocartilaginous **palmar ligament.**

The metacarpophalangeal joints of the fingers are condyloid joints which allow movement in two axes—flexion and extension—with a limited range of abduction and adduction. The interphalangeal joints and also the metacarpophalangeal joint of the thumb are hinge joints which allow movement (flexion and extension) through a single axis only.

It will be easier to examine a metacarpophalangeal joint if you now remove the middle finger. Detach it from the rest of the hand complete with its metacarpal bone and the second and third dorsal interosseous muscles.

The dorsal digital expansions

Study the dorsal digital expansion of this finger, which you first noted when you followed the insertion of the tendon of the extensor digitorum muscle [p.1.62]. The expansion is triangular and covers the dorsum of the proximal phalanx and the dorsum and sides of the metacarpophalangeal joint [Fig. 1.87], being attached at its proximal angles to a **deep transverse metacarpal ligament.** Note that the extensor tendon blends with the central part of the dorsal digital expansion and is prolonged to be attached to the bases of the middle and distal phalanges.

As you confirm these facts on your specimen, note that the tendon of the lumbrical muscle forms a thickened radial border for the expansion, and that an interosseous muscle is inserted into either side of the base of the expansion. Sometimes the interosseous muscles are also inserted into the base of the proximal phalanx [Fig. 1.88a].

Now flex the metacarpophalangeal joint and note how the expansion acts as a mobile hood, moving distally over the head of the metacarpal bone as flexion occurs, and proximally as the joint is extended again [Fig. 1.87b and c].

Pass the points of your dissecting forceps under the radial border of the dorsal expansion and gently separate it from the underlying bone. Then, with the metacarpophalangeal joint flexed, ease the expansion forwards, separating it from the dorsal part of the capsule of the joint. Be careful lest your tear the expansion, for parts of it are thin. You may find a small bursa between the capsule of the metacarpophalangeal joint and the expansion [Fig. 1.88a]. Occasionally you may find that the latter sends a small slip in front of the bursa into the base of the proximal phalanx.

The collateral ligaments

With the metacarpophalangeal joint flexed, a little blunt dissection proximal to the two sides of the dorsal expansion will quickly reveal the strong triangular collateral ligaments [Fig. 1.87c]. These are attached at their apices to the sides of the head of the metacarpal bone, whilst their bases are attached to the base of the proximal phalanx and the sides of the palmar ligament. In order to see these ligaments more clearly, separate one corner of the triangular expansion from the deep transverse metacarpal ligament and reflect the expansion from the capsule of the joint. Alternatively, flex and extend the finger, and note how its collateral ligaments tighten in flexion, and how they are responsible for the stability of the joint [Fig. 1.88].

Now incise the thinner dorsal part of the capsule and examine the articular surface. Finally, examine the **palmar ligament** and note how thick it is. Its palmar surface is grooved for the flexor tendons, and its edges are connected to the deep transverse metacarpal ligaments and the digital fibrous sheath.

Dissect on each side of an interphalangeal joint, and you will find a collateral ligament similar to but smaller than those of the metacarpophalangeal joints. Open the dorsum of the interphalangeal joint, after turning aside the dorsal expansion, and examine the articular surfaces. Note that these joints, too, have thick palmar ligaments.

The movements of the thumb

At this stage refer again to your dissection and review once more the movements of the thumb. Note again that they occur at the carpometacarpal, metacarpophalangeal, and interphalangeal joints.

Opposition is effected by the opponens pollicis and flexor pollicis brevis muscles which, together, medially rotate the first metacarpal bone upon the carpus.

Adduction is produced by the adductor pollicis and first

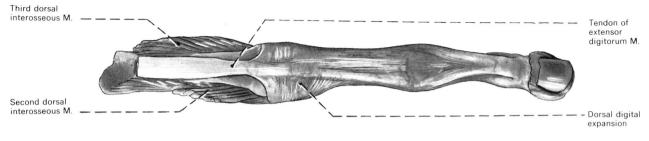

Third dorsal
interosseous M.

Tendon of
extensor
digitorum M.

Second dorsal
interosseous M.

Dorsal digital
expansion

a. *Viewed from above*

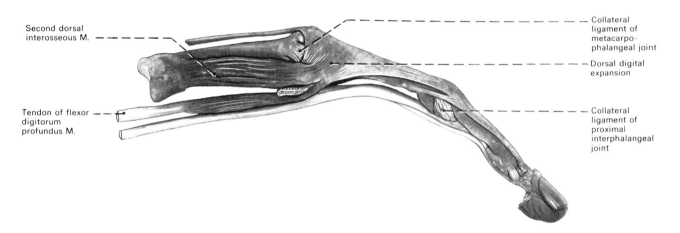

Second dorsal
interosseous M.

Collateral
ligament of
metacarpo-
phalangeal
joint

Dorsal digital
expansion

Tendon of flexor
digitorum
profundus M.

Collateral
ligament of
proximal
interphalangeal
joint

b. *Lateral view, with the finger extended*

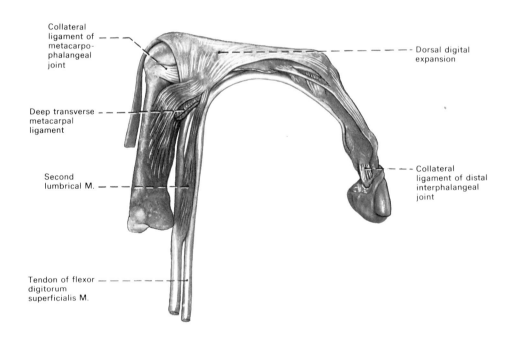

Collateral
ligament of
metacarpo-
phalangeal
joint

Dorsal digital
expansion

Deep transverse
metacarpal
ligament

Second
lumbrical M.

Collateral
ligament of distal
interphalangeal
joint

Tendon of flexor
digitorum
superficialis M.

c. *Lateral view, with the finger flexed* Compare with Fig. 1.87b where the finger is extended, and note that the proximal edge of the dorsal digital expansion has moved distally

Fig. 1.87   The dorsal digital expansion of the left middle finger.

1.70

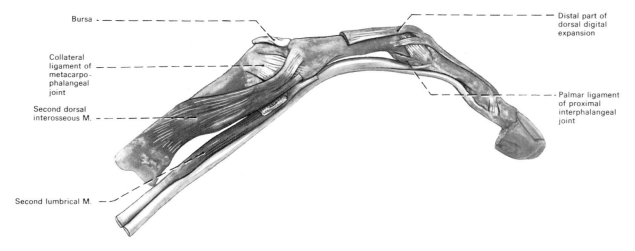

Bursa

Collateral ligament of metacarpo-phalangeal joint

Second dorsal interosseous M.

Second lumbrical M.

Distal part of dorsal digital expansion

Palmar ligament of proximal interphalangeal joint

a. *Lateral view* The proximal part of the dorsal digital expansion has been excised

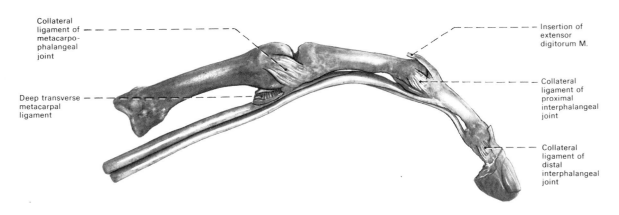

Collateral ligament of metacarpo-phalangeal joint

Deep transverse metacarpal ligament

Insertion of extensor digitorum M.

Collateral ligament of proximal interphalangeal joint

Collateral ligament of distal interphalangeal joint

b. *Lateral view* To show the collateral ligaments

Fig. 1.88 The joints of the left middle finger.

palmar interosseous muscles, and abduction by the abductor pollicis muscles, both actions occurring at the carpometacarpal and metacarpophalangeal joints.

Flexion is effected by the flexor pollicis brevis at the metacarpophalangeal joint and by the flexor pollicis longus at this joint and at the interphalangeal joint. Extension is produced by the extensor pollicis brevis at the metacarpophalangeal joint and by the extensor pollicis longus at both metacarpophalangeal and interphalangeal joints.

Combined movements of the fingers

Again study the combined movements of the fingers in your dissected specimen and in your own hand. Flexion at the metacarpophalangeal joints with simultaneous extension of the interphalangeal joints, as occurs in the upstroke movement in writing, is produced by the combined action of the long flexors and the interosseous and lumbrical muscles.

Flexion at the metacarpophalangeal joints with simultaneous flexion at the interphalangeal joints is effected by the long flexor muscles.

Extension at the metacarpophalangeal joints with flexion at the interphalangeal joints is produced by the combined action of the long extensor and flexor muscles. Move each finger in turn and note how the various tendons become prominent in turn.

Chart of contents of the lower limb

COMPONENTS	REGIONS			
	Hip **Gluteal**	**Thigh**	**Leg**	**Foot**
Bones	pelvis	femur	tibia fibula	tarsals metatarsals phalanges
Joints	sacroiliac hip pubic symphysis		knee ankle	foot
Muscles	extensors abductors flexors	extensors of knee extensors of hip flexors of knee adductors of hip	extensors flexors	intrinsic
Nerves	from lumbosacral plexus dorsal rami of lumbar and sacral nerves	femoral sciatic obturator	common peroneal tibial	terminal branches
Arteries	iliac	femoral popliteal	anterior tibial peroneal posterior tibial	dorsal digital plantar
Veins *superficial* *deep*	 iliac	 great saphenous femoral popliteal	 great saphenous small saphenous anterior tibial posterior tibial	 dorsal digital plantar
Lymph nodes	inguinal	popliteal		

Part 2

The lower limb

The lower limb is subdivided by the hip joint, knee joint, and ankle joint, into the regions of the buttock, thigh, leg, and foot. The movements which occur at the hip joint are similar to those that take place at the shoulder joint, but their range is much more limited. Those at the knee joint occur mainly in one plane. When the knee is bent it is said to be flexed; it is extended when the leg is straightened. The ankle joint is a more simple type of hinge joint than the knee joint. Bending the foot upwards dorsiflexes (or extends) the joint; while bending the foot downwards plantar-flexes (or flexes) the joint. The foot can also be turned inwards (inverted) or outwards (everted) at the ankle. This movement actually takes place at the joints between certain of the bones of the foot. The shape of the foot itself can be altered by movement between its constituent bones, but the toes have a small range of movement. This is particularly apparent when you compare the movements of the great toe and those of the thumb.

The dissection of the lower limb is begun with the subject lying face downwards, and the buttock (gluteal region) is the first part to be studied. This is not an easy part of the body to dissect, mainly because of the subcutaneous fat it contains. Beneath the fat are some large muscles, and also the biggest nerve in the body. Most of the blood vessels you will meet are branches to muscles.

Section 2.1

The gluteal region

Immediately beneath the subcutaneous fat of the buttock are three large muscles called, according to their size, the gluteus maximus, the gluteus medius, and the gluteus minimus. The gluteus maximus overlaps the other two gluteal muscles and to a large extent the gluteus medius overlaps the gluteus minimus. Deep to the gluteus maximus lies a group of small muscles which are lateral rotators of the thigh. From above down, they are the piriformis, and then three muscles, the obturator internus and the superior and inferior gemellus muscles, which have separate origins but a common tendon of insertion into the neck of the femur. Below these is another small lateral rotator, called the quadratus femoris, deep to which is the tendon of the obturator externus muscle. You dissect these small lateral rotators as a group after you have cleaned and reflected the gluteus maximus.

The large nerve in the buttock is the sciatic nerve. It begins within the cavity of the pelvis, and as it passes into the thigh after emerging from the greater sciatic foramen of the pelvis, it lies on the lateral rotator muscles. Its branches supply most of the skin and muscles of the lower limb.

The skeleton of the gluteal region consists of the hip-bone (which, with the sacrum posteriorly, bounds the pelvic cavity) and the upper end of the thigh bone or femur. The hip-bone not only gives attachment to the muscles of the lower limb, but also to those of the abdominal wall.

Osteology

Examine an articulated pelvis and also a separate hip-bone.

The pelvis and the hip-bone

The hip-bone [Fig. 2.1] is formed from three separate bones, the **ilium,** the **ischium,** and the **pubis,** which up to the time of puberty are united by a Y-shaped piece of cartilage in and around the **acetabulum.** The acetabulum is the cup-shaped cavity with which the head of the femur articulates on the lateral surface of the hip-bone, which becomes a single bone at puberty, when its three constituent elements fuse. Look at a skeleton and note that the two hip-bones articulate in front with each other, and behind with the **sacrum,** and that the three bones make up the pelvis [Fig. 2.2].

Note that the pelvis consists of a splayed-out part above, called the **greater pelvis,** and a smaller cavity below, called the **lesser pelvis.** The greater pelvis lacks an anterior wall. Its sides are formed by the broad plates of the two iliac bones and, in so far as it has a posterior wall, this is formed by the anterior edge of the base of the sacrum and by the body of the fifth lumbar vertebra.

The lesser pelvis is a complete but irregular bony canal. Its anterior wall is formed by the union of the two pubic bones at the **pubic symphysis.** On either side of the symphysis is the large **obturator foramen.** The anterior part of this foramen is formed by the pubis, and the posterior by the ischium. On the inner side of the lesser pelvis, above and behind the foramen, is a flat expanse of bone which posteriorly forms the anterior margin of a deep notch, called the **greater sciatic notch.** A backwardly-projecting **ischial spine** separates this greater notch from a **lesser sciatic notch** below it [Fig. 2.1].

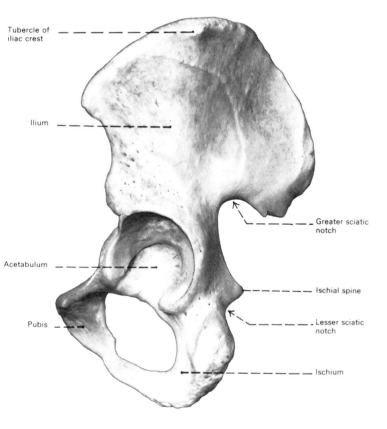

Tubercle of iliac crest

Ilium

Acetabulum

Pubis

Greater sciatic notch

Ischial spine

Lesser sciatic notch

Ischium

Fig. 2.1 The lateral aspect of the left hip-bone.

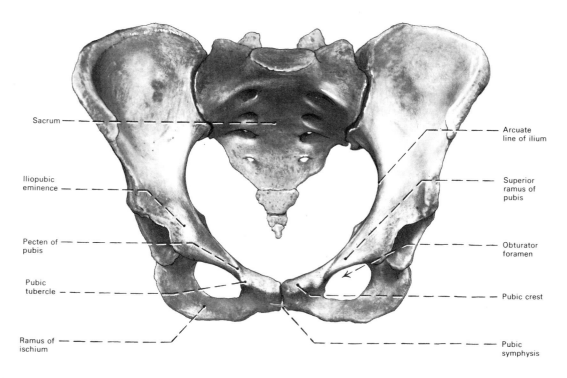

Fig. 2.2 The pelvis (anterior view).

The labels on the figure read (left side, top to bottom): Sacrum; Iliopubic eminence; Pecten of pubis; Pubic tubercle; Ramus of ischium. (right side, top to bottom): Arcuate line of ilium; Superior ramus of pubis; Obturator foramen; Pubic crest; Pubic symphysis.

The ilium

Now look at a disarticulated hip-bone. The upwardly-convex superior border of the ilium is known as the **iliac crest** [Fig. 2.3a], and has inner and outer lips separated by an intermediate line. The iliac crest begins at the **anterior superior iliac spine** and ends at the **posterior superior iliac spine,** which on a skeleton you will see marks the centre of the sacroiliac joint. You can feel both of these spines on your own body. Below the anterior superior spine define a smaller projection called the **anterior inferior iliac spine,** and below the posterior superior spine the **posterior inferior iliac spine.**

The prominence you see on the lateral aspect of the crest of the hip-bone about 5 cm behind the anterior superior spine is known as the **tubercle of the crest.**

The lateral surface of the upper expanded part or **ala of the ilium** is called the **gluteal surface.** On it you may be able to discern three ridges, which are called, according to their positions, the **posterior gluteal line,** the **anterior gluteal line,** and the **inferior gluteal line.** You will be able to understand their significance when you dissect the gluteal muscles.

The narrow part of the ilium below the gluteal surface forms part of the cup-shaped socket called the acetabulum.

The pubis

Below and medial to the anterior inferior iliac spine, and on the anterior aspect of the acetabulum, note a prominence called the **iliopubic eminence.** This marks the junction of the body of the ilium with the **superior ramus of the pubis.** The sharp upper border of this superior ramus, known as the **pecten of the pubis,** should next be defined [Fig. 2.2]. It continues laterally into a rounded border on the medial aspect of the ilium, called the arcuate line. At its medial end the pecten of the pubis meets the **pubic crest,** which is the superior border of the **body of the pubis,** at an angle that is marked by a sharp **pubic tubercle.**

The body of the pubis lies below the pubic crest and is the part of the bone adjacent to the pubic symphysis. The medial surface of the body is the **symphysial surface of the pubis.**

You can see that the inferior border of the superior ramus of the pubis bounds the obturator foramen. The border is sharp, and is known as the **obturator crest.**

The **inferior ramus of the pubis,** medial to and below the foramen, runs into the single ramus of the ischium, the point of union being difficult to define. The upper border of the stretch of bone which these two rami form is the medial and inferior rim of the obturator foramen. The lower border forms part of the **pubic arch** of the pelvis, beneath which lies the **subpubic angle.**

The ischium

Posteriorly the **ramus of the ischium** runs into the **ischial tuberosity** [Fig. 2.3b], which is a part of the **body of the ischium.** The tuberosity is a mass of bone which forms the most inferior part of the hip-bone, and which superiorly,

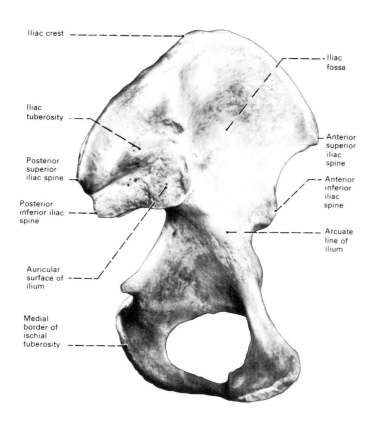

Iliac crest

Iliac fossa

Iliac tuberosity

Posterior superior iliac spine

Posterior inferior iliac spine

Auricular surface of ilium

Medial border of ischial tuberosity

Anterior superior iliac spine

Anterior inferior iliac spine

Arcuate line of ilium

a. *Medial aspect*

Fig. 2.3 The left hip-bone.

5. The sharp medial border of the ischial tuberosity. This gives attachment to a powerful sacrotuberous ligament [Fig. 2.4], which passes down from the sacrum and the posterior part of the gluteal surface of the ala of the ilium. Closely applied to the deep or pelvic surface of this ligament is the sacrospinous ligament, which is attached to the ischial spine. These two ligaments convert the greater and lesser sciatic notches into the **greater and lesser sciatic foramina.**

Orientation of the pelvis

Turn again to an articulated skeleton, and note that the pelvis is so orientated that from the front you look straight into the superior aperture of the (lesser) pelvis. In the standing position the plane of the linea terminalis (which runs from the upper margin of the pubic symphysis along the pecten of the pubis and arcuate line, and then along the anterior part of the base or promontory of the sacrum) is usually inclined at an angle of about 60° to the horizontal [Fig. 2.5]. Another measure of the forward tilt of the pelvis is the fact that in the standing position the anterior superior spine and the pubic symphysis are in approximately the same vertical plane.

reaches nearly to the acetabulum. The body of the ischium continues above the ischial tuberosity to form a large part of the acetabulum.

The ischial tuberosity gives origin to a group of muscles called the hamstring muscles, which lie on the posterior aspect of the thigh.

The **ischial spine** lies above and medial to the ischial tuberosity. Note again that it separates the greater sciatic notch above from the lesser sciatic notch below.

The sacropelvic aspect of the hip-bone

Examine the medial (sacropelvic) aspect of the hip-bone [Fig. 2.3a], and note:
1. A rough area of bone lying above the greater sciatic notch. This is called the **auricular surface.** It is here that the hip-bone articulates with the sacrum to form the sacroiliac joint.
2. A rough area, called the **iliac tuberosity,** for the attachment of ligaments to the articular surface.
3. The ridge, called the **arcuate line,** which extends upwards and backwards from the pecten of the pubis, and with it forms a major part of the **linea terminalis,** which is the boundary between the greater and lesser pelves.
4. The concave part of the ilium, called the **iliac fossa,** above the arcuate line.

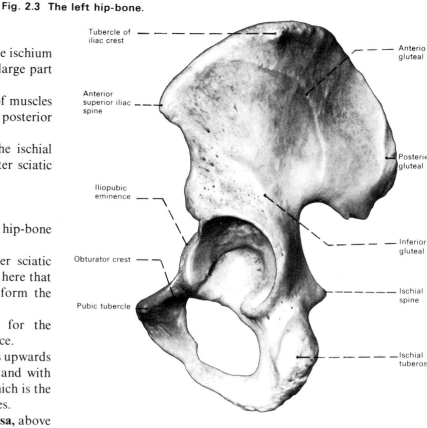

Tubercle of iliac crest

Anterior superior iliac spine

Iliopubic eminence

Obturator crest

Pubic tubercle

Anterio gluteal

Posterio gluteal

Inferior gluteal

Ischial spine

Ischial tuberos

b. *Lateral aspect*

2.4

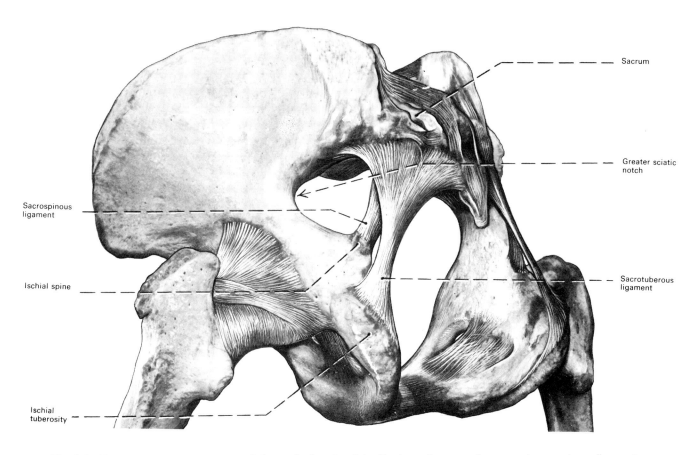

Sacrum

Greater sciatic notch

Sacrospinous ligament

Sacrotuberous ligament

Ischial spine

Ischial tuberosity

Fig. 2.4 The postero-lateral aspect of the articulated pelvis. To show the sacrotuberous and sacrospinous ligaments.

The femur

You will find it useful to keep these facts about the hip-bone in mind before you start dissecting the gluteal region. Before you begin dissecting it is also useful to get a general idea of the femur, which is the longest and strongest bone in the body. Its **head** articulates above with the acetabulum of the

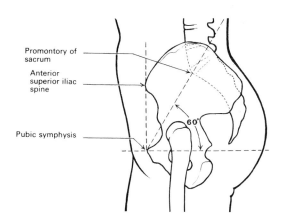

Promontory of sacrum

Anterior superior iliac spine

Pubic symphysis

60°

Fig. 2.5 The orientation of the pelvis in the standing position.

hip-bone, and its enlarged distal end consists of two **condyles** which articulate at the knee with the upper end of the tibia or shin-bone.

Examine a femur [Fig. 2.6], and note that its head forms two-thirds of a sphere. The head is characterized by a central depression called the **fovea capitis femoris. A neck** connects the head with the **shaft** of the femur at an angle of about 120° in the male (rather less in the female). The size of this angle is altered in certain diseases.

The zone of union of the neck and shaft is marked by two tuberosities called trochanters. Look at a femur from behind. The **greater trochanter** is a powerful quadrate process which ends above in a beak-like process that overhangs the base of the neck. The greater trochanter can be easily felt in the living body in the upper part of the lateral aspect of the thigh.

The **lesser trochanter** is the small knob on the medial side of the upper part of the shaft of the femur, into which a crest of bone, the **intertrochanteric crest,** passes from the overhanging beak at the top of the greater trochanter. The projection on the middle of the crest is the **quadrate tubercle,** and the cavity under the overhanging part of the trochanter the **trochanteric fossa.**

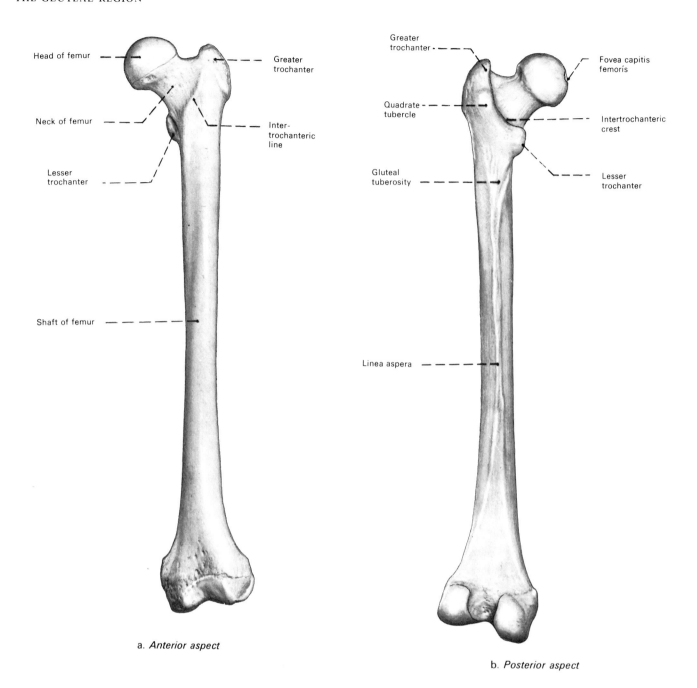

Head of femur

Greater trochanter

Neck of femur

Inter-trochanteric line

Lesser trochanter

Shaft of femur

a. *Anterior aspect*

Greater trochanter

Fovea capitis femoris

Quadrate tubercle

Intertrochanteric crest

Gluteal tuberosity

Lesser trochanter

Linea aspera

b. *Posterior aspect*

Fig. 2.6 The left femur.

If you now turn the bone over you will see that the two trochanters are joined in front by the **intertrochanteric line.**

The shaft of the femur is smooth and round, and is marked posteriorly by a rough ridge called the **linea aspera,** to which most of the muscles of the thigh are attached. Note how the margins of this ridge diverge from each other both above and below. The rough area into which the lateral border of the linea aspera runs above is called the **gluteal tuberosity.** It gives attachment to fibres of the gluteus maximus muscle.

The sacrum

Now examine the sacrum [Fig. 2.7]. Note that it is formed by the fusion of five vertebrae of decreasing size, so that its outline is triangular. You will see that its pelvic surface is concave and much smoother than the dorsal, on which you can see the spinous processes of the sacral vertebrae, fused to form the **median sacral crest.** The anterior projecting edge of the upper part of the first sacral vertebra is the **promontory of the sacrum.** The foramina on the pelvic sur-

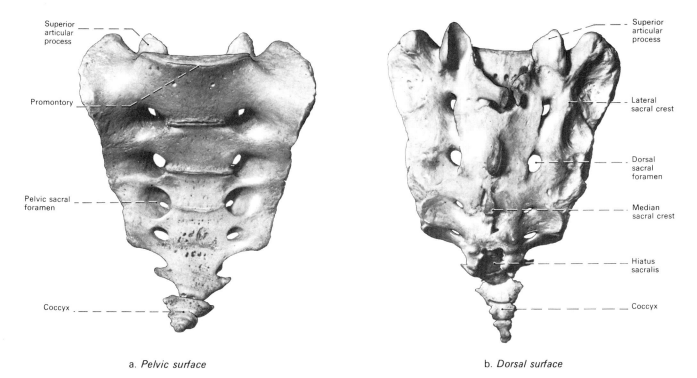

Superior
articular
process

Promontory

Pelvic sacral
foramen

Coccyx

a. *Pelvic surface*

Superior
articular
process

Lateral
sacral crest

Dorsal
sacral
foramen

Median
sacral crest

Hiatus
sacralis

Coccyx

b. *Dorsal surface*

Fig. 2.7 The sacrum and coccyx.

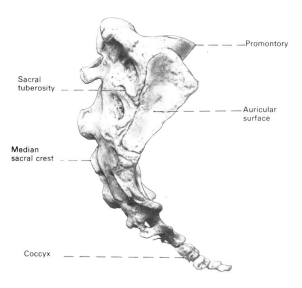

Promontory

Sacral
tuberosity

Auricular
surface

Median
sacral crest

Coccyx

c. *Lateral aspect*

face of the bone transmit the ventral rami of the sacral nerves and those on the dorsal surface, the dorsal rami.

On the upper part of the lateral surface of the sacrum you will see a rough articular facet, called the **auricular surface,** which articulates with the corresponding facet on the ilium. Below, the tip of the sacrum articulates with a small bone called the **coccyx.** This consists of a variable number of fused vestigial tail-vertebrae.

It is worth noting now that the ventral rami of the upper three sacral nerves (and also part of the fourth) join with those of the fifth and part of the fourth lumbar nerves to form the sacral plexus of nerves [Fig. 2.32]. This supplies most of the lower limb. The part of the lower limb the sacral plexus does not innervate is supplied by the lumbar plexus, which is formed immediately above the sacral plexus from the first four lumbar nerves. Both plexuses are situated on the posterior wall of the abdominal cavity, and so cannot be dissected till you come to study the abdomen.

Surface anatomy

Examine the superficial features of the gluteal region, both on your dissecting-room subject and, when you have an opportunity, on your own body, and try to relate to the body some of the facts about the pelvis and femur which you have just learnt [Fig. 2.8].

First run your finger forwards along the iliac crest till you locate the anterior superior iliac spine. About 5 cm behind it feel for the tubercle of the crest. Then identify the posterior superior iliac spine, the sacrum and coccyx, the ischial tuberosities and the greater trochanter of the femur, behind which you will usually find a well-marked depression. All these features are fairly easily defined, the posterior superior iliac spine being marked by a dimple about 5 cm from the midline and about the same distance below the vertex of the iliac crest.

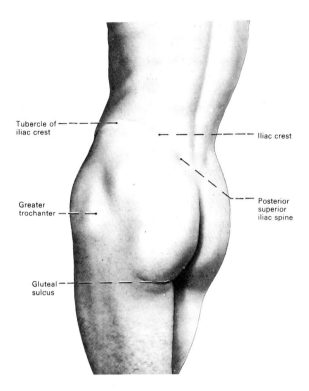

Fig. 2.8 The surface anatomy of the buttock.

The skin fold at the lower border of the buttock is called
the **gluteal sulcus.** Note now, and confirm later when you
dissect, that this does not correspond to the lower border
of the gluteus maximus muscle.

On the front of the body, in the midline in the lower part
of the abdomen, feel for the upper border of the body of
the pubis, the pubic crest. Run your fingers along this border
until the pubic tubercle is felt at its lateral end. Continue
laterally along the fold of the groin until the anterior
superior spine is reached. When you do this on your own
body you may be able to feel an important ligament called
the inguinal ligament.

Reflection of the skin

With the cadaver lying face downwards, make the following
incisions through the skin [Fig. 2.9]:

1. A transverse incision from the anterior superior iliac
   spine along the line of the iliac crest to the midline of
   the back. (If the upper limb has been dissected, this incision will have been made already.)
2. A vertical incision down the midline from the medial end
   of this last incision to the tip of the coccyx.
3. An oblique incision from the tip of the coccyx, across
   the gluteal sulcus, to a point on the lateral surface of the
   thigh, halfway between the greater trochanter and the
   knee joint.

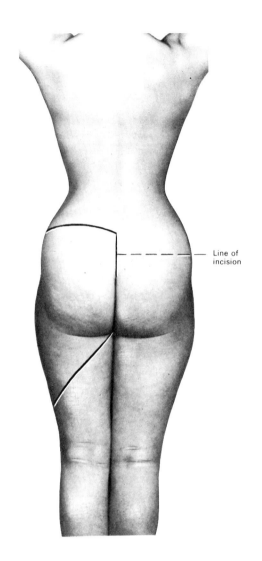

Fig. 2.9 Skin incisions of the gluteal region.

Reflect the skin from the structures beneath it and turn
it laterally. Because of the way the skin is tied to the underlying fat, you are not likely to do this as easily or as neatly
as you can reflect the skin of most other parts of the body.

The cutaneous nerves

As you turn the skin back you may come across certain
cutaneous nerves in the dense fat. You are more likely to
discover them if you first study a plan of the distribution
of the cutaneous nerves in this region [Fig. 2.10]. If you do
not readily find the nerves shown in this figure, do not waste
time looking for them. They are the **inferior nerves of the
buttocks,** branches of the fairly large posterior cutaneous
nerve of the thigh, and branches of the dorsal rami of the
lumbar and sacral nerves, which emerge near the midline
and pass obliquely downwards and laterally. The inferior
nerves of the buttock curl round the lower border of gluteus

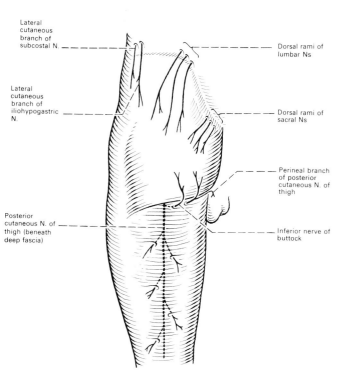

Lateral cutaneous branch of subcostal N.

Lateral cutaneous branch of iliohypogastric N.

Posterior cutaneous N. of thigh (beneath deep fascia)

Dorsal rami of lumbar Ns

Dorsal rami of sacral Ns

Perineal branch of posterior cutaneous N. of thigh

Inferior nerve of buttock

Fig. 2.10 The cutaneous nerves of the left buttock.

maximus to supply the skin of the buttock. Inferiorly you may also find the longest of the **perineal branches of the posterior cutaneous nerve of the thigh,** passing into the perineum to supply the external genitalia. Antero-superiorly, the **lateral cutaneous branches of the subcostal** and **iliohypogastric nerves** cross the iliac crest to enter the buttock.

Dissection of the buttock

The gluteus maximus muscle

The superficial fascia and fat, and the thin layer of deep fascia over the gluteus maximus, must now be removed in one sheet, starting from above and cutting downwards and laterally along the line of the muscle fibres, taking care to leave intact the deep fascia of the thigh, known as the **fascia lata.** Most of the gluteus maximus is inserted into a thickened part of this fascia which covers the lateral surface of the thigh, and which is called the **iliotibial tract.** This tract is attached above to the iliac crest and below to the lateral condyle of the tibia.

The upper and lower borders of the gluteus maximus should be carefully cleaned and defined [Fig. 2.11]. The muscle can now be seen to take origin from the posterior part of the ilium; from the adjacent dorsal surface of the sacrum; and from the sacrotuberous ligament, which you can feel by inserting a finger beneath the lower border of the muscle.

Look again at the gluteal surface of a hip-bone [Fig. 2.3b].

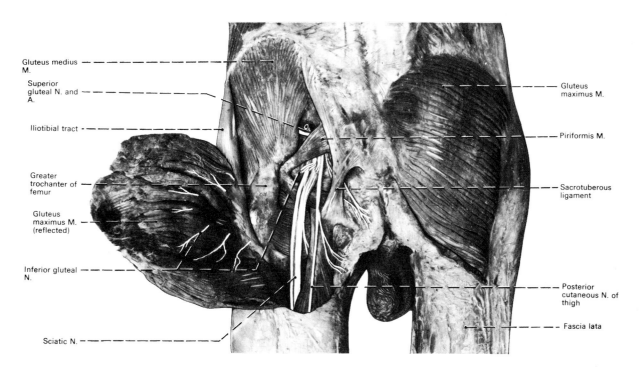

Gluteus medius M.

Superior gluteal N. and A.

Iliotibial tract

Greater trochanter of femur

Gluteus maximus M. (reflected)

Inferior gluteal N.

Sciatic N.

Gluteus maximus M.

Piriformis M.

Sacrotuberous ligament

Posterior cutaneous N. of thigh

Fascia lata

Fig. 2.11 The gluteal muscles. The left gluteus maximus muscle has been detached from its origin and turned laterally.

Note a short bony ridge that passes upwards from the posterior part of the superior rim of the greater sciatic notch to the posterior part of the iliac crest. This ridge, the posterior gluteal line, marks the anterior limit of the bony origin of the gluteus maximus muscle.

The gluteus maximus should be separated from the structures deep to it by gently pushing a finger under the lower border of the muscle and between it and the underlying deep fascia. Another finger should be pushed downwards under the upper border of the muscle, through the deep fascia beneath the muscle. The fascia is thin superiorly, and the strands you will feel leading from it to the undersurface of the muscle are the inferior gluteal artery and vein and the inferior gluteal nerve below, and the superficial branches and tributaries of the superior gluteal artery and vein above. Clean them as you proceed, and divide them as near to the gluteus maximus as you can.

The muscle should then be detached from its origin, beginning below and working upwards towards the iliac crest. Do not damage the sacrotuberous ligament. The gluteus maximus muscle is then turned laterally and the vessels and nerve entering it divided. Care should be taken not to damage the posterior cutaneous nerve of the thigh, which runs deep to the deep fascia.

Note that the major part of the gluteus maximus passes into the dense layer of fascia, the fascia lata, which clothes the lateral part of the thigh, and that only its deeper fibres are inserted into the gluteal tuberosity of the femur. At this stage confirm that the fascia lata extends upwards from the thigh over the muscles covering the gluteal aspect of the ilium, and that it becomes attached above to the iliac crest and behind to the sacrum.

Note the large bursa between the muscle and the greater trochanter.

The gluteus medius muscle

The muscles you have exposed by reflecting the gluteus maximus are the lesser gluteal muscles and the lateral rotators of the thigh. The gluteus medius, which is the largest and most superficial [Figs 2.12 and 2.14], overlaps most of the

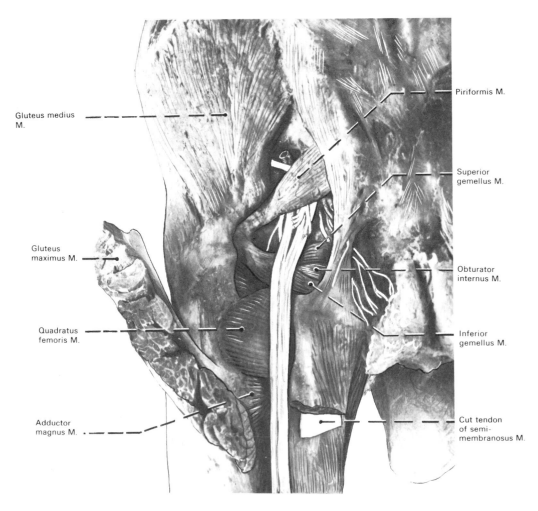

Gluteus medius M.

Gluteus maximus M.

Quadratus femoris M.

Adductor magnus M.

Piriformis M.

Superior gemellus M.

Obturator internus M.

Inferior gemellus M.

Cut tendon of semi-membranosus M.

Fig. 2.12 The lateral rotators of the left thigh. Most of the left gluteus maximus muscle has been excised; the remaining part is reflected laterally.

gluteus minimus, and the two muscles may blend so intimately that it will be difficult to separate them.

Clean the gluteus medius by detaching its covering of fascia lata from the iliac crest, as far anteriorly as the tubercle of the crest. Then reflect the fascia lata laterally. By referring to a hip-bone identify the area of origin of the muscle from the gluteal surface of the ilium between the anterior and posterior gluteal lines [Fig. 2.3b]. The anterior gluteal line is a ridge of bone on the gluteal surface of the ala of the ilium, which is sometimes poorly marked, and which arches forward from the greater sciatic notch to just in front of the tubercle of the iliac crest.

Trace the insertion of the gluteus medius into the lateral surface of the greater trochanter.

Structures deep to the gluteus maximus

Now that you have cleaned the gluteus medius, you will be able to define the small triangular **piriformis muscle,** which lies just below it [Fig. 2.11]. You will not be able to see its origin from the pelvic aspect of the sacrum, but you will see the muscle emerging through the greater sciatic foramen. As you clean the piriformis, verify that it is inserted into the upper border of the greater trochanter of the femur, just behind the insertion of the gluteus medius.

Follow the gluteus medius to its insertion into the oblique ridge on the lateral surface of the greater trochanter of the femur.

The leash of vessels and nerves which are emerging from the greater sciatic foramen between the piriformis and the gluteus medius are the **superior gluteal vessels** and the **superior gluteal nerve.** Clean them (removing the veins) as far as the present stage of the dissection will allow.

Identify the **sciatic nerve.** This is a very large flat cord that enters the field of your dissection from below the piriformis. It often divides high in the thigh and may be found in two parts [Fig. 2.11]. A very small artery accompanying (and supplying) the nerve is often identifiable.

Complete the cleaning of the **inferior gluteal nerve** and **artery,** which you divided [p. 2.10] at the point where they entered the deep surface of the gluteus maximus. As you trace them towards the sciatic nerve you will find, a little superficial and medial to the latter, another nerve, whose course is directed into the thigh. This is the **posterior cutaneous nerve of the thigh,** which you will remember gives branches to the skin of the buttock, perineum, and thigh [p. 2.8]. Clean this nerve, too.

The lateral rotator muscles of the thigh

The small muscles which are mainly responsible for the lateral rotation of the thigh can now be seen running transversely below the piriformis [Fig. 2.12]. They cover the posterior aspect of the hip joint and comprise, from above downwards, the **superior gemellus, obturator internus,** and **inferior gemellus** (the three are usually fused together at their

insertion), and the **quadratus femoris** muscles. The **obturator externus** cannot yet be seen, but after you have cleaned and defined the quadratus femoris you may be able to see below it the upper part of the biggest adductor of the thigh, the adductor magnus muscle. Clean these muscles, but carefully preserve all the nerves in the region.

The origins of the hamstring muscles

Now examine the region medial to the quadratus femoris and study the origins of the hamstring muscles from the ischial tuberosity [Fig. 2.13].

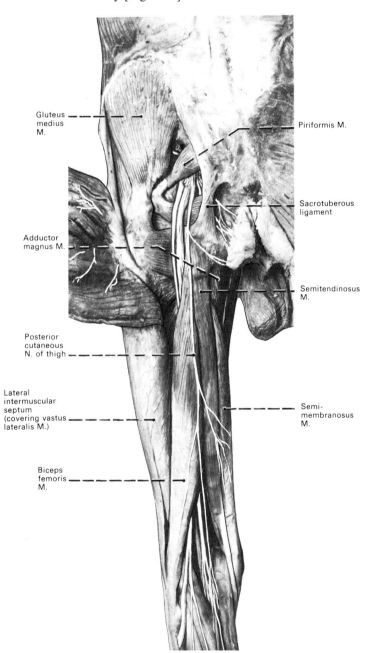

Fig. 2.13 The posterior aspect of the left thigh. The gluteus maximus muscle is turned laterally.

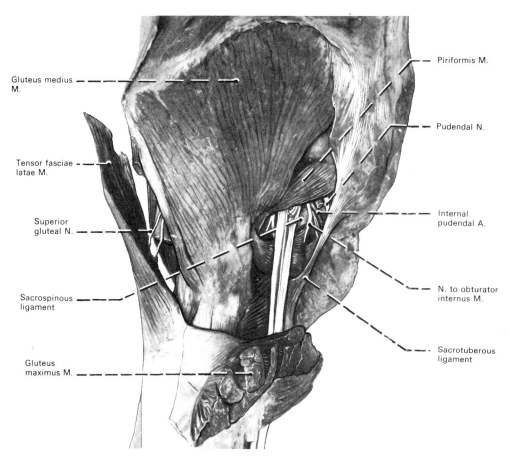

Gluteus medius M.

Tensor fasciae latae M.

Superior gluteal N.

Sacrospinous ligament

Gluteus maximus M.

Piriformis M.

Pudendal N.

Internal pudendal A.

N. to obturator internus M.

Sacrotuberous ligament

Fig. 2.14 Lateral view of the left buttock. Most of the left gluteus maximus muscle has been excised; the remaining part is reflected downwards and laterally. The tensor fasciae latae muscle has been detached from the ilium.

The most superficial structure you will see is the musculo-tendinous origin of the **biceps femoris muscle** and the **semitendinosus muscle,** with the hamstring part of the fleshy adductor magnus on its medial side. On a deeper plane, and on the lateral side, is the tendon of origin of the **semimembranosus muscle.**

Examine a hip-bone to define precisely the area of origin of these muscles. Note that the muscle which arises from the supero-lateral aspect of the posterior surface of the tuberosity, just medial to the origin of the quadratus femoris, is the semimembranosus. The tendon which is attached to the infero-medial aspect of the same surface is the conjoined tendon of the biceps femoris and semitendinosus muscles. The muscle which arises from the infero-lateral surface of the tuberosity is the **adductor magnus.**

Turn back to the cadaver and clean the ischial tuberosity and define the origins of these muscles. As you dissect, you will find that they are supplied by branches of the sciatic nerve.

The sacrotuberous ligament [Figs 2.12 to 2.14]

Now clean the sacrotuberous ligament. You will see that it becomes attached to the medial margin of the ischial

tuberosity. Deep, or anterior, to the sacrotuberous ligament identify, by feeling, the ischial spine and sacrospinous ligament, which is attached to it [Fig. 2.14].

As you saw when you examined the hip-bone, the ischial spine marks the upper boundary of the lesser sciatic foramen. Look again at the obturator internus tendon. You will see that it passes through this foramen from the interior of the pelvis.

There are three smaller structures to identify in this region [Fig. 2.14]. Each passes from the pelvis through both sciatic foramina into the perineum, i.e. into the space below the pelvic floor. Search medially to the point where the sciatic nerve emerges from the lower border of the piriformis, and find, closely applied to each other and to the sacrospinous ligament (or the adjacent ischial spine across which they pass) from the medial to the lateral side: the **pudendal nerve,** the **internal pudendal artery** and **vein,** and the **nerve to obturator internus.** The latter may be difficult to find, so do not spend time searching for it. The pudendal artery and nerve should be cleaned carefully and preserved, removing the veins as usual.

In the next stage of your dissection you divide several muscles in order to display the important structures which

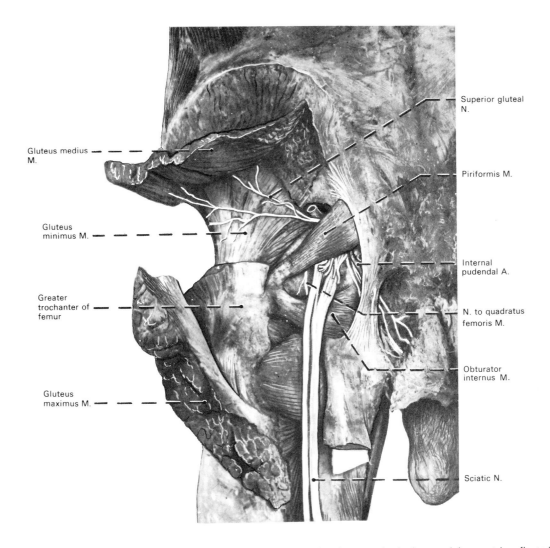

Gluteus medius M.

Gluteus minimus M.

Greater trochanter of femur

Gluteus maximus M.

Superior gluteal N.

Piriformis M.

Internal pudendal A.

N. to quadratus femoris M.

Obturator internus M.

Sciatic N.

Fig. 2.15 The lesser gluteal muscles. Most of the gluteus maximus muscle has been excised; the remaining part is reflected laterally. The gluteus medius muscle has been incised and turned upwards.

lie deep to them. Unless otherwise stated, these muscles should be completely divided about 3 cm from their insertions and, as each is reflected, its origin and insertion should be carefully examined and confirmed.

Reflection of the gluteus medius

Begin by dividing the posterior two-thirds of the gluteus medius, leaving the anterior (or lateral) margin of the muscle undivided. Do this by separating the posterior border of the muscle from the underlying gluteus minimus, and then make a transverse incision, starting at the posterior border, about 3 cm above the greater trochanter. If you divide the muscle completely you will almost certainly cut into another muscle, which you have not yet seen, on the lateral side of the thigh. This is the **tensor fasciae latae muscle,** and it lies superficial to the anterior part of the gluteus medius [Fig. 2.14].

Now turn the cut ends of the gluteus medius aside, as far as possible, so that the superior gluteal artery and nerve can be traced on the under-surface of the muscle [Fig. 2.15]. As you do this, clear away the accompanying veins. The superior gluteal nerve is distributed to the gluteus minimus, to the gluteus medius, and anteriorly to the tensor fasciae latae, which you will clean later. Again confirm the insertion of the gluteus medius into the oblique line on the lateral aspect of the greater trochanter.

If you look at two or three femurs you will see that the detailed markings on the lateral surface of the greater trochanter vary greatly. This reflects the variable way in which the gluteus medius may be inserted into the bone. Usually the oblique ridge on which it is inserted runs downwards and forwards, the gluteus minimus being inserted into the region in front of the line and to the front of the trochanter. Sometimes the gluteus medius and the gluteus minimus are so fused that their separate insertions cannot be defined.

The gluteus minimus muscle [Figs 2.15 and 2.17]

Clean the gluteus minimus. The anterior part of the muscle lies deep to the undivided portion of the gluteus medius. Note the origin of the muscle from the ilium between the anterior and inferior gluteal lines, and its insertion into the anterior surface of the greater trochanter of the femur, in front of the oblique line.

If you refer to a hip-bone [Fig. 2.16], you will see that the inferior gluteal line is an indistinct ridge of bone which passes from the apex of the greater sciatic notch posteriorly, more or less transversely forwards to the region of the anterior inferior iliac spine.

Return to the cadaver and divide the piriformis muscle about 3 cm from its insertion, and confirm that it passes into the superior border of the greater trochanter of the femur. Note that the piriformis is inserted above the obturator internus and the gemelli muscles.

The exposure of the hip joint

Turn the cut ends of the piriformis aside. Part of the articular capsule of the hip joint will then come into view. You will also now be able to trace the sciatic nerve upwards to the point where it emerges from the greater sciatic foramen. Carefully pull this nerve aside and look for a slender branch

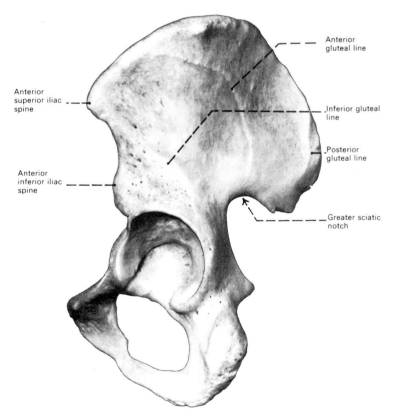

Fig. 2.16 The lateral aspect of the left hip-bone.

Anterior gluteal line

Anterior superior iliac spine

Inferior gluteal line

Posterior gluteal line

Anterior inferior iliac spine

Greater sciatic notch

deep to it. This is the **nerve to the quadratus femoris** and the inferior gemellus muscles [Fig. 2.15].

Your next step is to cut the conjoined tendons of the obturator internus and the gemelli muscles. If you do this very carefully and turn them out of the way, you may see the branch which the nerve to the quadratus femoris sends to the inferior gemellus. Do not spend time seeking this branch if you do not see it immediately. Trace the nerve to the quadratus femoris over the capsule of the hip joint into the muscle itself.

Now examine the origins of the gemelli muscles. You will see that the **superior gemellus** arises from the ischial spine, and the **inferior gemellus** from just above the ischial tuberosity [Fig. 2.17]. As already observed, the obturator internus muscle arises within the pelvic cavity, and its origin cannot be seen at this stage. Confirm the insertion of these muscles into the medial surface of the greater trochanter of the femur, below the insertion of the piriformis muscle.

The cutting of the conjoined tendons of the obturator internus and the gemelli brings more of the capsule of the hip joint into view. You will also be able to display the **obturator internus tendon** passing through the lesser sciatic foramen, and to find the bursa that lies between it and the underlying bone.

To complete the dissection of this region, the **quadratus femoris muscle** should be divided through its middle, and the two halves turned aside as far as possible. If the muscle is thick and well developed it will be difficult to separate the cut ends very much. Note that the muscle arises from the body of the ischium lateral to the ischial tuberosity, and that it is inserted into the quadrate tubercle on the intertrochanteric crest of the femur, and for a short distance into the bone below. Examine a hip-bone and a femur to confirm these points on the bones.

As you dissect below the quadratus femoris, you will come across the ramifying branches of an artery. This is the **medial circumflex femoral artery,** a branch of the profunda femoris artery, which you will expose later on the front of the thigh. The medial circumflex supplies adjacent muscles and the hip joint, and takes part in an anastomosis called the cruciate anastomosis, which will be described later.

Now try and identify the structures which lie beneath the quadratus femoris below the hip joint. You should easily be able to find the **obturator externus,** which is passing upwards and laterally to its insertion into the trochanteric fossa. By looking deep to the obturator externus you will find the distal portion of the **iliopsoas muscle,** which is formed from the combined distal parts of two muscles called iliacus and psoas major. The iliacus arises from the iliac fossa on the medial aspect of the hip-bone and the psoas from the bodies of lumbar vertebrae so that the main contractile mass of these muscles is only visible when the posterior abdominal wall has been exposed [see Fig. 4.63]. At this stage you may be able to see and feel the insertion of

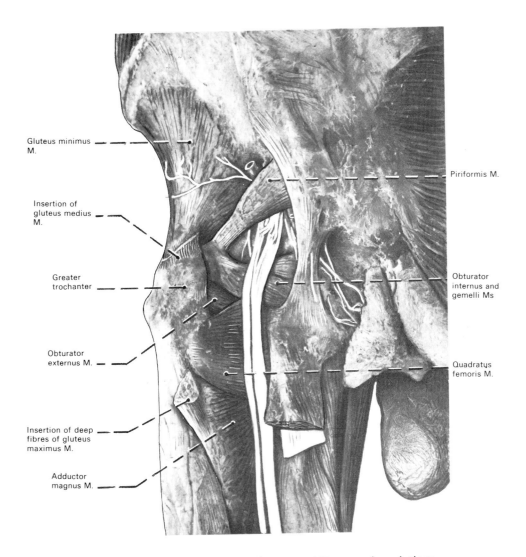

Gluteus minimus M.

Piriformis M.

Insertion of gluteus medius M.

Greater trochanter

Obturator internus and gemelli Ms

Obturator externus M.

Quadratus femoris M.

Insertion of deep fibres of gluteus maximus M.

Adductor magnus M.

Fig. 2.17 The left greater trochanter and its muscular relations.

the muscles on the lesser trochanter. If the subject you are dissecting has a well-developed quadratus femoris muscle, it may be awkward, if not impossible, to see the iliopsoas at this stage.

The actions of the gluteal muscles

Before leaving this part of the dissection, take a further look at the attachments of the important gluteal muscles, with the object of studying their action [Figs 2.11 and 2.14].

The line of pull of the gluteus maximus is behind the hip joint, and it is the main extensor of the thigh (i.e. it draws the lower limb backwards). The chief flexor of the thigh, whose insertion into the lesser trochanter you may have seen, is the iliopsoas, so that in their actions these two powerful muscles are directly antagonistic to each other. Another important function of the gluteus maximus is to help raise the trunk from the stooping position, and in these circumstances it acts in reverse, i.e. from its insertion to-

wards its origin. The gluteus maximus can also laterally rotate the thigh.

You should now try to understand how the gluteus maximus works on your own body. Keeping your knees extended, bend down and then raise the trunk. You will feel the muscle contracting and stiffening as you do so. Now stand as upright as you can. You will again feel the muscle contracting. Climb some steps and again note the muscle contracting. Walk around with your hands on your buttocks and note that both gluteus maximus muscles remain relaxed. In most individuals the muscle contracts only when you run, during the final phase of extension of the hip joint. When both gluteus maximus muscles are contracted, the anal opening becomes even more tightly closed than usual.

The gluteus medius, the gluteus minimus, and the tensor fasciae latae (which arises below the iliac crest in front of the gluteus medius, and which you will dissect later) work together as abductors and medial rotators of the thigh.

2.15

All the gluteal muscles and, to a lesser extent, the tensor fasciae latae, acting in reverse, help to steady the pelvis on the lower limb. The gluteus medius and minimus, therefore, have a most important function to perform in walking, for as each limb is successively raised from the ground, these two muscles pull or tilt the pelvis to the supported side of the body. If it were not for this, normal walking would be impossible. The tensor fasciae latae has other specialized functions, which will be described when your dissection has proceeded further [pp. 2.25–2.27].

In order to study the actions of gluteus medius and minimus place the tips of your fingers on the upper lateral side of your own thigh, halfway between the iliac crest above and the greater trochanter below. Then walk. You will feel these muscles contracting alternately on the left and right sides. When they contract on the side that bears the weight of your body, the pelvis is tilted off the opposite, raised, limb. Now stand still and move one limb away from your body. With the tips of your fingers still in the same position you will feel these two gluteal muscles contracting.

Remember the nerve supply of these muscles—the gluteus maximus from the inferior gluteal nerve; the gluteus medius, minimus, and tensor fasciae latae from the superior gluteal nerve.

Section 2.2

The front and medial side of the thigh

Turn the body over on to its back, in order to dissect the front of the thigh, which contains two important groups of muscles. On the anterior aspect is the extensor of the knee, the quadriceps femoris, which is composed of four muscles, the rectus femoris, the vastus lateralis, the vastus medialis, and the vastus intermedius. There is one further muscle on the front of the thigh which you will have to examine. This is a thin, strap-like muscle, called the sartorius, which arises from the region of the anterior superior iliac spine and which runs obliquely downwards and medially across the front of the thigh. It ends by being inserted into the tibia on the medial aspect of the leg. Its individual muscle fibres are the longest in the body.

On the medial aspect of the thigh are the adductor muscles, the adductor magnus, the adductor longus, the adductor brevis, the gracilis, and the pectineus. On the front of the thigh are also the main blood vessels, the femoral artery and femoral vein, which pass to and from the lower limb, and two main nerves, the femoral nerve, which supplies the extensor muscles of the knee joint, and the obturator nerve, which supplies the adductor muscles. These two nerves are the main branches of the lumbar plexus.

The **fascia lata,** whose intimate relations to the gluteus maximus and gluteus medius you have already studied, spreads out as a strong sheath to envelop the whole thigh. The fascia is particularly strong on the lateral aspect of the thigh, where it is thickened by the dense iliotibial tract, which extends from the iliac crest to the lateral condyle of the tibia. On the medial aspect of the thigh, just below the inguinal ligament (this is the ligament you felt when you were studying the surface anatomy of the groin [p. 2.8]) is a small aperture in the fascia lata, called the saphenous opening. This opening transmits the great saphenous vein, which is an important vessel that begins in the foot and which drains the major part of the superficial aspect of the lower limb. This vein and its tributaries are often permanently dilated (varicose).

The upper ends of the femoral vessels are enclosed in a fascial sheath called the femoral sheath.

Osteology

Begin by studying the bones to which all these structures are related.

The femur

You have already noted the general features of the upper part of the femur. Examine the lower part of the bone. The **lateral** and **medial condyles** are separated by an **intercondylar fossa** [Fig. 2.18]. Projecting from the condyles are two small prominences called the **medial** and **lateral epicondyles.** Above the medial epicondyle is the particularly prominent **adductor tubercle,** where the tendon of the large adductor magnus muscle becomes attached to the femur. Note that there is a groove on the lateral aspect of the lateral condyle. It gives attachment to a small but important muscle called the popliteus. The articular surface between and just above the condyles on the anterior surface of the shaft articulates with the patella, or knee-cap.

If you turn the femur over you will see that the **linea aspera** ends about two-thirds of the way down the bone, and that the lateral and medial lips of the linea aspera are continued as slightly raised ridges, called the **lateral** and **medial supracondylar lines,** which extend to the lateral condyle and adductor tubercle respectively. The triangular area between the two lines is the **popliteal surface** of the femur. Note that the medial supracondylar line is less distinct than the lateral.

The patella

Examine the patella. It is a sesamoid bone lying within the tendon of the quadriceps femoris muscle, the muscle of the front of the thigh. The posterior surface of the patella articulates with the patellar surface of the femur, which you have just examined. Because of the presence of the patella, the quadriceps pulls on the tibia at an angle in the later stages of extension of the knee joint, and the power of the muscle is thus increased.

Now study the general features of the upper ends of the bones of the leg—the tibia on the medial, and the fibula on the lateral side.

The tibia

The tibia is a massive bone which has to sustain the whole weight of the body, which is transmitted through the femur. The medial surface of the tibia is subcutaneous and easily felt. This part is called the shin. Refer to the skeleton and note that the upper surface of the proximal end of the tibia articulates with the condyles of the femur, and that on its lateral side the proximal end of the tibia also articulates with the head of the fibula.

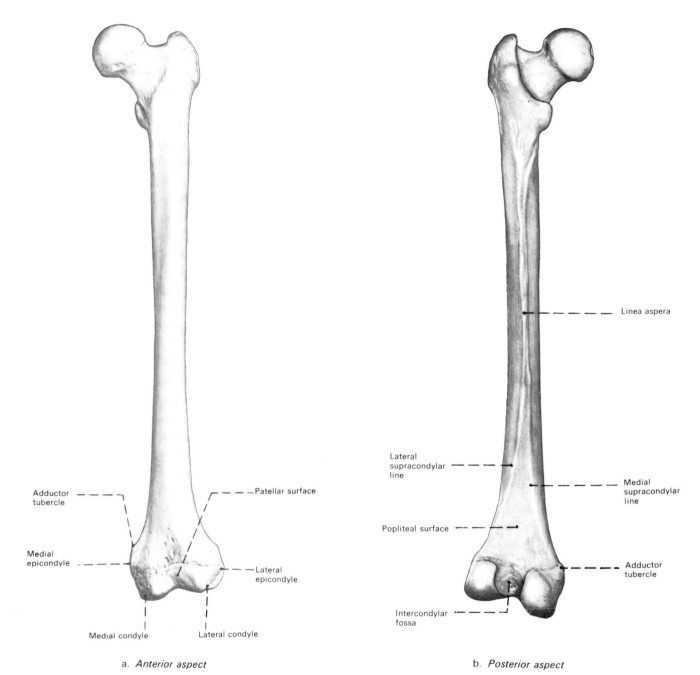

a. *Anterior aspect*

b. *Posterior aspect*

Fig. 2.18 The left femur.

You will see that the upper end of the tibia is divided into two articular **condyles** [Fig. 2.19]. Between these condyles note the prominent **intercondylar eminence** separating an **anterior intercondylar area** from a **posterior intercondylar area.** On the postero-lateral aspect of the lateral condyle, locate the round **fibular articular surface** with which the head of the fibula articulates. Note the groove on the posterior aspect of the medial condyle. Into it is inserted the semi-membranosus muscle, whose origin from the ischial tuberosity has already been dissected [p. 2.12].

At the proximal end of the shaft of the tibia, in the midline in front, find the **tuberosity of the tibia.** You can easily feel the tuberosity on your own leg. Into it is inserted the single tendon into which the quadriceps femoris muscle converges, and within which the patella lies. This tendon is called the patellar ligament. Expansions from it reinforce the capsule of the knee joint and are inserted into the tibial condyles.

The fibula [Fig. 2.19]

The fibula lies on the lateral aspect of the tibia and takes no part in the formation of the knee joint. The proximal end is the **head,** and you will see that it extends upwards

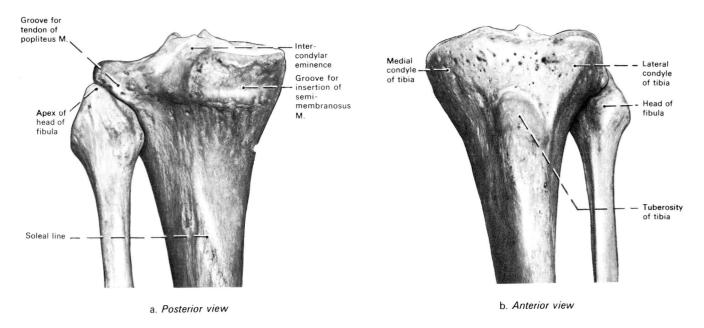

a. *Posterior view*

b. *Anterior view*

Fig. 2.19 The proximal ends of the left tibia and fibula.

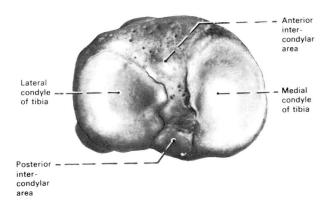

c. *Superior articular surface of tibia*

into the **apex of the head** of the fibula. No muscles on the front of the thigh are inserted into the fibula, which you need not, therefore, study further at this stage.

Surface anatomy

The surface anatomy of the thigh is best studied at a convenient moment on your own body. Feel the inguinal ligament in the groin. The pulsations you can feel below its centre are caused by the femoral artery, which at this point is passing out of the pelvis to enter the thigh.

Feel for a prominent tendon on the medial aspect of the thigh immediately below the groin. This is the tendon of a muscle called the adductor longus [Fig. 2.20]. If you follow the tendon upwards you will feel that it leads to the pubic tubercle on the body of the pubis.

Flex, abduct, and laterally rotate your thigh. The long narrow muscle which you can see forming a ridge all the way from the anterior superior spine of the ilium to the medial side of the knee is the sartorius. With your limb in this position, define the important **femoral triangle.** Its base is formed by the **inguinal ligament** (which is the lower border of the external oblique muscle of the abdomen and which passes from the anterior superior iliac spine to the pubic tubercle), its lateral margin by the sartorius, and its medial margin by the medial margin of the adductor longus. The triangle is covered only by skin and fascia, and so it will be felt as a depression in this region. The apex of the triangle is in the middle third of the thigh.

Now examine the knee. The patella and the patellar ligament will be most conspicuous. Define the condyles of the femur and distinguish them from the condyles of the tibia. Feel the head of the fibula just below the lateral condyle of the tibia.

Reflection of the skin

Begin your dissection of the thigh by making the following incisions through the skin [Fig. 2.21]:

1. From the anterior superior iliac spine to the pubic tubercle, along the line of the inguinal ligament. (In thin subjects you must take great care lest you include more than the skin in your incision.)
2. From the pubic tubercle downwards and posteriorly into the crease at the upper limit of the medial surface of the thigh, just skirting the external genitalia.

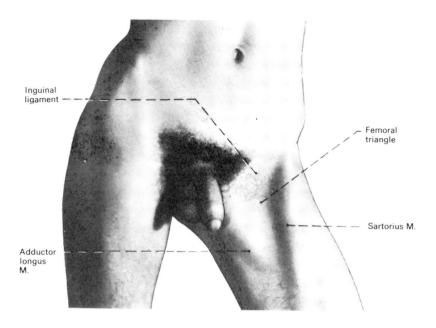

Fig. 2.20 Surface anatomy of the femoral triangle.

3. A vertical incision approximately along the line between the medial and posterior surfaces of the thigh, carrying your cut across the medial side of the knee and finishing at least 15 cm below the joint.
4. A transverse incision around the upper part of the leg starting at the end of the last incision.

Starting medially, dissect the large skin flap away from the superficial structures, and turn it laterally to hinge on the lateral border of the thigh.

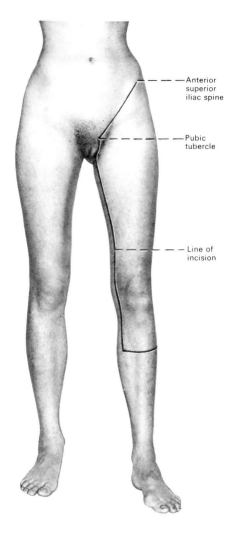

Fig. 2.21 Skin incisions on the front of the thigh.

Dissection of the front and medial side of the thigh

The cutaneous nerves

Figure 2.22 shows where the cutaneous nerves on the anterior aspect of the thigh usually appear through the deep fascia. There is little point in spending time on their dissection, but when you are dissecting in the superficial fascia, try to find the following two cutaneous nerves just below the inguinal ligament, starting medially and moving laterally:

1. The terminal branches of the **ilio-inguinal nerve,** which is a branch of the first lumbar nerve.
2. The **femoral branch of the genitofemoral nerve,** a nerve which is formed by branches from the first and second lumbar nerves.

The area of skin innervated by these two nerves is restricted to the upper part of the thigh and the external genitalia. On the front of the thigh below this area, find the **anterior cutaneous branches of the femoral nerve.** These are known as the medial and intermediate cutaneous nerves of the thigh. Next find the **lateral cutaneous nerve of the thigh,** which is formed from the ventral rami of the second and third lumbar nerves, independently of the femoral nerve.

Follow the latter three nerves to the patella. If you dissect carefully you may see that various branches they give off interconnect to form a plexus of cutaneous nerves around the patella. Do not spend time trying to define this plexus.

While dissecting in the region of the knee define the **subcutaneous prepatellar bursa.** It lies subcutaneously in front of the lower half of the patella and on the patellar ligament.

The superficial veins of the thigh

You will see a number of veins in the superficial fascia on the front of the thigh, and may notice that they run into the **great saphenous vein** on the medial aspect of the thigh.

2.20

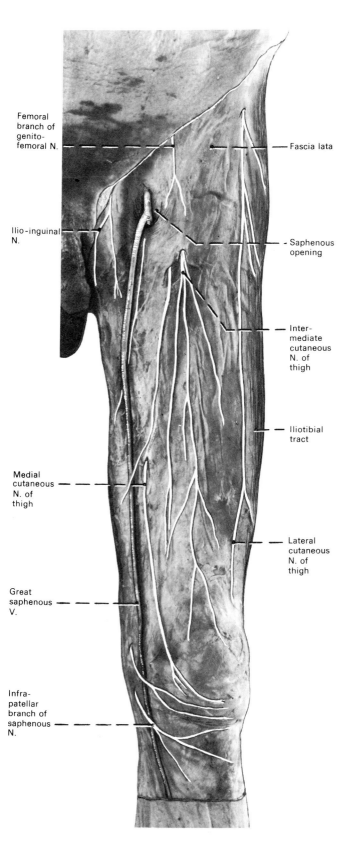

Femoral branch of genito-femoral N.

Ilio-inguinal N.

Medial cutaneous N. of thigh

Great saphenous V.

Infra-patellar branch of saphenous N.

Fascia lata

Saphenous opening

Inter-mediate cutaneous N. of thigh

Iliotibial tract

Lateral cutaneous N. of thigh

Fig. 2.22 The cutaneous nerves on the anterior surface of the left thigh.

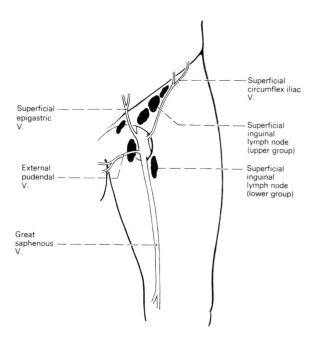

Superficial epigastric V.

External pudendal V.

Great saphenous V.

Superficial circumflex iliac V.

Superficial inguinal lymph node (upper group)

Superficial inguinal lymph node (lower group)

Fig. 2.23 The superficial inguinal veins and lymph nodes of the left thigh.

Follow this vein upwards. It will be found to enter the **saphenous opening** in the fascia lata; this small oval opening lies 3.5 cm below and lateral to the pubic tubercle. The fascia which covers the opening is called the **cribriform fascia,** and is part of the superficial fascia. Note that the sharp lateral **falciform margin** of the saphenous opening is attached above to the pubic tubercle, and that it is much more distinct than the ill-defined medial margin of the opening.

As it enters the saphenous opening you will see that the great saphenous vein receives three or more small tributaries, which you need not dissect [Fig. 2.23]. These tributaries drain the upper part of the thigh, the lower part of the anterior abdominal wall, and the external genitalia. These veins are accompanied by arteries which branch from the femoral artery.

The superficial lymph nodes of the thigh [Fig. 2.23]

You are likely to encounter some of the **superficial inguinal lymph nodes** near the termination of the great saphenous vein. You will also find some of this group of lymph nodes along the lower border of the inguinal ligament. These nodes of hard matted tissue are the most constant and easily demonstrated in a dissecting-room body, but they should be cleared away as they come into view. You may expose a few other lymph nodes when you come to the dissection of the back of the knee, but you will not be able to obtain from your dissection any clearer a picture of the lymphatic drainage of the lower limb than you did of the arm. For this you will have to refer to the Appendix.

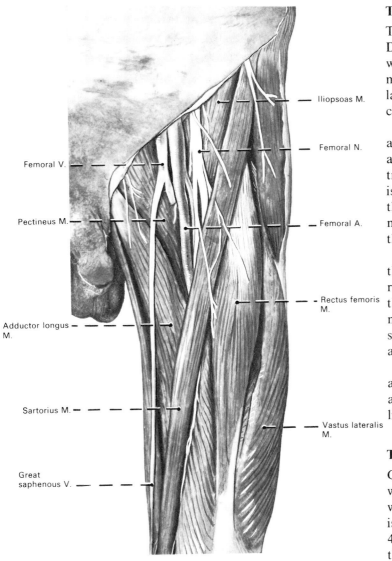

Iliopsoas M.

Femoral N.

Femoral V.

Pectineus M.

Femoral A.

Rectus femoris M.

Adductor longus M.

Sartorius M.

Vastus lateralis M.

Great saphenous V.

Fig. 2.24 The left femoral triangle.

The femoral triangle

Turn your attention to the femoral triangle [Fig. 2.24]. Define the medial margin of the **adductor longus muscle,** which forms the medial boundary of the triangle, and the medial margin of the **sartorius muscle,** which forms its lateral boundary. The triangle is deep and care must be exercised in its dissection.

Define the origin of the adductor longus, which is a triangular muscle whose apex is attached to the pubis in the angle between the pubic crest and the pubic symphysis. Also trace the sartorius to its origin. As you see, the sartorius is a long strap-like muscle that extends obliquely across the thigh from the anterior superior iliac spine and from the notch below it. At this stage you will not be able to define the insertions of either of these two muscles.

Carefully make a vertical incision in the fascia covering the floor of the lateral part of the femoral triangle, and then remove the fascia, being careful not to damage some nerves that lie immediately beneath the fascia. The muscle you have now exposed is the iliopsoas. Closely applied to its anterior surface you will find the femoral nerve as it descends vertically from behind the inguinal ligament.

Lying on the iliopsoas, on the medial side of the nerve, are the femoral vessels, invested by the femoral sheath. The artery is the central structure in the femoral triangle, and lies lateral to the vein.

The femoral nerve [Figs 2.24 to 2.27]

Clean the femoral nerve, and define the femoral sheath which, if the limb you are dissecting is not the one which was injected in the preparation of the cadaver, you will see is a funnel-shaped fascial tube that surrounds the uppermost 4 cm of the femoral vessels. (If it is the limb that was injected, the femoral sheath may have been cut into and its normal appearance disturbed.) The mouth of the funnel opens into the abdomen behind the inguinal ligament. The lower part of the funnel gradually closes upon, and fuses with the outer coat of the vessels [Fig. 2.26].

Notice that after a course in the triangle of only about 2 cm the main trunk of the femoral nerve starts dividing into branches. First find the **nerve to the pectineus.** This muscle forms part of the floor of the femoral triangle between the adductor longus and the iliopsoas muscles [Fig. 2.25]. The nerve comes off the main trunk of the femoral nerve and passes medially behind the femoral vessels to reach the pectineus. Find the **nerves to the sartorius,** and trace them to the muscle. You have already seen the **anterior cutaneous nerves of the thigh,** whose origin from the femoral nerve is associated with that of the motor nerves you are now dissecting.

Now define the muscular branches which arise from the femoral nerve on a deeper plane, and which pass to the component muscles of the quadriceps femoris, and also the

Turn your attention to the fascia lata on the lateral surface of the thigh. Remember that this dense and tendinous part of the deep fascia, which extends from the iliac crest to the tibia, is called the iliotibial tract [Fig. 2.22]. Trace the tract upwards. At a later stage you will be able to see that the tract splits to enclose the tensor fasciae latae muscle, which is inserted into it. You will dissect the muscle later.

Remove what remains of the superficial fascia and all the deep fascia from the thigh, except for the iliotibial tract and the fascia overlying the tensor fasciae latae muscle. As you do so, you will have to sacrifice most of the superficial vessels and nerves which you have already dissected, but take care not to damage the underlying femoral sheath.

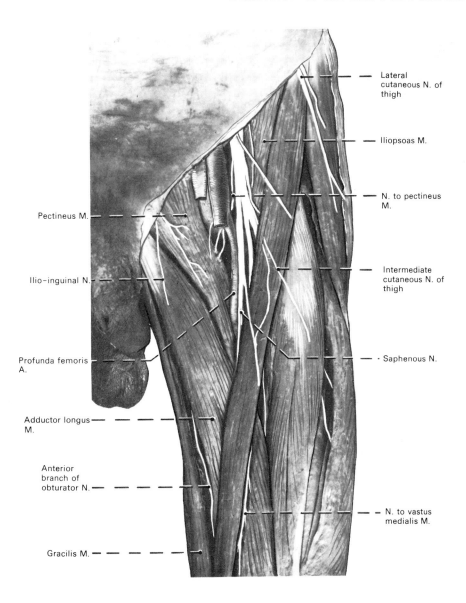

Lateral cutaneous N. of thigh

Iliopsoas M.

N. to pectineus M.

Intermediate cutaneous N. of thigh

Saphenous N.

N. to vastus medialis M.

Pectineus M.

Ilio-inguinal N.

Profunda femoris A.

Adductor longus M.

Anterior branch of obturator N.

Gracilis M.

Fig. 2.25 The left femoral triangle.

prominent **saphenous nerve.** The latter nerve will be found on the lateral side of the femoral artery. It is a sensory nerve which, as you will see later, passes down the thigh in close relationship with the artery. It ends by supplying the skin on the medial side of the leg and foot.

The artery which you may see ramifying in the femoral triangle, between the branches of the femoral nerve, is the lateral circumflex femoral artery. It is a branch of the profunda femoris artery, which is one of the main branches of the femoral artery.

The floor of the femoral triangle [Figs 2.25 and 2.33]

Now clean the muscles that form the floor of the femoral triangle, remembering that they lie deeply and that their dis-

section may prove difficult. From the lateral to the medial side the muscles comprise the **iliopsoas,** the **pectineus,** and the **adductor longus.** The part of the iliopsoas which you see is the distal part of two large and conjoined muscles, the **psoas major** and the **iliacus,** both of which arise within the abdomen, the former from the lumbar part of the vertebral column and the latter from the iliac fossa. Although the origin of these two muscles cannot be seen in this dissection, they must be followed to their insertion into the lesser trochanter. The iliopsoas, as has already been pointed out [p. 2.15], is the principal flexor of the hip joint.

The pectineus arises from the superior ramus of the pubis. If you follow the muscle downwards with your fingers you can feel that it is inserted just below the lesser trochanter.

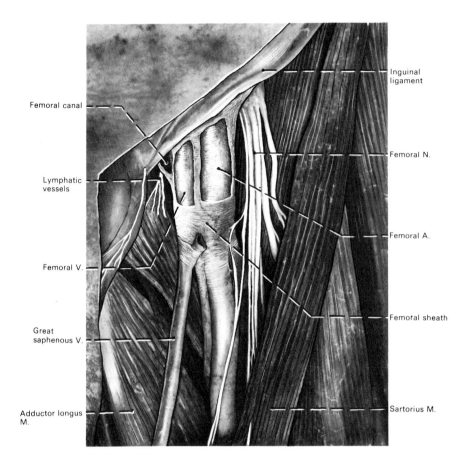

Femoral canal

Lymphatic
vessels

Femoral V.

Great
saphenous V.

Adductor longus
M.

Inguinal
ligament

Femoral N.

Femoral A.

Femoral sheath

Sartorius M.

Fig. 2.26 The left femoral sheath. The three compartments of the sheath have been opened by removing part of the anterior wall.

You should also trace the adductor longus to its insertion in the middle third of the linea aspera. The precise attachments of both these muscles to the femur will be seen more clearly at a later stage of the dissection.

The femoral sheath

Now open the femoral sheath by making vertical incisions into its anterior wall [Fig. 2.26]. Try to confirm that the sheath consists of three compartments. The lateral and middle compartments will be seen to be occupied by the femoral artery and femoral vein respectively. The medial compartment, called the **femoral canal,** is filled with fat and a lymph node, and transmits lymphatic vessels.

Clean the femoral vessels as far as the apex of the femoral triangle. Observe that the superior opening of the femoral canal is oval in shape. It is called the **femoral ring.** Note that its boundaries are anteriorly, the inguinal ligament; posteriorly, the pectineus muscle; medially, a reflected part of the inguinal ligament called the **lacunar ligament,** which passes back from the ligament itself to be attached to the pecten of the pubis; and laterally, the femoral vein. Through this opening a loop of intestine, or a piece of fatty tissue

called omentum, occasionally forms a femoral hernia by passing into the femoral canal from the abdominal cavity. Since the gut may become strangulated if this happens, the boundaries of the femoral ring are of some clinical importance.

Branches of the femoral artery

Look for a vessel behind the femoral canal, crossing the pectineus and the adductor longus on its way to the perineum and genital organs. This vessel is one of the **external pudendal arteries,** which branch from the femoral artery. Find a large artery that springs from the lateral aspect of the femoral artery, and almost immediately gives off two big branches. The large artery is the **profunda femoris,** and its branches the **medial** and **lateral circumflex femoral arteries.** The circumflex vessels are not constant in their origins; they sometimes arise directly from the femoral artery. In addition there are numerous muscular branches.

Trace the profunda femoris artery as it passes out of the femoral triangle deep to the adductor longus. The circumflex arteries pass between the muscles on either side of the femur and their branches join an anastomotic chain of

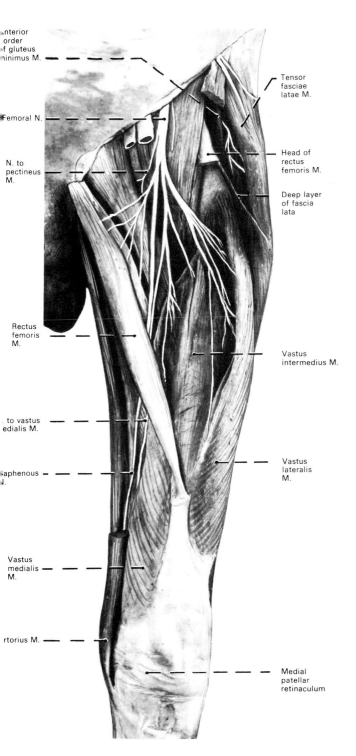

Anterior border of gluteus minimus M.

Femoral N.

N. to pectineus M.

Rectus femoris M.

to vastus medialis M.

Saphenous N.

Vastus medialis M.

Sartorius M.

Tensor fasciae latae M.

Head of rectus femoris M.

Deep layer of fascia lata

Vastus intermedius M.

Vastus lateralis M.

Medial patellar retinaculum

Fig. 2.27 The left quadriceps femoris muscle and the femoral nerve. The rectus femoris muscle has been divided near its origin and turned medially; most of the sartorius muscle has been excised.

vessels which you will see later on the back of the thigh. The veins you come across should be removed in order to display the arteries more clearly.

The quadriceps femoris muscle

You should now clean and study the quadriceps femoris muscle [Fig. 2.27]. The centrally-situated long and flat muscle in the midline of the thigh is the **rectus femoris.** The fibres of this muscle arise from a central tendon, and are arranged in a bipennate way. Cut the muscle transversely through its middle, and turn its upper end back on to its tendinous origin. The latter, as you will see later, consists of a straight head of origin from the anterior inferior iliac spine and a reflected head from a rough area of bone above the acetabulum. Turn the lower end of the muscle aside to see the other parts of the quadriceps femoris. In this way the **vastus intermedius,** which lies behind the rectus femoris, and the **vastus medialis** and **vastus lateralis,** which lie at its sides, will be exposed more fully. These three flat muscles, which you will be able to examine more clearly very shortly, envelop the femur. At this stage identify and clean the branches which pass to them from the femoral nerve.

The branches of the lateral circumflex femoral artery will also now come fully into view, and should be cleaned.

Trace the quadriceps femoris muscle to its insertion. The rectus femoris becomes tendinous and is inserted into the base of the **patella,** which in turn is attached by the **patellar ligament** to the tuberosity of the tibia. The vastus lateralis, medialis, and intermedius are inserted into the tendon of the rectus femoris, and into the borders of the patella. Fibrous expansions from the insertions of these muscles, called the **patellar retinacula,** reinforce the articular capsule of the knee joint on either side, and are attached to the medial and lateral condyles of the tibia. These retinacula should now be defined.

You can easily see from the arrangement of the muscle that the quadriceps femoris is an extensor of the knee joint. Verify this on your own body. Sit on a chair and attempt to straighten one leg while feeling the front of your thigh. You will note the quadriceps hardening as you unbend your knee.

The tensor fasciae latae muscle

Now examine the tensor fasciae latae muscle [Fig. 2.28], which you first encountered when you were dissecting the gluteal muscles. It arises from the tubercle of the iliac crest and the bone immediately in front of it, and forms a flat sheet on the lateral aspect of the superior part of the thigh.

Incise vertically the fascia lata over the anterior margin of the muscle and trace the latter to its insertion into the iliotibial tract. You can now see that the tract splits to enclose the muscle, which is supplied by a branch of the superior gluteal nerve which enters the muscle from behind.

The tensor fasciae latae, as has already been noted

2.25

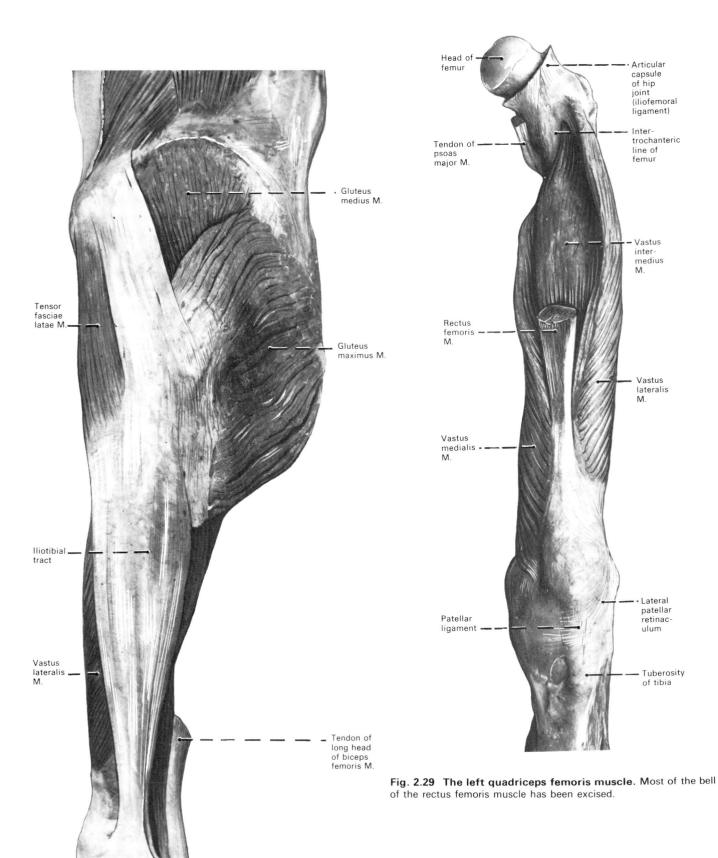

Gluteus
medius M.

Tensor
fasciae
latae M.

Gluteus
maximus M.

Iliotibial
tract

Vastus
lateralis
M.

Tendon of
long head
of biceps
femoris M.

Head of
femur

Articular
capsule
of hip
joint
(iliofemoral
ligament)

Tendon of
psoas
major M.

Inter-
trochanteric
line of
femur

Vastus
inter-
medius
M.

Rectus
femoris
M.

Vastus
lateralis
M.

Vastus
medialis
M.

Lateral
patellar
retinac-
ulum

Patellar
ligament

Tuberosity
of tibia

Fig. 2.29 The left quadriceps femoris muscle. Most of the bell
of the rectus femoris muscle has been excised.

Fig. 2.28 The left iliotibial tract.

[p. 2.15], assists in abduction of the thigh, and also helps the anterior parts of the gluteus medius and minimus to rotate the thigh medially. It also pulls on the fascia lata and so helps to steady the pelvis on the femur, and the femur on the tibia. It therefore plays a part in the maintenance of the erect posture.

The insertions of the gluteal muscles

Again examine the insertion of the gluteus maximus and note that all of its fibres except the deep ones of its distal part pass into the iliotibial tract. In consequence the tensor fasciae latae muscle may influence the action of the gluteus maximus by altering the obliquity of its pull.

Now, from the front, identify the anterior borders of the gluteus medius and the gluteus minimus [Fig. 2.27]. This can be done by dissecting deep to the tensor fasciae latae. Then, by turning the body on to its side as necessary, identify the gluteus medius and gluteus minimus in the buttock. Divide the iliotibial tract and the tensor fasciae latae (including the deep part of the sheath of the muscle, which you will find is attached to the capsule of the hip joint) close to their origins along the iliac crest. Turn the tensor fasciae latae muscle and iliotibial tract downwards and laterally, and as you do so, note the branch from the superior gluteal nerve by which the muscle is supplied [Fig. 2.14].

A good view of the gluteus medius and vastus lateralis is now obtained. Note again that only the anterior parts of the gluteus medius and minimus rotate the thigh medially. Then separate the anterior border of the gluteus medius from the underlying gluteus minimus, and complete the division of the gluteus medius. As you do so, note again that the layer of fascia on the deep aspect of the tensor fasciae latae blends with the capsule of the hip joint.

The vastus muscles

You can now study the full extent of the vastus lateralis. Begin by separating it from the lateral intermuscular septum which is still attached to the fascia lata. You will easily see that the vastus lateralis is the largest muscle of the quadriceps femoris group [Fig. 2.29], and that it has an extensive origin, beginning above in front of the insertion of the gluteus minimus, and extending down the lateral lip of the linea aspera. The vastus medialis has a corresponding origin from the medial lip of the linea aspera, and if you separate it from the vastus intermedius you will see that the latter arises from the front and lateral surfaces of the upper two-thirds of the femur.

The adductor canal [Fig. 2.30]

Examine the adductor canal. It is a continuation of the femoral triangle, and lies beneath the sartorius muscle on the medial aspect of the middle third of the thigh. Its roof and medial wall are formed by a fascial sheet that extends beneath the sartorius between the adductor longus and the

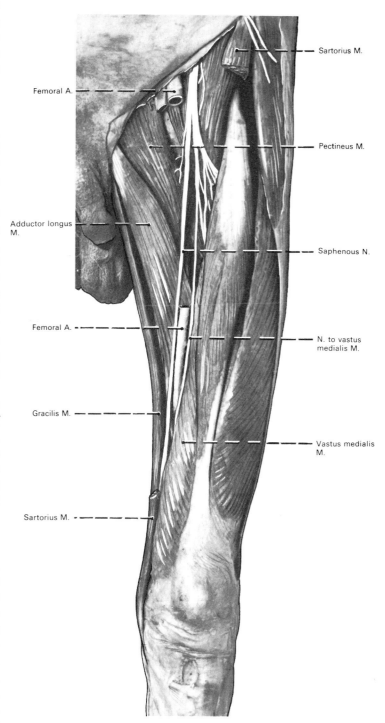

Fig. 2.30 The left adductor canal. Most of the sartorius muscle has been excised.

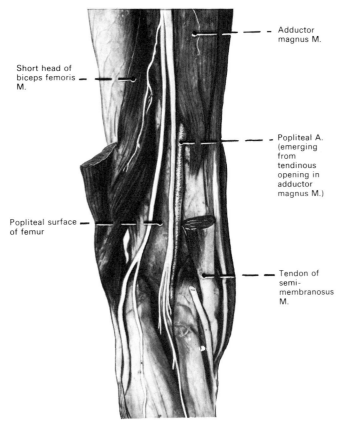

Fig. 2.31 The left adductor magnus muscle and the popliteal artery (posterior view).

adductor magnus medially and the vastus medialis laterally.

Turn the sartorius muscle aside. Open the adductor canal by cutting through the fascia beneath the sartorius, and clean its boundaries and contents. You will see that the canal contains the femoral vessels, the vein lying posterior to the artery in the upper half, and lateral to the artery in the lower.

The nerve that you will now see crossing the vessels superficially from the lateral to the medial side is the saphenous nerve.

Note that the vastus medialis forms the lateral wall of the canal. Find the nerve which passes into this muscle from the femoral nerve; it will be found lying on the muscle. Define the floor of the canal, which is formed by the adductor longus and adductor magnus muscles. The adductor magnus is a large muscle whose upper part lies behind the adductor longus. It forms the lower part of the floor of the adductor canal.

Trace the saphenous nerve as it leaves the canal by passing through the fascial roof. Also trace the femoral vessels as they enter a **tendinous opening in the adductor magnus.** The opening leads into the popliteal fossa, and is shown from behind in Fig. 2.31.

The obturator nerve

The obturator nerve is a branch of the lumbar plexus [Fig. 2.32], and arises in the abdomen from the ventral rami of

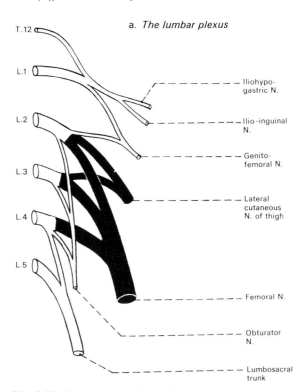

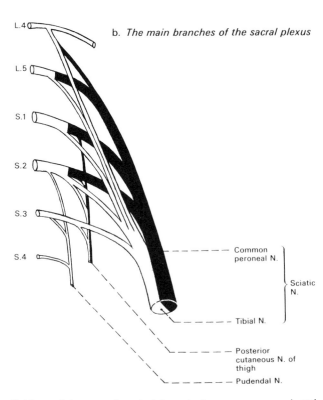

Fig. 2.32 Schemata of the left lumbar and sacral plexuses. The posterior divisions of the ventral rami of the spinal nerves concerned, and their derivatives, are shown black: the corresponding anterior divisions are shown in outline.

the second, third, and fourth lumbar nerves. It passes down the posterior wall of the abdomen and into the pelvis, which it leaves by passing through the upper part of the obturator foramen, within which it divides into an **anterior branch** and a **posterior branch.** As you will see in a moment, the anterior branch passes in front of the obturator externus, before descending in front of the adductor brevis and behind the pectineus and adductor longus muscles.

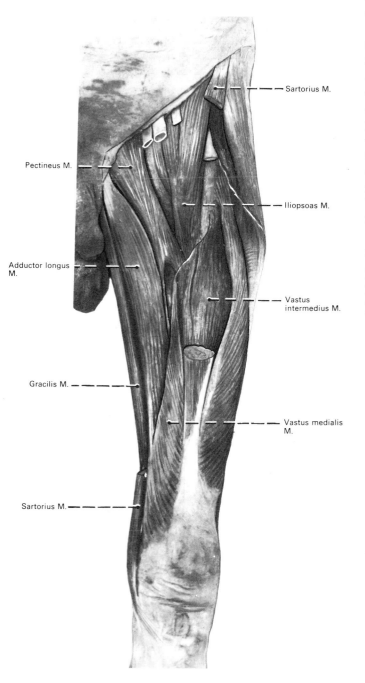

Pectineus M.

Adductor longus M.

Gracilis M.

Sartorius M.

Sartorius M.

Iliopsoas M.

Vastus intermedius M.

Vastus medialis M.

Fig. 2.33 The superficial adductor muscles of the left thigh. The greater parts of the rectus femoris and sartorius muscles have been excised.

Before moving on to the next stage of your dissection, again confirm the fact that the adductor canal connects the femoral triangle with the popliteal fossa through an opening in the insertion of the adductor magnus muscle.

The adductor muscles

Now clean and examine the adductor group of muscles, which lie on the medial aspect of the thigh [Fig. 2.33] Raise the foot of your specimen in order to facilitate your dissection.

First locate the narrow strap-like **gracilis muscle,** if necessary reflecting a further piece of skin. It is the most medial muscle on the anterior aspect of the thigh. Clean the muscle and examine its tendinous origin from the inferior ramus of the pubis and the ramus of the ischium. The muscle tapers as it descends. Note its tendinous insertion into the upper part of the medial surface of the tibia.

Turn your attention to the **adductor longus** and the **pectineus muscles** on the lateral aspect of the gracilis. Again confirm that the adductor longus rises by a rounded tendon from the angle between the pubic crest and pubic symphysis. Note that the pectineus has a fleshy origin from the superior ramus of the pubis.

Divide the adductor longus and pectineus muscles 2 cm from their origins and turn them downwards. Find the anterior branch of the obturator nerve behind the adductor longus and identify the branches it sends to the adductor longus, adductor brevis, gracilis muscles, and occasionally to the pectineus muscle [Fig. 2.34].

You can now confirm that the adductor longus is inserted into the medial lip of the linea aspera. Behind it is the profunda femoris artery.

Clean the **adductor brevis** and note that it is a large muscle which arises from the inferior ramus of the pubis. Cut it 2 cm below its origin and follow it to its insertion into the upper part of the linea aspera behind the pectineus muscle and the upper part of the adductor longus, and in front of the adductor magnus.

Search between the adductor brevis and adductor magnus for the posterior branch of the obturator nerve [Fig. 2.35]. This nerve pierces the obturator externus muscle and comes to lie on the adductor magnus, giving branches to both these muscles. It also gives an articular branch to the knee joint. This branch is, however, seldom found.

Look carefully behind the pectineus muscle. You may find an **accessory obturator nerve,** which is present in about a tenth of all subjects. While the main obturator nerve passes into the thigh through the obturator canal in the obturator foramen, the accessory obturator nerve passes over the superior ramus of the pubis. When present it gives branches to the pectineus and the hip joint.

At this stage of your dissection the medial circumflex femoral artery should be fully displayed.

Clean the **obturator externus muscle** and the anterior sur-

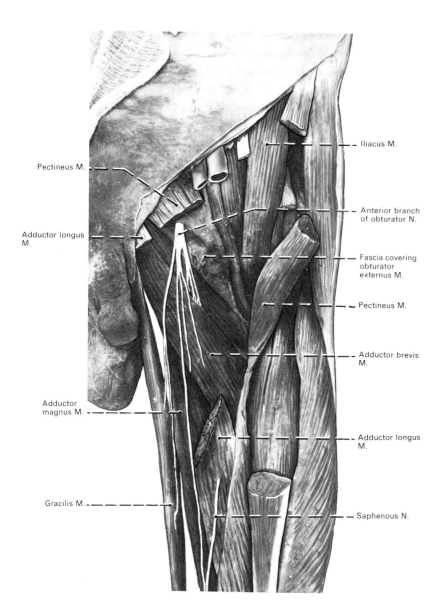

Fig. 2.34 The left adductor brevis muscle and the anterior branch of the obturator nerve. Parts of the rectus femoris, the sartorius, and the adductor longus muscles have been excised; the pectineus muscle has been divided and reflected laterally.

face of the adductor magnus muscle. Note that the obturator externus arises from the obturator membrane and the adjacent bone. The muscle passes behind the neck of the femur, and is inserted into the trochanteric fossa on the medial aspect of the greater trochanter of the femur.

You will now be able to verify that the large **adductor magnus muscle** arises from the side of the pubic arch and the lower part of the ischial tuberosity. Look at its extensive aponeurotic insertion into the gluteal tuberosity, along the linea aspera and the upper part of the medial supracondylar line, ending as a rounded tendon which becomes attached to the adductor tubercle just above the medial epicondyle of the femur. The opening through which the femoral vessels pass is situated between the attachment of the muscle to

the medial supracondylar line and its lower tendinous attachment to the adductor tubercle.

As you can easily deduce from their attachments, the three adductor muscles get their name because they adduct the thigh. Confirm their action on your own body by standing with your feet well apart. Push your fingers into the upper medial aspects of your thighs and try to adduct both limbs. You will feel the adductors contracting powerfully. While still trying to adduct, run your index finger upwards along the taut upper medial border of the adductor longus to its origin. Next move your finger slightly upwards and laterally to feel the pubic tubercle. The latter is an important landmark in the surgery of hernias.

Detach the obturator externus from its origin as much

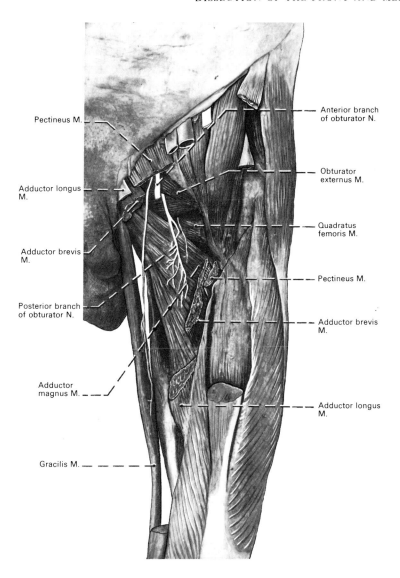

Pectineus M.

Adductor longus
M.

Adductor brevis
M.

Posterior branch
of obturator N.

Adductor
magnus M.

Gracilis M.

Anterior branch
of obturator N.

Obturator
externus M.

Quadratus
femoris M.

Pectineus M.

Adductor brevis
M.

Adductor longus
M.

Fig. 2.35 The left adductor magnus muscle and the posterior branch of the obturator nerve. The greater parts of the rectus femoris, sartorius, pectineus, adductor longus, and adductor brevis muscles have been excised.

as is necessary to display the obturator artery and obturator nerve emerging through the obturator canal.

Finally, cut the iliopsoas muscle near its insertion into the lesser trochanter, and lift it up in order to determine the position of the important **iliopectineal bursa** which lies between the psoas major muscle and the hip joint, with which the bursa usually communicates. At this stage the anterior aspect of the capsule of the hip joint is fully exposed.

Before doing anything further, again examine the profunda femoris artery and its branches.

Section 2.3

The back of the thigh and the popliteal fossa

Turn the body on to its face in order to dissect the posterior compartment of the thigh. This contains the hamstring group of muscles, which comprises the biceps femoris, semitendinosus, semimembranosus, and the hamstring part of the adductor magnus (the part that is inserted into the adductor tubercle). The skin in this region is innervated almost entirely by the posterior cutaneous nerve of the thigh, which you saw when you dissected the gluteal region. The sciatic nerve follows a vertical course beneath the biceps femoris muscle, before dividing in the lower third of the thigh into its two terminal branches, the tibial nerve and the common peroneal nerve. The division may take place higher up, even in the gluteal region. It is best to begin the dissection of this region by exploring the popliteal fossa, which lies behind the knee joint. Here you will find the tibial and common peroneal nerves, the popliteal vein, the popliteal artery, and perhaps some lymph nodes embedded in fat.

Osteology

Look again at a hip-bone and a femur. You have already dissected the origin of the hamstring muscles from the ischial tuberosity. The precise attachments of these muscles to this portion of the hip-bone should be verified once more [pp. 2.11–2.12]. At the same time, re-examine the extensive origin of the adductor magnus from the conjoined rami of the ischium and pubis. The biceps femoris, as its name suggests, has a second head. This arises from the lateral lip of the linea aspera just below the gluteal tuberosity.

Note again that the main insertion of the adductor magnus muscle is into the linea aspera, between its medial and lateral lips. The part that is inserted into the adductor tubercle above the medial epicondyle is related, as already observed, to the group of hamstring muscles. Notice that just below the division of the linea aspera into the medial and lateral supracondylar lines, the popliteal surface of the bone is smooth [Fig. 2.18b]. It is here that the femoral vessels descend into the popliteal fossa through the tendinous opening in the adductor magnus muscle.

Surface anatomy

The tendon of the biceps femoris can be felt without difficulty on the lateral aspect of the back of your knee [Fig. 2.36]. Trace it as it passes to its insertion into the head of the fibula. On the medial aspect of this tendon it is possible to feel the common peroneal nerve, which can also be felt as it winds round the fibula to enter the substance of a muscle, called the peroneus longus, in the lateral part of the leg. The nerve can be rolled between your finger and the bone immediately below the head of the fibula.

On the medial aspect of the popliteal fossa you can feel two tendons. The more superficial one is the tendon of the semitendinosus muscle. This will be found to lie on the broader tendon of the semimembranosus muscle.

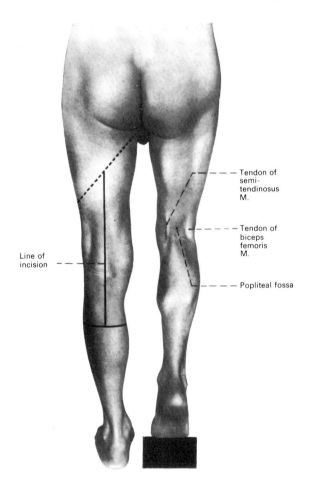

Line of incision

Tendon of semi-tendinosus M.

Tendon of biceps femoris M.

Popliteal fossa

Fig. 2.36 The posterior aspect of the lower limbs. The right knee is partly flexed to show the popliteal fossa; the skin incisions are marked on the left side.

Reflection of the skin

Begin the dissection of the posterior aspect of the thigh by making the following incisions through the skin [Fig. 2.36]:

1. A vertical incision through the centre of this region, extending down to a point 15 cm below the knee.
2. A transverse incision at the lower end of the above vertical incision.
3. An incision continuing the one you have already made around the external genitalia until it reaches the medial edge of the ischial tuberosity.

Then turn aside the flaps of skin.

Dissection of the back of the thigh and the popliteal fossa

The cutaneous nerves and vessels

In the superficial fascia below the knee you will find the centrally-situated **posterior cutaneous nerve of the thigh,** whose course in the gluteal region you have already examined. This nerve sends many branches, some of which may already have been cut, through the deep fascia into the superficial fascia of the thigh [Fig. 2.37]. Medially you will also come across the **saphenous nerve,** and on the lateral aspect of the popliteal fossa you may find the **lateral cutaneous nerve of the calf** piercing the deep fascia.

Identify a vein in the midline of the superficial fascia on the posterior aspect of the leg. It is the **small saphenous vein.** Then clean the deep fascia, noting again the position of the cutaneous nerves and vessels you have encountered.

Cut vertically through the deep fascia in the midline, and then make a transverse incision through it at the level of the transverse skin incision. Carefully turn the fascia aside.

On the lateral side look for a layer of fascia passing deeply from the fascia lata between the quadriceps and hamstring muscles. This is the **lateral intermuscular septum.** It is attached to the whole length of the linea aspera and also to its superior and inferior prolongations.

Follow and clean the insertions of the gracilis, sartorius, and semitendinosus muscles into the medial aspect of the upper part of the shaft of the tibia [Fig. 2.38], and note that they are also inserted into the deep fascia, and that the sartorius, which is the most anterior, has a more extensive attachment to the bone than the other two. The muscle that is inserted immediately posterior to the gracilis is the semitendinosus.

The boundaries of the popliteal fossa

Now clean and define the muscular boundaries of the diamond-shaped popliteal fossa [Fig. 2.39]. First dissect the tendon of the **semitendinosus.** You will see that it forms the supero-medial boundary, and that it lies superficially in the grooved surface of another muscle, the **semimembranosus.**

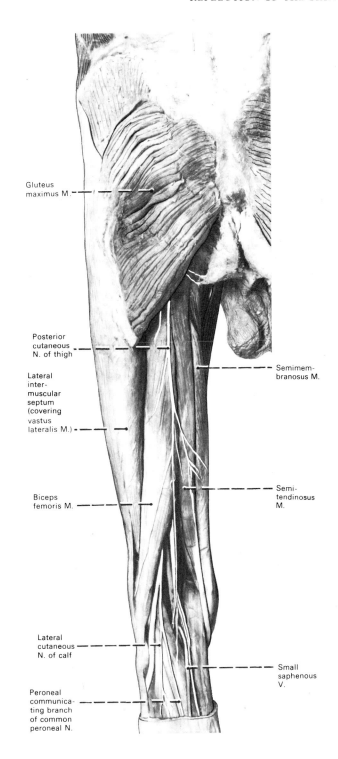

Fig. 2.37 The posterior cutaneous nerve of the thigh and the left hamstring muscles.

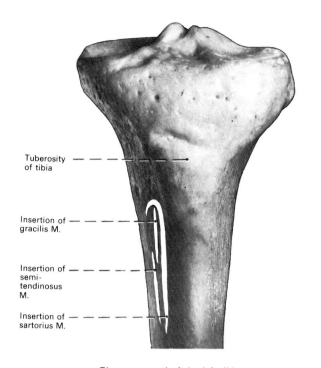

Tuberosity
of tibia

Insertion of
gracilis M.

Insertion of
semi-
tendinosus
M.

Insertion of
sartorius M.

a. The upper end of the left tibia

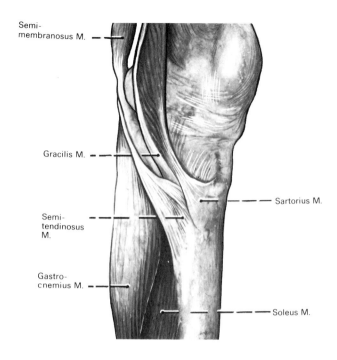

Semi-
membranosus M.

Gracilis M.

Semi-
tendinosus
M.

Gastro-
cnemius M.

Sartorius M.

Soleus M.

*b. The medial aspect of the knee and
upper end of the left leg*

Fig. 2.38 The insertions of the left semitendinosus, gracilis, and sartorius muscles.

The muscle forming the supero-lateral boundary of the fossa is the **biceps femoris.** It should be cleaned and followed to its insertion into the head of the fibula and the adjacent part of the lateral condyle of the tibia. You will see that at its insertion the tendon of the biceps femoris wraps round a cord-like ligament which is also attached to the head of the fibula. This is the fibular collateral ligament of the knee joint.

Define the lower boundaries of the popliteal fossa. These are formed by the **medial head** and the **lateral head** of origin of a large superficial muscle of the calf called the **gastro-cnemius.** The two heads of this muscle, which you must now clean, arise from the medial and lateral condyles of the femur. Note that some fibres at the medial margin of the lateral head can be separated from the main mass of the gastrocnemius. They constitute a small vestigial muscle called the **plantaris** [Fig. 2.40]. Occasionally this muscle may not be present.

The common peroneal nerve

Now dissect the contents of the popliteal fossa, removing the considerable amount of fat it contains. The nerve on the medial side of the tendon of the biceps, which you will recall can be felt easily on your own leg [p. 2.32], is the common peroneal nerve. Clean it and trace it inferiorly as it winds round the fibula just below its head, where the nerve becomes superficial. This nerve gives off four branches in

the popliteal fossa. The first two are small and will be found in the upper part of the fossa; they supply the knee joint. If they do not spring immediately into view, do not spend time searching for them. A little lower down you will find two bigger branches, which may come off together. They are the **lateral cutaneous nerve of the calf** and the **peroneal communicating branch** [Fig. 2.39]. Without spending too much time on the task, trace them downwards as far as you can within the present field of dissection. The lateral cutaneous nerve of the calf supplies the skin of the anterior, posterior, and lateral surfaces of the proximal part of the leg, whilst the peroneal communicating branch, as you may see later, usually joins the medial cutaneous nerve of the calf, a branch of the tibial nerve, in the middle of the leg, to form the sural nerve.

The tibial nerve [Fig. 2.39]

Now find the tibial nerve. It occupies a central and relatively superficial position in the popliteal fossa. Trace its branches. It gives off the **medial cutaneous nerve of the calf,** which will be found as it descends superficially between the two heads of the gastrocnemius, and also three articular branches to the knee joint, which you may have difficulty in finding; do not spend time searching for them. The medial cutaneous nerve of the calf, which is joined by the peroneal communicating branch of the common peroneal nerve to form the sural nerve, supplies the skin of the lateral and posterior

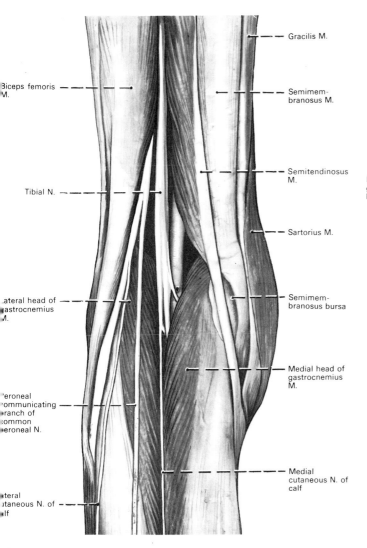

Gracilis M.

Biceps femoris M.

Semimem- branosus M.

Semitendinosus M.

Tibial N.

Sartorius M.

Semimem- branosus bursa

Lateral head of gastrocnemius M.

Medial head of gastrocnemius M.

Peroneal communicating branch of common peroneal N.

Medial cutaneous N. of calf

Lateral cutaneous N. of calf

Fig. 2.39 The boundaries of the left popliteal fossa.

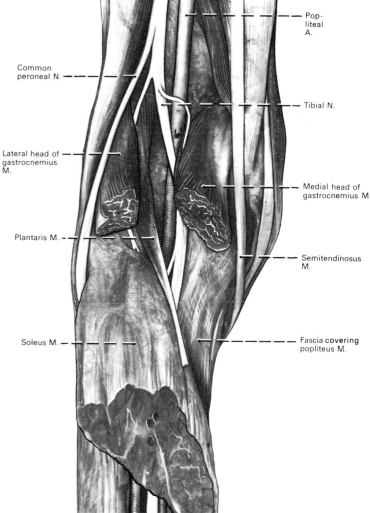

Pop- liteal A.

Common peroneal N.

Tibial N.

Lateral head of gastrocnemius M.

Medial head of gastrocnemius M.

Plantaris M.

Semitendinosus M.

Soleus M.

Fascia covering popliteus M.

Fig. 2.40 The left popliteal fossa. The distal parts of the gastro- cnemius, plantaris, and soleus muscles have been excised.

surfaces of the lower third of the leg. The sural nerve supplies the skin of the lateral side of the foot.

Trace the muscular branches of the tibial nerve to the gastrocnemius, the soleus (a large muscle of the calf lying deep to the gastrocnemius), and the plantaris muscle [Fig. 2.40]. The tibial nerve, as you will see later, also supplies the popliteus muscle.

The popliteal vein

Deep to the tibial nerve find the popliteal vein running upwards and a little medially. The popliteal vein becomes the **femoral vein** when it passes into the anterior part of the thigh through the tendinous opening in the adductor magnus muscle. Pick up and define the **small saphenous vein,** which you saw at the start of your dissection of the popliteal fossa. This vein drains the superficial structures on the pos-

tero-lateral aspect of the foot and leg, and as you can now see, passes into the popliteal vein. The other tributaries of the popliteal vein should be removed in order to obtain a freer view of the popliteal fossa.

You will have noticed already that the fossa contains a large quantity of fat. This makes it difficult to locate the lymph nodes which are situated in this region; do not spend time on their dissection.

The popliteal artery [Fig. 2.40]

Deep to the popliteal vein you will find the popliteal artery. Clean it and trace it upwards to the point where it appears through the tendinous opening in the adductor magnus muscle, and where it becomes the continuation of the **femoral artery.**

The popliteal artery gives off a series of small branches

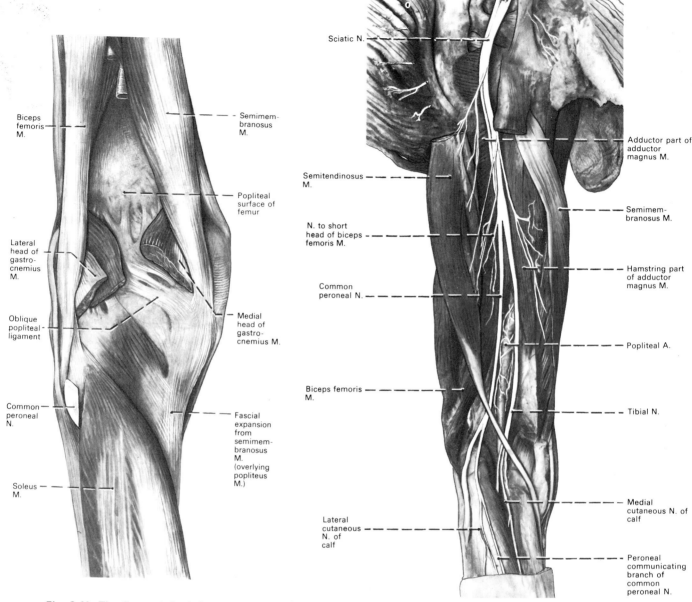

Fig. 2.41 The floor of the left popliteal fossa.

Fig. 2.42 The left sciatic nerve and its branches. The semi-tendinosus muscle and the long head of the biceps femoris muscle have been divided below their origin and displaced laterally; the semi-membranosus muscle has been displaced medially.

to adjacent muscles and to the knee joint, all of which can be sacrificed in order to expose the floor of the popliteal fossa fully. When these small obstructions have been cleared away, separate the muscles that bound the fossa as widely as possible and examine its floor. This will be made easier if, in addition to separating the two heads of the gastro-cnemius from each other, they are also separated from the underlying soleus muscle.

The floor of the popliteal fossa

The floor of the popliteal fossa [Fig. 2.41] will be seen to

comprise, from above down, the popliteal surface of the femur, the articular capsule of the knee joint (this is streng-thened by a fascial expansion, called the **oblique popliteal ligament,** which springs from the insertion of the semi-membranosus muscle), and the fascia covering a small flat triangular muscle. This is the **popliteus muscle.** The fascia covering the muscle is also reinforced by tendinous fibres from the insertion of the semimembranosus muscle. You can see that the popliteus is attached to the back of the upper part of the tibia. You will study it more fully at a later stage of your dissection.

Now clean the popliteal artery [Fig. 2.40] and follow it from its origin at the tendinous opening in the adductor magnus to its termination at the lower border of the popliteus muscle, where it divides into the anterior and posterior tibial arteries. The division cannot be seen at this stage.

The hamstring muscles

Extend the area of your dissection upwards, and clean the hamstring muscles as far upwards as their origins. Note again that the **semimembranosus, semitendinosus,** and the **long head of the biceps femoris muscle** arise from the ischial tuberosity, and that the origin of the semimembranosus is above and lateral to that of the other two muscles [Fig. 2.43]. You will see that the biceps femoris is reinforced by a sheet of muscle fibres which arise from the linea aspera of the femur and the lateral supracondylar line. This is the **short head of the biceps femoris muscle.** Trace the tendon of the biceps femoris to the head of the fibula, and the semitendinosus tendon to the upper part of the medial surface of the tibia, where you have already noted its relation to the insertion of the gracilis and sartorius muscles [p. 2.33]. You will find that the semimembranosus muscle is inserted into a groove and into the adjacent bone on the back of the medial condyle of the tibia. At this stage of your dissection you should not try to define the various fascial expansions which may be seen extending from the insertion of the semimembranosus muscle.

The hamstring muscles extend the hip joint and flex the knee joint. You should verify this on your own body. Feeling the back of your thigh as you walk around, note that the hamstring muscles contract when the hip joint is extended. Sit on a chair with one leg forward, then try to flex the knee against resistance. As you feel the back of the thigh, note that the hamstring muscles are firm and contracted. Note also that when you flex both your knee and hip joints you may be able to make the anterior surface of your thigh touch your anterior abdominal wall. On the other hand, when you extend the knee, you can only partially flex the hip. This is because the extended hamstring muscles prevent full flexion of the hip joint.

The sciatic nerve

Turn the hamstring muscles aside and clean the remainder of the sciatic nerve [Fig. 2.42]. Trace the branches it sends to the semitendinosus, semimembranosus, the long head of the biceps, and the adductor magnus muscles. (Remember that the main part of the adductor magnus muscle is supplied by the posterior branch of the obturator nerve.) All these branches arise from the **tibial division of the sciatic nerve,** and will be seen to emerge from the medial side of the sciatic nerve. Find the nerve to the short head of the biceps femoris as it emerges from the lateral side of the sciatic nerve. It is a branch of the **common peroneal division**

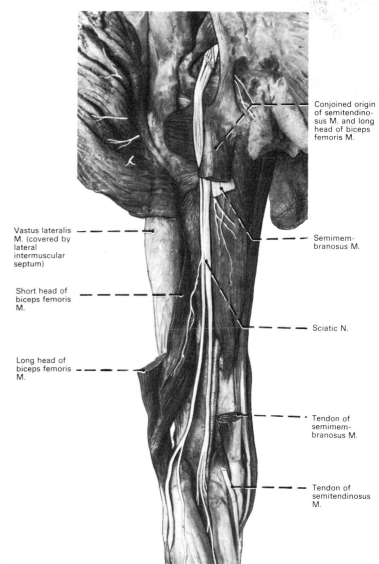

Labels on figure:
- Conjoined origin of semitendinosus M. and long head of biceps femoris M.
- Vastus lateralis M. (covered by lateral intermuscular septum)
- Short head of biceps femoris M.
- Long head of biceps femoris M.
- Semimembranosus M.
- Sciatic N.
- Tendon of semimembranosus M.
- Tendon of semitendinosus M.

Fig. 2.43 The short head of the left biceps femoris muscle. The bellies of the semitendinosus and semimembranosus muscles have been excised, together with the greater part of the long head of the biceps femoris muscle.

of the sciatic nerve. As already noted, the sciatic nerve may divide into its two main divisions at any level of the thigh.

Divide the hamstring muscles about 5 cm below their origins from the ischial tuberosity, and turn them aside. The adductor magnus with its adductor and hamstring portions will now be fully exposed. Again confirm the origin of the muscle from the conjoined rami of the pubis and ischium, and from the ischial tuberosity. Also follow the extensive insertion of the muscle from the gluteal tuberosity of the femur above to the adductor tubercle below.

2.37

The perforating arteries

Note that the adductor magnus is pierced, very close to its insertion, by four small arteries that are given off in the front of the thigh. These are the perforating arteries which spring from the **profunda femoris artery.** These perforating arteries wind round the back of the femur and end in the vastus lateralis muscle, giving branches to the muscles of the thigh and anastomosing with one another.

The first perforating artery also takes part in an anastomosis which is formed by the transverse branches of the medial and lateral circumflex femoral arteries, and by a branch from the inferior gluteal artery. This anastomosis, being in the form of a cross, is called the **cruciate anastomosis** [p. 2.14]. Unless you see it immediately, do not spend time in trying to define the anastomosis. As the four perforating arteries anastomose with one another, and since the fourth perforating artery also anastomoses with branches of the

popliteal artery, they provide an important alternative route by which the lower limb could receive its blood supply if the femoral artery were obstructed by disease or trauma, say in the lower part of the femoral triangle.

Again examine the large opening in the adductor magnus muscle through which the femoral vessels pass into the popliteal space.

Bursae around the knee joint

As the hamstring muscles are traced to their insertions, some bursae may come into view between their tendons. At this stage note especially the **semimembranosus bursa** between the medial head of the gastrocnemius and the semi-membranosus muscle [Fig. 2.39]. Try to establish whether the bursa communicates with the synovial cavity of the knee joint.

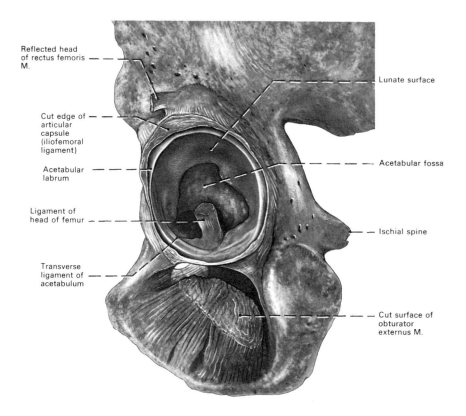

Reflected head
of rectus femoris
M.

Cut edge of
articular
capsule
(iliofemoral
ligament)

Acetabular
labrum

Ligament of
head of femur

Transverse
ligament of
acetabulum

Lunate surface

Acetabular fossa

Ischial spine

Cut surface of
obturator
externus M.

Fig. 2.44 The left acetabulum.

Section 2.4
The hip joint

You should now dissect the hip joint. To make your task easier, it is useful to get a general picture of the joint before you start, with a femur and the hip-bone by your side for reference.

Osteology

The joint is an articulation between the hemispherical **head of the femur** and the cup-shaped **acetabulum** on the hip-bone [Fig. 2.44]. It is a synovial ball-and-socket joint. The **acetabular notch** at the lower part of the acetabulum is bridged by the transverse ligament of the acetabulum, and to the rim of the acetabulum is firmly attached a fibrocartilaginous

ring, the acetabular labrum, which deepens the acetabulum and clasps the head of the femur. Visualize these facts as you examine a hip-bone and a femur.

On the hip-bone the articular capsule is attached to the margin of the acetabulum outside the labrum, and to the transverse ligament. On the femur the capsule is attached anteriorly to the **intertrochanteric line** [Fig. 2.45]; above to the medial aspect of the base of the **greater trochanter**; posteriorly to the **neck of the femur** 1.5 cm medial to the **intertrochanteric crest**; and below to the base of the **lesser trochanter.** Articulate the femur with the hip-bone, and try to visualize the attachments of the capsule to these bones. The precise attachment of the capsule to the femur is especially important.

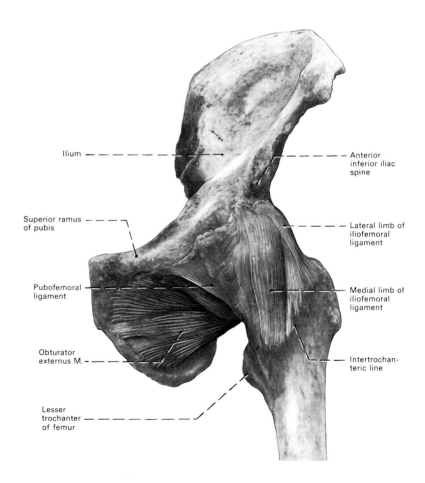

Fig. 2.45 The anterior aspect of the left hip joint. The iliopectineal bursa did not communicate with the joint.

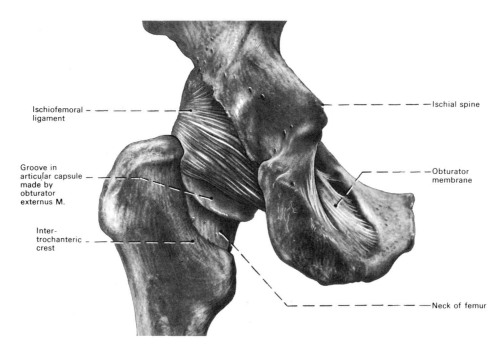

Fig. 2.46 The posterior aspect of the left hip joint.

The capsule is reinforced in front by a powerful ilio-femoral ligament [Fig. 2.45]. This is a triangular ligament, with its apex attached to the lower part of the **anterior inferior iliac spine,** between the two heads of the rectus femoris muscle. As the ligament descends it divides into two bands. One passes to the upper and the other to the lower part of the intertrochanteric line of the femur. The medial band blends with another triangular ligament, called the pubofemoral ligament. The pubofemoral ligament also strengthens the capsule. Its base is attached to the **superior ramus of the pubis,** while its apex is attached to the lesser trochanter of the femur. Posteriorly the capsule is strength-ened by a band called the ischiofemoral ligament [Fig. 2.46]. This is attached to the **body of the ischium** near the acetabu-lar margin, and sweeps upwards and laterally over the back of the neck of the femur in a spiral manner. There is usually a gap in the capsule between the pubofemoral and ilio-femoral ligaments through which a pouch of synovial mem-brane herniates to form the iliopectineal bursa.

Dissection of the hip joint

Turn the body on its back and cut through the femoral vessels and nerve just below the inguinal ligament and tie them together. Divide the sartorius and gracilis muscles close to their origins from the hip-bone, and then divide the adductor part of the adductor magnus muscle close to the rami of the ischium and pubis. At this stage the obturator externus muscle is displayed fully [Fig. 2.45], and you should take this opportunity to re-examine its origin from the obturator membrane and the adjacent bone, and its inser-tion into the trochanteric fossa on the medial aspect of the greater trochanter. Cut the obturator nerve and then divide the obturator externus muscle near its middle. Re-examine the origin of the rectus femoris muscle from the anterior inferior iliac spine and from the rough area of bone above the acetabulum, for both heads are now displayed fully.

The anterior aspect of the hip joint

The **articular capsule** of the hip joint should now be exam-ined from the front [Fig. 2.45]. First, note its attachment to the intertrochanteric line and to the bases of the greater and lesser trochanters. Then define the **iliofemoral ligament.** Note that its apex is attached to the ilium between the two heads of the rectus femoris muscle. Define the two limbs of the ligament, one passing to the base of the greater tro-chanter and the other to the base of the lesser trochanter. Dissect one of the limbs of the ligament away from the capsule and note its thickness.

Then expose the **pubofemoral ligament** on the infero-medial aspect of the capsule. Clean the ligament and follow it to its attachment to the base of the lesser tro-chanter, and examine its wide attachment to the superior ramus of the pubis just above the obturator foramen.

Note the **iliopectineal bursa** between the iliofemoral and pubofemoral ligaments.

The posterior aspect of the hip joint [Fig. 2.46]

Turn the body over, and divide the gluteus minimus trans-versely across its middle. Turn the two parts aside and con-firm that the muscle arises from the ilium between the anterior gluteal line and the inferior gluteal line; also note again its insertion into the anterior surface of the greater trochanter of the femur, in front of the oblique line.

The glistening fibrous tissue beneath the gluteus minimus muscle is the upper part of the capsule of the hip joint.

Cut through the sciatic nerve close to the point where it enters the buttock from under the piriformis muscle, and divide the hamstring part of the adductor magnus muscle close to its origin from the ischial tuberosity. Take this further opportunity to confirm the insertions of the gluteus medius and gluteus minimus muscles into the greater trochanter. Note again that the gluteus minimus lies in front of the gluteus medius [Fig. 2.17].

Now examine the back of the capsule of the hip joint and clean it sufficiently to define the fibres of the **ischiofemoral ligament** as they sweep over the neck of the femur [Fig. 2.46]. Note particularly the loose attachment of the capsule to the neck of the femur posteriorly, and confirm that it does not extend as far as the intertrochanteric crest. The head of the femur receives its blood supply from small vessels which reach it by running up the neck of the bone after passing under the attachment of the capsule.

The interior of the hip joint [Fig. 2.44]

Cut through the capsule of the hip joint just beyond the margin of the acetabulum, and lever the head of the femur out of its socket. You will feel the grip the **acetabular labrum** has on the bone. As you do this you will find that a ligament attaches the head of the femur to the acetabulum. This ligament is the **ligament of the head of the femur** [Fig. 2.44]. Note that the ligament is attached to a small pit, the **fovea capitis femoris,** on the head of the femur, to the margin of the acetabular notch on the hip-bone, and to the **transverse ligament of the acetabulum.** It lies within the joint and is ensheathed by **synovial membrane.**

Cut the ligament of the head near its femoral attachment.

The lower limb should then be completely detached from the body.

Examine the acetabular labrum and the transverse ligament, both of which serve to deepen the cup-shaped acetabulum. You will see that the transverse ligament is continous with the labrum, and that it is attached to the margin of the acetabular notch, converting it into a tunnel through which blood vessels and nerves supply the joint. Look at the smooth **lunate surface** of the articular part of the acetabulum, and at the deep central **acetabular fossa,** which is filled with fat.

You may not be able to make out the following points clearly, but note that the synovial membrane lines the capsule, and that it covers both surfaces of the acetabular labrum and also the fat which lies in the acetabular fossa. It also ensheathes the ligament of the head of the femur and herniates to form the iliopectineal bursa.

The movements of the hip joint

The movements which take place at the hip joint are flexion, mainly due to contraction of the iliopsoas muscle; extension, chiefly by the gluteus maximus muscle; abduction, by the gluteus medius and minimus muscles; adduction, by the adductor muscles; lateral rotation, by the gluteus maximus, quadratus femoris, piriformis, obturator internus, gemelli, and obturator externus muscles; and medial rotation, chiefly by the anterior part of the gluteus minimus and medius, and tensor fasciae latae muscles.

Note that the hip joint is innervated by branches from the femoral, obturator, and sciatic nerves, by the nerve to the quadratus femoris and also by branches which it receives directly from the sacral plexus.

From now on you will be concerned with the dissection of the detached limb. Before you start, take a further opportunity of studying the numerous muscles that are attached to the upper part of the femur.

Section 2.5

The leg and the foot

In the articulated skeleton the space in the leg between the massive tibia and the slender fibula is bridged by a ligamentous sheet called the interosseous membrane of the leg, which corresponds to the similarly-named membrane which joins the radius and ulna in the forearm [p. 1.41].

Look at the extensive **medial surface of the tibia** (the shin). If you feel your own leg you will appreciate that this surface is subcutaneous, and that the fleshy part of the leg lies lateral to, and behind it. As you will see later, the non-osseous parts of the leg are enveloped by a sheath of deep fascia which is attached both to the anterior border and to the sharp medial border of the tibia.

Now look at the sharp **anterior border of the fibula.** An intermuscular fascial septum connects it to the sheet of fascia which envelops the leg [Fig. 2.47]. Another fascial septum is attached to the smoother and somewhat twisted posterior border of the bone. In this way the leg becomes subdivided into anterior, lateral, and posterior compartments [Fig. 2.49].

The anterior compartment contains the muscles which move the foot upwards at the ankle joint (a movement called dorsiflexion as opposed to the opposite movement of plantar-flexion). These muscles also extend the toes. The anterior compartment also contains the anterior tibial artery (a terminal branch of the popliteal artery) and the deep peroneal nerve (a terminal branch of the common peroneal nerve). The lateral compartment contains two muscles which evert the foot (that is to say, twist the foot so that its lateral border is pulled from the floor), and also the superficial peroneal nerve (the other terminal branch of the common peroneal nerve) which supplies them. The muscles which fill the posterior compartment are the plantar-flexors of the ankle joint and the flexors of the toes.

All of these muscles become tendinous near the ankle, and are inserted into the bones of the foot. In the ankle region their tendons are bound down by thickened bands of deep fascia called retinacula.

Osteology

The tibia

The general features of the upper ends of the tibia and fibula have already been described [pp. 2.17–2.19]. Examine the two bones again, and note these further points about the tibia [Fig. 2.48]. The sharp anterior border of the bone becomes rounded where it passes into the **tuberosity** below the con-

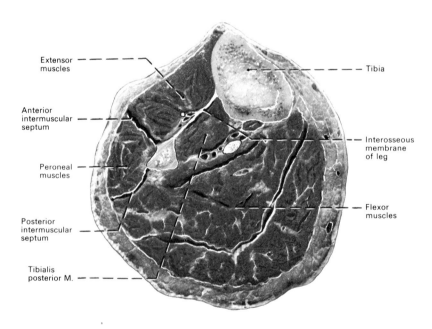

Fig. 2.47 The upper part of the left leg (transverse section; viewed from above).

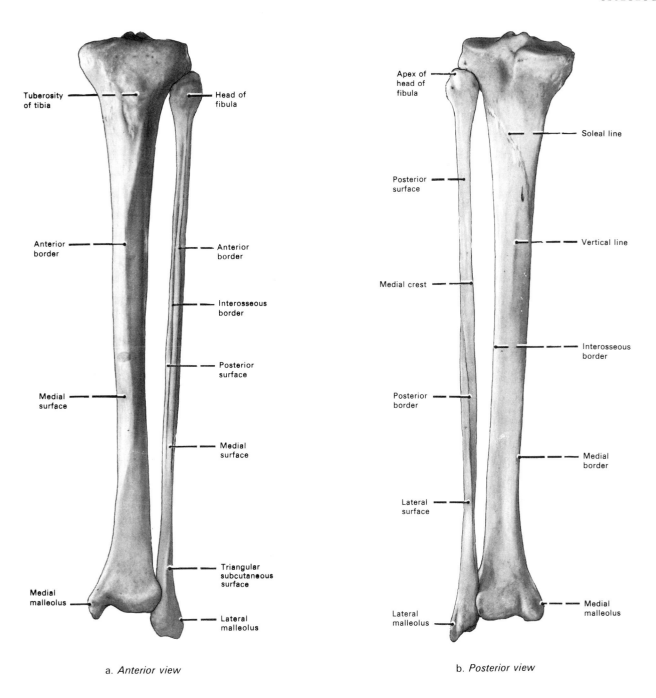

a. *Anterior view*

b. *Posterior view*

Fig. 2.48 The left tibia and fibula.

dyles. On the upper part of the posterior surface is a ridge called the **soleal line**, which passes obliquely from behind the lateral condyle to the upper part of the medial border of the bone. The popliteus muscle is attached to the triangular area above the line, and from the line the soleus muscle, which you have already noted deep to the gastrocnemius, takes origin [p. 2.35]. From the midpoint of the soleal line an indistinct **vertical line** descends to divide the posterior

surface of the shaft into two areas. There is usually a large nutrient foramen close to this ridge.

At its distal end the tibia articulates with the fibula and with the talus, which is one of the main bones of the foot. Note that the distal end of the tibia is prolonged downwards to form a bony prominence on the medial side of the ankle joint, called the **medial malleolus.** Also note a large groove on the posterior surface of the medial malleolus.

2.43

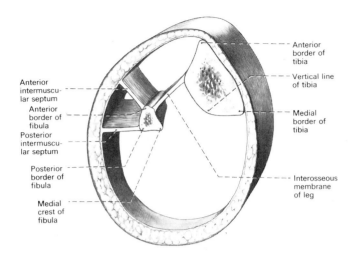

Fig. 2.49 The fascial septa of the left leg (schematic transverse section; viewed from above).

The fibula [Fig. 2.48]

Now turn to the fibula, and look again at the way the proximal end, or **head** of the fibula, articulates with a fibular articular facet on the posterior surface of the lateral condyle of the tibia, and once more note the prominent **apex of the head** of the bone.

The lower end of the fibula is flattish and triangular, and forms the prominence on the lateral side of the ankle joint called the **lateral malleolus.**

On the medial aspect of the lateral malleolus is a smooth **malleolar articular surface,** and immediately behind this a deep **lateral malleolar fossa.**

Examine the two ends of the fibula carefully. Note again that the distal extremity is somewhat flatter than the enlarged proximal end; and that the articular surface on its medial surface is bigger than that on the proximal end, and that it faces more medially. Taken together, all these features allow you to tell which is the proximal and which the distal end of the bone, and to which side the bone belongs.

Now look at the shaft of the fibula. It has three borders and a crest which bound four surfaces. Articulate the bone with the tibia and try and define the anterior, interosseous, and posterior borders, and the **medial crest** [Figs 2.48 and 2.49] (their exact disposition varies greatly from bone to bone).

The anterior border is sharp, and below splits to enclose a triangular area of bone above the lateral malleolus. This area is subcutaneous. A variable distance behind the anterior border you will see, on the medial surface of the shaft, the **interosseous border** to which the interosseous membrane is attached. Between these two borders is the narrow medial surface of the bone.

Posterior to the interosseous border, and running into it below, is the medial crest of the bone. The posterior border

is fairly sharp, and passes from the region of the apex of the head of the fibula above, to the posterior surface of the distal end of the bone. The lateral surface of the fibula lies between the anterior and posterior borders. The posterior surface of the bone lies between the interosseous and posterior borders, and is divided into two parts by the medial crest.

Look at the lateral malleolus on an articulated specimen of the lower limb, and note that it forms a joint with the lateral surface of the talus.

Although you will be doing this again later in your dissection, you will find it useful to study Figs 2.47 and 2.49 at this stage, so that you can get an idea of the way the borders and surfaces of the tibia and fibula, and the intermuscular septa attached to them, divide the leg into separate anatomical compartments.

Now turn to the bones of the foot, which to some extent correspond with those of the hand. Examine them both in an articulated foot [Fig. 2.50] and also separately in so far as you find this necessary.

The tarsal bones

The tarsal bones comprise the calcaneum or heel-bone, the talus or ankle-bone, and five other bones named the navicular bone, the cuboid bone, and the three cuneiform bones.

The calcaneum

First examine the calcaneum [Fig. 2.51]. It is the relatively big bone which forms the heel, and which articulates above with the talus, and in front with a smaller bone called the cuboid.

The posterior surface of the calcaneum forms the prominence of the heel. You will see a transverse ridge on this surface. The smooth area above the ridge is in contact with a bursa which separates the bone from the tendon of the heel (tendo calcaneus), which becomes attached to the ridge. On the lateral surface of the calcaneum, near its anterior end, you will see a projection. This is the **peroneal trochlea,** which can often be felt in the living body. It separates the tendons of the two muscles (the peroneus longus and the peroneus brevis) which are found in the lateral compartment of the leg as they pass to the foot.

The medial surface of the calcaneum presents a well-marked shelf of bone, known as the **sustentaculum tali,** on which part of the talus lies. The superior surface of the calcaneum is largely articular, but note the rough area on its antero-lateral aspect. From it arises the small extensor muscle of the toes (extensor digitorum brevis). This is the only muscle that arises from the dorsum of the foot.

Examine the three articular facets on the upper surface of the calcaneum. All are for the talus, and the posterior one is separated from the others by a groove, called the **groove of the calcaneum.** On the inferior, or plantar, surface look for **medial** and **lateral processes of the tuberosity of the**

calcaneum at the junction of the posterior and plantar surfaces, and for a prominence in the midline anteriorly (the **anterior tubercle**).

The talus [Fig. 2.52]

You will see that the talus articulates with the tibia both above and medially, and with the fibula laterally. Below it articulates with the calcaneum and with a strong and important ligament called the plantar calcaneonavicular ligament, which connects the sustentaculum tali with the plantar surface of the navicular bone. Anteriorly the talus articulates with the navicular bone.

Define the **head, neck** and **body** of the talus. On the body there is a superior articular surface which articulates with the tibia. Note that it is wider in front than behind. On the lateral aspect of the body of the talus look for the large triangular facet which articulates with the lateral malleolus.

On its medial aspect find a smaller lunate facet, which articulates with the medial malleolus. On the small posterior surface of the body look for a deep groove which lodges the tendon of one of the deeper muscles of the calf (the flexor hallucis longus) as it passes to the plantar surface of the big toe.

On the anterior surface of the head of the talus note the convex articular facet which fits into the posterior surface of the navicular bone. This is continuous on the plantar surface with small anterior and middle facets which are separated by a deep groove, called the **groove of the talus,** from a larger posterior articular facet. All three of these plantar facets articulate with different parts of the calcaneum. Part of the head of the talus also articulates with the plantar calcaneonavicular ligament. When the two bones are articulated the grooves of the talus and calcaneum together form the **tarsal sinus.**

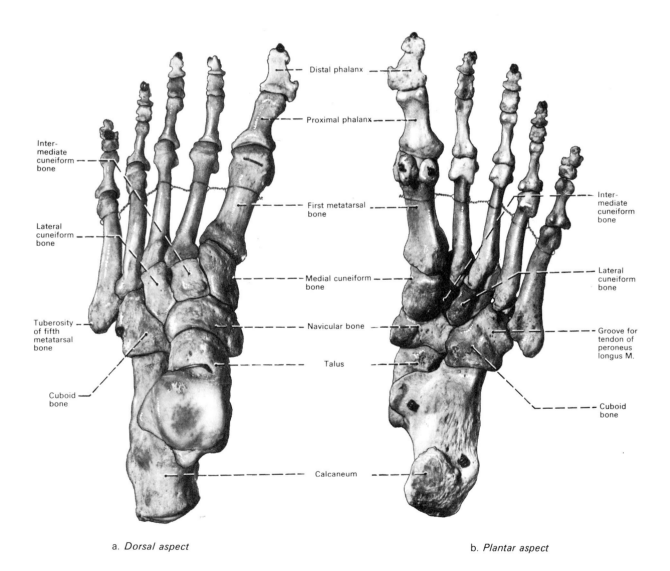

Inter-mediate cuneiform bone

Lateral cuneiform bone

Tuberosity of fifth metatarsal bone

Cuboid bone

Distal phalanx

Proximal phalanx

First metatarsal bone

Medial cuneiform bone

Navicular bone

Talus

Calcaneum

Inter-mediate cuneiform bone

Lateral cuneiform bone

Groove for tendon of peroneus longus M.

Cuboid bone

a. *Dorsal aspect*

b. *Plantar aspect*

Fig. 2.50 The bones of the left foot.

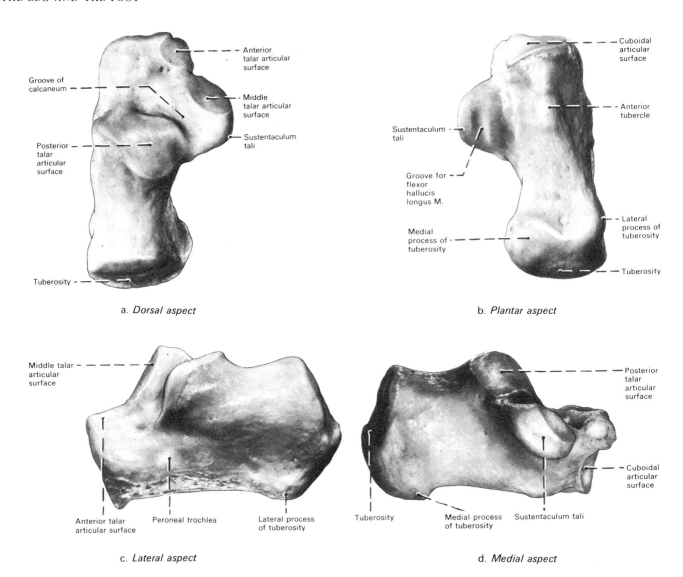

Anterior
talar articular
surface

Groove of
calcaneum

Middle
talar articular
surface

Sustentaculum
tali

Posterior
talar
articular
surface

Tuberosity

a. *Dorsal aspect*

Cuboidal
articular
surface

Sustentaculum
tali

Anterior
tubercle

Groove for
flexor
hallucis
longus M.

Medial
process of
tuberosity

Lateral
process of
tuberosity

Tuberosity

b. *Plantar aspect*

Middle talar
articular
surface

Posterior
talar
articular
surface

Cuboidal
articular
surface

Anterior talar
articular surface

Peroneal trochlea

Lateral process
of tuberosity

Tuberosity

Medial process
of tuberosity

Sustentaculum tali

c. *Lateral aspect*

d. *Medial aspect*

Fig. 2.51 The left calcaneum.

The cuboid

Now study the cuboid bone [Fig. 2.50]. On the plantar surface of the cuboid, near the front, you will find a groove which lodges the tendon of the peroneus longus muscle. Note the articular surfaces of this bone. Posteriorly there is one for the calcaneum. Anteriorly there are facets for the bases of the fourth and fifth metatarsal bones. Medially there is a facet for the lateral cuneiform bone.

The navicular

Identify the **tuberosity** at the medial extremity of the navicular bone [Fig. 2.53]. This can sometimes be seen and felt on the medial border of the living foot. Note that the navicular bone always articulates with the three cuneiform bones anteriorly and with the talus posteriorly. Laterally it frequently articulates with the cuboid.

The cuneiform bones

The three cuneiform bones [Fig. 2.50] are referred to, according to their positions in the foot, as the **medial cuneiform bone,** the **intermediate cuneiform bone,** and the **lateral cuneiform bone.** Note the articulations of these bones with the bases of the first, second, and third metatarsal bones respectively. The lateral cuneiform also articulates with the cuboid, and all three articulate with the navicular bone posteriorly.

The metatarsal bones and the phalanges

These are arranged in a manner similar to those of the hand. The base of the fifth metatarsal bone bears a **tuberosity** which can be easily seen and felt in the living body [Fig. 2.50].

2.46

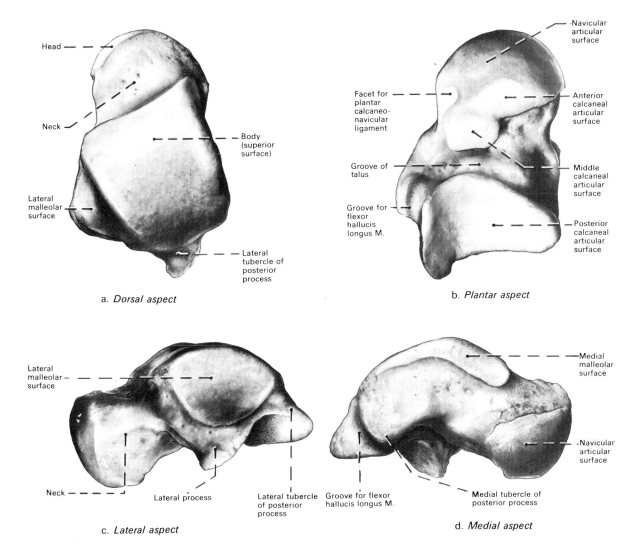

Head

Neck

Lateral malleolar surface

Body (superior surface)

Lateral tubercle of posterior process

a. *Dorsal aspect*

Navicular articular surface

Facet for plantar calcaneonavicular ligament

Anterior calcaneal articular surface

Groove of talus

Middle calcaneal articular surface

Groove for flexor hallucis longus M.

Posterior calcaneal articular surface

b. *Plantar aspect*

Lateral malleolar surface

Neck

Lateral process

Lateral tubercle of posterior process

c. *Lateral aspect*

Medial malleolar surface

Navicular articular surface

Groove for flexor hallucis longus M.

Medial tubercle of posterior process

d. *Medial aspect*

Fig. 2.52 **The left talus.**

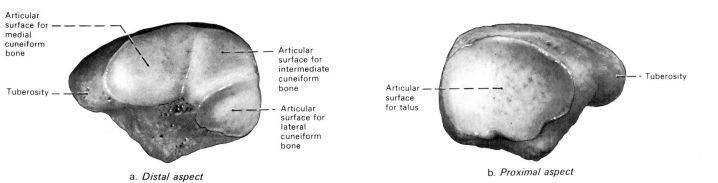

Articular surface for medial cuneiform bone

Tuberosity

Articular surface for intermediate cuneiform bone

Articular surface for lateral cuneiform bone

a. *Distal aspect*

Articular surface for talus

Tuberosity

b. *Proximal aspect*

Fig. 2.53 **The left navicular bone.**

Surface anatomy

Examine the foot of the cadaver you are dissecting, and when you have a suitable opportunity, your own foot as well. If need be, refer to a skeleton as well to orientate bony features.

First define the lateral and medial malleoli, noting that the former extends a little less than 1.5 cm more distally than the latter. Find the tuberosity of the navicular bone about 2.5 cm in front of, and below the medial malleolus [Fig. 2.54]. It is the most prominent bony point on the medial aspect of the foot. Immediately below the medial malleolus find the sustentaculum tali. The bone between it and the tuberosity of the navicular is the head of the talus. On the medial aspect of the foot locate the metatarsophalangeal joint of the great toe. An inflammation of the bursa over this joint gives rise to a bunion.

Define the tuberosity of the fifth metatarsal bone on the lateral aspect of the foot. This is a prominent landmark. The bone immediately behind this is the cuboid. Immediately below the lateral malleolus you may be able to define the peroneal trochlea of the calcaneum. Feel the bone imme-diately in front of the lateral malleolus. This is the cal-caneum. Now invert the foot (i.e. turn the sole inwards) and note that the head of the talus stands out prominently.

In front of the ankle joint you will be able to see and feel a number of tendons as they pass forward on the dorsum of the foot. They stand out prominently if the foot is dorsi-flexed, and can be more easily distinguished from one another if the foot is then alternately inverted and everted. You will be able to identify all of them after you have dis-sected the anterior compartment of the leg.

Reflection of the skin

Make the following incisions through the skin [Fig. 2.55]:

1. A vertical midline incision down the front of the leg and along the dorsum of the foot to the base of the third toe.
2. An incision across the ankle joint from one side of the heel to the other.
3. A transverse incision across the dorsum of the foot at the bases of the toes.
4. A vertical incision on the dorsum of one or more toes.

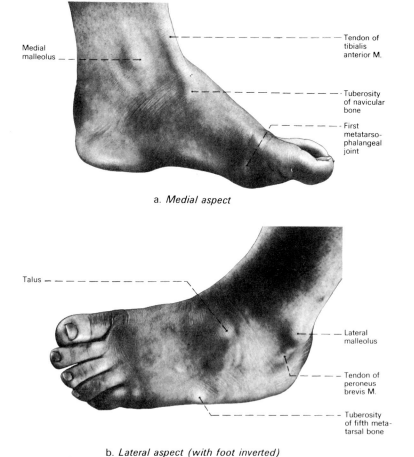

Medial malleolus —

Tendon of tibialis anterior M.

Tuberosity of navicular bone

First metatarso-phalangeal joint

a. *Medial aspect*

Talus —

Lateral malleolus

Tendon of peroneus brevis M.

Tuberosity of fifth meta-tarsal bone

b. *Lateral aspect (with foot inverted)*

Fig. 2.54 The left foot and ankle.

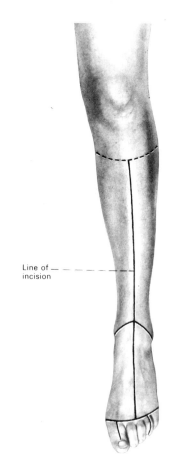

Line of incision

Fig. 2.55 Skin incisions on the leg and foot.

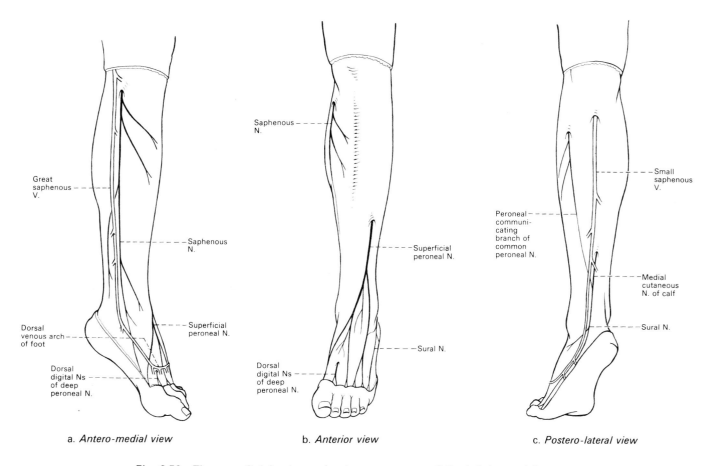

a. *Antero-medial view*   b. *Anterior view*   c. *Postero-lateral view*

Fig. 2.56   The superficial veins and cutaneous nerves of the left leg and foot.

Remove the skin from the whole of the front and sides of the leg, turning the skin flaps aside. Do the same on the dorsum of the foot and on the dorsal surfaces of those toes which you have incised.

Dissection of the front of the leg and dorsum of the foot

The superficial veins [Fig. 2.56]

First note the veins in the superficial fascia which you have exposed on the dorsum of the foot, but do not dissect them. They form the **dorsal venous network of the foot.** Sometimes you can see that two main veins spring from this network. The vein you will find on the medial border of the foot is the **great saphenous vein,** and that on the lateral border the **small saphenous vein.** You should be able to see that the great saphenous vein ascends in front of the medial malleolus and on the medial side of the leg, and that the small saphenous vein ascends behind the lateral malleolus and to the back of the calf. Do not dissect the veins at this stage.

The cutaneous nerves [Fig. 2.56]

In close relationship with each of the saphenous veins you should find a cutaneous nerve. The **saphenous nerve,** a branch of the femoral nerve, whose proximal course you have already followed, accompanies the great saphenous vein. Trace it now to the ball of the great toe. When you have done this you will have dissected the entire course of the nerve from its origin in the thigh. The **sural nerve** accompanies the small saphenous vein and can be traced along the lateral border of the foot and behind the lateral malleolus. Later you will see that it is formed in the middle of the calf of the leg by the union of the **medial cutaneous nerve of the calf** and the **peroneal communicating branch of the common peroneal nerve** [p. 2.57].

Between the saphenous and sural nerves you will find an important cutaneous nerve which pierces the deep fascia in the lower third of the front of the leg. This is the **superficial peroneal nerve,** one of the terminal branches of the common peroneal nerve. It should be followed to the dorsum of the foot, where its branches can be seen supplying the skin not

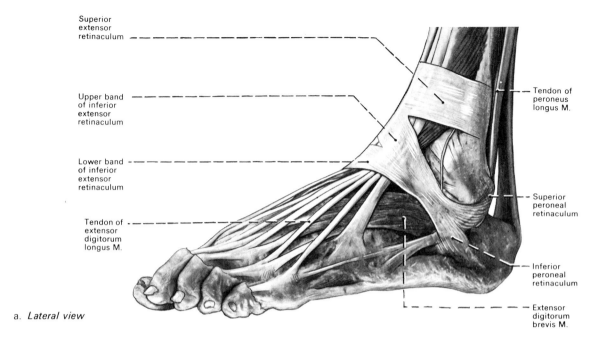

Superior extensor retinaculum

Upper band of inferior extensor retinaculum

Lower band of inferior extensor retinaculum

Tendon of extensor digitorum longus M.

Tendon of peroneus longus M.

Superior peroneal retinaculum

Inferior peroneal retinaculum

Extensor digitorum brevis M.

a. *Lateral view*

Fig. 2.57 The retinacula around the left ankle joint.

only of the foot itself, but also of the toes (except for the adjacent sides of the great and second toes and the lateral side of the little toe).

Dissect the superficial fascia of the first metatarsal space, and try to find a nerve which divides to supply the skin of the great and second toes. This nerve is the termination of the medial branch of the **deep peroneal nerve.** Later you will see that the latter nerve begins at the proximal end of the fibula, and that its main branches are distributed to the muscles of the front of the leg.

Now clean the deep fascia on the front of the leg and on the dorsum of the foot. Note that the deep fascia over the subcutaneous medial surface of the tibia blends with the periosteum.

The extensor retinacula

Examine the fascia around the ankle joint and note that it is thickened to form bands, called retinacula, which hold down the muscles and tendons that are crossing the joint. You will see that one band stretches between the distal ends of the tibia and fibula. This is the **superior extensor retinaculum** [Fig. 2.57]. Distal to it is a better-defined Y-shaped band whose main stem is attached to the upper part of the calcaneum. You can see that the proximal limb of the Y is attached to the medial malleolus, and that the distal end continues into the fascia on the medial side of the foot. This is the **inferior extensor retinaculum.**

The flexor retinaculum

Now examine the region between the medial malleolus and the calcaneum. Between the two bones you can define the

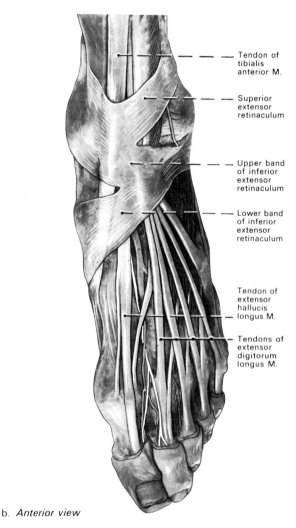

Tendon of tibialis anterior M.

Superior extensor retinaculum

Upper band of inferior extensor retinaculum

Lower band of inferior extensor retinaculum

Tendon of extensor hallucis longus M.

Tendons of extensor digitorum longus M.

b. *Anterior view*

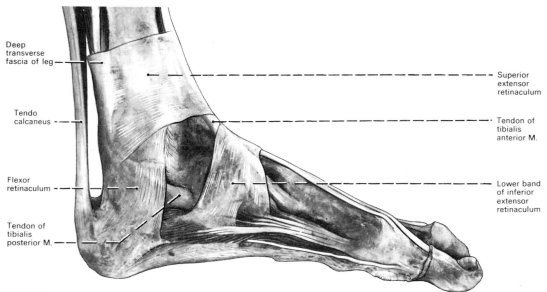

Fig. 2.57 c. *Medial view*

flexor retinaculum, which binds down the flexor tendons [Fig. 2.57c] and passes from the tibial malleolus above to the medial margin of the calcaneum below.

The peroneal retinacula

On the lateral side of the ankle joint look for the peroneal retinacula, which hold down the tendons of the peroneal muscles. Between the lateral malleolus and the calcaneum you should be able to define a **superior peroneal retinaculum** and, on the side of the calcaneum, towards its anterior end, an **inferior peroneal retinaculum** [Fig. 2.57a]. Try to establish that the upper end of the latter is continuous with the main stem of the inferior extensor retinaculum, and that its lower end is attached to the peroneal trochlea of the calcaneum.

You may have difficulty in defining exactly the proximal and distal borders of the various retinacula, but you should have none in recognizing the bands themselves. Having made your own decision as to where they begin and end (it does not matter if you make a mistake of 1 cm either way), make transverse incisions in the fascia along their presumed borders. Then remove the intervening deep fascia, leaving the retinacula intact.

The intermuscular septa of the leg

Now make a vertical incision in the deep fascia on the front of the leg from the knee above to the ankle below, about 2 cm lateral to the anterior border of the tibia, and reflect the fascia to either side from the underlying muscles, taking care not to cut the superficial peroneal nerve which you have already seen. Note that the medial flap of deep fascia becomes attached to the anterior border of the tibia, and that the lateral flap of deep fascia passes deeply between

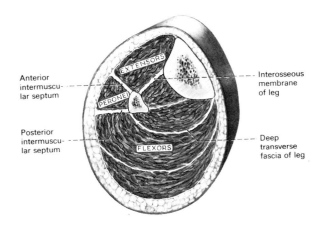

Fig. 2.58 A schematic transverse section through the left leg (viewed from above).

some muscles to become attached to the anterior border of the fibula, so forming an **anterior intermuscular septum**. Between the two attachments of these fascial flaps is the anterior compartment of the leg [Fig. 2.58].

Make another vertical incision in the fascia, lateral to the anterior intermuscular septum, and reflect the deep fascia in order to expose the muscles on the lateral side of the leg. You will find that the flap of fascia you turn forwards runs into the anterior intermuscular septum, and that the posterior flap joins the **posterior intermuscular septum** which is attached to the posterior border of the bone [Fig. 2.58].

The anterior and posterior intermuscular septa deepen the anterior and lateral compartments of the leg, and provide additional surfaces of origin for the muscles you will now dissect. But first neatly trim the fascia which you have reflected.

The muscles in the anterior compartment of the leg

Begin with the muscles in the anterior compartment. They are closely packed, but it is easy to define each muscle belly by following the tendons at the ankle upwards.

The muscle you will see lying on the lateral aspect of the upper part of the shaft of the tibia is the **tibialis anterior** [Fig. 2.59]. The tendon of this muscle emerges in the lower third of the leg, and should be followed to its insertion into the medial surface of the medial cuneiform bone and the adjacent part of the first metatarsal bone. As the tendon passes over the ankle joint, it lies under the superior extensor retinaculum. Incise the latter over the line of the tendon. You will see that the tendon lies in a compartment of its own, surrounded by a synovial sheath. Also incise the inferior extensor retinaculum along the line of the tendon. You can examine your own tibialis anterior by crossing your legs and then inverting and dorsiflexing the foot of the leg that is resting on your knee. This makes the tendon stand out so that it can be traced to its insertion by palpation.

Just lateral to the belly of the tibialis anterior is the belly of a muscle called the **extensor digitorum longus.** By blunt dissection verify that it arises from the upper two-thirds of the narrow medial surface of the fibula, as well as from the interosseous membrane which stretches between the shafts of the tibia and fibula throughout the whole of their extent. The fibres of this muscle run into a tendon which passes under the extensor retinacula, which you should again incise along the line of the tendon. You will see that the tendon subdivides into four tendons under the inferior retinaculum, and that the four tendons are contained in a common synovial sheath. Follow them over the dorsum of the foot to their insertions into the phalanges of the lateral four toes. You will easily see that they join a **dorsal digital expansion** of the extensor tendon over the proximal part of each toe, the general arrangement being similar to that found in the fingers [p. 1.69].

Clean the fascia from the dorsum of the foot. Under the long extensor tendons you will see the belly of a small muscle which splits into four tendons [Fig. 2.59]. This is the **extensor digitorum brevis,** which you will examine a little later in your dissection. For the moment note that its four tendons run to the medial four toes, where they unite with the long extensor tendons.

Examine the lateral aspect of the distal part of the extensor digitorum longus, and try to define a small muscle which arises from the distal part of the fibula. This is the **peroneus tertius.** Follow its tendon of insertion into the dorsum of the fifth metatarsal bone.

Deep to, and between, the tibialis anterior muscle and the extensor digitorum longus muscle you will find the stout tendon of another muscle. This is the **extensor hallucis longus.** Follow the tendon to its insertion into the base of the distal phalanx of the great toe, from the dorsum of which you

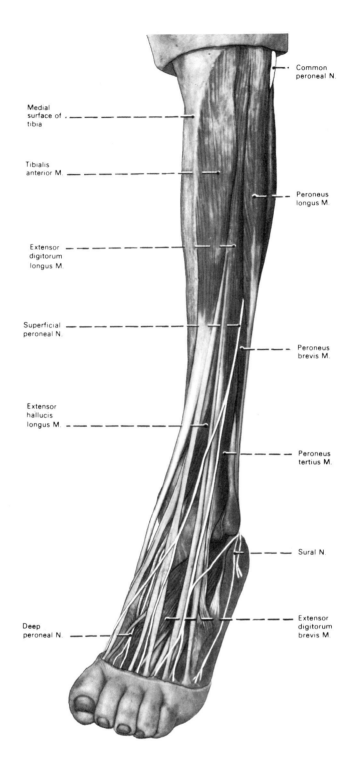

Fig. 2.59 The left leg and foot (antero-lateral aspect).

should reflect the skin. Slit the retinacula over the tendon, and note the tendon's separate synovial sheath. Examine the origin of the extensor hallucis longus muscle and verify that it arises from the middle of the medial surface of the fibula and from the adjacent part of the interosseous membrane.

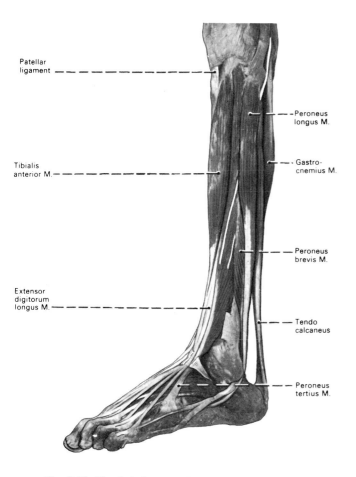

Fig. 2.60 The left leg and foot (lateral aspect).

Patellar ligament

Peroneus longus M.

Gastrocnemius M.

Tibialis anterior M.

Peroneus brevis M.

Extensor digitorum longus M.

Tendo calcaneus

Peroneus tertius M.

Try to feel the long and short extensor tendons by dorsiflexing your own foot.

The muscles in the lateral compartment of the leg

In the lateral compartment of the leg, immediately lateral to the extensor digitorum longus, is a muscle called the **peroneus longus,** whose belly gives way to a tendon about the middle of the leg [Fig. 2.60]. Beneath the tendon of the peroneus longus you will find the belly of another muscle. This is the **peroneus brevis,** whose tendon you will see passes in front of the tendon of the peroneus longus. Follow the tendons of both muscles behind the lateral malleolus on to the lateral aspect of the calcaneum. Note that the tendon of the peroneus brevis is in direct contact with the lateral malleolus, with the tendon of the peroneus longus behind it, and that on the lateral aspect of the calcaneum the tendon of the peroneus brevis lies above the peroneal trochlea, with the tendon of the peroneus longus below it. Trace the peroneus brevis to its insertion into the base of the fifth metatarsal bone. At this stage you will not be able to trace the tendon of the peroneus longus further than the lateral side of the foot, whence it passes into the sole.

Examine the origins of the peroneal muscles, and note that the peroneus longus arises from the proximal two-thirds of the lateral surface of the fibula, and the peroneus brevis from the distal two-thirds of the same surface. You can see the two tendons in your own foot by raising it from the floor and then dorsiflexing and everting it.

The muscles of the dorsum of the foot

Now examine the small **extensor digitorum brevis,** which you have already seen between the tendons on the dorsum of the foot [Fig. 2.61]. When you clean the muscle you will see

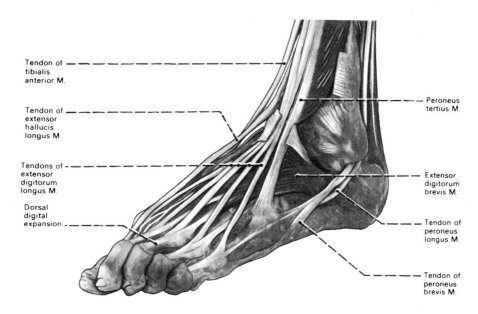

Tendon of tibialis anterior M.

Tendon of extensor hallucis longus M.

Tendons of extensor digitorum longus M.

Dorsal digital expansion

Peroneus tertius M.

Extensor digitorum brevis M.

Tendon of peroneus longus M.

Tendon of peroneus brevis M.

Fig. 2.61 The dorsum of the left foot.

2.53

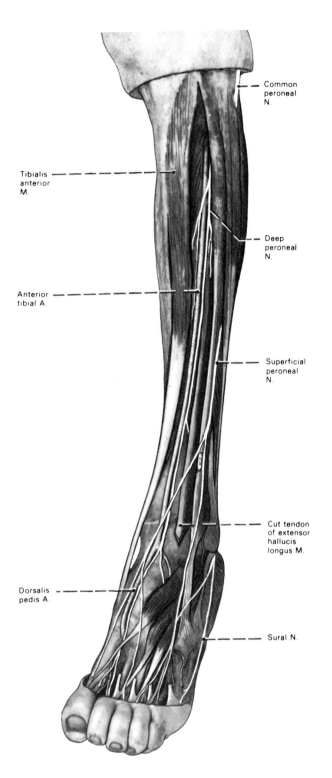

Common
peroneal
N.

Tibialis
anterior
M.

Deep
peroneal
N.

Anterior
tibial A.

Superficial
peroneal
N.

Cut tendon
of extensor
hallucis
longus M.

Dorsalis
pedis A.

Sural N.

Fig. 2.62 The anterior tibial artery and peroneal nerves.

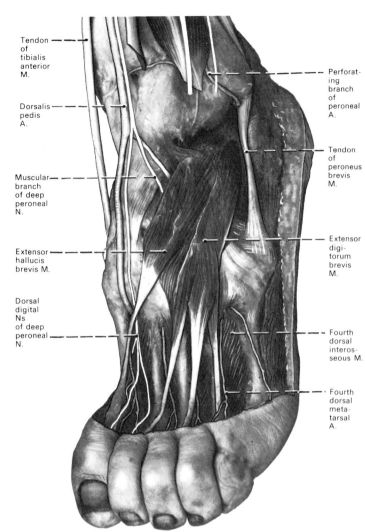

Tendon
of
tibialis
anterior
M.

Dorsalis
pedis
A.

Muscular
branch
of deep
peroneal
N.

Extensor
hallucis
brevis M.

Dorsal
digital
Ns
of deep
peroneal
N.

Perforat-
ing
branch
of
peroneal
A.

Tendon
of
peroneus
brevis
M.

Extensor
digi-
torum
brevis
M.

Fourth
dorsal
interos-
seous M.

Fourth
dorsal
meta-
tarsal
A.

Fig. 2.63 The left dorsalis pedis artery and the extensor digitorum brevis muscle. The arcuate artery is absent.

that it arises from the rough area of bone on the front of the dorsal surface of the calcaneum. Trace the four tendons of the extensor digitorum brevis forwards. The most medial, often called the **extensor hallucis brevis,** passes to the base of the proximal phalanx of the great toe. Clean and examine the three lateral tendons. You will see that they join the long extensor tendons to the second, third, and fourth toes.

The anterior tibial vessels

By blunt dissection in the upper part of the leg separate the belly of the tibialis anterior from that of the extensor digitorum longus. This will allow you to see the **anterior tibial artery,** accompanied by two companion veins, piercing the upper part of the interosseous membrane [Fig. 2.62]. The artery is one of the two terminal branches of the **popliteal artery.** Superficial (lateral) to it you will find the deep peroneal nerve, which you will remember is one of the terminal branches of the common peroneal nerve, emerging through the fibres of the extensor digitorum longus muscle.

Clean and trace the anterior tibial artery and the deep peroneal nerve downwards, removing the accompanying veins. The tendon of the extensor hallucis longus muscle will be seen to cross them superficially. You will find that the anterior tibial artery gives off many small branches (e.g. branches to an anastomosis around the knee joint, muscular branches, and branches to an anastomosis around the ankle joint), but they are variable in their origin and can be sacrificed as you encounter them in your dissection.

The dorsalis pedis artery

Midway between the two malleoli, the anterior tibial artery becomes the dorsalis pedis artery [Fig. 2.63]. This vessel usually plays an important part in maintaining the blood supply to the foot, but sometimes it is very small. Clean the artery and try to trace it to its termination. You will find that it runs forwards on the talus, navicular, and intermediate cuneiform bones to the first intermetatarsal space. Here it disappears from view by piercing the first dorsal interosseous muscle on its way into the sole.

Just before the dorsalis pedis artery disappears from view, you will find (if your specimen is well injected) that it gives off a branch which arches under the extensor tendons, proximal to the clefts between the toes. This branch is called the **arcuate artery.** As you clean the artery you will find that it sends branches to the toes.

When the dorsalis pedis artery is small or absent, the dorsum of the foot receives its blood supply from one of the branches of the posterior tibial artery [see pp. 2.65–2.66].

The peroneal nerves

As you clean the **deep peroneal nerve** [Fig. 2.64] you may find the branches it sends to the extensor digitorum longus, peroneus tertius, tibialis anterior, and extensor hallucis longus muscles. In front of the ankle joint you will find that the nerve divides into medial and lateral branches. Follow the medial branch. You will see that it splits into terminal branches which supply the skin of the adjacent sides of the great and second toes. The lateral branch of the deep peroneal nerve passes under the extensor digitorum brevis, which it supplies. It also supplies the intertarsal joints.

Now look behind the head of the fibula and pick up the termination of the **common peroneal nerve.** Cut transversely through the upper part of the peroneus longus at the point where you see the nerve disappearing into the muscle, and expose the nerve fully [Fig. 2.64]. You will find that it almost immediately divides into its terminal branches. One of them, as you have seen, is the deep peroneal nerve [p. 2.50]. Trace this nerve through the substance of the peroneus longus and extensor digitorum longus into the anterior compartment of the leg.

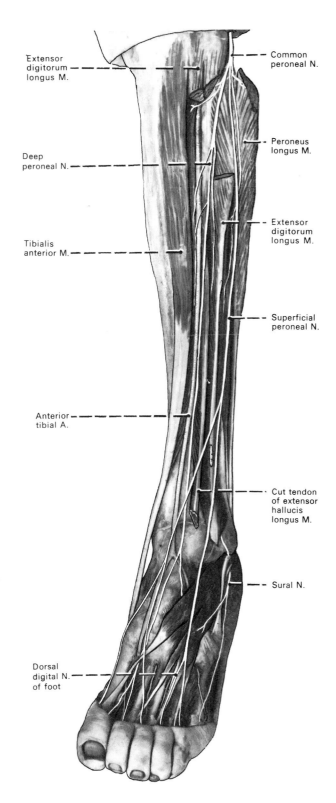

Fig. 2.64 The left common peroneal nerve and its branches. A section of the upper part of the extensor digitorum longus muscle has been excised. The peroneus longus muscle has been partially divided at its upper end and turned laterally.

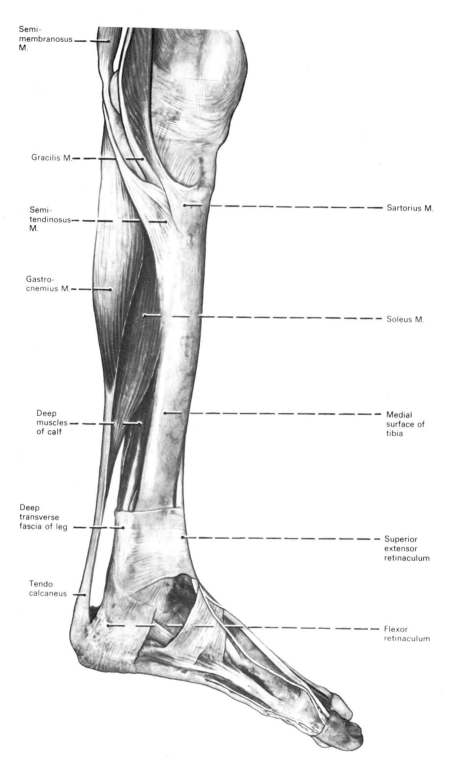

Semi-
membranosus
M.

Gracilis M.

Semi-
tendinosus
M.

Gastro-
cnemius M.

Deep
muscles
of calf

Deep
transverse
fascia of leg

Tendo
calcaneus

Sartorius M.

Soleus M.

Medial
surface of
tibia

Superior
extensor
retinaculum

Flexor
retinaculum

Fig. 2.65 The medial aspect of the left leg.

The other branch of the common peroneal is the **superficial peroneal nerve.** By dividing the more superficial fibres of the peroneus longus, follow this nerve in its course through the muscle to the point where it becomes superficial. As you do so you may find the branches it sends to the peroneus longus and brevis muscles.

Complete the dissection of the dorsum of the foot by dividing the tendons of the extensor digitorum longus and peroneus tertius muscles at the level of the ankle joint. Reflect them towards their insertion. Then complete the cleaning of the extensor digitorum brevis and verify its origin from the calcaneum. Detach the muscle close to the bone and turn it distally.

The dorsal interosseous muscles

Now dissect the four dorsal interosseous muscles between the metatarsal bones [Figs 2.63 and 2.87]. They are bipennate muscles and each arises by two heads from adjacent metatarsal bones and, as in the upper limb [p. 1.58], each is inserted into the proximal phalanx and into the dorsal digital expansion of the extensor digitorum longus muscle. The tendon of the first dorsal interosseous passes to the

medial side of the second toe, and that of the second to the lateral side of the same toe. The third and fourth muscles pass to the lateral sides of the third and fourth toes. The action of the dorsal interosseous muscles is to abduct the toes from the axis of the foot. This axis passes through the second metatarsal bone and the second toe.

Pick up the medial branch of the deep peroneal nerve and see if you can find the nerve it sends into the first dorsal interosseous muscle. The lateral branch sends one to the second dorsal interosseous muscle. You will see later, however, that the main nerve supply of all the interosseous muscles is from the lateral plantar nerve in the sole of the foot [p. 2.66].

Dissection of the back of the leg

You must now dissect the calf of the leg. The muscles of the calf act both on the ankle joint and the joints of the foot, and between them are the posterior tibial vessels and tibial nerve as these descend into the sole.

The swelling of the calf is formed by a fusion of the medial and lateral heads of the gastrocnemius muscle, which you have already seen, and by the belly of the soleus muscle which lies deep to them [Fig. 2.65]. The tendons of both muscles fuse to form the tendo calcaneus, which is easily seen and felt, and which becomes inserted into the back of the calcaneum. This is by far the largest and strongest tendon in the body. On a deeper plane are three muscles whose tendons pass into the sole of the foot behind the medial malleolus.

Before you proceed with your dissection, turn back to pages 2.42 to 2.48 and re-read the sections dealing with the bones and with the surface anatomy of the leg and foot.

The cutaneous nerves

Extend the reflection of the skin flaps you have already lifted from the front and sides of the leg and remove all the skin from the back of the leg. If the small saphenous vein, the upper part of which you have already seen in the popliteal fossa, is prominent, pick it up and follow it downwards through the superficial fascia in the midline of the calf. Accompanying its lower part you will find the **sural nerve** [Fig. 2.66]. Clean the nerve and follow it upwards to the point where it emerges from the deep fascia about halfway down the calf. Close to the point of its emergence you should pick up the **peroneal communicating branch of the common peroneal nerve,** which, as you have already been told [p. 2.49], joins the medial cutaneous nerve of the calf to form the sural nerve.

Between the medial malleolus and the heel see if you can find a cutaneous nerve which pierces the flexor retinaculum, and which supplies the skin over the heel. This is the **medial calcanean branch of the tibial nerve.** If you do not find it easily, do not spend time searching for it.

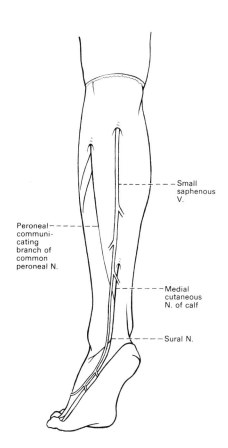

Peroneal communicating branch of common peroneal N.

Small saphenous V.

Medial cutaneous N. of calf

Sural N.

Fig. 2.66 The cutaneous nerves on the back of the left leg.

The superficial muscles of the calf [Figs 2.65 and 2.67]
Clean away the whole of the superficial fascia, preserving such cutaneous nerves as you can, but removing the small saphenous vein, and expose the deep fascia. Divide the deep fascia by a vertical midline incision, and turn it aside so that the superficial muscles of the calf are fully exposed.

Now follow the medial cutaneous nerve of the calf upwards to its origin from the tibial nerve. Re-examine the two heads of the gastrocnemius muscle, and if necessary continue the cleaning of their origins from the medial and lateral condyles of the femur and from the capsule of the knee joint [see p. 2.67].

Pull the **lateral head of the gastrocnemius** laterally to display the **plantaris muscle** fully. Clean this muscle, and follow its slender tendon downwards as it passes between the medial head of the gastrocnemius and the soleus muscle [Fig. 2.67].

Cutting transversely with your scalpel, divide the heads of the gastrocnemius and plantaris muscles 5 cm below their origins. Turn the attached part of the **medial head of the gastrocnemius** upwards. Between it and the medial femoral condyle you will find a bursa, which may communicate with the cavity of the knee joint.

The **soleus muscle** will be fully exposed if you turn the lower part of the gastrocnemius downwards. Try to establish that it arises from the upper third of the posterior surface of the fibula; from the soleal line on the posterior surface of the tibia; and from the medial border of the tibia. You should be able to see that the muscle also arises from a strong fibrous band, the **tendinous arch of soleus,** which stretches between the proximal ends of the shafts of the tibia and fibula.

Pick up and clean the popliteal vessel and the tibial nerve, and trace them downwards as far as the origin of the soleus. You will see that they pass into the deeper part of the calf, under the tendinous arch of the soleus muscle.

Now detach the soleus muscle from its origin. First separate the tibial origin of the muscle, from below upwards, and then reflect the muscle laterally, when the tendinous arch between the tibia and fibula will be exposed more fully. Complete the operation by separating the muscle from the fibula.

Turn the detached soleus muscle towards the heel, and in doing so pick up and then divide the branches of the tibial nerve which supply it. Note that the soleus continues as muscle beyond the point where the gastrocnemius becomes tendinous.

Now examine and clean the powerful **tendo calcaneus** into which the gastrocnemius and soleus muscles run [Fig. 2.67]. Trace the tendon of the plantaris to its insertion on the medial side of the posterior surface of the calcaneum. Trace the tendo calcaneus to its insertion into the horizontal ridge on the posterior surface of the calcaneum. Remove the fat which lies deep to the tendon and try to identify the

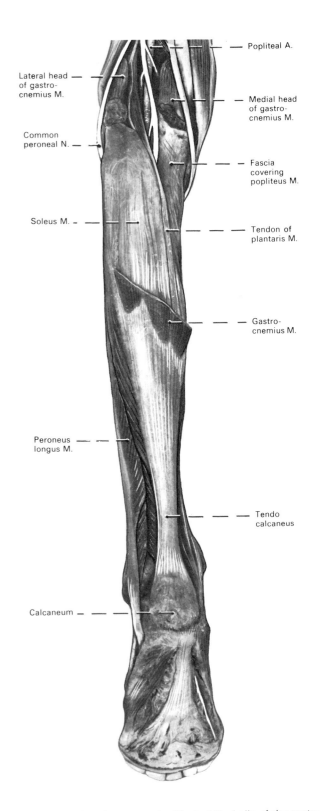

Fig. 2.67 The left soleus muscle. Most of the belly of the gastrocnemius muscle has been excised.

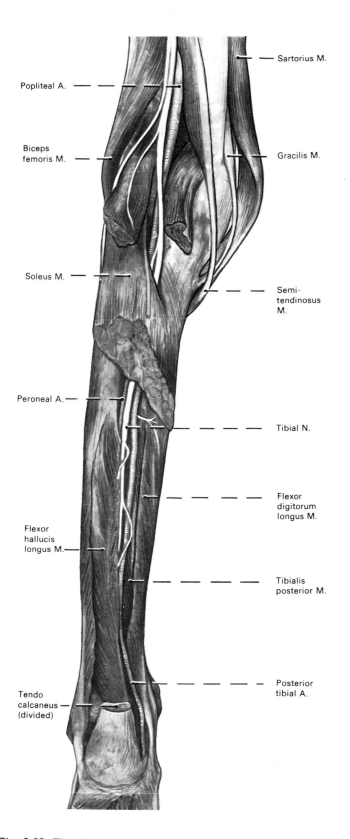

Popliteal A.

Biceps femoris M.

Soleus M.

Peroneal A.

Flexor hallucis longus M.

Tendo calcaneus (divided)

Sartorius M.

Gracilis M.

Semi-tendinosus M.

Tibial N.

Flexor digitorum longus M.

Tibialis posterior M.

Posterior tibial A.

Fig. 2.68 The deep muscles of the left calf. The bellies of the gastrocnemius and soleus muscles have been excised.

bursa which lies between the tendon and the calcaneum.

Both the gastrocnemius and soleus muscles are plantar flexors of the foot. The gastrocnemius also flexes the knee joint. When standing you can feel the contraction of these muscles by grasping the calf of your leg and then transferring your weight on to your toes.

The deep transverse fascia of the leg

The structures of the calf deep to the reflected soleus muscle will be seen to be covered by a layer of fascia. This layer is called the deep transverse fascia of the leg. Incise it in the midline and reflect it to either side. You will find that it is attached to the medial border of the tibia and to the posterior border of the fibula [Fig. 2.58]. Above, it will be seen to be attached to the soleal line of the tibia, and to be continuous here with the fascia over the popliteus muscle. Follow the deep fascia downwards and note that it thickens and becomes continuous with the **flexor** and **superior peroneal retinacula** [Fig. 2.65]. Divide the flexor retinaculum through its middle.

The deep structures of the calf

Under cover of the deep transverse fascia of the leg are the deep muscles of the calf, the flexor hallucis longus, the flexor digitorum longus, and the tibialis posterior muscles, together with the posterior tibial artery and the tibial nerve, all of which you now have to examine [Fig. 2.68].

The tibial nerve [Fig. 2.68]

Pick up the tibial nerve in the upper part of the calf, medial to the popliteal vessels. Find the **nerve to the popliteus muscle.** It runs across the popliteal vessels before turning round the lower border of the popliteus muscle to enter its deep surface.

Clean and follow the tibial nerve the whole way through the calf, noting the branches it sends to the deep muscles of the calf. At the ankle you may be able to confirm that the **medial calcanean nerve,** already dissected in the superficial fascia of the heel [p. 2.57], is one of its branches.

The posterior tibial artery [Fig. 2.68]

Clean the popliteal artery just above the lower border of the popliteus muscle so as to define its division into the anterior and posterior tibial arteries. Trace the former as it passes to the front of the leg below the popliteus muscle, above the tibialis posterior muscle and through the upper part of the interosseous membrane.

Clean the posterior tibial artery and its branches, as usual removing the associated veins. Trace the vessel downwards under cover of the soleus muscle to the interval between the medial malleolus and the calcaneum. Note that in the distal half of the leg the artery, having moved medial to the tendo calcaneus, becomes superficial and that it is covered by skin and fascia only.

The posterior tibial artery gives off small muscular branches throughout its course. These should be removed, together with branches the artery contributes to an anastomosis around the ankle joint. Just below the popliteal fossa you will find that the posterior tibial artery gives off a large branch which enters the belly of a muscle. The muscle is the flexor hallucis longus, and the branch, whose further course will be followed later, is the **peroneal artery.**

Structures behind the medial malleolus

Note the relative positions of the structures which lie behind the medial malleolus and beneath the flexor retinaculum [Fig. 2.69]. Most anteriorly and in contact with the medial malleolus is the tendon of the tibialis posterior muscle. Immediately behind it is the tendon of the flexor digitorum longus muscle. Behind the latter you will find the posterior tibial vessels and the tibial nerve. Behind them, and on a much deeper plane, you will see the tendon of the flexor hallucis longus muscle. The flexor hallucis longus, the tibialis posterior, and flexor digitorum longus, constitute the deep muscles of the calf.

Complete the removal of the deep transverse fascia of the leg so as to expose the underlying muscles.

The deep muscles of the calf

The muscle which lies immediately medial to the peroneus longus and peroneus brevis muscles is the **flexor hallucis longus** [Fig. 2.68]. Clean this muscle and verify its origin from the middle third of the posterior surface of the fibula. Trace its tendon, which emerges near the ankle, behind the talus and under the flexor retinaculum. Incise the latter for about 3 cm along the line of the tendon, which you will see lies in a separate fibrous tunnel within its own synovial sheath.

Return to the peroneal artery, which you saw springing from the origin of the posterior tibial artery, and follow it distally, if necessary incising the flexor hallucis longus muscle, to the back of the ankle joint. You will find that the peroneal artery terminates here by giving branches to the arterial anastomosis around the joint.

Now clean the bellies of the two muscles which lie medial to the flexor hallucis longus. They are the **flexor digitorum longus** and the **tibialis posterior,** the latter lying between the other two deep muscles of the calf, and on a somewhat deeper plane. As you clean the tibialis posterior you will see that it is covered by a layer of fascia which separates it from the other two muscles. Clear away this fascia. Note the origin of the flexor digitorum longus from the middle third of the posterior surface of the shaft of the tibia; and having done so, establish that the tibialis posterior arises from the proximal half of the posterior surface of the fibula, from the interosseous membrane and, lateral to the origin of flexor digitorum longus, from the middle third of the posterior surface of the tibia. The vertical line you noted running downwards from the soleal line on the back of the tibia marks the line of separation of these two muscles [p. 2.43].

Follow the tendons of the flexor digitorum longus and tibialis posterior muscles behind the medial malleolus where they will be found to lie in tunnels under the flexor retinaculum, which you should slit as far as is possible at present,

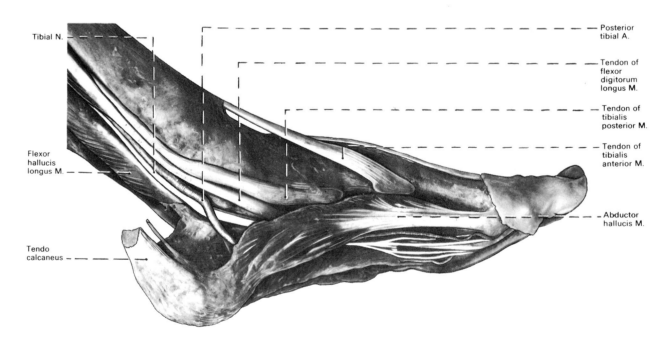

Fig. 2.69 Structures behind the left medial malleolus.

along the lines of the tendons. At a later stage you will follow the tendons in the sole of the foot. Note now that the tendon of the tibialis posterior passes forwards deep to the flexor digitorum longus, to lie in front of it [Fig. 2.69].

Dissection of the sole of the foot

The skin of the sole and toes should now be removed. This is a difficult operation which must be carried out with care.

Begin at the heel and reflect the skin forwards in a single sheet, which you can remove when the bases of the toes are reached. Then incise the skin of each toe centrally, reflect it laterally and remove it.

The plantar aponeurosis

The superficial fascia of the sole is nodular and fatty. Dissect and scrape it from the central part of the deep fascia. This forms a thick and strong plantar aponeurosis, which is almost ligamentous in texture [Fig. 2.70]. Clean and trace the aponeurosis backwards. You will find that it is attached to the medial process of the tuberosity of the calcaneum. Trace the aponeurosis forwards and you will see that it divides into five processes, which pass to the toes. Carefully clear away the less dense fascia between these processes. By so doing you expose the lumbrical muscles and also arteries and nerves passing to each of the toes [Fig. 2.70].

By dissecting further you can demonstrate that each process of the plantar aponeurosis splits to enclose a flexor tendon, and that it then becomes attached deeply at the bases of the toes. Later you may be able to see that each process also merges with a **deep transverse metatarsal ligament** which connects the plantar ligaments of adjoining metatarsophalangeal joints to one another.

Note that the deep fascia on the lateral and medial borders of the foot is very thin compared to the central part of the plantar aponeurosis.

Deep to the plantar aponeurosis are the layers of small or intrinsic muscles of the sole of the foot. In the first and most superficial layer are the abductor hallucis, the abductor digiti minimi, and the flexor digitorum brevis. The second layer consists of the flexor accessorius, the tendons of the flexor digitorum longus and the flexor hallucis longus, and the four lumbrical muscles, which lie between the flexor tendons. The third layer consists of the flexor hallucis brevis, the adductor hallucis, and the flexor digiti minimi brevis. The fourth and deepest layer consists of the dorsal and plantar interosseous muscles.

The first layer of the sole [Fig. 2.71]

Divide the plantar aponeurosis near its calcaneal attachment, and very carefully reflect it forwards from a small muscle, the **flexor digitorum brevis** which partly arises from the aponeurosis [Fig. 2.71]. Continue turning the aponeurosis forwards towards the toes, detaching it from the intermuscular septa which separate the flexor digitorum brevis from other small muscles which lie to its sides. Completely remove the aponeurosis when you reach the bases of the toes, again noting how strong it is. It plays a big part in maintaining the arches of the foot [see p. 2.78].

Now remove the deep fascia from the medial and lateral sides of the sole. This fascia is sometimes described as the medial and lateral parts of the plantar aponeurosis. Under cover of the medial part you will find a muscle called the **abductor hallucis.** Clean it and follow its tendon towards the base of the great toe. Under the lateral part you will find a muscle called the **abductor digiti minimi.** As you clean these small muscles be careful not to cut any nerves.

The plantar nerves and arteries [Figs 2.71 and 2.72]

In the interval between the flexor digitorum brevis and the abductor hallucis carefully clean the **medial plantar nerve**

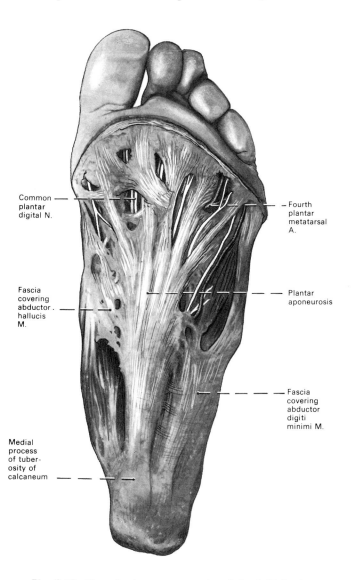

Common plantar digital N.

Fourth plantar metatarsal A.

Fascia covering abductor hallucis M.

Plantar aponeurosis

Fascia covering abductor digiti minimi M.

Medial process of tuberosity of calcaneum

Fig. 2.70 The plantar aponeurosis of the left foot.

and the **medial plantar artery.** Note that both emerge near the heel from under the belly of the abductor hallucis muscle. The nerve is one of the terminal branches of the tibial nerve. Trace it distally and clean the **plantar digital nerves** into which it divides. Note that the plantar digital nerves supply the medial three toes, and the medial side of the fourth toe. The artery, which also emerges from under cover of the abductor hallucis, is the smaller of the two terminal branches of the posterior tibial artery, and gives off a variable number of superficial branches, which accompany the digital branches of the nerve.

As you cleaned the abductor digiti minimi you should have seen the plantar digital nerves which pass to the lateral side of the little toe and the adjacent sides of the fourth and little toes. Clean these nerves now and trace them back to-

wards the heel [Fig. 2.72]. They will lead you to the **superficial branch of the lateral plantar nerve,** from which they spring.

If the specimen you are dissecting is well injected, you should be able to see that the superficial digital branches of the medial plantar artery unite near the bases of the clefts between the toes with the **plantar metatarsal arteries** [Fig. 2.71].

Turn now to the lateral side of the foot and find the **lateral plantar artery,** the other terminal branch of the posterior tibial artery. The lateral plantar artery, which runs with the lateral plantar nerve, is larger than the medial plantar artery, and you will find it emerging from under cover of the flexor digitorum brevis about the middle of the sole. Clean as much of it as you can see at this stage. Its main

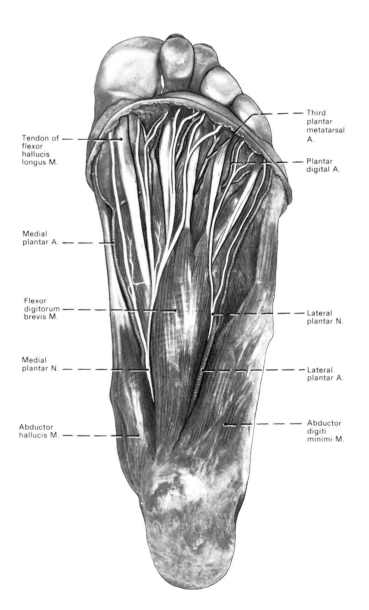

Fig. 2.71 The first layer of muscles of the sole.

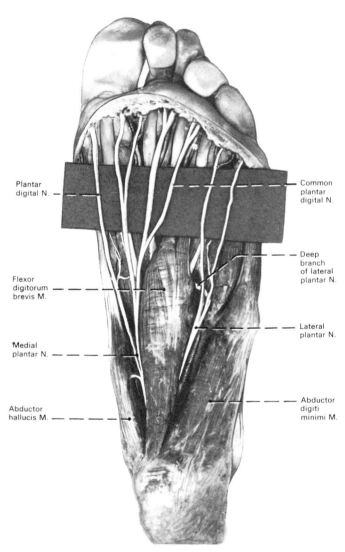

Fig. 2.72 The plantar nerves of the left foot.

part lies deeply, under the flexor tendons, but between the heads of each metatarsal bone you should find a plantar metatarsal artery which it sends to the cleft between each pair of toes. At this stage you will not be able to trace these vessels to their points of origin. If your specimen is well injected you should follow and clean one or two of the plantar metatarsal arteries to see how each divides into **plantar digital arteries** for the adjacent sides of the toes. You will also be able to find the plantar digital artery to the lateral side of the little toe, as it arises independently from the lateral plantar artery. The digital artery to the medial side of the great toe is a branch of the first plantar metatarsal artery.

The medial and lateral plantar nerves are the two terminal branches of the tibial nerve, which divides beneath the flexor retinaculum. Their distribution in the foot is comparable to that of the median nerve and ulnar nerve in the hand, and if you remember your dissection of the hand clearly [pp. 1.48 sqq.], you need not spend too much time on their dissection. Establish, however, that the lateral plantar nerve divides into a superficial and a deep branch in the same way as does the ulnar nerve. The deep branch disappears from view under cover of the flexor digitorum brevis [Fig. 2.72].

The superficial muscles of the sole

Dissect and follow the four slender tendons of the **flexor digitorum brevis** to the middle phalanges of the second, third, fourth, and little toes [Fig. 2.71]. As you do this, examine and open the **digital fibrous sheaths** on the plantar aspect of the toes. You will then be able to see that each tendon is inserted by two slips into the middle phalanx, and that the corresponding tendon of flexor digitorum longus passes between these slips to its insertion into the distal phalanx of the toe.

Using your scalpel, separate the flexor digitorum brevis from its origin from the medial process of the tuberosity of the calcaneum, and turn it forwards towards the toes. As you do so, you will see that it is supplied by a small branch of the medial plantar nerve. Divide this branch.

The small muscle that you will find exposed beneath the belly of the flexor digitorum brevis is the flexor accessorius [Fig. 2.73]. In the fascia by which the flexor accessorius is covered you can see the medial and lateral plantar nerves and arteries as they emerge from beneath the belly of the abductor hallucis. Clean the nerves and arteries and remove the fascia. As you do so, you may find the nerve which passes to the flexor accessorius from the lateral plantar nerve.

Now complete the cleaning of the **abductor hallucis muscle.** Cut it away from its origins from the medial process of the tuberosity of the calcaneum and the flexor retinaculum. Turn the muscle towards its insertion into the great toe, and as you do so note that, like the plantar nerves and vessels, the tendons of the flexor hallucis longus and the flexor digitorum longus pass into the sole deep to the abductor hallucis [Fig. 2.69]. As you reflect the abductor hallucis

you are bound to pick up its nerve, which is a branch from the medial plantar nerve. Divide it. The muscle fibres of the abductor hallucis run into a tendon about two-thirds of the way along the sole. Trace the tendon forwards to its insertion into the medial aspect of the base of the proximal phalanx of the great toe.

Continue the cleaning of the branches of the plantar nerves and arteries which you have exposed, and then turn to the **abductor digiti minimi muscle** on the lateral aspect of the sole. You will see that this muscle is surprisingly big relative to the size of the abductor hallucis. Sever it at its origin from the medial and lateral processes of the tuberosity of the calcaneum, and turn it towards its insertion into the lateral side of the proximal phalanx of the little toe. As you do so, pick up, and then divide the nerve which the lateral

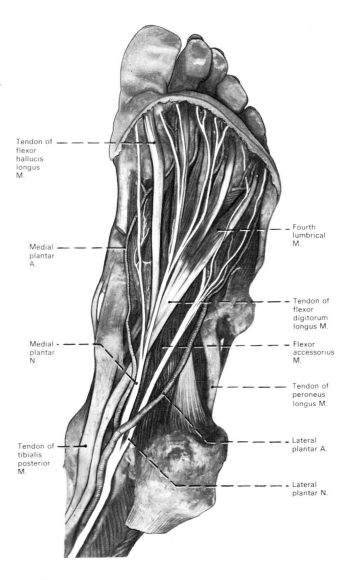

Fig. 2.73 The second layer of muscles of the sole.

plantar nerve sends to the muscle. Note also that the reflection of the abductor digiti minimi has exposed the tendon of the peroneus longus as it turns round the cuboid bone to enter the sole. A fibrocartilaginous nodule or sesamoid bone develops in the tendon as it crosses the lateral border of the bone. You may see or feel this as a hard swelling in the tendon.

The second layer of the sole [Figs 2.73 and 2.74]

Clean and define the attachments of the **flexor accessorius** [Fig. 2.74]. Note that it arises by two heads, a large medial head from the medial surface of the calcaneum, and a much smaller lateral head from the lateral margin of the plantar surface of the calcaneum. Follow the muscle to its insertion into the lateral aspect of the tendon of the flexor digitorum longus. Trace the latter back to the flexor retinaculum and also forwards to the point of its union with the flexor acces-

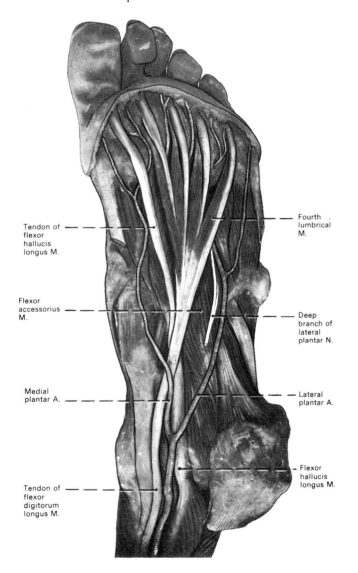

Tendon of
flexor
hallucis
longus M.

Flexor
accessorius
M.

Medial
plantar A.

Tendon of
flexor
digitorum
longus M.

Fourth
lumbrical
M.

Deep
branch of
lateral
plantar N.

Lateral
plantar A.

Flexor
hallucis
longus M.

Fig. 2.74 The lumbrical muscles of the left foot.

sorius, where it divides into four tendons, one of which should be traced into its insertion into the base of the distal phalanx of a toe. You have already opened the digital fibrous sheaths of the foot in order to study the insertion of the flexor digitorum brevis.

Now clean and define the attachments of the **lumbrical muscles** [Fig. 2.74]. They are arranged in much the same way as the corresponding muscles of the hand [p. 1.55]. The first arises from the medial side of the first tendon of the flexor digitorum longus, the second, third, and fourth from the adjacent sides of the first and second, second and third, and third and fourth tendons respectively.

The long flexor tendons of the toes [Fig. 2.74]

Trace the **flexor hallucis longus** to its insertion into the base of the distal phalanx of the great toe and open its digital fibrous sheath. Note that soon after it has emerged in the sole from under the flexor retinaculum, the tendon of the flexor hallucis longus crosses deep to the tendon of the **flexor digitorum longus.** Separate the two tendons and note that they are connected at their point of crossing by a fibrous slip.

Follow the tendons of both the long flexors back to the ankle joint, and completely open their canals in the flexor retinaculum so as to see their synovial sheaths, taking care not to damage the plantar arteries and nerves.

The third layer of the sole [Fig. 2.75]

Divide the tendon of the flexor digitorum longus just distal to the point where it is joined by the flexor accessorius. Divide the tendon of the flexor hallucis longus at the same level. Separate the cut ends of both tendons and look for a nerve which arises from the lateral plantar nerve and runs distally and medially until it disappears beneath a small muscle. This is the **deep branch of the lateral plantar nerve**; the muscle is the oblique head of the adductor hallucis [Fig. 2.75]. On the medial side of this small muscle you will find the smaller flexor hallucis brevis. These two muscles, together with a third on the lateral side of the foot (called the flexor digiti minimi brevis), form the third layer of muscles of the sole.

Note that the tendon of the flexor hallucis longus runs along the midline of the **flexor hallucis brevis** [Fig. 2.75], which, after being cleaned, should be separated from its origin from the cuboid and lateral cuneiform bone, and from the tendon of the tibialis posterior, to which it is joined by some tendinous slips. Trace the flexor hallucis brevis muscle to its insertion. You will see that near the base of the great toe it divides into two tendons, in each of which there is a sesamoid bone. Follow each tendon into the base of the proximal phalanx of the great toe. You may have seen the nerve supply to the muscle when you cleaned the plantar digital nerve to the medial side of the great toe.

Now examine the **adductor hallucis** [Fig. 2.75]. This is the largest muscle in the third layer of the sole, and it arises by two heads. Clean and define the **oblique head** which comes from the bases of the second, third, and fourth metatarsal bones, and the **transverse head** which takes origin from the plantar ligaments of the third and fourth (sometimes also the fifth) metatarsophalangeal joints, and also from the deep transverse metatarsal ligaments. Detach both heads of the muscle from their origins, and follow them as they converge into their insertion into the base of the proximal phalanx of the great toe.

Turn the adductor hallucis aside, and as you do so note the nerve which passes to it from the deep branch of the lateral plantar nerve. Also note that the plantar metatarsal arteries run deep to the transverse head of the muscle.

At this stage of your dissection the muscle on the lateral side of the foot is the **flexor digiti minimi brevis.** Clean it and detach it from its origin from the base of the fifth meta-

tarsal bone. Then turn it towards its insertion into the base of the proximal phalanx of the little toe, taking care not to damage the third plantar interosseous muscle which lies medial and deep to it. When you dissected the superficial branch of the lateral plantar nerve you may have found the small branch this nerve sends to the flexor digiti minimi brevis muscle.

The lateral plantar artery [Fig. 2.76]

You have already cleaned most of the lateral plantar artery. You can now deal with that part of the artery which disappeared from view by passing deep and medially under what you can now see is the oblique head of the adductor hallucis [Fig. 2.75]. You will see that the artery and the deep branch of the lateral plantar nerve run across the interosseous muscles, which form part of the fourth and deepest layer of the sole of the foot, the remaining part being the

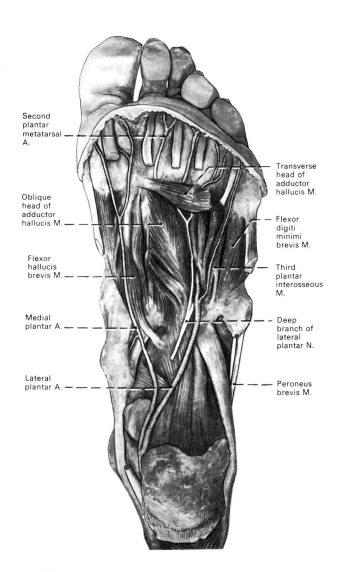

Fig. 2.75 The third layer of muscles of the sole.

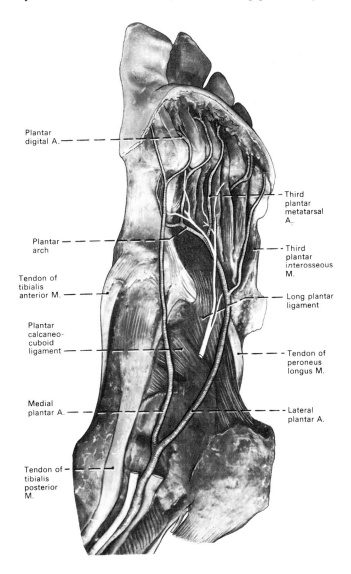

Fig. 2.76 The fourth layer of muscles of the sole.

tendons of the tibialis posterior and peroneus longus muscles [Fig. 2.76].

Clean the lateral plantar nerve and note that it sends branches to the interosseous muscles. Clean the lateral plantar artery and note that it continues as the **plantar arch,** which runs obliquely across the sole, at the same level as the deep branch of the lateral plantar nerve. At the base of the great toe you may be able to demonstrate that the artery joins the **deep plantar branch of the dorsalis pedis artery,** which you previously saw disappearing from view on the dorsum of the foot [p. 2.55].

Trace the **plantar metatarsal arteries** from the convexity of the plantar arch. Follow them distally as they pass deep to the transverse head of the adductor hallucis. You have already seen that they break up into the **plantar digital arteries** [p. 2.63].

The fourth layer of the sole [Figs 2.76 and 2.77]

The interosseous muscles

In order to define the individual interosseous muscles, carefully remove the fascia by which they are covered [Fig. 2.77]. Divide the deep transverse metatarsal ligaments between the bases of the toes and slightly separate the metatarsal bones, so as to expose the muscles more fully. The tendons that are inserted into the medial sides of the bases of the proximal phalanges of the third, fourth, and little toes (and into the corresponding dorsal digital expansions) belong to the three **plantar interosseous muscles.** Note the origins of these muscles from the third, fourth, and fifth metatarsal bones. They adduct the third, fourth, and little toes towards the axis of the foot, which runs through the second toe. The remaining muscles are the **dorsal interosseous muscles,** which you saw when you dissected the dorsum of the foot [p. 2.57]. The tendons of the dorsal interossei pass to the two sides of the base of the second toe, and to the lateral sides of the base of the third and fourth toes. As you will have already noted, the dorsal interossei abduct the toes from the axis of the foot.

The plantar ligaments

Look for and clean the **long plantar ligament** and the **plantar calcaneocuboid ligament** which lie deep to the muscles of the fourth layer of the sole. The long plantar ligament will be seen stretching from the calcaneum to the cuboid and to the bases of the second, third, and fourth metatarsal bones [Fig. 2.76]. The plantar calcaneocuboid ligament, which reaches from the calcaneum to the cuboid, lies on the deep aspect of the long plantar ligament.

The tendons of the peroneus longus and tibialis posterior muscles

You can now follow the whole course of the **tendon of the peroneus longus muscle** in the sole. Note that it lies in the groove on the under-surface of the cuboid bone, which in

part is converted into a tunnel by the long plantar ligament. Cut this ligament to demonstrate this point [Fig. 2.77]. Follow the tendon of the peroneus longus to its insertion into the lateral aspect of the base of the first metatarsal bone and the medial cuneiform bone.

Now return to the region of the flexor retinaculum and pick up the **tendon of the tibialis posterior.** Trace it into the tuberosity of the navicular bone. Try also to define at least some of the tendinous slips that pass from this tendon to the cuboid bone, to the sustentaculum tali, to the intermediate and lateral cuneiform bones, and to the bases of the second, third, and fourth metatarsal bones. These further insertions of the tibialis posterior muscle are important in helping to bind the tarsal bones together, and so in preserving the arches of the foot [see p. 2.78].

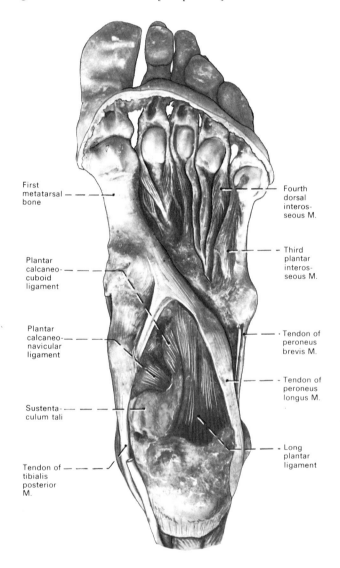

Fig. 2.77 The tendons of the peroneus longus and tibialis posterior muscles. The distal part of the long plantar ligament has been excised to expose the tendon of the peroneus longus muscle as it lies in its groove on the cuboid bone.

Section 2.6

Joints of the lower limb

The knee joint

The next step in your dissection is to examine the knee joint. Before you begin you will find it useful to get a general idea of the joint, which is the most complicated joint in the body. Read the following pages with an articulated skeleton at your side for reference.

The articular surfaces

The knee joint is an articulation between the condyles of the **femur** and of the **tibia** on the one hand, and between the lower end of the femur and the **patella** on the other. The articulation between the femur and the tibia is essentially a hinge joint which works in one plane, only a minor degree of rotation being possible. The articulation between the femur and the patella is a plane joint which allows the patella to glide on the femur. You will see that the articular surfaces on the femur are confined chiefly to the inferior and posterior aspects of the condyles, but that they also ascend on to the anterior aspect of the condyles, especially of the lateral condyle. Correspondingly, you will see that the lateral articular surface on the patella is larger than the medial one.

The superior surfaces of the **condyles of the tibia** are the articular surfaces. They are separated from each other by a central **intercondylar eminence,** and by centrally-situated **anterior** and **posterior intercondylar areas** [Fig. 2.19]. Lying on each tibial articular surface is a fibrocartilaginous meniscus. These you will see later.

The articular capsule

A complicated articular capsule which is reinforced by powerful ligaments ensheathes the joint and, with important exceptions, is attached to the margins of the articular surfaces of the femur and tibia. Since the knee joint is a synovial joint, the inner surface of the capsule, and much of the non-articular bone and other structures within the capsule, are lined by a synovial membrane.

You have already seen that many muscles take origin from or are inserted into bone in the neighbourhood of the knee joint. Turn to your specimen and look again at the insertion of the quadriceps femoris, noting that the muscle belly of the vastus medialis descends to a lower level than that of the vastus lateralis [Fig. 2.78]. The anterior part of the capsule of the knee joint is formed by the tendon of the quadriceps femoris muscle, by the patella into which it is

inserted, and by the **patellar ligament.** Note again that tendinous fibres from the lower ends of the vastus medialis and vastus lateralis reinforce the capsule on either side of the patella and patellar ligament. Look at the insertions of the **iliotibial tract** on the lateral, and of the sartorius on the medial side of the joint. You will be able to see that they, too, reinforce the capsule of the joint. The capsular reinforcements on either side of the patella and its ligament are called the **medial** and **lateral patellar retinacula.**

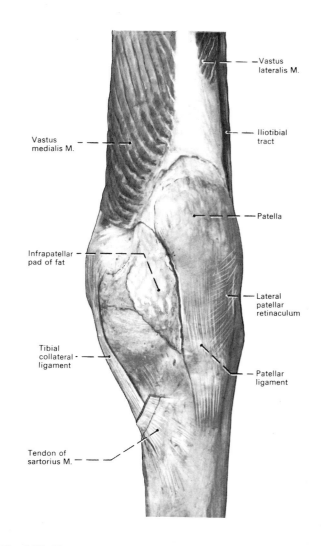

Fig. 2.78 The antero-medial aspect of the left knee joint. The medial patellar retinaculum has been excised to reveal the infrapatellar pad of fat.

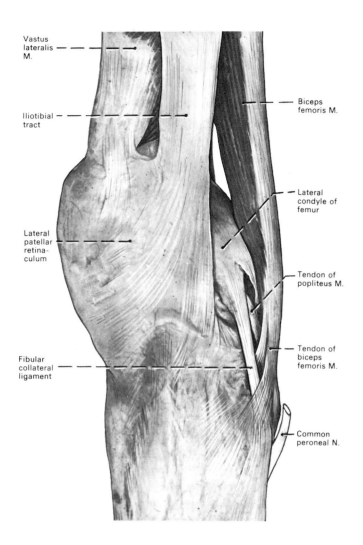

Vastus
lateralis
M.

Iliotibial
tract

Lateral
patellar
retina-
culum

Fibular
collateral
ligament

Biceps
femoris M.

Lateral
condyle of
femur

Tendon of
popliteus M.

Tendon of
biceps
femoris M.

Common
peroneal N.

Fig. 2.79 The lateral aspect of the left knee joint.

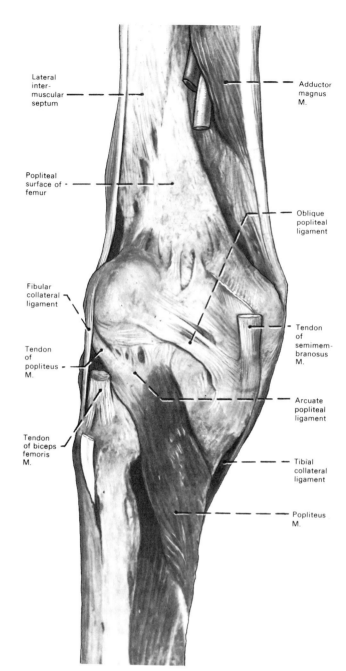

Lateral
inter-
muscular
septum

Popliteal
surface of
femur

Fibular
collateral
ligament

Tendon
of
popliteus
M.

Tendon
of biceps
femoris
M.

Adductor
magnus
M.

Oblique
popliteal
ligament

Tendon
of
semimem-
branosus
M.

Arcuate
popliteal
ligament

Tibial
collateral
ligament

Popliteus
M.

Fig. 2.80 The posterior aspect of the left knee joint.

The fibular collateral ligament

Turn now to the lateral side of the joint and examine the insertion of the biceps femoris muscle [Fig. 2.79]. Divide the tendon of the muscle at the level of the upper border of the lateral epicondyle of the femur and turn it downwards. The long and rounded fibular collateral ligament will come into view, in close relationship with the tendon of the biceps femoris. By blunt dissection make the fibular collateral ligament stand out as a cord. Between it and the more deeply lying capsule you should find the remains of the lateral genicular vessels. Confirm that the fibular collateral ligament is attached to the lateral femoral epicondyle above and to the head of the fibula below. Note, too, that the insertion of the tendon of the biceps femoris muscle is wrapped round the fibular attachment of the collateral ligament.

The popliteal ligaments

The part of the capsule on the deep aspect of the fibular collateral ligament is weak, but you should be able to make out that it is attached to the proximal end of the tibia. Turn the leg over, and note that the popliteus muscle is covered by a ligamentous band, called the **arcuate popliteal ligament,** which arches upwards and medially over the popliteus from the head of the fibula [Fig. 2.80]. Note also that the tendon of the popliteus muscle is attached to the lateral epicondyle just below the upper attachment of the fibular collateral ligament. The arcuate popliteal ligament reinforces the lower lateral part of the capsule of the joint.

Cut away the 5 cm or so of the lateral head of the gastrocnemius muscle that still remains attached to the lateral epicondyle of the femur, in order to make the latter point clear, but do not spend valuable time in trying to define the limits of the arcuate popliteal ligament. Do the same to the medial head of the gastrocnemius muscle. Now cut away all but about 2.5 cm of the attachment of the semimembranosus to the back of the medial condyle of the tibia, and remove all the vessels and nerves from the back of the knee joint.

You can now see the central part of the posterior part of the capsule of the knee joint. Clean it sufficiently to note that most of its ligamentous fibres run obliquely from the lateral side above to the medial side below, and that they end in the attachment of the semimembranosus tendon. These oblique fibres are called the **oblique popliteal ligament** [Fig. 2.80].

The tibial collateral ligament

Turn the specimen so that the medial side of the knee faces you. You will see that on this aspect the capsule is reinforced by a broad flat ligamentous band called the tibial collateral ligament [Fig. 2.78], which is attached above to the medial epicondyle of the femur, and below to the medial condyle of the tibia and the adjacent part of the shaft of the bone. You will see later that, unlike the fibular collateral ligament, which is well separated from the lateral meniscus, the medial ligament is attached to the medial meniscus. Note that the tendons of the sartorius, gracilis, and semitendinosus muscles are in direct contact with the tibial collateral ligament. You may be able to see a large bursa between the tendon of the semitendinosus muscle and the ligament.

The bursae around the knee joint

Again turn the specimen so that its anterior surface is uppermost. Cut through the quadriceps femoris muscle 8 cm above the patella. Your incision should go right through the vasti muscles. Turn down the lower part of the muscle mass. As you do so you should see some muscle fibres, known as the **articularis genus muscle** [Fig. 2.81], which are inserted into a thick pouch of synovial membrane under the tendon of the quadriceps femoris. This pouch, which should be incised, is the **suprapatellar bursa.** It is continuous with the synovial cavity of the knee joint. The muscle fibres inserted into it are part of the vastus intermedius, and arise from the shaft of the femur.

Turn the specimen over again, and pull the lower part of the semimembranosus towards its insertion behind the medial condyle of the tibia. You may be able to see another pouch of synovial membrane called the **semimembranosus**

bursa [Fig. 2.39]. This bursa also communicates with the joint [see p. 2.38].

Examine the popliteus muscle and the strong fascia by which it is covered. Cut through the muscle about its middle, and confirm that it is attached to the medial two-thirds of the triangular area above the soleal line of the tibia. Turn the upper part of the muscle upwards and laterally. You should be able to see a fold of synovial membrane, called the **subpopliteal recess,** separating the tendon from the upper end of the tibia, below the meniscus. Open this recess and try to confirm that it communicates with the knee joint. It also sometimes communicates with the synovial cavity of the tibiofibular joint.

Your dissection will have demonstrated to you that there are certain large gaps in the articular capsule of the knee joint through which the synovial membrane herniates.

The interior of the knee joint

You have seen that on the front of the femur the insertion of the quadriceps femoris and the patella together form the anterior part of the capsule. If you examine your specimen now, with the articulated bones of the lower limb available for reference, you will see that on the lateral epicondyle of the femur the capsule is attached above the popliteal groove, and that on the medial epicondyle it is attached below the adductor tubercle. Thus the popliteus tendon lies within the capsule of the joint and the tendon of the adductor magnus outside. You can see that posteriorly the capsule is attached to the posterior margin of the intercondylar fossa. This margin is called the intercondylar line. On the tibia the capsule is attached anteriorly to the margins of the tuberosity of the tibia and posteriorly to the margin of the posterior intercondylar area.

With your scalpel separate both sides of the patellar ligament from the patellar retinacula, by means of vertical incisions. If you now lift the patellar ligament from the bone you will see that a mass of fat, called the **infrapatellar pad of fat** [Fig. 2.78], separates the synovial membrane from the ligament.

The iliotibial tract should now be cut away from its attachments in this area. Turn down the patella, open the suprapatellar bursa fully, and flex the joint gently in order to put slight tension on a slender synovial band called the **synovial infrapatellar fold,** which will be seen passing to the intercondylar fossa on the femur from the patellar ligament [Fig. 2.81a]. At the base of this fold you will see pouches of synovial membrane filled with fat. These are the **alar folds.**

Cut the synovial infrapatellar fold close to the intercondylar fossa and flex the joint fully. If necessary, extend the incisions on each side of the patella in order to get a wider view. This will expose the **cruciate ligaments of the knee,** the **menisci,** and the **transverse ligament of the knee** by which the anterior margins of the menisci are joined.

The cruciate ligaments

The cruciate ligaments of the knee [Fig. 2.81b] are two powerful intracapsular ligaments which cross each other within the joint cavity. The **anterior cruciate ligament** is attached to the anterior intercondylar area of the tibia and passes upwards, backwards, and laterally to be attached to the posterior part of the medial surface of the lateral condyle of the femur. The **posterior cruciate ligament** is attached to

the posterior intercondylar area of the tibia and passes upwards, forwards, and medially to be attached to the anterior part of the lateral surface of the medial condyle of the femur.

The ligaments are tense in most positions of the knee and prevent excessive movement of the tibia in an antero-posterior direction. They tie the femur and tibia together, and rupture of one or both of these ligaments results in an unstable joint.

The menisci [Figs 2.81b and 2.82]

At this stage you can get only a partial view of the menisci, but the following points will become clear as you proceed with your dissection. The menisci are rings of compressed fibrous tissue (they contain very little cartilage), which lie on, and are attached to, the upper surface of the tibia [Fig. 2.82]. The tibial surface of each meniscus is flat, the femoral surface is concave. The menisci are about 1 cm wide and are triangular on section, the base of the triangle being situated at the periphery, and being about 3 to 5 mm thick.

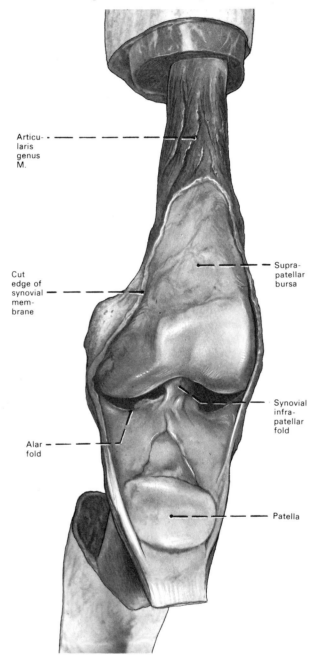

Articularis genus M.

Cut edge of synovial membrane

Suprapatellar bursa

Synovial infrapatellar fold

Alar fold

Patella

a. *The synovial folds*. (The quadriceps femoris muscle has been divided transversely above the patella, and the patella and its ligament have been turned down; the articularis genus muscle has been left *in situ*.)

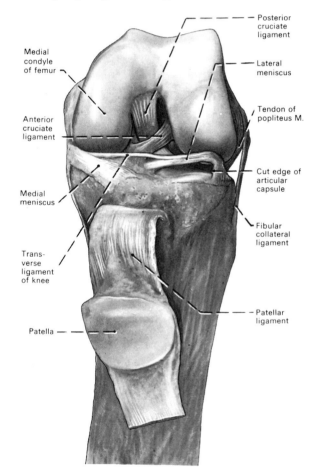

Medial condyle of femur

Anterior cruciate ligament

Medial meniscus

Transverse ligament of knee

Patella

Posterior cruciate ligament

Lateral meniscus

Tendon of popliteus M.

Cut edge of articular capsule

Fibular collateral ligament

Patellar ligament

b. *The ligaments*. (The synovial membrane and the infrapatellar pad of fat have been removed. The joint is flexed and part of the articular capsule between the menisci and the head of the tibia has been excised.)

Fig. 2.81 The left knee joint (opened from the front).

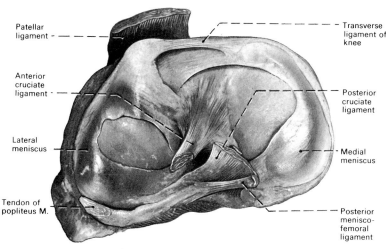

Patellar ligament
Transverse ligament of knee
Anterior cruciate ligament
Posterior cruciate ligament
Lateral meniscus
Medial meniscus
Tendon of popliteus M.
Posterior menisco-femoral ligament

Fig. 2.82 The superior articular surface of the left tibia with the menisci.

The **lateral meniscus** is nearly circular, and is attached by its anterior horn to the anterior intercondylar area of the tibia, immediately in front of the intercondylar eminence, and by its posterior horn to the posterior intercondylar area immediately behind this eminence. Its posterior border is attached to fibres from the popliteus muscle. Some fibres from the posterior border of the lateral meniscus usually pass into and become part of the posterior cruciate ligament.

The **medial meniscus** is semilunar in shape and is attached by its anterior horn to the anterior intercondylar area on the tibia, in front of the anterior cruciate ligament. It is attached by its posterior horn to the posterior intercondylar area on the tibia, in front of the posterior cruciate ligament, and behind the attachments of the lateral meniscus.

The **transverse ligament of the knee** is the name given to a variable amount of fibrous tissue which connects the anterior margins of the menisci.

The attachments of the menisci

It is important to realize that while the menisci are firmly attached to the tibia and must move with it, the peripheral edge of the medial meniscus is also attached to the tibial collateral ligament, and indirectly, therefore, to the femur. Because of this, the periphery of this meniscus moves when the joint is bent. Sometimes, when the femur is suddenly rotated medially with the knee flexed and the tibia fixed, the meniscus may be torn. The edge of the lateral meniscus is not attached to the femur, and is drawn back during flexion of the knee by the contraction of the popliteus muscle, some of whose fibres pass into it.

Many of these points can be demonstrated if you now turn your dissection over and make a transverse incision in the posterior surface of the capsule across the back of the

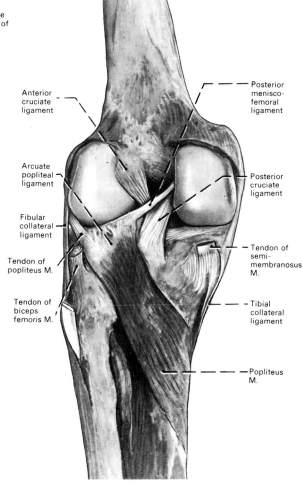

Anterior cruciate ligament
Arcuate popliteal ligament
Fibular collateral ligament
Tendon of popliteus M.
Tendon of biceps femoris M.
Posterior menisco-femoral ligament
Posterior cruciate ligament
Tendon of semi-membranosus M.
Tibial collateral ligament
Popliteus M.

Fig. 2.83 The ligaments of the left knee joint (posterior view). Most of the posterior part of the articular capsule has been excised.

condyles of the femur, and above the menisci. As you open the joint from this aspect, the **posterior meniscofemoral ligament,** a strong fasciculus from the lateral meniscus to the medial condyle, will come into view behind the posterior cruciate ligament. The attachments of both ligaments should be verified [Fig. 2.83]. Look for the attachment of the anterior cruciate ligament to the medial surface of the lateral condyle of the femur. Try to make out the connection of some fibres of the popliteus muscle to the lateral meniscus, and trace the tendon of this muscle to its attachment in the groove on the lateral epicondyle of the femur. Note again that it runs deep to the fibular collateral ligament of the joint.

Now detach the tibial collateral ligament from the medial epicondyle of the femur and turn it downwards in order to demonstrate its attachment to the medial side of the medial meniscus.

Next, divide the anterior and posterior cruciate ligaments

through their middles. You will discover that they are very tough.

Open the medial part of the capsule fully, and splay the joint open so that you can look into it from this aspect. The menisci are now completely exposed [Fig. 2.82]. You can see that the lateral meniscus is nearly circular. Cut through the menisci and verify that they are wedge-shaped on transverse section, with the base of the wedge lying at the periphery of the joint. Examine their extremities, or horns, by which the menisci are attached to the intercondylar area on the tibia. Confirm the laxity of the attachment of the menisci to the upper end of the tibia by moving them on the tibial condyles. Confirm the fact that if the popliteus muscle is pulled the lateral meniscus moves backwards. Note again the precise attachments of the cruciate ligaments on the tibia.

Do not spend too much time in trying to visualize the continuity of the synovial membrane within the joint. Remember that the synovial membrane lines the articular capsule to a limited extent only, that it herniates under the attachments of the quadriceps femoris and popliteus muscles (and sometimes the semimembranosus) to form bursae, and that the subpopliteal recess under the tendon of the popliteus may communicate with the cavity of the tibiofibular joint. Remember, too, that the infrapatellar pad of fat intervenes between the synovial membrane behind and the patellar ligament in front.

The movements of the knee joint

Although the only movements at the knee of which one is aware are flexion and extension about a transverse axis (as in a hinge joint), the action of the joint is very much more complex than this.

In extreme flexion there is contact between the posterior surface of the condyles of the femur and the posterior part of the menisci on the upper end of the tibia, and also, to a certain extent, with the upper end of the tibia itself. With the tibia fixed (e.g. with your foot on the ground), the condyles of the femur glide and roll upon the top of the tibia as the knee straightens. During this movement the condyles of the tibia and femur increase the area of their mutual contact, and as they do so, the menisci open up slightly.

If you examine the lower end of the femur, you will see that the antero-posterior axis of the lateral condyle is very nearly straight, whereas that of the medial is curved [Fig. 2.81b]. Because of this, the range of movement of the lateral condyle, as the knee extends, becomes exhausted before that of the medial condyle, which then starts rotating medially round a vertical axis. This rotation occurs around a vertical axis which is prolonged upwards along the line of the tibia between the condyles of the femur. This rotation 'locks' the joint, and tightens most of the ligaments, particularly the tibial and fibular collateral ligaments. When the knee flexes, the reverse movement has to take place, lateral rotation of

the medial condyle of the femur 'unlocking' the joint. This lateral twist is brought about by the pull of the popliteus muscle.

When the knee is bent with the foot on the ground, some rotation of the distal end of the femur is possible on the upper end of the tibia. In general, such voluntary rotation is possible only when the joint is flexed, for this is the only position in which the tibial collateral, fibular collateral, and cruciate ligaments of the joint are not tense. If you try to visualize the connections of the cruciate ligaments, it is easy to see why they play the important part they do in preventing the tibia from being displaced anteriorly or posteriorly.

The movement of the patella also needs to be noted. In maximal flexion of the joint there is no contact between the facets on the patella and the articular patellar surface on the anterior aspect of the lower end of the femur. In this position only the narrow vertical facet you can see on the medial aspect of the articular surface of the patella is in contact with a crescentic facet on the anterior end of the lower surface of the medial condyle of the femur. As the knee straightens, the anterior patellar surface on the lower end of the femur comes into contact first with the middle and then with the lower facets of the articular surface of the patella.

Several muscles are concerned in bringing about flexion of the knee joint (the hamstring muscles, the sartorius and gracilis, and also the gastrocnemius). The main extensor is, of course, the quadriceps femoris muscle. As already observed, the lateral rotation which takes place in the unlocking of the knee joint is brought about by the popliteus. Medial rotation is mainly a passive movement which occurs because of the shape of the medial condyle. Remember again that the iliotibial tract and the muscles inserted into it (e.g. the tensor fasciae latae and the gluteus maximus) play a very important part in keeping the knee stable. Try to analyse these various movements and the muscles responsible for them on yourself.

The interosseous membrane of the leg

The origins of the muscles of the leg

Remove the tendon of the biceps femoris from its insertion into the head of the fibula, and note again how it is wrapped around the fibular collateral ligament of the knee joint. Confirm the origins of the **peroneus longus** and **peroneus brevis** muscles from the lateral surface of the fibula, and remove them from their attachments. Cut the tendons of the two muscles just above the level of the lateral malleolus, and remove the bellies of the muscles. Confirm the origins of the **extensor hallucis longus,** the **extensor digitorum longus,** and the **peroneus tertius** muscles from the medial surface of the fibula and remove them from the bone. Divide their tendons at the level of the ankle joint and then remove the

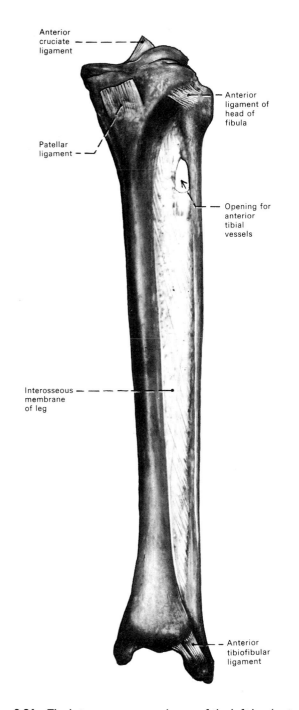

Anterior
cruciate
ligament

Anterior
ligament of
head of
fibula

Patellar
ligament

Opening for
anterior
tibial
vessels

Interosseous
membrane
of leg

Anterior
tibiofibular
ligament

Fig. 2.84 The interosseous membrane of the left leg (anterior view).

bellies of the muscles. Confirm the origin of the **tibialis anterior muscle** from the lateral surface of the tibia and the interosseous membrane of the leg [Fig. 2.84]. Remove the muscle, but take care not to injure the underlying membrane. Divide the tendon of the muscle at the level of the ankle joint, again completely removing the belly of the muscle.

Now divide the tendo calcaneus 5 cm above its insertion into the calcaneum, and remove the superficial muscles of the calf and the vessels and nerves deep to them. Confirm that the **flexor digitorum longus muscle** arises from the posterior surface of the shaft of the tibia, and the **tibialis posterior muscle** from the posterior surface of the shaft of the tibia, lateral to the flexor digitorum longus, and from the posterior surface of the fibula, anterior to the medial crest, as well as from the intervening interosseous membrane.

Confirm, too, that the **flexor hallucis longus muscle** arises from the posterior surface of the body of the fibula (behind the medial crest) and from the interosseous membrane.

Remove first the flexor digitorum longus, then the flexor hallucis longus, and finally the tibialis posterior muscle, again taking care not to damage the interosseous membrane. Divide their tendons at the level of the ankle joint and remove the bellies of the muscles.

The interosseous membrane

Note that the fibres of the interosseous membrane run downwards and laterally from the tibia to the fibula [Fig. 2.84]. The large oval opening you can see through the membrane transmits the anterior tibial vessels as they pass to the front of the leg. Below, you may see the opening for the perforating branch of the peroneal artery. Note now that the membrane is continuous below with the interosseous tibiofibular ligament of the tibiofibular syndesmosis (or distal tibiofibular joint), which will be examined later.

The ankle joint

Now turn your attention to the ankle joint, which is an articulation between the lower ends of the tibia and fibula, and the talus. The ankle joint is a synovial hinge joint allowing two movements only, plantar-flexion and dorsiflexion, which take place around a transverse axis. Plantar-flexion is brought about by gastrocnemius, soleus, tibialis posterior, and the two long flexors, and dorsiflexion by the tibialis anterior and the two long extensors. Confirm this on yourself.

The articular capsule and ligaments of the ankle joint

Clean the surface of the joint in order to demonstrate the articular capsule. Note that this is attached to the margins of the articular surfaces, which you should examine on the skeleton. You can see that the anterior and posterior surfaces of the capsule are weak. Examine the lateral surface [Fig. 2.85]. By blunt dissection you should make out that this is strengthened by three ligaments which are attached to the lateral malleolus. You should be able to make out an anterior ligamentous band, the **anterior talofibular ligament,** which passes horizontally forwards from the lateral malleolus and is attached to the neck of the talus; and a middle band, the **calcaneofibular ligament,** which passes

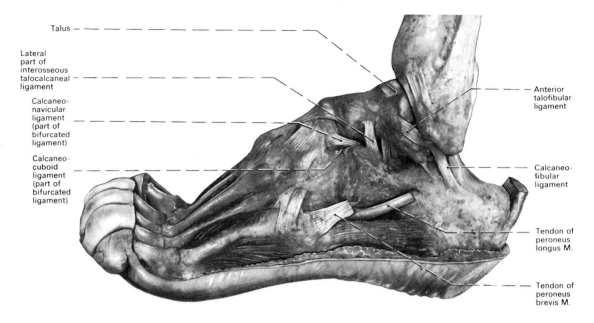

Talus

Lateral part of interosseous talocalcaneal ligament

Calcaneo-navicular ligament (part of bifurcated ligament)

Calcaneo-cuboid ligament (part of bifurcated ligament)

Anterior talofibular ligament

Calcaneo-fibular ligament

Tendon of peroneus longus M.

Tendon of peroneus brevis M.

Fig. 2.85   The lateral aspect of the left ankle joint.

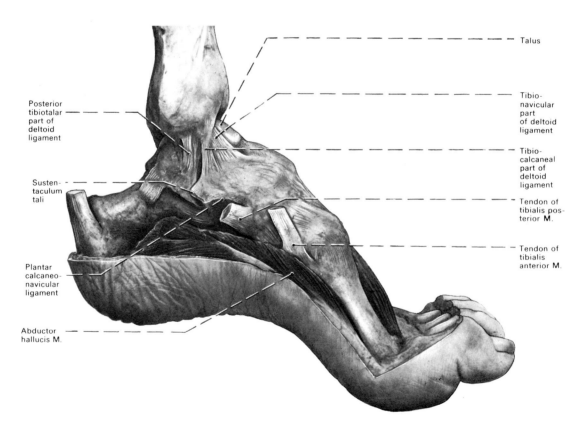

Posterior tibiotalar part of deltoid ligament

Susten-taculum tali

Plantar calcaneo-navicular ligament

Abductor hallucis M.

Talus

Tibio-navicular part of deltoid ligament

Tibio-calcaneal part of deltoid ligament

Tendon of tibialis pos-terior M.

Tendon of tibialis anterior M.

Fig. 2.86   The medial aspect of the left ankle joint.

downwards to be attached to the calcaneum. The posterior band, the **posterior talofibular ligament** [Fig. 2.88] lies more deeply, and passes horizontally backwards from the lateral malleolar fossa, on the medial aspect of the lateral malleolus behind the articular facet, to become attached to the body of the talus. Examine these ligaments carefully and especially note the position and attachments of the anterior talofibular ligament. Some of the fibres of this ligament are torn in the common condition of sprained ankle.

Now examine the medial aspect of the ankle [Fig. 2.86]. Blunt dissection and teasing with your scalpel will show you that here the capsule is strengthened by a strong triangular ligament, called the **deltoid ligament,** which is attached by its apex to the medial malleolus. The ligament has two sets of fibres, superficial and deep. The superficial set consists of three bands of fibres which, unlike the lateral ligaments, are continuous with each other. Trace the fibres of the anterior band, called the **tibionavicular part** of the ligament, to the tuberosity of the navicular bone. Some also run into an important ligament which bridges the gap between the

sustentaculum tali of the calcaneum and the plantar surface of the navicular bone. This is a thick triangular ligament, with articular cartilage on its upper surface, which is called the plantar calcaneonavicular ligament. Trace the middle band of the superficial fibres, the **tibiocalcaneal part,** to the sustentaculum tali, and the posterior band, the **posterior tibiotalar part,** to the medial side of the talus.

Dissect deep to the anterior superficial fibres and follow the deeper fibres of the deltoid ligament, the **anterior tibiotalar part,** to the non-articular part of the medial surface of the talus.

The tibiofibular joints

The tibiofibular syndesmosis

Now turn to the distal tibiofibular joint, or tibiofibular syndesmosis, which usually lacks a synovial cavity and is a fibrous joint or syndesmosis. You will see that an **anterior tibiofibular ligament** [Fig. 2.87] extends obliquely downwards and laterally between the adjacent margins of the tibia and fibula on the front of the joint.

Examine the posterior surface of the joint [Fig. 2.88]. By teasing with the point of your scalpel you should be able to make out the **posterior tibiofibular ligament.** The lower fibres of this ligament form the **inferior transverse ligament,** which runs transversely from the upper part of the lateral malleolar fossa on the fibula to the posterior border of the articular surface of the tibia. Next examine the inferior border of the interosseous membrane. It is thickened to form the **interosseous tibiofibular ligament.**

Now cut the anterior part of the articular capsule of the ankle joint, as well as the anterior talofibular and the calcaneofibular ligaments [Figs 2.85 and 2.87]. Open the joint and examine the articular surfaces of the bones, noting their shapes. Confirm that the superior articular surface of the talus is wedge-shaped, the wide end of the wedge being directed forwards. This arrangement prevents the leg moving too far forwards on the foot. It is also a limiting factor in dorsiflexion.

The tibiofibular joint

Now examine the proximal tibiofibular joint which is a synovial joint. Note that its capsule is strengthened by the **anterior** and **posterior ligaments of the head of the fibula** [Fig. 2.84]. Incise the capsule and separate the head of the fibula from the tibia. Try to determine whether the joint cavity in your specimen communicates with the subpopliteal recess.

Divide the interosseous membrane as far down as the interosseous tibiofibular ligament, and cut through the anterior tibiofibular ligament. You can now see that the interosseous ligament is very strong. Incise it, and examine the articular surfaces of the tibiofibular syndesmosis, noting the cartilage at their lower ends.

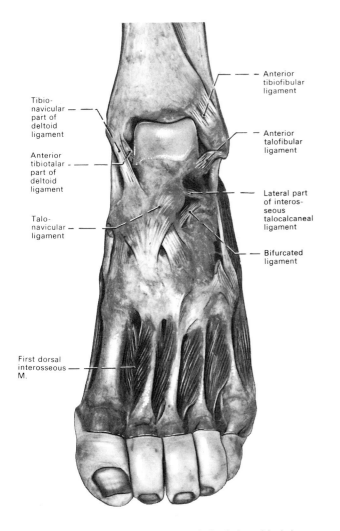

Tibio-navicular part of deltoid ligament

Anterior tibiotalar part of deltoid ligament

Talo-navicular ligament

First dorsal interosseous M.

Anterior tibiofibular ligament

Anterior talofibular ligament

Lateral part of interosseous talocalcaneal ligament

Bifurcated ligament

Fig. 2.87   The anterior aspect of the left ankle joint.

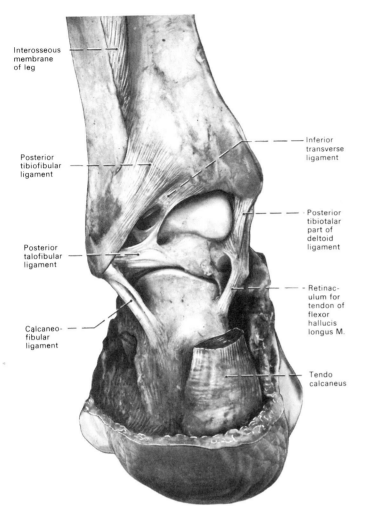

Interosseous
membrane
of leg

Posterior
tibiofibular
ligament

Posterior
talofibular
ligament

Calcaneo-
fibular
ligament

Inferior
transverse
ligament

Posterior
tibiotalar
part of
deltoid
ligament

Retinac-
ulum for
tendon of
flexor
hallucis
longus M.

Tendo
calcaneus

Fig. 2.88 The posterior aspect of the left ankle joint.

The joints of the foot

Turn your attention to the joints of the foot. The intertarsal joints are synovial plane joints allowing gliding movements, as well as some degree of rotation. The latter movements are associated with inversion and eversion. The articular capsules between the tarsal bones are thickened to form **dorsal tarsal ligaments** and **plantar tarsal ligaments,** and the bones are also held together by strong **interosseous tarsal ligaments.**

As in the case of the corresponding joints of the hand, the tarsometatarsal joints are synovial plane joints; the metatarsophalangeal joints are synovial condyloid joints; and the interphalangeal joints of the foot are synovial hinge joints.

The subtalar joint

Divide the deltoid ligament [Fig. 2.86] and the remaining ligaments of the ankle joint below their upper attachments,

thereby removing the tibia and fibula from the foot. Next demonstrate the movements of inversion and eversion of the foot by holding the body of the talus and turning the foot outwards and inwards. Try to determine for yourself the joints at which these movements take place. You will see that they take place mainly at the subtalar and talo-calcaneonavicular joints. Note that inversion is caused by the contraction of the tibialis anterior and tibialis posterior muscles, and eversion by that of the peroneus longus and brevis muscles. Try to analyse these movements on yourself.

With an articulated skeleton and separate tarsal bones available for reference, define the **interosseous talocalcaneal ligament** [Fig. 2.89]. It is attached above to the groove of the talus and below to the groove of the calcaneum [see p. 2.44]. Remove the talus by incising the posterior part of the capsule of the posterior talocalcaneal joint, which is called the subtalar joint, the deep fibres of the deltoid ligament, the dorsal talonavicular ligament [Fig. 2.87], and finally the interosseous talocalcaneal ligament. The latter is best divided by carrying the blade of the scalpel in a postero-medial direction, first cutting its most anterior fibres. Now examine the articular surfaces of the talus again.

When the talus has been removed, examine the articular surfaces of the subtalar joint [Fig. 2.89]. This joint is an articulation between the posterior concave articular facet on the inferior surface of the talus and the convex facet on the posterior aspect of the superior articular suface of the calcaneum. The capsule is reinforced by a **lateral talo-calcaneal ligament,** a **medial talocalcaneal ligament,** as well as by weak anterior and posterior ligaments. The two bones, however, are mainly held together by the interosseous talo-calcaneal ligament, which you have already seen. This ligament separates the subtalar joint posteriorly from the talo-calcaneonavicular joint anteriorly, and is common to both.

The talocalcaneonavicular joint

Now examine the articular surfaces of the talocalcaneo-navicular joint. This joint is a ball and socket joint in which the hemispherical head of the talus articulates with the pos-terior concave articular surface on the navicular bone, with the anterior articular facet on the superior surface of the calcaneum, and with the upper or dorsal surface of the plantar calcaneonavicular ligament. The joint, which allows considerable rotatory and gliding movements, has a thin capsule which is strengthened posteriorly by the interosseous talocalcaneal ligament.

Examine the articular cartilage on the important **plantar calcaneonavicular ligament** to which the deltoid ligament is attached, and the remains of the interosseous talocalcaneal ligament in the tarsal sinus [p. 2.45], noting again that the latter ligament separates the subtalar joint from the talo-calcaneonavicular joint. Clean the plantar surface of the plantar calcaneonavicular ligament [Fig. 2.90] and note that it connects the anterior margin of the sustentaculum tali of

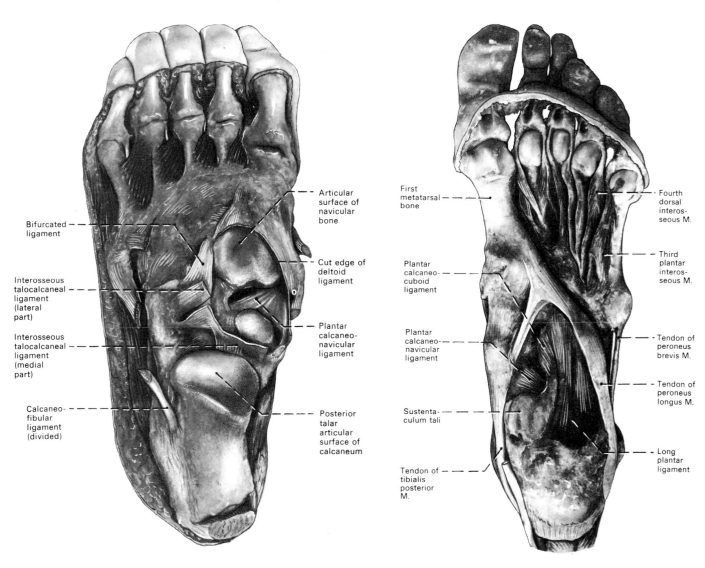

Fig. 2.89 The left subalar and talocalcaneonavicular joints. The talus has been excised.

Fig. 2.90 The plantar ligaments of the left foot. The distal part of the long plantar ligament has been excised to expose the tendon of the peroneus longus muscle as it lies in its groove on the cuboid bone.

the calcaneum to the plantar surface of the navicular bone. Confirm that the ligament is supported by the tendons of the deep calf muscles which are in contact with it, and especially by the tendons of the tibialis posterior and flexor hallucis longus muscles, which lie beneath it. The plantar calcaneonavicular ligament helps to support the head of the talus. It also limits eversion and so plays a part in preventing 'flat-foot'.

Next clean a strong Y-shaped band which is attached by its stem to the anterior part of the upper surface of the calcaneum. This is the **bifurcated ligament** [Fig. 2.89]. The medial limb of the Y forms part of the socket of the talo-calcaneonavicular joint, and is fixed to the lateral surface of navicular bone. The lateral limb of the Y is attached to the medial surface of the cuboid bone [Fig. 2.85].

The calcaneocuboid joint

Divide the bifurcated ligament and the dorsi-lateral part of the articular capsule of the calcaneocuboid joint and examine that joint. The calcaneocuboid joint is a synovial plane joint between the anterior surface of the calcaneum and the posterior surface of the cuboid bone. The articular capsule is strengthened by the lateral limb of the bifurcated ligament dorsally and by the **long plantar ligament** and the **plantar calcaneocuboid ligament** on the plantar surface of the foot [Fig. 2.90]. The joint allows limited rotatory and gliding movements. The calcaneocuboid and talocalcaneo-navicular joints extend across the foot, and are sometimes collectively referred to as the **transverse tarsal joint.** Most of the movement of inversion or eversion takes place in the transverse tarsal and subtalar joints.

Re-examine the long plantar ligament and the plantar calcaneocuboid ligament and the tendon of the peroneus longus muscle distal to them. Divide the long plantar ligament across its middle in order to get a more complete view of the plantar calcaneocuboid ligament. Note the relation of the latter to the calcaneocuboid joint.

The small joints of the foot

Examine the other **intertarsal, tarsometatarsal,** and **intermetatarsal joints,** noting that the first tarsometatarsal joint is isolated. The arrangement of these joints is similar to the corresponding ones in the hand.

Finally, examine the **metatarsophalangeal** and **interphalangeal joints,** and note that the dorsal digital expansions are similar to those you found in the fingers [p. 1.69]. Demonstrate the **articular capsules** and the **plantar** and **collateral ligaments** of these joints; they are also similar to those of the hand.

The arches of the foot

When one is standing, the sole of the foot does not make contact everywhere on the ground [Fig. 2.91]. The normal foot is arched both longitudinally and transversely, the arching being caused primarily by the conformation of the bones of the foot and the ligaments which bind them together, and secondarily, by the muscles which act upon the bones. The **longitudinal arch of the foot** is higher on the medial side, where it forms the instep [Fig. 2.91]. On the lateral side, the foot is in contact with the ground. The **transverse arch of the foot** can be most easily seen in a section which passes through the cuneiform and cuboid bones, or through the bases of the metatarsal bones. The shape of the arches depends primarily on the way the bones of the foot articulate with each other, but since a small amount of movement can take place at their articulations, the arches undergo minor degrees of deformation as the load they can bear is altered.

Every ligament that connects the bones of the foot plays a part in the maintenance of the arches, but some which pass across two or more articulations are especially important. Among these are the long plantar ligament, the plantar calcaneocuboid ligament, and the plantar calcaneonavicular ligament, on which the head of the talus rests [Fig. 2.90]. Whilst the normal tone of the small intrinsic muscles of the foot also plays an essential part in keeping the arches intact, the long muscles which are inserted by tendons into the bones of the foot have an even more important role. Thus, the tendon of the tibialis anterior muscle is inserted into the medial cuneiform bone and the base of the first metatarsal bone, both of which will consequently be kept elevated because of the tonic contraction of the muscle. Similarly, the tendon of the tibialis posterior muscle passes across the sustentaculum tali and the plantar calcaneonavicular ligament, thus supporting the talus, before being inserted not only into the tuberosity of the navicular bone but also into each of the other tarsal bones, with the exception of the talus. By means of its multiple insertions the tonic contraction of the tibialis posterior tends to draw the bones of the foot together, thus maintaining the arches. The peroneus

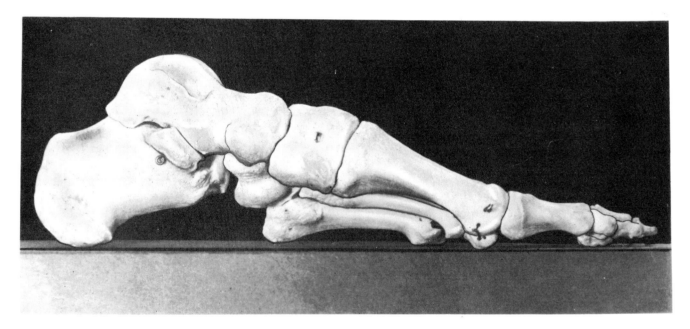

a. *The skeleton of the left foot (viewed from the medial side).* (Note the relative heights of the medial and lateral parts of the longitudinal arch.)

Fig. 2.91 The arches of the foot.

longus muscle, again, passes around the lateral side of the foot and runs transversely across the sole to the base of the first metatarsal and medial cuneiform bones [Fig. 2.90]. This muscle, therefore, acts as a sling to maintain the longitudinal arch, and as it passes transversely across the sole it strengthens the transverse arch. Finally, the tendons of the flexor hallucis longus and the flexor digitorum longus pass beneath the talus and run longitudinally through the sole. To some extent, therefore, they too help to maintain the integrity of the instep.

The fact that the medial side of the foot bears the greatest strain in walking and standing, and that its arch is higher and more resilient, can be related to its more powerful muscular support. When the balance of power shifts to the lateral muscles of the calf, and the action of the evertors thus becomes dominant, the condition of 'flat-foot' may result.

Movements such as adduction and abduction of the toes are very limited, in contrast to what occurs in monkeys and apes. Thus, although the abductor hallucis is a large and powerful muscle, few adults can abduct the great toe (the great toe is more mobile in children). The lumbrical and interosseous muscles in the foot are correspondingly less important than their counterparts in the hand. On the other hand, the interosseous muscles of the foot help to control the position of the toes and therefore help to propel the body forward in walking. The intrinsic muscles also help to maintain the arches of the foot, which they span.

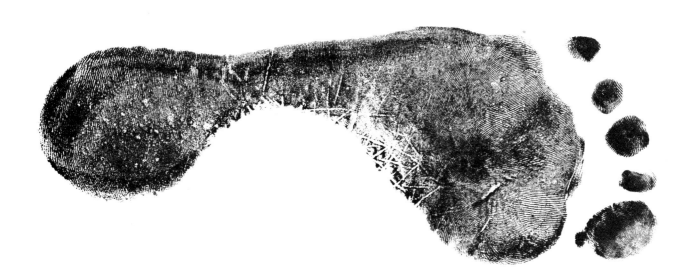

Fig. 2.91 b. *The print of the left foot* (*when standing*). (Note that the heel, the lateral border of the sole, the ball of the foot, and the pads of the toes are in contact with the ground.)

Chart of contents of the thorax

Thoracic wall

COMPONENTS	REGIONS	
	Pectoral	**Back**
Bones	sternum, costal cartilages, ribs	ribs, vertebrae, [scapula]
Joints	sternocostal costochondral interchondral	costovertebral costotransverse intervertebral
Muscles	intercostal related upper limb muscles	spinal extensors related upper limb muscles
Nerves	ventral rami of thoracic nerves [intercostal nerves]	dorsal rami of thoracic nerves
Vessels	intercostal	spinal
Organs	breast	spinal medulla

Thoracic cavity

	REGIONS				
		Mediastinum			
	Pleuropulmonary	**Superior**	**Inferior**		
			Anterior	Middle	Posterior
CONTENTS	pleura lungs, bronchi pulmonary vessels lymph nodes	thymus oesophagus vagus nerves sympathetic trunks phrenic nerves trachea arch of aorta brachiocephalic Vs thoracic duct	fat lymph nodes	phrenic nerves pericardium heart pulmonary trunk ascending aorta coronary arteries veins of heart venae cavae	oesophagus vagus nerves sympathetic trunks descending aorta azygos veins thoracic duct
Superior boundary	superior aperture of thorax	plane of sternal angle			
Inferior boundary	diaphragm	plane of sternal angle	diaphragm		

Part 3

The thorax

The main organs which you will examine in your dissection of the thorax are the lungs and heart. The aorta, which is the channel by which arterial blood leaves the heart, arches above the heart and then descends on the posterior thoracic wall. Also leaving the heart is the pulmonary trunk carrying venous blood to be oxygenated in the lungs. Entering the heart are the pulmonary veins, which return the oxygenated blood from the lungs to the heart. Above the heart are the large veins that drain the head and neck and upper limbs, converging into right and left brachiocephalic veins, which unite to form the superior vena cava. This large vein opens directly into the heart, as does also the inferior vena cava, which drains the lower half of the body.

On the posterior wall of the thoracic cavity, the oesophagus descends from the neck into the abdomen. In front of the oesophagus is the trachea, which divides into left and right main bronchi. These enter the lungs through the roots of the lungs. The space between the lungs in the midline of the chest, which is occupied largely by the heart and great vessels, is called the mediastinum.

Below, the thoracic cavity is shut off from the abdominal cavity by a large dome-shaped muscle called the diaphragm. This not only forms the floor of the thorax but is also the principal muscle of respiration.

Section 3.1
The chest wall

Osteology

Before you start dissecting, you should study the bones which make up the thoracic cage, beginning with the vertebrae.

The vertebral column

The vertebral column consists of thirty-three vertebrae, made up of seven **cervical vertebrae,** twelve **thoracic vertebrae,** five **lumbar vertebrae,** five **sacral vertebrae,** and four **coccygeal vertebrae.**

The **bodies of the vertebrae** are united to one another by fibrocartilaginous **intervertebral discs,** except in the sacral and coccygeal regions, where they are fused together. You will study the sacrum when you dissect the abdomen.

The curves of the vertebral column

Look at the vertebral column of an articulated skeleton [Fig. 3.1]. You will see that it has four curves. The thoracic and sacral curves are convex backwards, and are called **primary curves,** because they are present at birth. The cervical and lumbar curves are convex forward. The first is acquired when the infant begins to hold up its head and neck, and the second when the baby sits and later stands. The cervical and lumbar curves are, therefore, known as **secondary curves.**

The parts of a vertebra

All vertebrae are constructed on the same general plan. As an example of this plan, examine a vertebra from the mid-thoracic region [Fig. 3.2]. It consists of a **body** from which two bars of bone, called the **pedicles of the vertebral arch,** project backwards. The borders of the pedicles are notched, and in the articulated vertebral column the notches on contiguous vertebrae help to form the **intervertebral foramina,** through which pass the spinal nerves.

From the pedicles two thin plates of bone called the **laminae of the vertebral arch** pass medially and posteriorly. These are united in the midline behind. A prominent **spinous process** projects posteriorly from the united laminae. At the junction of the pedicle and lamina a bar

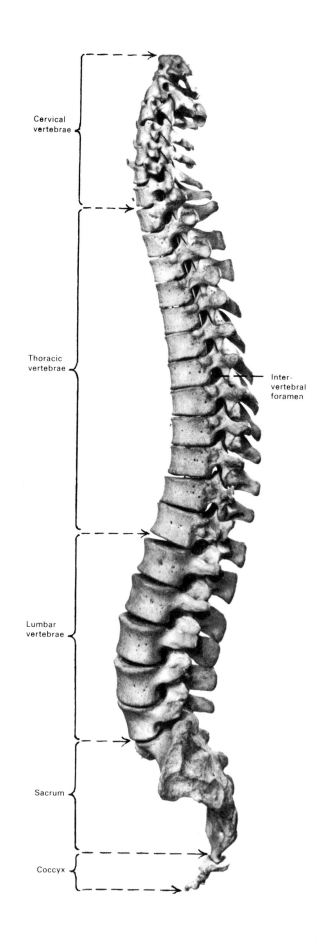

Cervical vertebrae

Thoracic vertebrae

Intervertebral foramen

Lumbar vertebrae

Sacrum

Coccyx

Fig. 3.1 The vertebral column (viewed from the left side).

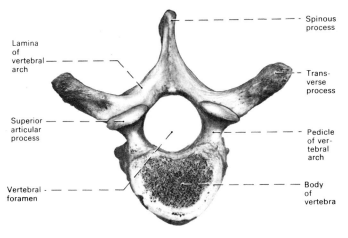

a. Viewed from above

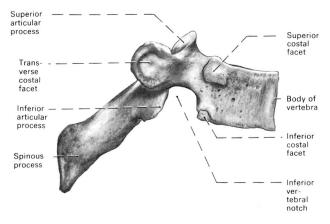

b. Viewed from the right side

Fig. 3.2 The fifth thoracic vertebra.

of bone, called the **transverse process,** projects laterally. From the same region **superior** and **inferior articular processes** project superiorly and inferiorly. These articulate with the reciprocal processes of adjacent vertebrae. The vertebral body, pedicles, and laminae bound a space, called the **vertebral foramen,** which is occupied by the spinal medulla and its coverings. Pedicles and laminae together form the vertebral arch.

The cervical vertebrae

Now examine a vertebra from the mid-cervical region [Fig. 3.3]. It has the same general features, but can be readily distinguished by the following characteristics. The spinous process is bifid; there is a foramen, the **foramen transversarium,** in each transverse process; the vertebral foramen is triangular; the body is small and the lateral margins of its upper surface are turned upwards. The lower

surface is concavo-convex. In the cervical region the intervertebral discs do not extend to the lateral extremities of the bodies. Here synovial joints intervene beween adjacent vertebrae.

The first and second cervical vertebrae are atypical, and are discussed in the section dealing with the head and neck [see p. 5.3].

The thoracic vertebrae

Now again examine a typical thoracic vertebra [Fig. 3.2]. Note that among its distinguishing features are half-facets on the supero-lateral and infero-lateral aspects of the body, and a whole facet on each transverse process. The former are for articulation with the heads of ribs, and the latter for articulation with the tubercle of the rib [see p. 3.5].

Look at the first thoracic vertebra and note that it has a whole facet on the upper part of its body for the first rib (which does not articulate with the seventh cervical vertebra), and a half-facet on the lower part of its body for the upper facet on the head of the second rib. Examine the tenth, eleventh, and twelfth thoracic vertebrae, and you will see that each of them has only one facet on the body, and that in addition the eleventh and twelfth vertebrae have no facets on their transverse processes.

The lumbar vertebrae

Examine a vertebra from the mid-lumbar region [Fig. 3.4]. You will see that it is characterized by a large kidney-shaped body, short pedicles, long and slender transverse processes, thick laminae, a triangular vertebral foramen, and a horizontally-directed quadrate spinous process. You can immediately tell that a vertebra belongs to the lumbar series by the absence of facets for ribs, as occur in the thoracic vertebrae, and by the absence of foramina in the transverse processes, as occur in the cervical vertebrae. Although lumbar vertebrae are larger than those from any other part of the vertebral column, this is not a feature that can be relied upon when identifying individual vertebrae.

The sternum

Refer again to the sternum, which you examined when dissecting the upper limb [Fig. 3.5]. It consists of the **manubrium** of the sternum, the **body** of the sternum, and the **xiphoid process.** On the upper border of the manubrium is the **jugular notch.** At the junction of the manubrium with the body is the **sternal angle.** From above down the lateral border of the sternum articulates with the clavicle and with the costal cartilages, which join the upper seven ribs to the sternum. Apart from the first sternocostal joint, all these articulations are synovial joints.

The ribs

Examine the ribs on an articulated skeleton [Fig. 3.6]. Note that there are twelve pairs. The upper seven, which are

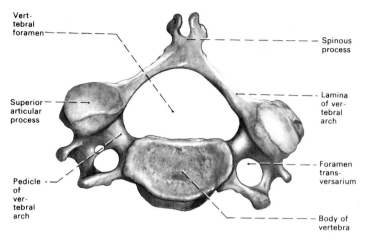

a. *Viewed from above*

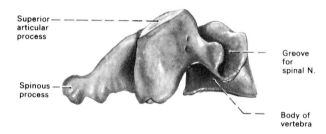

b. *viewed from the right side*

Fig. 3.3 A typical cervical vertebra.

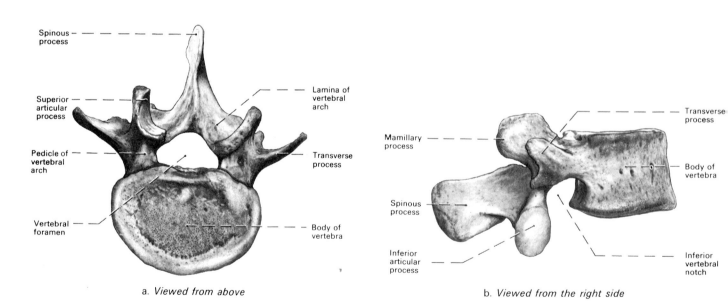

a. *Viewed from above*

b. *Viewed from the right side*

Fig. 3.4 The third lumbar vertebra.

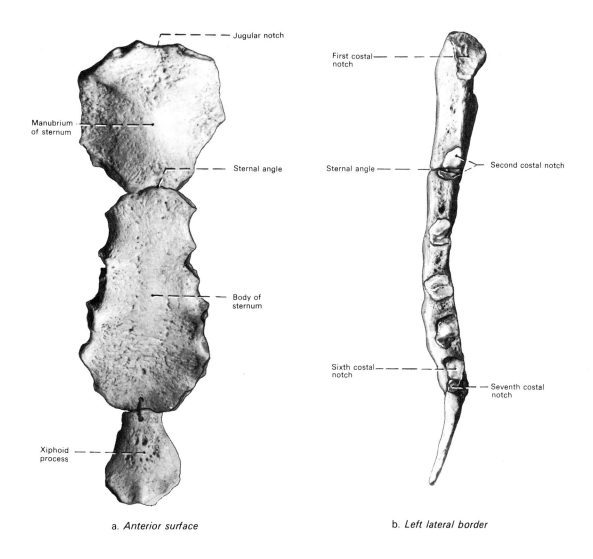

a. *Anterior surface*   b. *Left lateral border*

Fig. 3.5 The sternum.

known as **true ribs,** will be seen to be attached by their costal cartilages to the sternum. The lower five are known as **false ribs.** The costal cartilages of the eighth, ninth, and tenth ribs articulate with the cartilage immediately above, and hence these three ribs are attached to the sternum indirectly. The lowest two ribs end in free extremities: they are known as **floating ribs.**

The parts of a rib

Examine a typical rib, and note that it presents a **head,** a **neck,** a **tubercle,** and a **shaft** [Fig. 3.7]. The head will be seen to be divided by the **crest of the head** of the rib into an upper and a lower facet. Articulate a typical rib (one from about the middle of the thorax) with two typical thoracic vertebrae. You will see that the lower facet on the head articulates

with a half-facet on the supero-lateral aspect of the body of the corresponding vertebra, and the upper facet with a similar facet on the infero-lateral aspect of the vertebra above. The crest between the two facets, which fits between the vertebral bodies, is attached by the intra-articular ligament of the head of the rib to the intervertebral disc.

The tubercle of the rib will be seen to articulate with the transverse process of the corresponding vertebra.

On the lower part of the internal surface of the shaft of a typical rib is a deep groove. This **costal groove** lodges the intercostal vessels and nerve, the vein above the artery, and the nerve below it.

Note that the shaft of a typical rib is bent forwards and also twisted a short distance lateral to the tubercle, at what is called the **angle of the rib.**

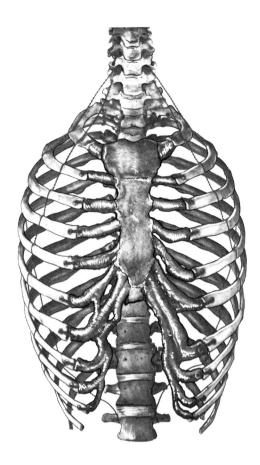

Fig. 3.6 The skeleton of the thorax (anterior view).

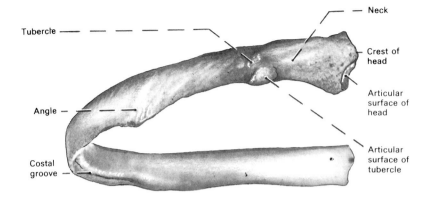

Fig. 3.7 The left fifth rib (viewed from behind).

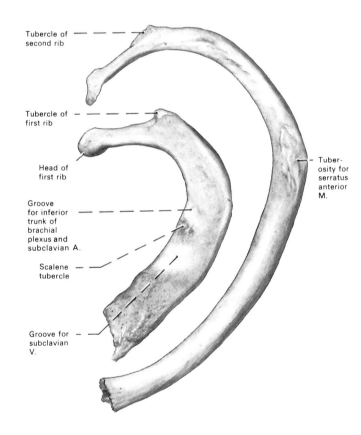

Fig. 3.8 The left first and second ribs (viewed from above).

The first rib

The first, second, tenth, eleventh, and twelfth ribs are atypical. Examine a first rib [Fig. 3.8]. It will be found to be short, flat, and more sharply curved than any of the others. It has upper and lower surfaces, with outer and inner borders, and on its head there is one articular facet only. This articulates with the body of the first thoracic vertebra. On the inner border of this rib is a small projection called the **scalene tubercle.** In front of the tubercle you will see a groove. This lodges the subclavian vein. Behind it is another groove for the inferior trunk of the brachial plexus [see p. 5.15]. The depth of the grooves varies from specimen to specimen.

The second rib

Now examine the second rib [Fig. 3.8]. It is markedly curved and is characterized by a rough area on its outer border from which a powerful part of the serratus anterior muscle arises.

The lowest three ribs

Look at the tenth rib. It usually has one facet only on the head. The eleventh and twelfth ribs are small, the twelfth more so than the eleventh, and both lack tubercles and necks. The twelfth is further distinguished by the fact that it has no angle.

You will notice that in all these atypical ribs the costal groove is either poorly marked or is absent altogether.

The thoracic cage

Look again at a skeleton. Note that the adult thorax is kidney-shaped on transverse section (it is more rounded in children), and that the posterior wall extends much more inferiorly than does the anterior. The xiphisternal junction lies level with the medial end of the seventh costal cartilage, and opposite the intervertebral disc between the ninth and tenth thoracic vertebrae [Fig. 3.6]. Note that the sternal angle is at the level of the second costal cartilage in front. Now look at the **superior aperture of the thorax.** You will see that its plane is oblique, with its posterior margin at a higher level than the anterior, and that it is bounded in front by the jugular notch, at the sides by the first ribs, and behind by the body of the first thoracic vertebra. Note the narrowness of the opening, although through it the blood vessels (some of which are very large), nerves, and lymphatics, as well as the trachea and oesophagus, enter or leave the **thoracic cavity.** In addition the superior aperture of the thorax accommodates the apices of the lungs. These ascend for 3 cm into the neck, reaching as high as the necks of the first ribs.

Examine the way the ribs lie in the skeleton. They pass obliquely downwards and forwards from the vertebral column. Note that the **intercostal spaces** are wider in front than behind.

The thoracic cage not only protects the thoracic viscera, but also the liver, spleen, and suprarenal glands, and to a lesser extent, the stomach and kidneys.

Surface anatomy

Feel on your own chest and identify the sternal angle at the junction of the manubrium with the body of the sternum. A line projected horizontally backwards from the sternal angle, where the second costal cartilage joins the sternum, would pass through the intervertebral disc between the fourth and fifth thoracic vertebrae. This plane can be conveniently called the **plane of the sternal angle.** Note, too, that the sternal angle is a useful reference point from which to count the ribs. You will find that the first rib is scarcely palpable. The first intercostal space can, however, be readily identified between the first and second ribs.

Dissection of the chest wall

Begin by examining the remains of the pectoralis major, pectoralis minor, serratus anterior, and latissimus dorsi muscles [Figs 3.9 and 3.10], which were divided when the upper limb was removed [p. 1.23]. As the remains of each

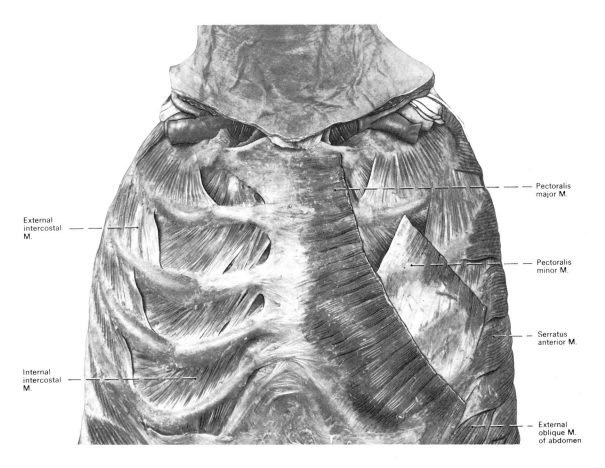

External intercostal M.

Internal intercostal M.

Pectoralis major M.

Pectoralis minor M.

Serratus anterior M.

External oblique M. of abdomen

Fig. 3.9 The anterior chest wall. On the right side the pectoral muscles, the serratus anterior muscle, and the external intercostal membranes have been excised.

3.7

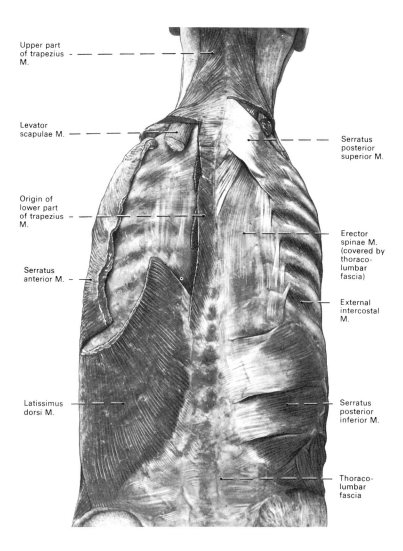

Upper part
of trapezius
M.

Levator
scapulae M.

Origin of
lower part
of trapezius
M.

Serratus
anterior M.

Latissimus
dorsi M.

Serratus
posterior
superior M.

Erector
spinae M.
(covered by
thoraco-
lumbar
fascia)

External
intercostal
M.

Serratus
posterior
inferior M.

Thoraco-
lumbar
fascia

Fig. 3.10 The posterior chest wall. On the right side the latissimus dorsi and serratus anterior muscles have been excised.

muscle are identified they should be removed entirely from the chest wall. In removing the lower half of the serratus anterior take care not to cut the slips of origin of the external oblique muscle of the abdomen, one of the muscles of the abdominal wall with which the serratus anterior is in very close relation.

As you clear away the muscles, identify, but do not spend undue time dissecting, the lateral cutaneous branches of the intercostal nerves, which you will encounter emerging from the lateral surface of the chest wall, the small perforating branches of the internal thoracic arteries, and the anterior cutaneous branches of the intercostal nerves, which you will find piercing the pectoralis major near the lateral margin of the sternum. On the posterior aspect of the trunk you will see the serratus posterior superior and the serratus posterior inferior [Fig. 3.10], two thin muscles which extend between the vertebrae and the ribs. In the undissected body

the former is covered by the upper part of trapezius and by the levator scapulae. Having identified the muscles, do not spend further time on their dissection.

The external intercostal muscles [Figs 3.9 and 3.10]

Now clean the superficial muscles which fill the spaces between any two or three pairs of ribs. They are called the external intercostal muscles. Observe that their fibres run downwards, forwards, and medially. Anteriorly the muscles are absent, being replaced by a band of shiny fascia called the **external intercostal membrane.**

Dissect away the external intercostal membrane from the upper four intercostal spaces, and then, cutting carefully with a scalpel, separate the external intercostal muscle from its upper attachment in two of the spaces you have cleaned. Begin anteriorly and continue backwards as far as the angle of the rib. You will see that the muscle is very thin anteriorly

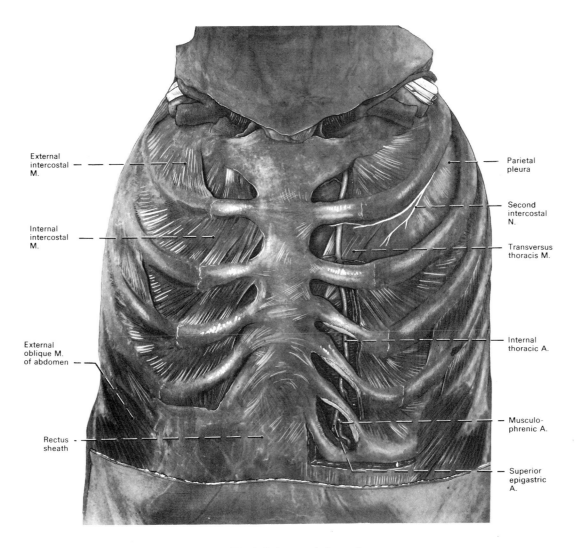

External
intercostal
M.

Internal
intercostal
M.

External
oblique M.
of abdomen

Rectus
sheath

Parietal
pleura

Second
intercostal
N.

Transversus
thoracis M.

Internal
thoracic A.

Musculo-
phrenic A.

Superior
epigastric
A.

Fig. 3.11 The left internal thoracic artery.

and that it thickens as you proceed posteriorly. Turn the muscle down, taking care not to damage the underlying lateral cutaneous branch of the intercostal nerve. Then separate the muscle from its lower attachment, again beginning anteriorly. Remove the strip of muscle you have isolated from its attachments.

The internal intercostal muscles

The muscle you have now exposed is the internal intercostal muscle [Fig. 3.11]. You will see that its fibres run at right angles to those of the external intercostal muscles, and that it reaches no further posteriorly than the angles of the ribs.

You should now detach the upper ends of two muscles of the anterior abdominal wall from the fifth and sixth ribs and costal cartilages. These muscles are the rectus abdominis, which has a well-marked fibrous sheath called the rectus sheath, and the external oblique muscle of the abdomen [Fig. 3.11]. Before doing this you may find it an advantage to reflect the skin downwards for a further 5 cm. Reflecting the skin will be easier if you first make a 5 cm vertical midline incision from the cut edge of the skin towards the umbilicus. Turn down the upper ends of the rectus abdominis and external oblique muscles, so that the underlying intercostal muscles are exposed.

The internal thoracic vessels [Figs 3.11 and 3.12]

Now remove the thin internal intercostal muscles from the anterior parts of the upper six intercostal spaces. You will then see an artery and its accompanying veins running deep to the costal cartilages, roughly parallel to the edge of the sternum, and between 1 and 2 cm from it. These are the **internal thoracic artery** and **veins** [Fig. 3.11]. You may also see one or two small lymph nodes in the uppermost spaces. These are the **parasternal lymph nodes.** Remove the veins

3.9

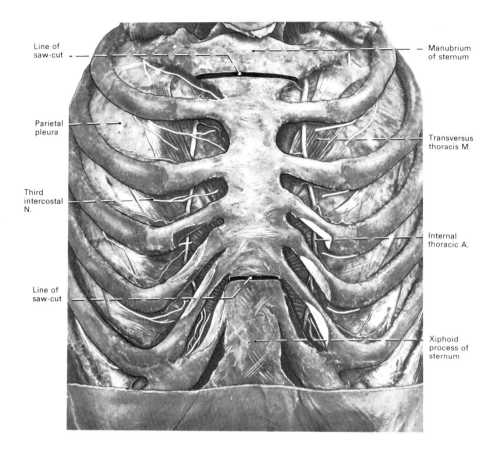

Line of saw-cut

Parietal pleura

Third intercostal N.

Line of saw-cut

Manubrium of sternum

Transversus thoracis M.

Internal thoracic A.

Xiphoid process of sternum

Fig. 3.12 The removal of the anterior chest wall (anterior view of thorax).

and nodes and follow the artery downwards to the sixth intercostal space. Now pare away the adjacent edges of the fifth, sixth, and seventh costal cartilages on one side. You will then be able to see that the internal thoracic artery divides in the sixth intercostal space into the **superior epigastric artery** and the **musculophrenic artery.** The former passes vertically downwards into the abdominal wall; the latter supplies the periphery of the diaphragm and the adjacent trunk wall. Do not follow these vessels further.

Deep to the internal thoracic artery in each intercostal space you will see some muscle fibres running obliquely upwards and laterally from the back of the sternum to the costal cartilages. These are fibres of the thin **transversus thoracis muscle** [Fig. 3.12].

The intercostal nerves [Figs 3.12 and 3.14]

Examine two or three intercostal nerves, arteries, and veins in the posterior part of their course. You will do this most easily by dissecting just under the lower border of the third, fourth, or fifth ribs near their angles. In each intercostal space trace the nerve forwards until it disappears beneath the posterior end of the internal intercostal muscle. You will find the vessels lying above the nerve, but if you trace them

forwards you may easily tear them, for they are small. Now follow the intercostal nerve towards the edge of the sternum by incising the internal intercostal muscle. As you do so, you may find the small **collateral branch** of the nerve which arises near the angle of the rib; in each space it runs forward on the upper border of the rib below. Further forwards you should find the **lateral cutaneous branch** springing from the main nerve. This branch, as you have already seen [p. 1.16], is relatively large in the second and third spaces, for it runs to the medial surface of the arm.

The muscle fibres you can see deep to the intercostal nerves, with their fibres running in the same direction as those of the internal intercostal muscles, are the **intercostales intimi.** The fibres of these muscles often span more than one intercostal space.

Each intercostal nerve supplies the intercostal muscles of the corresponding intercostal space. The distal ends of the lower six intercostal nerves extend into the abdominal wall, whose musculature they also supply. Each intercostal nerve, through its cutaneous branches, also supplies the anterior and lateral parts of an area of skin called a dermatome. Typically, each dermatome extends around the trunk from the posterior to the anterior median line, the posterior part of the dermatome being innervated by cutaneous branches of the dorsal ramus of the corresponding spinal nerve. The dermatomes of consecutive spinal nerves overlap to a considerable extent.

In addition, each intercostal nerve supplies the underlying parietal pleura, the membrane which lines each half of the thoracic cavity. Those nerves which extend on to the abdominal wall also supply the parietal peritoneum, the lining membrane of the abdominal cavity.

The intercostal muscles

After tracing two or three intercostal nerves, remove the remaining parts of both the external and internal intercostal muscles from the upper six intercostal spaces [Fig. 3.12], using the same incisions as before, and extending as far back as the angles of the ribs. You will then obtain an adequate view of the deepest layer of muscles of the chest wall (consisting anteriorly of the transversus thoracis muscle, and more laterally of the intercostales intimi). The intercostales intimi should be removed. As you do so, try not to tear the underlying pleura, which covers the lungs and lines the inside of the thorax.

Now consider the intercostal muscles as a whole [Fig. 3.11]. There are eleven **external intercostal muscles** on each side. Each muscle arises from the lower border of one rib and is inserted into the upper border of the rib below. Its fibres run downwards, forwards, and medially. The muscle extends to the tubercle of the rib posteriorly, but stops anteriorly at the junction of the ribs and costal cartilages, where it is replaced by the **external intercostal membrane.**

On a deeper plane are the eleven **internal intercostal muscles,** each arising from the floor of the costal groove of the rib forming the upper border of an intercostal space, to be inserted into the upper border of the rib below. The fibres of the internal intercostal muscles run downwards and backwards at right angles to those of the external intercostal muscles. Anteriorly each internal intercostal muscle extends to the medial end of the costal cartilage. Posteriorly it ends at the angle of the rib, where it becomes continuous with an **internal intercostal membrane.**

Deep to these muscles on the inside of the chest wall is a thin sheet of muscle, subdivided into the **transversus thoracis muscle** anteriorly [Fig. 3.12], the **subcostal muscles** near the angles of the ribs, and, between these two, the **intercostales intimi muscles.** All the intercostal muscles are concerned with respiration [see p.3.51] and are supplied by the intercostal nerves. You will have seen that these nerves run between the middle and innermost layers of muscle.

The pleura and mediastinum

The removal of the anterior chest wall

With rib shears or a saw, cut through the second to the sixth ribs, just in front of their angles [Fig. 3.14]. Take great care not to injure either the underlying pleura or the diaphragm. With a saw, cut through the manubrium of the sternum transversely just below the attachment of the first costal cartilage, first pushing back the underlying soft parts from the bony skeleton to ensure that they are not harmed [Fig. 3.12]. Divide each internal thoracic artery in the first intercostal space.

Now pull the upper end of the detached sternum from the underlying soft parts, and divide the strands of fibrous tissue, called **sternopericardial ligaments,** which attach the pericardium (the sac that covers the heart) to the posterior surface of the sternum. At the same time, carefully separate the ribs and the attached transversus thoracis muscle from the pleura and intercostal nerves. With a scalpel separate the sixth from the seventh costal cartilage on each side of the thorax. You will see they articulate together by means of a small synovial joint. Divide the superior epigastric and musculophrenic arteries in each sixth intercostal space, and then, with a saw, cut through the sternum transversely between the sixth and seventh costal cartilages. Divide the transversus thoracis muscle at its attachment to the seventh rib and costal cartilage. Having done all this, carefully lift the detached portion of the thoracic cage, leaving behind the intercostal nerves lying on the parietal pleura, to which they send sensory fibres too small for you to see.

Examine the posterior aspect of the sternum and detached ribs. You will obtain a good picture of the transversus thoracis muscle and its relation to the internal thoracic artery.

The contents of the thorax can now be studied.

The pleural cavities

First examine the pleura [Fig. 3.13]. It consists of an outer layer called the **parietal pleura,** which is normally in contact with a thin inner layer called the **pulmonary pleura.** The latter is adherent to the surface of the lung, and dips into the fissures between the lobes of the lungs. The potential space between the parietal and pulmonary layers of pleura is called the pleural cavity.

Make a large cruciate incision in the anterior part of the parietal pleura on both sides, and turn aside the flaps you form [Fig. 3.15]. Then explore the boundaries and extent of the pleural cavities with your hand. In the living body the pressure of the air in the lungs is that of the atmosphere outside, and that in the pleural 'cavity' subatmospheric, so that no real cavity exists. The pleural cavity is, however, a potential space, which normally contains a film of lymph that acts as a lubricant for the moving surfaces of the lungs. In the condition called pleurisy, fluid collects within the space, and fibrous adhesions may be formed between the two layers of pleura. If you encounter any such adhesions in your specimen, break them with your fingers.

Free the lung from the parietal pleura and pull it laterally from the mediastinum in order to expose the **root of the lung.** The parietal and pulmonary layers of pleura become continuous here [Fig. 3.13]. Below the root you will feel a small fold of pleura. This, the **pulmonary ligament,** is merely an empty extension of the pleura of the root of the lung [Fig. 3.43]. This ligament is reflected from the lung on to the pericardium, and ends below in a free border just above the diaphragm. It is of no importance.

Note that almost all the mobile viscera of the body, such as the lungs, heart, and the stomach, have a double serous coating. The principle in each case is the same. Imagine that you are pushing a finger into a rubber balloon that has only been partially filled with air. One layer of the rubber will be in contact with your finger; then there will be some air; and then an outer layer of rubber. In the case of the lungs, the outer layer of rubber is represented by the parietal pleura; the inner layer is the pulmonary pleura; while the air is represented by a thin film of tissue-fluid.

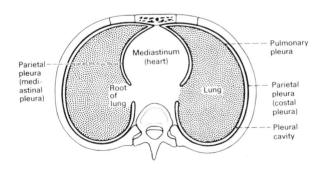

Fig. 3.13 Schematic transverse section of the thorax to show the pleura.

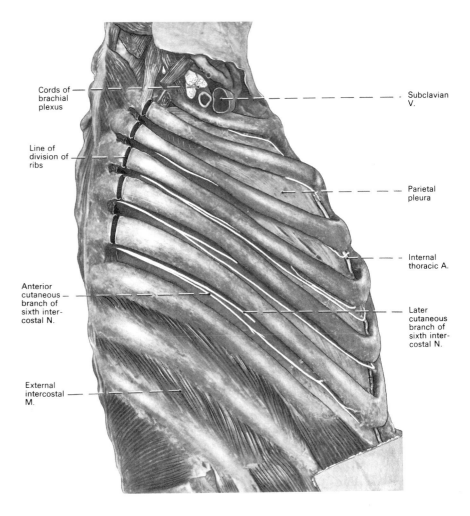

Cords of brachial plexus

Line of division of ribs

Anterior cutaneous branch of sixth intercostal N.

External intercostal M.

Subclavian V.

Parietal pleura

Internal thoracic A.

Later cutaneous branch of sixth intercostal N.

Fig. 3.14 The removal of the anterior chest wall (lateral view of thorax).

The parietal pleura

Now consider the parietal pleura. Note that it can be subdivided into a **costal pleura** which is in contact with the ribs; a **diaphragmatic pleura,** which covers the diaphragm; and a **mediastinal pleura** which forms the lateral wall of the mediastinum. Note especially that part of the mediastinal pleura blends with the pericardium which envelops the heart. The **dome of the pleura** is that part of the parietal layer which ascends into the neck and overlies the apex of the lung.

The lines of pleural reflection [Fig. 3.16]

Because the heart and mediastinum project more to the left than to the right, the pleural cavities are not symmetrical, and 'the lines of pleural reflection', which indicate the boundaries of the pleural cavities as projected on the surface of the body, consequently differ on the two sides. Try and visualize, even if you cannot verify, the following points on your dissection, with a skeleton available for reference.

Note first that the apex of the lung, covered by pleura, reaches, in an undissected body, 3 cm above the medial third of the clavicle. The medial edge of the parietal pleura then runs obliquely downwards to the sternoclavicular joint, and the margins of the parietal pleura of the two sides come together at the sternal angle and remain together until the level of the fourth costal cartilage [Fig. 3.16]. Note that at this level the pleura on the left side sweeps obliquely downwards and laterally, and that, at the level of the eighth costal cartilage, it reaches a vertical line, called the mid-clavicular line, projected downwards from the middle of the clavicle. In contrast, it will be seen that on the right side the pleura descends vertically to the level of the sixth or seventh costal cartilage, and then passes obliquely downwards and laterally to reach a corresponding point on the mid-clavicular line at the level of the eighth costal cartilage. Because of this arrangement, the heart and pericardium are exposed behind the sternum from the fourth to the sixth costal cartilages.

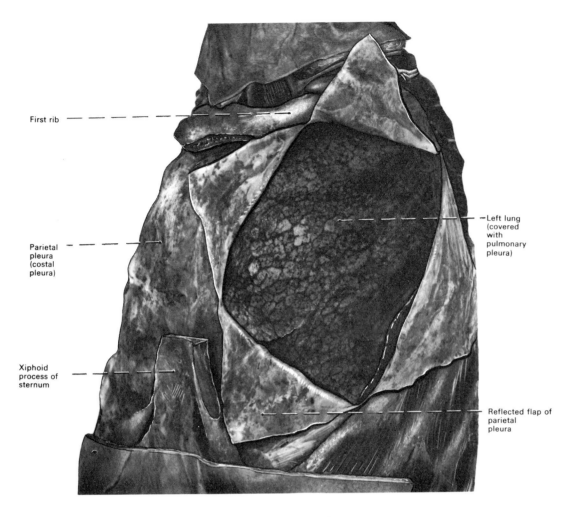

First rib

Parietal
pleura
(costal
pleura)

Xiphoid
process of
sternum

Left lung
(covered
with
pulmonary
pleura)

Reflected flap of
parietal
pleura

Fig. 3.15 The incision of the parietal pleura.

From the mid-clavicular line the parietal pleura follows the same line of reflection posteriorly on the two sides. It crosses the tenth rib in the axillary line, the eleventh rib in the line of the inferior angle of the scapula, and the twelfth rib at the lateral border of the erector spinae muscle, before continuing medially towards the spinous process of the twelfth thoracic vertebra. Since the twelfth rib lies obliquely, the line of pleural reflection is inferior to the posterior (medial) half of the rib. As you will see later [p. 4.77], the pleura in consequence forms a posterior relation to the upper part of the kidneys, with the diaphragm intervening.

The lungs *in situ*

Now define the position of the lungs, remembering that in your specimen the lung is certainly not in a fully-expanded condition [Fig. 3.17]. The margins of the upper parts of the lungs correspond to the lines of pleural reflection. Look at the right lung, and note that its **anterior border** follows the line of pleural reflection to the level of the sixth or seventh costal cartilage, but that its **inferior border** does not extend as far down as does the pleura [Fig. 3.16]. The level of this border depends, of course, on the degree of inflation of the lungs. The important point to remember is that there is an appreciable space, called the **costodiaphragmatic recess,** between the pulmonary pleura covering the inferior border of the lung and the lowest part of the parietal pleura. In certain diseases fluid collects in this recess. Posteriorly the space extends below the twelfth rib.

Now look at the left lung. Its anterior border will be seen to follow the line of pleural reflection downwards as far as the level of the fourth costal cartilage, and then to pass for a short distance laterally along the lower border of this cartilage before turning downwards to the sixth costal cartilage in the mid-clavicular line, thus forming the **cardiac notch of the left lung** [Figs 3.16 and 3.17]. Confirm that the level of the inferior border corresponds to that of the right lung.

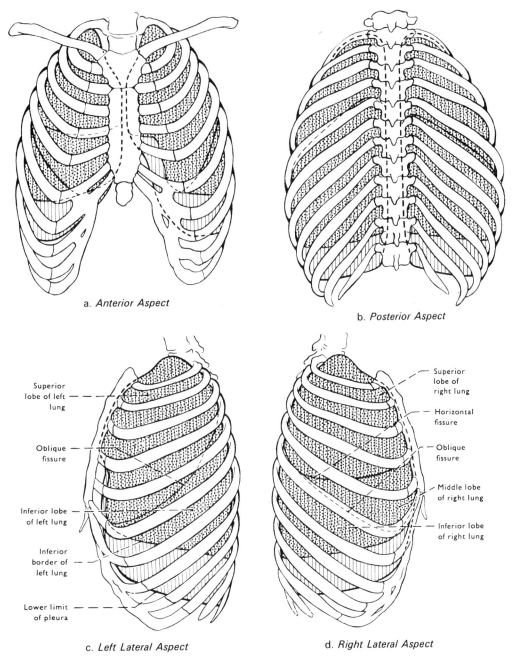

a. *Anterior Aspect*

b. *Posterior Aspect*

Superior
lobe of left
lung

Oblique
fissure

Inferior lobe
of left lung

Inferior
border of
left lung

Lower limit
of pleura

c. *Left Lateral Aspect*

Superior
lobe of
right lung

Horizontal
fissure

Oblique
fissure

Middle lobe
of right lung

Inferior lobe
of right lung

d. *Right Lateral Aspect*

Fig. 3.16 Surface projection of the lungs and pleurae on the thoracic wall. The extent of the lungs is indicated by dotted shading, and that of the pleurae by vertical shading.

The removal of the lungs

With a scalpel cut carefully and firmly through the root of the lung. Your blade will sever several big structures. Remove both lungs from the body, and keep them for later examination.

The root of the right lung

Examine the lateral aspect of the mediastinum. On the right side, identify the structures which you severed where they entered the root of the lung [Fig. 3.18]. They are, from above downwards, the **right superior lobe bronchus,** the **right pulmonary artery,** the **right inferior lobe bronchus,** and the **right superior** and **inferior pulmonary veins.** All of these structures will be seen in transverse or oblique section, and all are large in calibre. The veins have a thinner wall than the artery, and both veins and artery may contain clots. The bronchi have cartilage in their walls. Since all these are branching structures, their precise relationships to one another depend

3.15

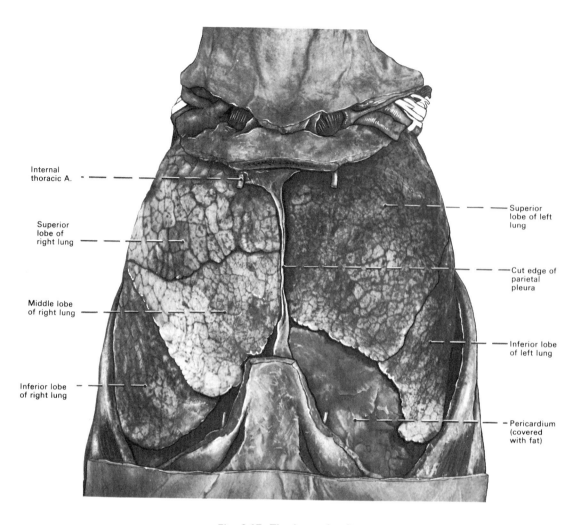

Fig. 3.17 The lungs *in situ*.

to some extent on the plane of the incision which you made when the lung was removed. In general, the veins lie more anteriorly than the artery, and the latter more anteriorly than the bronchi.

Between all these structures in the root of the lung you will see lymph nodes which are always black in colour, and one of which usually extends into the upper part of the pulmonary ligament.

The right phrenic nerve

Identify the right phrenic nerve on the side of the heart, accompanied by the small pericardiacophrenic artery and vein (the artery is a branch of the internal thoracic artery), and free it by dissection from the mediastinal pleura. Trace the nerve downwards into the diaphragm, which it supplies, and note now that it lies successively on the right brachio-cephalic vein, the superior vena cava, and the pericardium covering the right atrium of the heart [Fig. 3.18].

You will re-examine these relations later. Note, too, that the nerve descends in front of the root of the lung between the mediastinal pleura and the pericardium.

On the right side strip away the mediastinal and costal parts of the parietal pleura, together with the dome of the pleura, and identify and clean a vein which is closely applied to the mediastinum. You will find it arching over the root of the right lung as it passes from the posterior thoracic wall to enter the superior vena cava. This is the azygos vein [Fig. 3.18]. You will complete its dissection later.

The root of the left lung

On the left side, identify the structures you severed as they entered the lung root [Fig. 3.19]. From above downwards they are the **left pulmonary artery,** the **left main bronchus,** and the **left superior** and **inferior pulmonary veins.**

The left phrenic nerve

Define and isolate the left phrenic nerve in front of the root of the lung [Fig. 3.19]. Follow it downwards to the dia-phragm which it supplies, and upwards to the arch of the aorta, which you will recognize as a rounded swelling at the upper end of the heart. Here you will see that the phrenic nerve crosses a larger nerve, the left vagus nerve. If you

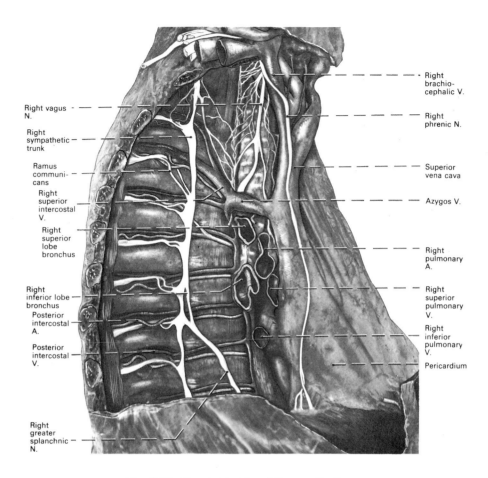

Right vagus N.

Right sympathetic trunk

Ramus communicans

Right superior intercostal V.

Right superior lobe bronchus

Right inferior lobe bronchus

Posterior intercostal A.

Posterior intercostal V.

Right greater splanchnic N.

Right brachio-cephalic V.

Right phrenic N.

Superior vena cava

Azygos V.

Right pulmonary A.

Right superior pulmonary V.

Right inferior pulmonary V.

Pericardium

Fig. 3.18 The right side of the mediastinum.

isolate and dissect the vagus you will find that it descends behind the root of the lung, to the anterior aspect of which it also sends branches.

You will see a vein between the left phrenic and the left vagus nerves, on or above the arch of the aorta. This is the left superior intercostal vein. It passes into the left brachiocephalic vein and drains the posterior parts of the second and third intercostal spaces.

As on the right side, strip away the mediastinal and costal pleura, and the dome of the pleura, and then note the positions of the heart, the arch of the aorta and the descending aorta, relative to the other structures so far displayed.

Continue your examination of the mediastinum. It lies between the two pleural cavities, and for purposes of description is divided into a superior part and an inferior part.

The mediastinum

The **superior mediastinum** is that part of the mediastinum which lies above the plane of the sternal angle, which passes through the intervertebral disc between the fourth and fifth thoracic vertebrae [Fig. 3.20]. It contains the arch of the aorta and three large vessels which arise from the arch, the

brachiocephalic trunk, which soon divides into the right common carotid artery and the right subclavian artery, and the left common carotid and left subclavian arteries.

The **inferior mediastinum** is that part of the mediastinum which lies below the horizontal plane of the sternal angle. It is subdivided into an **anterior mediastinum** in front of the pericardium, which contains only the internal thoracic vessels, the sternopericardial ligaments (which you tore away when you removed the sternum), and some lymph nodes; a **middle mediastinum** containing the pericardium and its contents; and a **posterior mediastinum** behind the pericardium.

The superior mediastinum [Fig. 3.21]

The most superficial structure you may see in the superior mediastinum is a flat, fatty, grey mass. This is a remnant of the **thymus,** a structure which is fairly prominent up to the age of puberty. Clear it away. It is not attached to any important structure.

To facilitate your further dissection of the superior mediastinum, you may need to saw the remains of the manubrium of the sternum carefully down the midline, so that the two halves, each attached to the first rib, may be

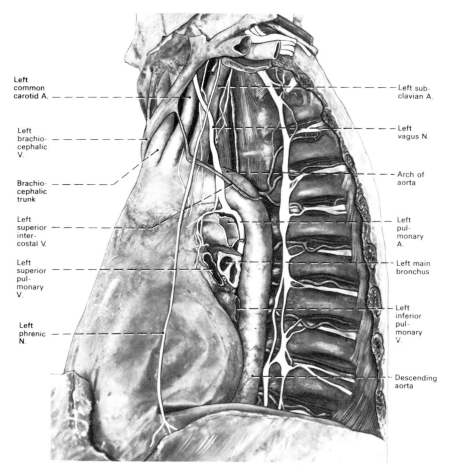

Left common carotid A.

Left brachio-cephalic V.

Brachio-cephalic trunk

Left superior inter-costal V.

Left superior pul-monary V.

Left phrenic N.

Left sub-clavian A.

Left vagus N.

Arch of aorta

Left pul-monary A.

Left main bronchus

Left inferior pul-monary V.

Descending aorta

Fig. 3.19 The left side of the mediastinum.

1 Superior mediastinum
2 Anterior mediastinum
3 Middle mediastinum (heart)
4 Posterior mediastinum

Fig. 3.20 The mediastinum; a schematic median section of the thorax.

gently lifted upwards and outwards. Do not do this, however, unless it is necessary to demonstrate the various structures, for in lifting the manubrium the first rib is very likely to be broken.

Now identify the large left brachiocephalic vein which passes obliquely across the three branches of the aorta just above the aortic arch [Fig. 3.21]. It is thin-walled, about 1.5 cm wide, and will almost certainly be filled with clots. You will soon see that it joins the shorter right brachiocephalic vein to form the superior vena cava.

Behind these large vessels you should be able to identify the trachea with the oesophagus deep to it. These structures, together with the phrenic and vagus nerves, and the thoracic duct, which will not be fully seen until later, constitute the main contents of the superior mediastinum.

The superior vena cava [Fig. 3.21]

The superior vena cava is the very large and thin-walled vein which you will find at the upper right-hand corner of the heart. It is about 2.5 cm wide. Clean and trace it upwards to its formation by the union of the right and left brachiocephalic veins behind the first right costal cartilage. Then follow it downwards to the point where it enters the peri-

cardium. It is about 7 cm long but its inferior half is within the pericardium. The large vessel behind its termination is the right pulmonary artery. It will be obvious to you that in its normal state the superior vena cava is overlapped by the right lung.

Note that the ascending aorta and the commencement of the brachiocephalic trunk are on the immediate left of the superior vena cava, and that the right phrenic nerve is on its right. Behind its lower end is the root of the right lung.

Again examine the **azygos vein.** Note that it enters the superior vena cava after arching over the root of the right lung [Fig. 3.18].

The brachiocephalic veins [Fig. 3.21]

Complete the cleaning of the right and left brachiocephalic veins. You will find that the **right brachiocephalic vein,** which is about 1.5 cm wide, is formed in the lower part of the neck behind the right sternoclavicular joint, by the union of the **right internal jugular vein** and **right subclavian vein.** Note the short course of the right brachiocephalic vein; it is no more than 2.5 cm long. You will see that the phrenic nerve is first posterior and then lateral to the vein.

Now examine the **left brachiocephalic vein.** It is nearly

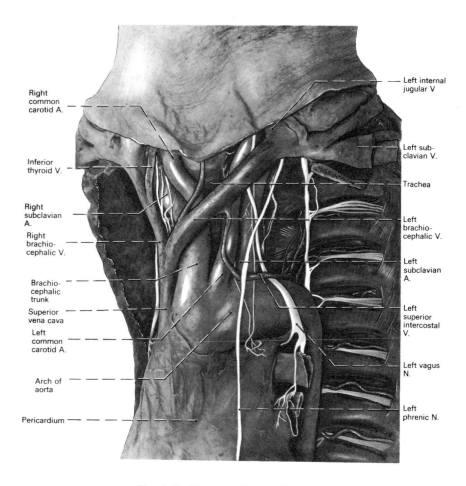

Right common carotid A.

Inferior thyroid V.

Right subclavian A.

Right brachio- cephalic V.

Brachio- cephalic trunk

Superior vena cava

Left common carotid A.

Arch of aorta

Pericardium

Left internal jugular V

Left sub- clavian V.

Trachea

Left brachio- cephalic V.

Left subclavian A.

Left superior intercostal V.

Left vagus N.

Left phrenic N.

Fig. 3.21 The superior mediastinum.

three times as long as the right one. It begins in the lower part of the neck behind the left sternoclavicular joint, where, as you will see when you dissect the head and neck, it is formed by the union of the **left internal jugular** and **left sub-clavian veins.** As you will also see later, the brachiocephalic vein receives the **thoracic duct** at its point of origin. This duct is a relatively small vessel which, in spite of its size, is the main collecting duct of the lymph of the body. In appearance it resembles an empty vein.

Note again that the left brachiocephalic vein passes obliquely downwards and to the right across the origins of the left subclavian and left common carotid arteries and the brachiocephalic (arterial) trunk, from the arch of the aorta. You will find that the vein also crosses the left phrenic and vagus nerves and the trachea, and that it is often joined by **inferior thyroid veins,** which descend in front of the trachea. Again note that the left brachiocephalic vein ends behind the first right costal cartilage, where it joins the right brachiocephalic vein to form the superior vena cava.

Clean the **left superior intercostal vein,** which you have already seen between the left vagus and phrenic nerves. You will see that it enters the left brachiocephalic vein, and you may be able to determine that it drains the posterior part

of the second and third left intercostal spaces. Its position relative to the aortic arch is very variable, but the vein always passes superficial to the vagus nerve and deep to the phrenic nerve.

The right side of the mediastinum

On the right side complete the cleaning of the phrenic nerve and trace it upwards as it passes into the root of the neck on the lateral side of the superior vena cava and the right brachiocephalic vein.

The right vagus nerve

Now clean and trace the right vagus nerve as it descends in the superior mediastinum on the right of the trachea [Fig. 3.22]. Gently pull the vagus away from the subclavian artery, and try to identify a branch which it sends behind the artery. This is the **right recurrent laryngeal nerve.** Do not try to follow this branch further at this stage.

As you stretch the vagus by pulling it from the medias-tinum, you will see slender branches that pass medially and downwards to a plexus of nerves between the trachea and the heart. These are the **cardiac branches** of the vagus and

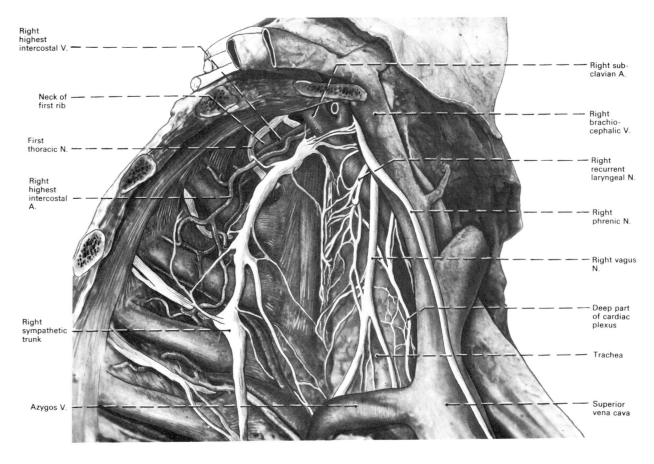

Right highest intercostal V.

Neck of first rib

First thoracic N.

Right highest intercostal A.

Right sympathetic trunk

Azygos V.

Right sub-clavian A.

Right brachio-cephalic V.

Right recurrent laryngeal N.

Right phrenic N.

Right vagus N.

Deep part of cardiac plexus

Trachea

Superior vena cava

Fig. 3.22 The right vagus nerve.

right recurrent laryngeal nerves going to the **cardiac plexus,** which you will examine later. Other nerves, the cardiac branches of the cervical part of the sympathetic trunk, pass into this plexus from the neck. In front of the vagus and lying against the trachea you will almost certainly find some lymph nodes.

The brachiocephalic trunk [Fig. 3.21]

Clean the brachiocephalic (arterial) trunk, and trace the vessel upwards to its division into the **right common carotid** and **right subclavian arteries.** Carefully note that these vessels lie medial to the phrenic and vagus nerves and to the apex of the lung. Also note the origin of the internal thoracic artery from the subclavian artery.

The azygos vein

Next complete the cleaning of the azygos vein [Fig. 3.18], but be careful not to damage the thin and small thoracic duct medial to it. Note that some small veins pass into the azygos vein after running over the sides of the vertebral bodies from the right posterior chest wall. These are the **posterior intercostal veins** and the **right superior intercostal vein.** The former are accompanied by the posterior intercostal

arteries, which pass behind the azygos vein from the descending aorta. (The azygos vein also receives the bronchial vein from the right bronchus, but you are most unlikely to identify this vessel.)

Remove the fascia from the right side of the vertebral column and the posterior part of the thorax, and then trace two or three of the right posterior intercostal vessels laterally. At this stage do not dissect the vessels in the upper two intercostal spaces. You will see that the vessels pass behind a vertically-directed nerve, which is characterized by a series of ganglionic swellings. This is the right sympathetic trunk. Continue to follow the posterior intercostal vessels laterally in the intercostal spaces as they lie on the internal intercostal membranes, until they disappear behind the intercostales intimi muscles. Below them lie the intercostal nerves, which emerge from the intervertebral foramina.

The right sympathetic trunk

Carefully clean the right sympathetic trunk and its **ganglia,** and follow it as it descends obliquely in front of the necks of the ribs to the sides of the bodies of the vertebrae [Fig. 3.18]. You will see that it leaves the thorax by passing behind the diaphragm into the abdomen.

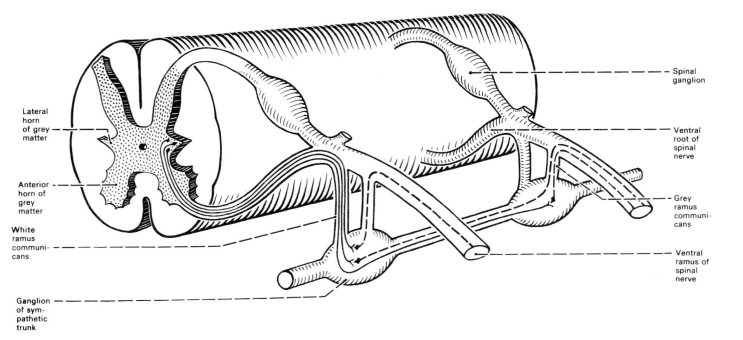

Fig. 3.23 Schema of a section of the spinal medulla and sympathetic trunk to show their interconnections. Preganglionic fibres are shown as solid lines in the white rami communicantes; typical postganglionic fibres are shown as interrupted lines.

The thoracic part of the sympathetic trunk is made up of a series of ganglia, usually twelve in number, joined together by nerve fibres [Fig. 3.23]. The ganglia consist mainly of nerve cells, which are also dispersed in the intervening strands of nerve fibres.

Although the disposition of the ganglia varies from subject to subject, they are typically disposed segmentally, each ganglion being joined to a spinal nerve by two **rami communicantes.** One of these communicating branches is a **white ramus communicans,** which consists of myelinated preganglionic nerve fibres that arise in the spinal medulla and pass to the sympathetic trunk from the intercostal nerve, to synapse in the ganglia. The other is a **grey ramus communicans,** which consists of postganglionic unmyelinated nerve fibres. These arise in the cells of the ganglion and pass into the intercostal nerve to be distributed with its branches.

By dissecting behind the sympathetic trunk, using a probe or the points of fine dissecting forceps, try to make out the rami communicantes of two or three ganglia [Fig. 3.18]. It will be difficult to distinguish the white (myelinated) from the grey (unmyelinated) rami, and you may also discover that more than two rami are associated with one ganglion.

Not only the arrangement but also the branches of the sympathetic trunk are very variable. As a rule, the second, third and fourth ganglia send branches to the cardiac plexus (part of which you have already seen), and to the root of the lungs, where they help form the posterior part of the pulmonary plexus.

The splanchnic nerves

Try to trace branches which rise from the fifth, sixth, seventh, eighth, and ninth ganglia or the intervening nerve trunks, and which pass anteriorly and downwards on the side of the vertebral column. They join together to form the right **greater splanchnic nerve** [Fig. 3.18]. Corresponding branches from the tenth and eleventh ganglia may form a right **lesser splanchnic nerve,** and sometimes a branch from the twelfth ganglion forms the **lowest splanchnic nerve.** These splanchnic nerves pass obliquely downwards and forwards over the vertebral bodies and pierce the diaphragm to enter the abdomen, where you will trace them later.

The neck of the first rib

Now turn to the neck of the right first rib [Fig. 3.22]. By removing the fascia and dissecting in this region you will identify on the neck of the rib the sympathetic trunk medially (sometimes swollen to form a ganglion, called the **stellate ganglion,** which extends into the neck); the **first thoracic nerve** laterally (passing to the inferior trunk of the brachial plexus); and between the two, the **highest intercostal artery** and the **highest intercostal vein.** The artery, a branch of the costocervical trunk of the subclavian artery, supplies the first and second intercostal spaces posteriorly. It is unnecessary to trace these vessels.

As you dissected the posterior intercostal vessels and splanchnic nerves, you will have noticed the oesophagus lying behind the trachea and the pericardium. You may also

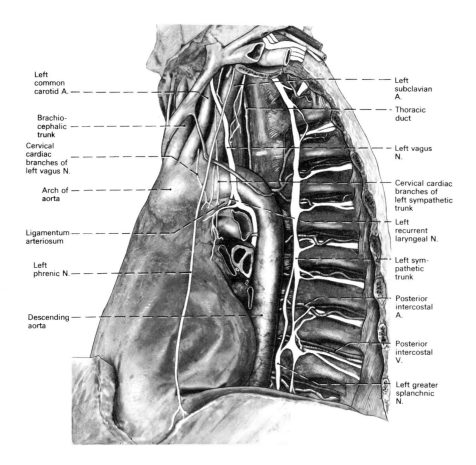

Left common carotid A. —

Brachio-cephalic trunk —

Cervical cardiac branches of left vagus N. —

Arch of aorta —

Ligamentum arteriosum —

Left phrenic N. —

Descending aorta —

Left subclavian A.

Thoracic duct

Left vagus N.

Cervical cardiac branches of left sympathetic trunk

Left recurrent laryngeal N.

Left sympathetic trunk

Posterior intercostal A.

Posterior intercostal V.

Left greater splanchnic N.

Fig. 3.24 The left side of the mediastinum.

have come across the thin-walled thoracic duct in the posterior mediastinum behind the oesophagus and medial to the azygos vein. Do not, however, clean any of these structures at this stage.

The left side of the mediastinum

Now turn to the left side of the thorax and trace the phrenic nerve to the root of the neck, as on the right side. Clean the arch of the aorta and carefully define the origins of the great vessels which spring from it [Fig. 3.24].

Note again that the phrenic nerve crosses the vagus either on or above the arch, and that the two nerves are separated by the left superior intercostal vein. If you tease the fascia on the arch, between the two nerves, you may find two smaller nerves which run parallel to them. They are **cervical cardiac branches** of the left vagus and left sympathetic trunk. Do not spend more than a few minutes searching for them if they do not immediately come into view. If you find them, trace them downwards until they enter a network of fine nerves, the superficial part of the **cardiac plexus,** which lies in the concavity of the aortic arch.

The ligamentum arteriosum [Fig. 3.24]

If you dissect below the concavity of the arch of the aorta, you will find a thick rounded fibrous cord called the ligamentum arteriosum, which is attached at its upper end to the under-surface of the aorta, and at its lower to the left pulmonary artery. This is the remains of the obliterated **ductus arteriosus,** which in the foetus conveys venous blood from the pulmonary trunk to the descending part of the arch of the aorta. Lift the left vagus away from the aorta and note that it sends a branch, the **left recurrent laryngeal nerve,** around the ligament. Clean the ligament, but do not trace the left recurrent laryngeal nerve at this stage.

The left vagus nerve

Clean and trace the vagus nerve upwards as far as you can into the root of the neck, and note that in the superior mediastinum it lies between the left common carotid and left subclavian arteries [Fig. 3.24]. Then trace the vagus downwards as far as the root of the lung. Complete, if necessary, the cleaning of the left common carotid and left subclavian arteries, and find the point where the internal thoracic artery springs from the latter.

The arch of the aorta

Now study the arch of the aorta, and note the following points [Fig. 3.24].

The arch is a continuation of the **ascending aorta,** which lies within the pericardium. It commences behind the second right sternocostal joint, ascends to within 2 cm of the upper border of the manubrium of the sternum, and ends on the left of the vertebral column at the level of the lower border of the fourth thoracic vertebra, where it becomes the **descending aorta.** You will see that the arch is directed not only to the left but also backwards. This is an important point to appreciate, otherwise the relationships of the arch to adjacent structures will not be understood. Note that the beginning of the arch lies on the trachea, but that more superiorly both the latter and the oesophagus have the arch on their left side. You have already identified the left phrenic and vagus nerves crossing each other on or above the arch, and you may have seen the cardiac branches of the vagus and sympathetic trunk crossing the arch to form the superficial part of the cardiac plexus in the concavity of the arch.

Another feature of this part of the aorta is that the root of the left lung lies inferior to the arch, as also does the ligamentum arteriosum, with the left recurrent laryngeal nerve hooking round it and the superficial part of the cardiac plexus lying in front of it.

Immediately below the arch of the aorta you will find the left pulmonary artery. Do not attempt to clean it at this stage. You will see that the arch is overlapped by both lungs, and particularly by the left. In the living body the arch is covered in front of the lungs by the thymus and the manubrium of the sternum.

The left posterior intercostal arteries

Continue dissecting the left side of the thorax by removing the fascia from the descending aorta and its branches, and from the adjacent parts of the ribs [Fig. 3.24]. As you do so, you will see that the aorta sends branches (the posterior intercostal arteries) into each intercostal space, and you may also see that it gives off bronchial branches to the bronchi, as well as a variable number of small branches to the oesophagus, pericardium, and diaphragm.

The hemiazygos veins

If you clean one or two of the veins that are associated with the left posterior intercostal arteries, you will find that they join to form vertically-disposed hemiazygos veins, which lie on the left of the vertebral column. If the veins are not full they will be difficult to dissect. The hemiazygos veins correspond to the azygos vein on the right side, and end by crossing the midline to join it.

The left sympathetic trunk [Fig. 3.24]

Clean the intercostal nerves in two or three spaces. Then clean the left sympathetic trunk and the splanchnic nerves in the same way as you cleaned those of the right side. Now dissect out and identify the structures crossing the neck of the left first rib. You will find that they are arranged in a similar way to those of the right side [p. 3.21].

Section 3.3

The heart

The examination of the heart *in situ*

You must now proceed to study the **heart,** about which you should first note the following facts. It consists of four chambers, of which two, the atria, receive, and two, the ventricles, distribute the blood. The **right atrium** receives the venous blood of the body by way of the superior and inferior venae cavae, and pumps it into the **right ventricle.** This, a more muscular chamber, pumps the blood through the pulmonary trunk into the lungs. Here the blood is re-oxygenated. The blood then returns by four pulmonary veins to the **left atrium,** from which it is pumped into the most powerful of the four chambers, the **left ventricle.** When this contracts, the oxygenated blood passes into the ascending aorta to be distributed by the arteries to all parts of the body. The contraction of the four chambers occurs in a co-ordinated sequence, and the blood is pumped through the small pulmonary and the extensive systemic circulations in a succession of pulsations which reflect the rhythmic beat of the heart.

The heart lies obliquely in the thoracic cavity, so that the left and right atria lie above, somewhat to the right of and behind the ventricles.

The whole heart is usually shaped like a flattened cone, with an apex, a base, and three surfaces (a sternocostal surface, a diaphragmatic surface, and a pulmonary surface). The sternocostal surface is limited by the four borders of the heart—left, right, upper, and lower. The apex points downwards and to the left, while the base of the heart is directed backwards towards the vertebral column.

The pericardium

The heart lies in the pericardium, which consists of an outer fibrous sac and a double inner layer of serous membrane. The inner layer of serous membrane in contact with the heart muscle is called the **visceral layer of the serous pericardium;** the outer layer is the **parietal layer of the serous pericardium,** and between the two is a thin film of serous fluid or lymph, which acts as a lubricant. A reference to Fig. 3.25 will help you realize that the heart does not lie inside the serous sac. It invaginates the sac from the outside. As a result of this arrangement and the presence of a thin film of lymph, the heart, covered by a visceral layer of serous membrane, can move freely and without friction within the parietal layer. The visceral layer is so firmly adherent to the heart that it is also called the **epicardium.**

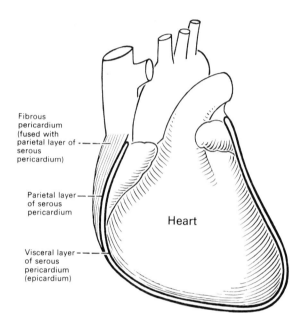

Fig. 3.25 A schematic section of the pericardium.

The pericardium differs from the serous membranes which cover other viscera, in that it possesses an outer tough layer of fibrous tissue, called the **fibrous pericardium,** on to which the mediastinal pleura is reflected. The fibrous pericardium is connected with the sternum in front by the **sterno-pericardial ligaments.** These you tore through when you removed the sternum. Inferiorly you can see that the fibrous pericardium blends with the diaphragm (with a part known as the **central tendon of the diaphragm).** Look at the posterior surface of the fibrous pericardium, and note that on each side it is pierced by two pulmonary veins. Above, on the right, you will see that it is pierced by the superior vena cava, and below, and again on the right, by the inferior vena cava. Above and in front, the pericardium is pierced by the pulmonary trunk and ascending aorta.

The surface relations of the heart [Fig. 3.26]

Now replace the bony plate consisting of sternum and ribs which you removed and, by referring both to your specimen and to a skeleton, try to visualize that the surface projection of the heart falls within an area which is defined by the following landmarks:

1. A point at the level of the lower border of the second left costal cartilage 2 cm to the left of the lateral border of the sternum.
2. A point at the upper border of the third right costal cartilage at its junction with the sternum.
3. A point at the level of the sixth right costal cartilage 2 cm to the right of the lateral border of the sternum.
4. A point, which marks the **apex of the heart,** in the fifth left interspace in the mid-clavicular line.

By uniting these points as shown in Fig. 3.26 the outline of the heart can be mapped out. When standing upright the surface markings of the heart will be slightly lower. The clinician is particularly concerned with the size of the heart and with the position of the apex beat, which he can usually feel.

If, as is often the case, the heart of your cadaver does not coincide with these dimensions, it may be either enlarged, as sometimes occurs in old age, or as occasionally happens, it may have been accidentally ruptured after death because of the pressure with which the preservative was injected into the arterial system.

The incision of the pericardium

With this general description of the heart in mind, make two parallel vertical incisions in the pericardium immediately anterior to the lines of the phrenic nerves, each about 8 cm long, and a transverse incision joining their lower ends. Open the pericardial sac by turning the pericardial flap you have made upwards.

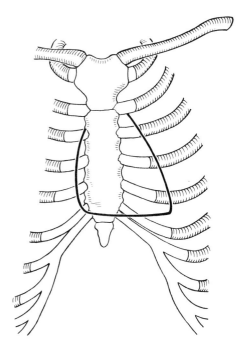

Fig. 3.26 The surface projection of the heart on to the anterior chest wall.

Examine the attachments of the pericardium to the roots of the great vessels. After you have done this, but before proceeding further, note the following facts about the serous pericardium.

The serous pericardium lies within the fibrous pericardium and consists of a single layer of mesothelial cells resting on some loose areolar tissue. The parietal layer of serous pericardium lines the fibrous pericardium and is adherent to it. The visceral layer covers the surface of the heart and is so much a part of the heart that it is called the epicardium.

The sinuses of the pericardium

Reflections of the serous pericardium around the vessels entering and leaving the heart form two recesses, called the **transverse sinus** of the pericardium and the **oblique sinus** of the pericardium [Figs 3.27 and 3.28]. The former lies on the upper aspect of the heart and is bounded in front by the serous pericardium, which encloses the pulmonary trunk and aorta, and behind by the reflection of this part of the pericardium on to the atria.

Study the boundaries of the transverse sinus on your dissection by slipping your finger from the left side into the pericardial sac behind the pulmonary trunk, and so into the sinus. In front of your finger are the pulmonary trunk and ascending aorta; behind it are the atria and the superior vena cava. You can see the other pericardial recess, the oblique sinus of the pericardium, if you lift and turn the heart from its bed and examine its posterior aspect. The boundary of the oblique sinus is shaped like an inverted J. The serous pericardium enclosing the left pulmonary veins forms the smaller limb of the J. The reflection of the pericardium across the left atrium to the right side of the heart forms the base of the J (and also the posterior wall of the transverse sinus). The larger limb of the J is formed by the reflection of pericardium being continued to enclose the superior vena cava, the right pulmonary veins and the inferior vena cava. The anterior wall of the sinus is the posterior wall of the left atrium.

Insert fingers into both sinuses simultaneously and feel the upper part of the left atrium between them. Note the posterior position of most of the left atrium.

The surfaces of the heart *in situ*

Now examine the surfaces of the heart as the organ lies *in situ* [Fig. 3.28]. Note that about two-thirds of the organ lie to the left of the midline. Look at the right convex border of the heart. It is formed by the right atrium, which ends superiorly in a slightly ridged or serrated appendix called the right auricle (or auricular appendage). Note that the anterior or **sternocostal surface** of the heart is formed chiefly by the right ventricle, and to a lesser extent by the left ventricle. The **pulmonary surface,** including the apex of the

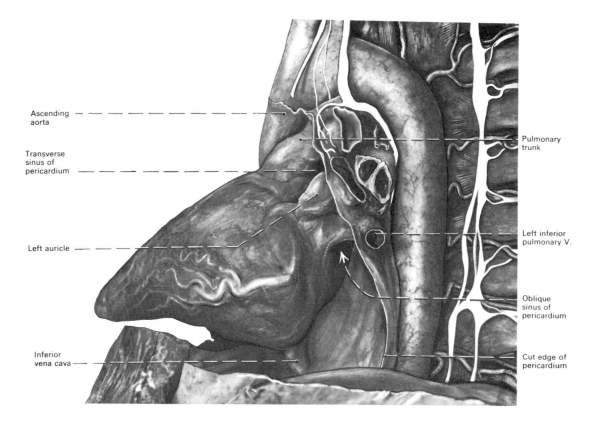

Ascending aorta

Transverse sinus of pericardium

Left auricle

Inferior vena cava

Pulmonary trunk

Left inferior pulmonary V.

Oblique sinus of pericardium

Cut edge of pericardium

Fig. 3.27 The sinuses of the pericardium. The heart has been turned to the right and is seen from the left side.

heart, is formed entirely by the left ventricle except at the extreme upper end, where you will see the tip of the left auricle.

If you gently lift up the apex of the heart you will see the surface that rests on the diaphragm. This is the inferior or **diaphragmatic surface,** and it is formed chiefly by the left ventricle, and to a lesser extent by the right ventricle. The diaphragmatic surface is separated from the sternocostal surface by the sharp lower border. The part of the heart that is directed towards the vertebral column is the **base.** It lies opposite the bodies of the fifth, sixth, seventh, and eighth thoracic vertebrae, and is formed largely by the left atrium and to a lesser extent by the right atrium.

You will see a set of vertically-disposed vessels on the left side of the sternocostal surface, usually surrounded by fat. The main artery of this group, which is a branch of the **left coronary artery,** sends branches downwards and to the left over the surface of the left ventricle. The vertically-disposed vessels mark the line of division of the two ventricles [Fig. 3.28].

You will sometimes see another set of vessels, of which the artery is the **right coronary artery,** lying on the right side of the sternocostal surface of the heart. Usually, however, these vessels, which lie obliquely between the right atrium

and right ventricle in the anterior part of a groove, called the **coronary groove,** are covered by too much fat to be clearly defined. If they are not immediately obvious, do not dissect either of these sets of vessels at this stage.

Now look at the superior part of the sternocostal surface. The big vessel that lies anteriorly and which emerges from the upper part of the right ventricle is the **pulmonary trunk.** The larger vessel behind it at its origin is the **ascending aorta.** Note that the pulmonary trunk almost immediately runs to the left of the ascending aorta.

You can see that the ascending aorta starts from the base of the left ventricle of the heart, at the level of the third left costal cartilage and behind the left half of the sternum. Its direction is obliquely upwards and to the right. At the level of the plane of the sternal angle it turns obliquely backwards and to the left to form the **arch of the aorta.** Note that the ascending aorta lies wholly within the pericardium.

Note that the **superior vena cava** passes behind the right auricle and ends in the upper part of the right atrium. Examine the lower end of the right border of the heart, and find the **inferior vena cava** as it pierces the central tendon of the diaphragm. Note that after a very short course in the thorax it enters the lower part of the right atrium.

Cut through the inferior vena cava and then lift up the

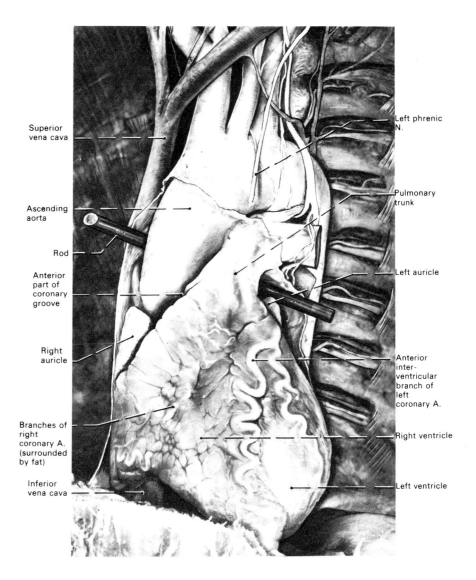

Superior
vena cava

Ascending
aorta

Rod

Anterior
part of
coronary
groove

Right
auricle

Branches of
right
coronary A.
(surrounded
by fat)

Inferior
vena cava

Left phrenic
N.

Pulmonary
trunk

Left auricle

Anterior
inter-
ventricular
branch of
left
coronary A.

Right ventricle

Left ventricle

Fig. 3.28 The heart *in situ*. Most of the fibrous pericardium has been excised. A rod has been placed in the transverse sinus of the pericardium.

heart and identify the four **pulmonary veins** entering the left atrium.

The removal of the heart

Your next step is to remove the heart from its bed in the thoracic cavity so that you can examine it in detail.

First pass a pair of forceps into the transverse sinus, and with a scalpel cut through the aorta and pulmonary trunk down on to the forceps. This will give you a good view of the sinus. Again examine its boundaries, all of which are covered by serous pericardium, and note that anteriorly are the ascending aorta and pulmonary trunk; posteriorly, the right and left atria and the superior vena cava; superiorly,

the inferior surface of the right pulmonary artery; and inferiorly, the reflection of serous pericardium from the atria to the aorta and pulmonary trunk.

Examine the position of the transverse and oblique sinuses relative to each other. If you place a finger in the oblique sinus and another in the transverse sinus behind the cut aorta and pulmonary trunk, you will be able to feel the pericardial reflection and the upper part of the left atrium between your two fingers.

Now insert a pair of forceps behind the superior vena cava and cut down on to it. The vena cava should be divided within the pericardium and therefore below the point of entry of the azygos vein. Then carefully divide the two left pulmonary veins within the pericardial sac, midway between the parietal pericardium and their entry into the

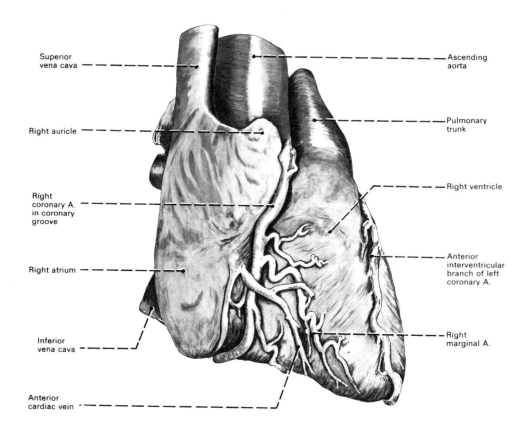

Superior
vena cava

Right auricle

Right
coronary A.
in coronary
groove

Right atrium

Inferior
vena cava

Anterior
cardiac vein

Ascending
aorta

Pulmonary
trunk

Right ventricle

Anterior
interventricular
branch of left
coronary A.

Right
marginal A.

Fig. 3.29 The right atrium and ventricle.

left atrium. Cut through the pericardial reflection on to the left atrium between the oblique and transverse sinuses. Divide the right pulmonary veins in the same way as you did the left, and then lift the heart out of the body and begin its dissection.

The surface of the heart

First identify the **coronary groove** [Fig. 3.29]. This marks the separation, on the surface, of the two atria from the two ventricles. The groove is fairly distinct on the posterior surface and, with the heart in roughly the position it occupies in the body, runs obliquely downwards from the left above to the right below. The pulmonary trunk and ascending aorta lie in front of the left end of the anterior part of the groove; fat beneath the epicardium (i.e. the visceral layer of serous pericardium) often fills and obscures the right end. Behind, the groove is filled by a thin-walled vein called the coronary sinus, which is the main vessel draining the heart wall.

Look at the sternocostal surface of the heart and note that the coronary groove appears to be interrupted by the origins of the pulmonary trunk and aorta. Further inspection will

reveal that these large vessels actually lie in front of the groove [Fig. 3.29].

If you now examine the diaphragmatic surface of the heart near its middle, you may see a ridge caused by a set of vessels lying in the **posterior interventricular groove.** The artery of this group of vessels is the posterior interventricular branch of the right coronary artery [Fig. 3.30]. It runs down towards the apex of the heart where it anastomoses with the anterior interventricular branch of the left coronary artery. This branch crosses the sternocostal surface in the **anterior interventricular groove.** You will dissect these vessels later.

If you now examine the base of the heart, you may be able to discern a shallow **interatrial groove,** lying just in front of the entrances of the right pulmonary veins into the left atrium. This groove marks the position of the interatrial septum, which separates the atria.

General anatomy of the heart

A general picture of the anatomy of the heart is provided in the following few paragraphs which you should study closely before going on with your dissection.

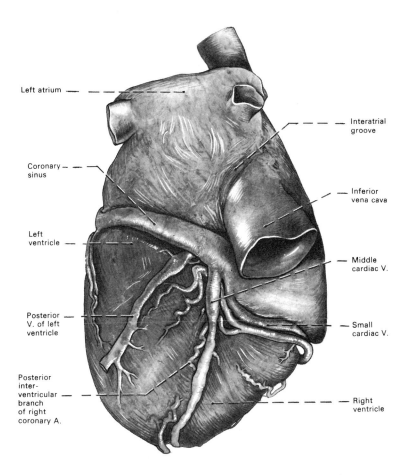

Left atrium

Coronary sinus

Left ventricle

Posterior V. of left ventricle

Posterior interventricular branch of right coronary A.

Interatrial groove

Inferior vena cava

Middle cardiac V.

Small cardiac V.

Right ventricle

Fig. 3.30 The base and diaphragmatic surface of the heart.

The visceral pericardium, or **epicardium**, covers the heart and deep to it is a variable amount of fat. Most of the substance of the heart is muscle known as **myocardium.** It consists of a highly-specialized meshwork of involuntary striped muscle fibres. The four chambers which make up the interior of the heart, the two atria and two ventricles, are lined by a layer of endothelial cells which forms the **endocardium.**

On the surface the line separating the atria from the ventricles is indicated by the coronary groove, which you have just identified. The groove also marks the position, in the interior of the heart, of the **atrioventricular valves** which control the openings of the right and left atria into their respective ventricles. The interior of the heart is completely divided into right and left halves. The two atria are separated by the **interatrial septum,** and the two ventricles by the **interventricular septum.**

The atrioventricular valves are folds of the endocardium which enclose fibrous tissue. The base of each valve is attached to a **fibrous ring** that surrounds the atrioventricular orifice. The atrioventricular valve between the right atrium

and right ventricle has three cusps, and hence is known as the **tricuspid valve.** The atrioventricular valve on the left side has two cusps, and is known as the **mitral valve.** Each cusp is roughly triangular in shape, with its base, as already stated, attached to the rim of the opening between the atrium and the ventricle. To the ventricular side of the periphery of each triangular cusp are attached a number of tendinous cords called **chordae tendineae,** which are anchored to the apices of nipple-like muscular projections of the ventricular walls known as the **papillary muscles.**

Opening into the right atrium are the superior and inferior venae cavae, which you have already seen, and the **coronary sinus,** into which drain the veins of the heart wall. The blood is then pumped from the atrium through the tricuspid valve into the right ventricle, which it leaves through the pulmonary trunk. The commencement of this vessel is guarded by the **pulmonary valve,** consisting of three semilunar valves.

Opening into the left atrium are four pulmonary veins which bring to the heart oxygenated blood from the lungs. This blood is then pumped through the mitral valve into the left ventricle, which it leaves by way of the aorta, whose opening is guarded by an **aortic valve** consisting, like the pulmonary valve, of three semilunar valves.

The heart wall is supplied with arterial blood by two very important vessels, the **right** and **left coronary arteries,** which arise from the beginning of the ascending aorta.

The arteries of the heart [Figs 3.29 and 3.31]

Return to your dissection and clean away the epicardium and fat from the root of the ascending aorta; this will reveal the two main arteries of the heart muscle, the right and left coronary arteries, coming from small dilatations, the **aortic sinuses,** at the base of the ascending aorta. As you dissect the coronary arterial tree you will find accompanying veins. Clean these also and leave them in position for later examination.

Follow the left coronary artery from its origin at the **left aortic sinus,** which lies not only to the left but also posteriorly. The artery passes behind the pulmonary trunk and in front of the left auricle and divides into two main branches. The anterior branch is called the **anterior interventricular branch** of the left coronary artery. You will see it on the anterior surface of the heart in the anterior interventricular groove which on the surface marks the separation of the right and left ventricles. Note that this anterior interventricular artery is accompanied by a vein, the **great cardiac vein,** the complete connections of which you will see later. The artery gives many branches to both ventricles and to the anterior part of the interventricular septum.

Now trace the posteriorly-directed branch of the left coronary artery. This is the **circumflex branch** which curves around the left border of the heart into the posterior part of the coronary groove. This branch of the artery is much

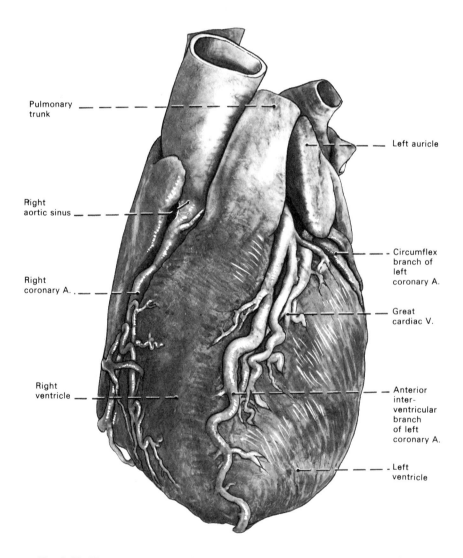

Pulmonary trunk

Left auricle

Right aortic sinus

Circumflex branch of left coronary A.

Right coronary A.

Great cardiac V.

Right ventricle

Anterior inter- ventricular branch of left coronary A.

Left ventricle

Fig. 3.31 The coronary arteries on the sternocostal surface of the heart.

smaller than the anterior interventricular branch, and it gives branches to the adjacent atrial and ventricular walls. Take care not to damage the upper part of the great cardiac vein which you should clean as it accompanies the circumflex artery along the coronary groove to the back of the heart.

Now return to the anterior aspect of the root of the aorta, and establish that the right coronary artery arises from the **right aortic sinus.** With the heart in its normal position in the body, this sinus lies on the anterior aspect of the aorta. Trace the artery downwards in the anterior part of the coronary groove; follow it as it passes around the lower part of the right border of the heart to enter the posterior part of the coronary groove. It gives off a **right marginal artery** which runs along the lower border of the right ventricle. More posteriorly you will find the **posterior interventricular branch** of the right coronary artery. It runs in a groove, the posterior interventricular groove, on the diaphragmatic surface of the heart, and supplies both ventricles and the posterior part of the interventricular septum. This posterior groove corresponds to the anterior interventricular groove, and marks the line of separation of the two ventricles on the posterior aspect of the heart.

At the apex of the heart the posterior interventricular and right marginal branches of the right coronary artery anastomose with the anterior interventricular branch of the left coronary artery, which you have traced down the anterior interventricular groove. A corresponding anastomosis is found between the right coronary artery and the circumflex branch of the left coronary artery in the posterior part of the coronary groove. Take care not to damage the large venous collecting vessel, the coronary sinus, which lies superficial to these anastomosing arteries.

The coronary arteries supply not only the muscle which constitutes the walls of the ventricles, atria, and septa of the heart, but also the bases of the large vessels entering and leaving the heart.

The coronary vessels are of the greatest clinical importance because when they narrow (a process called stenosis) or become blocked (occluded) because of a thickening of their lining endothelium or as a result of a blood clot, or because of a collapse of their walls, the cardiac muscle is damaged. Heart attacks follow. These range all the way from the minor form of 'angina' to sudden death. If a large branch of the coronary artery becomes blocked, the anastomoses of the coronary arterial system are rarely adequate to ensure an efficient collateral circulation. The smaller branches of the coronary system are in fact end-arteries. Appropriate cases of coronary stenosis or occlusion are now dealt with in 'open-heart' surgery by grafting a piece of great saphenous vein [p. 2.20] to bypass the diseased section or sections of the affected vessels.

The veins of the heart [Figs 3.30 and 3.31]

Now complete the examination of the venous drainage of the heart. Note again the large thin-walled **coronary sinus** in the posterior part of the coronary groove. The coronary sinus is covered only by epicardium, and is closely applied to the heart muscle. You will find that the sinus suddenly ends by penetrating the wall of the right atrium. Note the vein which you have already seen accompanying the anterior interventricular branch of the left coronary artery. This is the **great cardiac vein.** It passes upwards and turns to the left in the coronary groove and then follows the groove posteriorly to enter the coronary sinus. Pick up the corresponding vein in the posterior interventricular groove, the **middle cardiac vein,** and note that it ascends to enter the coronary sinus near its termination. In the right part of the coronary groove identify the **small cardiac vein** which accompanies the right coronary artery. This vein also terminates in the coronary sinus. Joining the small cardiac vein is a small venous tributary, the **right marginal vein,** which accompanies the right marginal artery. There are also a variable number of smaller veins entering the coronary sinus. In addition to the blood which is drained through the coronary sinus, the blood from the walls of the right atrium and ventricle enters the right atrium directly through the **anterior cardiac veins. Venae cordis minimae,** which are minute channels too small to dissect, also open independently into the subjacent chambers, but mainly into the right atrium.

The interior of the heart

The right atrium [Figs 3.32 and 3.33]

Pass the blade of a long knife through the superior vena caval opening down into the right atrium and out through the inferior vena caval opening. Cut laterally to open the right atrium. Then use scissors to make a second incision through the anterior wall of the right atrium at right angles to the first cut. Extend this into the apex of the right auricle as in Fig. 3.32. Remove any clots from the atrial cavity and thoroughly wash out the atrium so that its internal features are clearly displayed.

Examine the **opening of the inferior vena cava** below, and note a small semilunar endothelial fold which forms the **valve of the inferior vena cava.** Note the smooth **opening of the superior vena cava** above. In the middle of the **interatrial septum** separating the two atria you will find an oval depression above and to the left of the opening of the inferior vena cava. This is the **fossa ovalis** which in the foetus was an opening between the left and right atria called the **foramen ovale.** The valve of the inferior vena cava is relatively large in the foetus in which it directs blood from the inferior vena cava

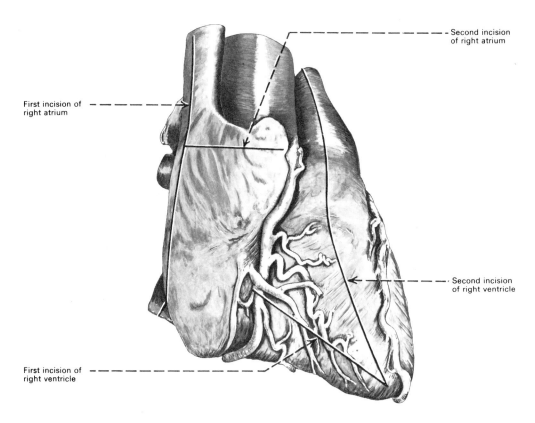

First incision of
right atrium

Second incision
of right atrium

Second incision
of right ventricle

First incision of
right ventricle

Fig. 3.32 The right atrium and ventricle (showing lines of incision).

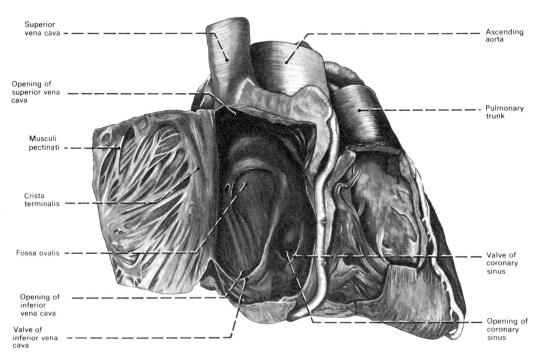

Superior
vena cava

Opening of
superior vena
cava

Musculi
pectinati

Crista
terminalis

Fossa ovalis

Opening of
inferior
vena cava

Valve of
inferior vena
cava

Ascending
aorta

Pulmonary
trunk

Valve of
coronary
sinus

Opening of
coronary
sinus

Fig. 3.33 The interior of the right atrium and ventricle (antero-lateral view). This dissection is different from the one described in the text. The wall of the right atrium has been reflected laterally; part of the wall of the right ventricle has been excised.

into the left atrium by way of the foramen ovale. This opening in the septum closes soon after birth, and the valve becomes vestigial. Occasionally, however, you may find that a small opening persists in the upper part of the fossa ovalis.

Between the valve of the inferior vena cava and the atrioventricular opening find the smaller **opening of the coronary sinus.** This too is guarded by a somewhat rudimentary valve, the **valve of the coronary sinus,** which prevents regurgitation of blood into the sinus during the contraction of the atrium.

On the lateral wall of the atrium, between the openings of the two venae cavae note a ridge, called the **crista terminalis.** It is sometimes indicated on the exterior of the atrium by a groove called the **sulcus terminalis.** From the crista terminalis you will see a series of muscular ridges which extend forwards into the anterior wall of the atrium and into the auricle of the atrial cavity. These ridges are the **musculi pectinati.**

Now examine the **right atrioventricular opening** which, in a healthy heart, should admit three fingers. You will see that it is guarded by a valve called the **tricuspid valve.** Its three cusps are named the **anterior cusp** (which is the largest), the **septal cusp,** and the **posterior cusp,** according to the positions they occupy.

The right ventricle [Figs 3.32, 3.34, and 3.35]

To open the right ventricle pass a pointed, long-bladed knife through the atrioventricular valve between the anterior and septal cusps until it emerges through the apex of the right ventricle. When the knife is in this position, open the ventricle by cutting antero-laterally to the left. Next pass the knife from the lower end of the ventricular incision upwards through the pulmonary valve and out of the cut end of the pulmonary trunk. Now cut anteriorly, thus increasing the exposure of the interior of the right ventricle and at the same time opening the pulmonary trunk. Remove any clots and wash out the ventricle under a tap.

First examine the ventricular aspect of the tricuspid valve. The bases of its cusps are attached to the fibrous ring which forms a rim to the atrioventricular opening. Attached to the margins and ventricular surfaces of the cusps are the chordae tendineae. Trace these to their attachments to the papillary muscles in the right ventricle. The latter are conical projections from the ventricular wall. Notice that there is an **anterior papillary muscle** arising from the anterior (sterno-costal) wall, and a smaller **posterior papillary muscle** arising from the inferior (diaphragmatic) wall of the ventricle. The incision with which you opened the ventricle may have cut through the anterior papillary muscle. On the septum between the two ventricles you may also find small muscular papillae which are collectively named **septal papillary muscles** to which some chordae tendineae are also attached. Note that the chordae tendineae attached to a given papillary muscle always pass to two adjacent cusps.

In the interior of the ventricle is a mesh of muscular ridges, the **trabeculae carneae.** Some of these are separated from the ventricular wall except at their ends. The papillary

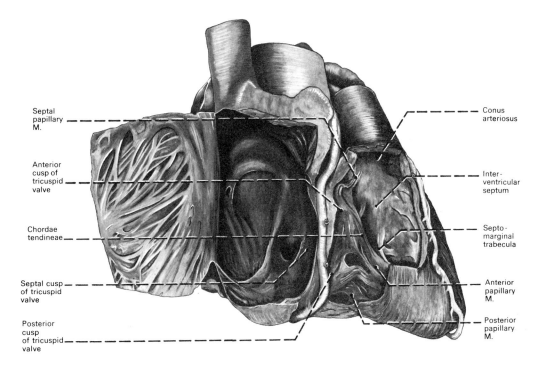

Septal papillary M.

Anterior cusp of tricuspid valve

Chordae tendineae

Septal cusp of tricuspid valve

Posterior cusp of tricuspid valve

Conus arteriosus

Inter-ventricular septum

Septo-marginal trabecula

Anterior papillary M.

Posterior papillary M.

Fig. 3.34 The interior of the right atrium and ventricle (antero-lateral view). This dissection is different from the one described in the text. The wall of the right atrium has been reflected laterally; part of the wall of the right ventricle has been excised.

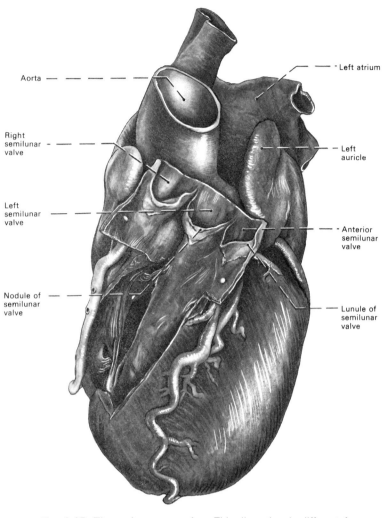

Aorta

Right
semilunar
valve

Left
semilunar
valve

Nodule of
semilunar
valve

Left atrium

Left
auricle

Anterior
semilunar
valve

Lunule of
semilunar
valve

Fig. 3.35 The pulmonary valve. This dissection is different from the one described in the text. The pulmonary trunk has been opened to display the valve.

muscles are specialized trabeculae carneae which are attached at one end to the heart wall and at the other to the chordae tendineae. A band of muscle, not invariably present, called the **septomarginal trabecula,** passes between the interventricular septum and the base of the anterior papillary muscle. As you will see later it is associated with part of the specialized conducting system of muscle-fibres of the heart wall.

The upper part of the right ventricle, from which the pulmonary trunk springs, is called the **conus arteriosus.** Note its smooth wall. Note, too, that the **opening of the pulmonary trunk** is guarded by the **pulmonary valve,** which consists of three separate semilunar valves. With the heart in its normal position in the body, two of these valves are anterior and one posterior. The semilunar valves are, however, named in relation to their relative positions when the heart is orientated with the interventricular septum in the midline. When so disposed, there is an **anterior semilunar valve** and two posterior semilunar valves called the **right semilunar** and the **left**

semilunar valves. On each semilunar valve look for a central **nodule.** The thin crescentic area on either side of this nodule is called the **lunule.** After blood is pumped into the pulmonary trunk by the contraction of the ventricle the three semilunar valves come together and completely shut off the vessel from the cavity of the heart.

The left atrium [Fig. 3.36]

Two right and two left pulmonary veins enter the left atrium (before entering the atrium, two of the veins may sometimes unite as they emerge from the lung). Make a vertical cut through the wall of the atrium so as to join the two right pulmonary openings. Do the same with the two left pulmonary veins. Make a transverse cut to join these two small vertical incisions and so open the left atrium posteriorly. Then extend this cut as far as the apex of the left auricle. Wash out the interior of the atrium.

Examine the interior of the left atrium and also its auricular appendage. Note the smooth lining of the atrium itself and the pectinate muscles in the auricle. Also note the **openings of the pulmonary veins** in the atrium.

Examine the **left atrioventricular opening** and its two-cusped **mitral valve.** Note that in the normal subject this opening is smaller than the atrioventricular opening on the right side, and that it admits only two fingers.

The left ventricle [Figs 3.37–3.41]

To open the left ventricle first pass a pointed, long-bladed knife through the mitral valve until it emerges through the apex of the left ventricle. When the knife is in this position, open the left ventricle by cutting laterally to the left [Fig. 3.37]. Next pass the knife from the lower end of this incision upwards, between the cusp of the mitral valve and the interventricular septum, through the aortic valve and out through the cut end of the aorta. Now cut posteriorly to expose the interior of the left ventricle and the ascending aorta [Fig. 3.38]. Clean out any clots that may still be present.

First examine the ventricular aspect of the left atrioventricular opening and note the two triangular cusps of the mitral valve [Fig. 3.39]. The **anterior cusp** is larger than the **posterior cusp.** You will see that their chordae tendineae are arranged exactly as are those on the right side. Small intermediate cusps may be present.

Note the two large papillary muscles in the left ventricle. The **anterior papillary muscle** is attached to the anterior wall and the **posterior papillary muscle** to the wall which rests on the diaphragm. Note that the trabeculae carneae in the interior of the left ventricle are similar to those of the right, but that there is no septomarginal trabecula.

Examine the **opening of the aorta** in the upper part of the left ventricle [Figs 3.40 and 3.41]. It is guarded by the **aortic valve** formed by three semilunar valves which are disposed differently from those of the pulmonary trunk, with one posteriorly, the **posterior semilunar valve,** and two anteriorly.

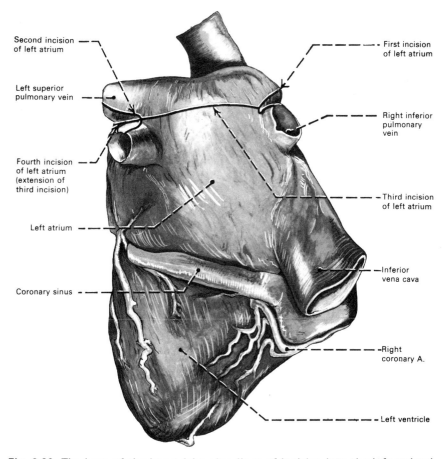

Fig. 3.36 The base of the heart (showing lines of incision into the left atrium).

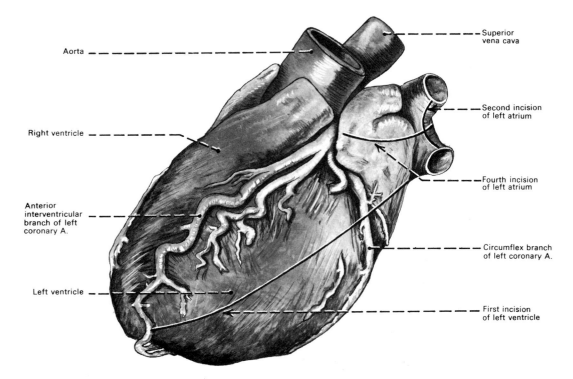

Fig. 3.37 The left ventricle (showing lines of incision).

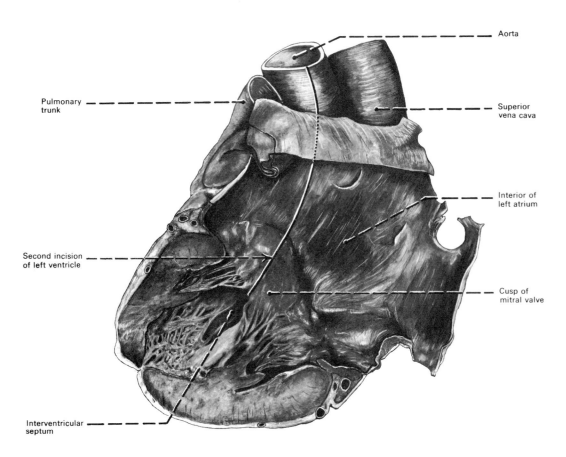

Pulmonary trunk

Aorta

Superior vena cava

Interior of left atrium

Second incision of left ventricle

Cusp of mitral valve

Interventricular septum

Fig. 3.38 The interior of the left atrium and ventricle (showing line of incision into the aorta).

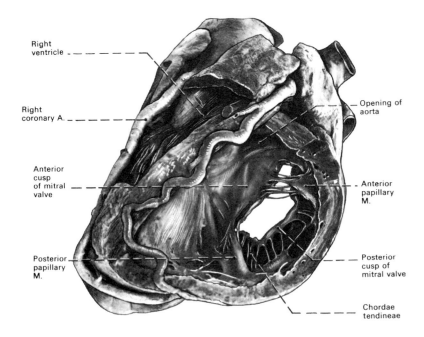

Right ventricle

Right coronary A.

Anterior cusp of mitral valve

Posterior papillary M.

Opening of aorta

Anterior papillary M.

Posterior cusp of mitral valve

Chordae tendineae

Fig. 3.39 The interior of the left ventricle (viewed from the left). This dissection is different from the one described in the text. The sternocostal wall of the left ventricle has been excised, together with part of the diaphragmatic wall.

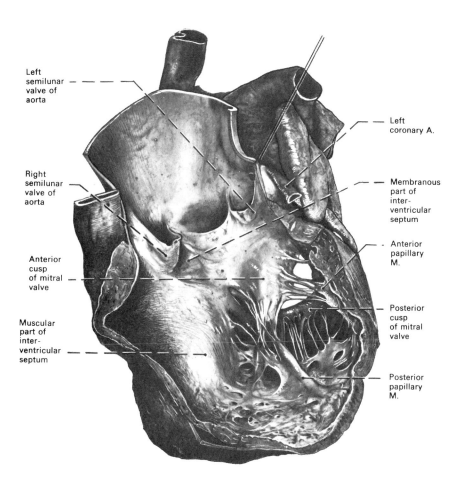

Left
semilunar
valve of
aorta

Left
coronary A.

Right
semilunar
valve of
aorta

Membranous
part of
inter-
ventricular
septum

Anterior
papillary
M.

Anterior
cusp
of mitral
valve

Posterior
cusp
of mitral
valve

Muscular
part of
inter-
ventricular
septum

Posterior
papillary
M.

Fig. 3.40 The mitral and aortic valves. This dissection is different from the one described in the text. The ascending aorta has been incised and the left ventricle opened widely, after the excision of part of its wall.

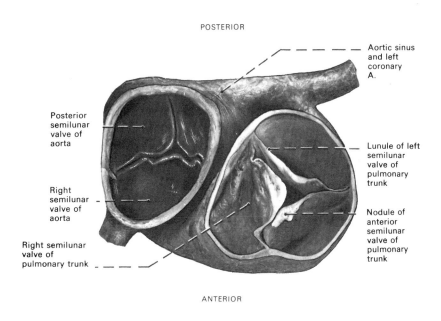

POSTERIOR

Aortic sinus
and left
coronary
A.

Posterior
semilunar
valve of
aorta

Lunule of left
semilunar
valve of
pulmonary
trunk

Right
semilunar
valve of
aorta

Nodule of
anterior
semilunar
valve of
pulmonary
trunk

Right semilunar
valve of
pulmonary trunk

ANTERIOR

Fig. 3.41 The aortic and pulmonary valves (viewed from above). The dissection is different from the one described in the text.

The two anterior semilunar valves are called the **right** and **left semilunar valves.** Observe that the position of the semilunar valves is marked internally by three slight excavations. These are the aortic sinuses, which you have already seen from the exterior. Examine the openings of the coronary arteries. They are the two small openings which you see immediately above the level of attachment of the aortic semilunar valves. The right coronary artery arises from the right sinus, and the left from the left sinus. With the heart in its normal position in the body, the right coronary artery springs from the anterior and the left from the left posterior aspect of the aorta.

Clean the origins of the aorta and pulmonary trunk. Separate them from each other, and separate the atria from the aorta. This will allow you to examine the external surface of the aortic sinuses again, and to appreciate that the atria lie entirely on the posterior aspect of the heart. Note that the aortic, pulmonary, and both atrioventricular valves all lie in the plane of the coronary groove.

The walls of the heart

Note that the ventricles have much thicker walls than the atria, and that the wall of the left ventricle is much thicker than that of the right. Also note again that, with the exception of the auricles, which are ridged, the atria have smooth walls, as compared with the ventricles, whose walls are roughened by trabeculae carneae.

Now look again at the septa between the right and left halves of the heart. First examine the **interatrial septum.** Note that this is placed so obliquely that the right atrium lies almost directly in front of the left. The principal feature of the interatrial septum is the fossa ovalis. Next look at the **interventricular septum.** Note that it is almost entirely muscular except for a small **membranous part** just below the aortic opening. The septum also lies obliquely and bulges slightly into the right ventricle.

The conducting system of the heart

The wall of the heart is made up of a unique meshwork of muscle fibres, and also of a special conducting system which is called the **neuromyocardium.** The study of this system is usually impracticable in a dissecting-room cadaver, but the following facts should be noted.

In the upper part of the sulcus terminalis, near the opening of the superior vena cava into the right atrium, is a small **sinuatrial node,** formed by neuromyocardial cells. This node is sometimes called the 'pacemaker', for it governs the rate at which the heart beats. Both the vagus nerves, which slow the heart, and the sympathetic nerves, which accelerate it, influence the 'pacemaker'. The impulse which initiates each heart-beat starts in this node and then radiates over the atria to another mass of neuromyocardium called the **atrioventricular node,** which is situated in the right atrium near the opening of the coronary sinus. From here the impulse passes along a tract of specialized neuromuscular tissue called the **atrioventricular bundle.** This divides into two branches, one for each ventricle, and these pass down on either side of the interventricular septum to link up with a plexus of specialized subendocardial muscle-fibres, called the **Purkinje fibres.** The fibres of the **left branch** of the atrioventricular bundle are distributed mainly to the anterior and the posterior papillary muscles of the left ventricle. The **right branch** terminates in the papillary muscles of the right ventricle, much of it traversing the septomarginal trabecula when this is present. This arrangement allows the cardiac impulse to reach all parts of the ventricles rapidly and in an ordered succession starting at the apex of the heart. The arrangement of the conducting system ensures the contraction of the papillary muscles which control the movement of the cusps of the valves between the atria and the ventricles.

Note again the blood supply to the conducting system. The atrioventricular node, the atrioventricular bundle and its right branch are supplied by the right coronary artery. The sinuatrial node and the left branch of the atrioventricular bundle are supplied by both right and left coronary arteries.

The heart-beat

The conducting system is responsible for the various phases of the heart-beat (cardiac cycle). The contraction of the atria (atrial systole) comprises the first phase of the heart-beat. As a result, blood is pumped into the ventricles. During this phase, the edges of the flaps of the mitral and tricuspid valves, which are non-contractile, are directed towards the ventricular cavities because of the flow of blood. The ventricles then contract (ventricular systole), and drive blood from the right side of the heart into the pulmonary trunk and so to the lungs, and from the left side by way of the aorta to the body as a whole. As the ventricles contract, the cusps of the tricuspid and mitral valves are pulled together, partly because the papillary muscles attached to them contract with the ventricular walls and partly because of the pressure of blood on their ventricular surfaces. Since the papillary muscles are attached by the chordae tendineae to the periphery of the cusps, the latter cannot be forced back into the atria as the pressure of blood in the ventricles rises. The atrioventricular openings are thus closed, and blood cannot be regurgitated into the atria. Correspondingly, immediately after the blood is pumped from the ventricles and the ventricles begin to relax, the pulmonary and aortic valves close because the pressure of blood in the ventricles drops below that in the pulmonary trunk and aorta, and regurgitation of blood into the ventricles is thereby prevented.

Systole is followed by a phase of relaxation called diastole, during which the heart is filled.

Section 3.4

The lungs

The surfaces of the lungs

Now turn to the lungs of your specimen, bearing in mind that they have been hardened by the preserving fluid, and that their hard rubbery texture is entirely different from that of the living lung, which is light and spongy. The lungs will be seen to be a dark mottled grey owing to discoloration by carbon deposits inhaled in the air we breathe. The natural colour of the lung, as seen in the foetus and in children, is pink.

You will see that each lung is conical in shape [Fig. 3.42]. Replace them in the thorax and confirm that, in both, the **apex of the lung** would have extended into the neck for about 3 cm above the clavicle. Note the large concave **base of the lung** which rests on the diaphragm. On the right side the diaphragm separates the base of the right lung from the superior part of the convex **diaphragmatic surface** of the right lobe of the liver, so that the base of the lung is deeply concave. The base of the left lung is shallower, since the diaphragm separates it only from the smaller left lobe of the liver and the softer stomach and spleen.

On both lungs note the rounded lateral or **costal surface** on which you may see impressions made by the ribs. This surface ends in front in a sharp anterior border. Behind, the thick and rounded posterior border separates the costal surface from the **vertebral part of the medial surface**. The **mediastinal part of the medial surface** of each lung should be studied separately.

The lobes and fissures of the lungs [Fig. 3.42]

Compare the two lungs and note their fissures, which are very variable in their disposition. If your specimen follows the more usual pattern, you will find on the left lung an extensive **oblique fissure** which divides the substance of the lung into two (so that it is visible both on the costal surface and also on the medial surface, both above and below the **hilum of the lung**). The fissure divides the lung into a **superior lobe** and an **inferior lobe**. Note that the superior lobe is the anterior lobe, since it lies mainly in the front of the thoracic cavity, and that the inferior lobe lies mainly in the back of the thoracic cavity. Note also that much of the inferior lobe extends above the lower part of the superior lobe. The apex of the left lung is part of the superior lobe, and the base is part of the inferior lobe.

Now examine the right lung and note that it, too, is divided by an oblique fissure into two main lobes. Note also that the upper of these two lobes is usually cut in two by a **horizontal fissure,** whose level is roughly parallel to the lower border of the fourth rib. That part of the lung which lies between the oblique and horizontal fissures is called the **middle lobe.**

On both sides the upper part of the oblique fissure passes through the posterior border 6 cm below the apex, and transects the inferior margin 6 cm behind the antero-inferior angle. You may be able to see that the upper limit of this fissure corresponds to the spinous process of the third or fourth thoracic vertebra, and that it lies at the level of the fourth intercostal space or fifth rib.

The right lung is larger than the left, into which the heart projects. If you look at the anterior border of the left lung you will see that it is marked by a wide notch. This is the **cardiac notch of the left lung** [Fig. 3.17]. A large part of the sternocostal surface of the heart is not covered by lung.

The medial surface of the right lung [Fig. 3.43a]

Now examine the medial surface of the right lung [Fig. 3.43a], and replace it in the body from time to time in order to visualize the relations it would have had in the undisturbed thorax. First, look at the **root of the lung.** It is the fixed part of the lung and lies opposite the bodies of the fifth, sixth, and seventh thoracic vertebrae. You may have difficulty in defining the cut edge of the **pulmonary ligament** at the lower extremity, but you should have none in distinguishing the **pulmonary artery** from the **pulmonary veins** and the **bronchi.** Use your forceps to pick out a number of black or dark-grey lymph nodes which lie between these structures. Try to find the small **bronchial artery** which you may see closely applied to the wall of the bronchus. Locate the groove for the azygos vein immediately above the lung root.

In front of the lung root, and extending upwards as far as the anterior border, you will see a wide groove. This groove would have been in contact with the superior vena cava and the right brachiocephalic vein. You may see a shorter groove extending from the anterior border of the lung and leading to this wider groove. It lodged the left brachiocephalic vein. Posterior to the groove for the right brachiocephalic vein the apex of the lung may be marked by a groove caused by the right subclavian artery. Below the groove for the superior vena cava and in front of the lung root is a concavity which accommodated the right atrium

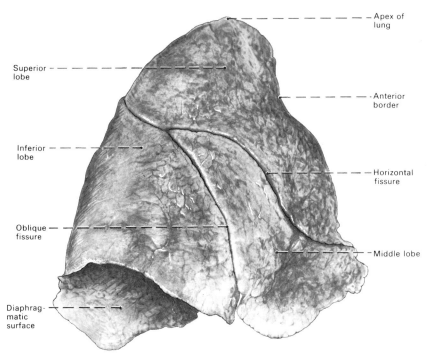

Apex of
lung

Superior
lobe

Anterior
border

Inferior
lobe

Horizontal
fissure

Oblique
fissure

Middle lobe

Diaphrag-
matic
surface

a. *The right lung*

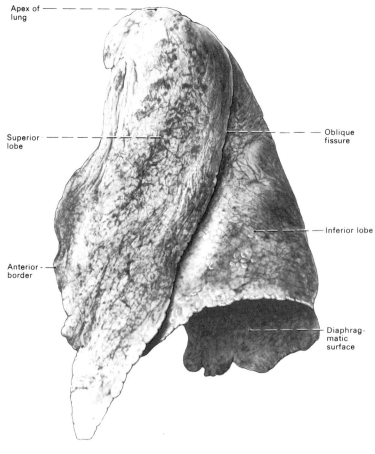

Apex of
lung

Superior
lobe

Oblique
fissure

Inferior lobe

Anterior
border

Diaphrag-
matic
surface

b. *The left lung*

Fig. 3.42 The costal surfaces of the lungs.

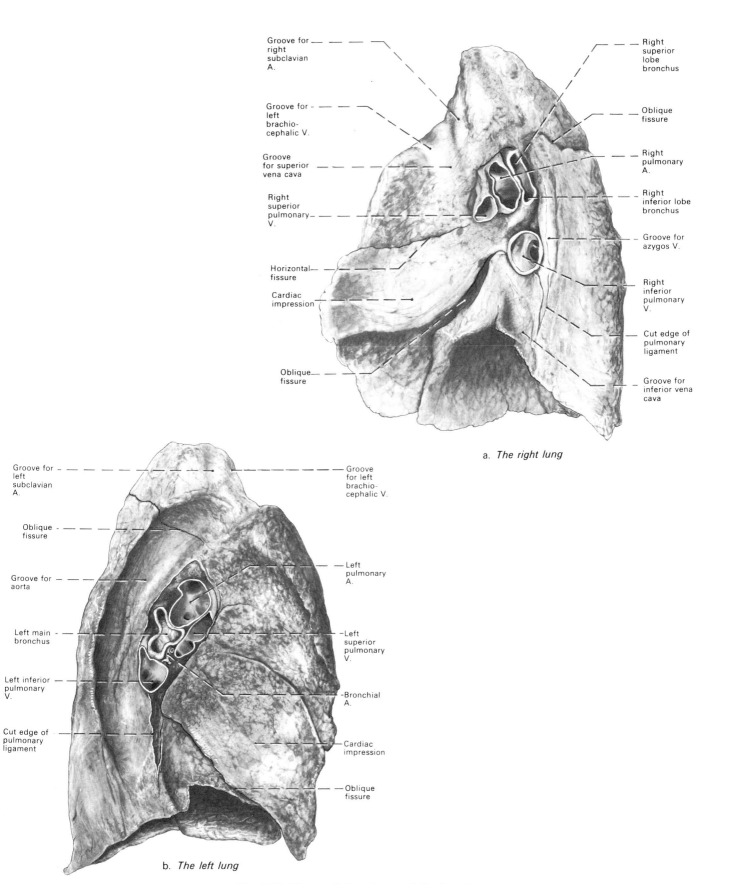

Groove for right subclavian A.

Groove for left brachio-cephalic V.

Groove for superior vena cava

Right superior pulmonary V.

Horizontal fissure

Cardiac impression

Oblique fissure

Right superior lobe bronchus

Oblique fissure

Right pulmonary A.

Right inferior lobe bronchus

Groove for azygos V.

Right inferior pulmonary V.

Cut edge of pulmonary ligament

Groove for inferior vena cava

a. *The right lung*

Groove for left subclavian A.

Oblique fissure

Groove for aorta

Left main bronchus

Left inferior pulmonary V.

Cut edge of pulmonary ligament

Groove for left brachio-cephalic V.

Left pulmonary A.

Left superior pulmonary V.

Bronchial A.

Cardiac impression

Oblique fissure

b. *The left lung*

Fig. 3.43 The medial surfaces of the lungs.

and part of the right ventricle. On the inferior border of the medial surface, below this cardiac concavity, you may be able to discern a short shallow groove produced by the inferior vena cava.

Note the position of the trachea in relation to the right lung. It lies above the root of the lung, and behind the groove for the right brachiocephalic vein. The vertical groove behind the root was made by the right side of the oesophagus.

The medial surface of the left lung [Fig. 3.43b]
Now look at the medial surface of the left lung [Fig. 3.43b]. Examine the **root** and again identify the **pulmonary artery,** the **main bronchus,** the **superior** and **inferior pulmonary veins,** and, if possible, the cut edges of the **pulmonary ligament.** On the posterior surface of the left main bronchus look for two **bronchial arteries,** both of which usually arise from the descending aorta. Note the black lymph nodes in the root, and pick them out with your dissecting forceps.

The extensive concavity in front of the root and the pulmonary ligament, which is bisected by the oblique fissure, lodges the left, and to a lesser extent the right, ventricle of the heart. Replace the lung and try to appreciate that the wide groove you will see above the root of the lung lodged the aortic arch, and the one behind the root the descending aorta. The vertical groove you will see above the root of the lung lodged the left subclavian artery. In front of the groove for the subclavian artery you may see a shallow groove made by the left brachiocephalic vein. Finally, examine the inferior border of the lung in front of the groove for the descending aorta. You may find a shallow groove here produced by the oesophagus.

Dissection of the lungs

The root of the right lung
You should now try to dissect into the substance of the lung sufficiently far to demonstrate the disposition of the main subdivisions of the bronchi and pulmonary vessels. Identify once more the structures which comprise the root of the right lung, and which were cut when you removed the lung. You probably divided the **right main bronchus** after it had divided into a branch to the superior lobe, called the **right superior lobe bronchus,** and branches to the middle and inferior lobes, called the **right middle lobe bronchus** and the **right inferior lobe bronchus.** If you did, you will find that the pulmonary artery lies between the superior lobe bronchus and the lower part of the main bronchus, and that the two pulmonary veins lie anterior to and below them. Try to find the small right bronchial artery lying immediately behind the main bronchus. This artery arises either from the third right posterior intercostal artery, or from one of the left bronchial arteries.

These three lobar bronchi divide into **segmental bronchi** which supply definable subdivisions, or **bronchopulmonary segments,** of lung tissue. Each bronchus is accompanied by a corresponding branch of the pulmonary artery and by a tributary of the pulmonary vein.

The root of the left lung
Now examine the left lung, and note first that the left main bronchus does not divide until it is well inside the lung. Identify the pulmonary artery above the bronchus, and the two pulmonary veins, one anterior to the bronchus and the other below it. You should find two small left bronchial arteries on the posterior surface of the bronchus. They usually arise from the descending aorta. You will again find lymph nodes in the lung root.

Repeat on the left lung the dissection that you carried out when tracing the bronchi of the right lung. The **left main bronchus** is longer than the right, and does not descend so steeply as it passes into the lung. It divides into a **left superior lobe bronchus,** which leads off in an antero-lateral direction, and a **left inferior lobe bronchus,** which continues postero-inferiorly in line with the main bronchus.

The lobar bronchi of the left lung subdivide segmentally, in the same way as those of the right side.

Section 3.5

The posterior and the superior mediastinum

Your next step is to complete the dissection of the posterior mediastinum and the deeper parts of the superior mediastinum. These contain the descending aorta, the trachea and bronchi, the oesophagus, the thoracic duct, the azygos vein, and the sympathetic trunks.

Divide the superior vena cava just above the level where it is joined by the azygos vein [Fig. 3.44]. This will allow the upper part of the superior vena cava and the brachio-cephalic veins to be turned up out of the way. Dissect away the pericardium from the front of the ascending aorta and the pulmonary trunk. Divide the brachiocephalic trunk close to its origin and turn the arch of the aorta to the left. Clean away all the fibrous pericardium from the back of the ascending aorta, the upper part of the arch of the aorta, and the upper surfaces of the pulmonary arteries.

The cardiac plexus

This dissection will have exposed the deep part of the cardiac plexus lying on the lower part of the trachea, near its bifurcation, and the lymph nodes in this region. If you tease the tissue on the right antero-lateral aspect of the trachea, you will find nerve strands from the cervical parts of the sympathetic trunks which pass to the deep part of the plexus of sympathetic and parasympathetic nerves called the cardiac plexus [pp. 3.19–3.21]. Trace some of these small

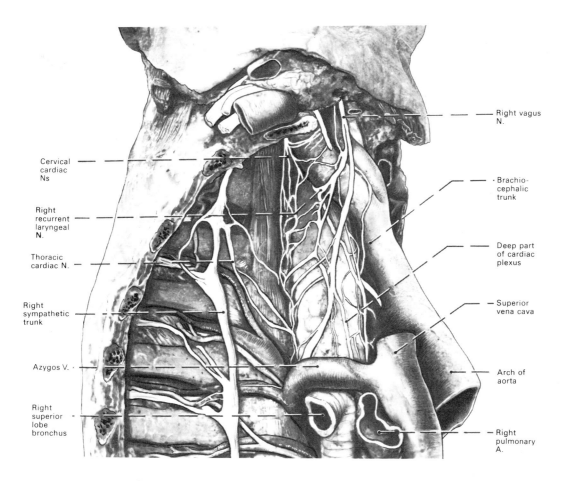

Fig. 3.44 The right side of the deep part of the cardiac plexus.

nerves upwards as far as is possible. On the right side try to find branches from the vagus nerve, and from the **right recurrent laryngeal nerve,** which also pass to this plexus [Fig. 3.44].

Also try to find branches passing from the deep part of the cardiac plexus to a plexus of nerves beginning in front of the root of the lung. This is the anterior part of the **pulmonary plexus.** Do not spend more time on this part of your dissection than is necessary to provide you with a general idea of the disposition of the cardiac plexus.

The nerves to the heart come from the cardiac plexus and comprise branches of both sympathetic trunks and parasympathetic and afferent branches of both vagus nerves. A **superficial part** of the cardiac plexus lies in the concavity of the aortic arch in front of the ligamentum arteriosum [Fig. 3.45]. The larger, **deep part** of the cardiac plexus [Figs 3.44 and 3.47] lies behind the aortic arch in front of the bifurcation of the trachea.

The cardiac plexus sends branches to the anterior parts of the left and right pulmonary plexuses and to the corresponding coronary arteries for distribution to the atria and ventricles of the heart and to the sinuatrial and atrioventricular nodes.

Now investigate the structures lying on the left of the trachea. To do this remove the arch of the aorta by dividing

it along the lines indicated in Fig. 3.45, noting that the incision commences proximal to the attachment of the ligamentum arteriosum and that the left common carotid and subclavian arteries remain attached to the arch at their origins.

Clean the left common carotid and left subclavian arteries and turn them, too, out of the way. This will allow you to dissect on the left side of the trachea, where you should find more nerve strands passing to the deep part of the cardiac plexus from the left sympathetic trunk and the left vagus nerve. It should be easy to demonstrate connections between the deep part of the cardiac plexus and the superficial part of the plexus, lying below the arch of the aorta.

You will also see lymph nodes in the vicinity of the trachea and main bronchi. Remove these.

The vagus nerves [Figs 3.44 and 3.45]

Pick up the origin of the **left recurrent laryngeal nerve** as it hooks round the ligamentum arteriosum and trace it upwards as far as possible. Trace the main trunk of the left vagus nerve behind the root of the lung, identify some of the branches it sends to the **pulmonary plexus** which, were the lungs in place, would be found lying on the anterior and posterior aspects of the root; and continue to trace the main

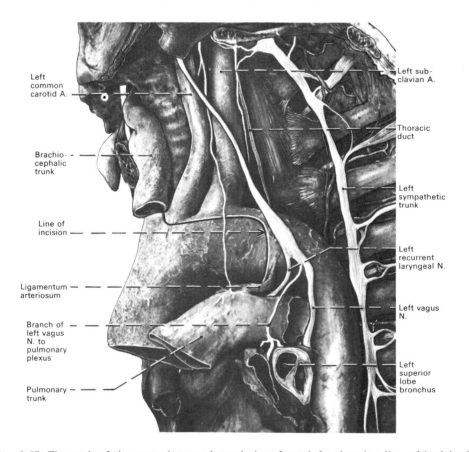

Left common carotid A.

Brachio-cephalic trunk

Line of incision

Ligamentum arteriosum

Branch of left vagus N. to pulmonary plexus

Pulmonary trunk

Left sub-clavian A.

Thoracic duct

Left sympathetic trunk

Left recurrent laryngeal N.

Left vagus N.

Left superior lobe bronchus

Fig. 3.45 The arch of the aorta (antero-lateral view from left, showing line of incision).

3.44

trunk of the vagus behind the pericardium to the front of the oesophagus, on which you will see it breaks up into a plexus. Trace the right vagus nerve similarly. At this stage of your dissection do not try to follow the **oesophageal plexus** right down the oesophagus.

The thoracic duct [Fig. 3.46]

Dissect behind the origin of the left subclavian artery and find the thoracic duct [Fig. 3.45]. This is the small and thin-walled grey vessel which is running upwards from behind the arch of the aorta. Trace it upwards as far as you can behind and to the left of the oesophagus. You may find small efferent vessels from lymph nodes at the side of the trachea joining the duct. Follow the lower part of the thoracic duct downwards into the right side of the posterior mediastinum. It crosses behind the oesophagus to lie on the left of the azygos vein, where, with care, it may be found.

The duct commences in the abdomen from a dilated sac called the **cisterna chyli.** This you will see when you dissect the abdomen. Lift up the lower end of the oesophagus and dissect behind it. You will find the duct on the left side of the azygos vein, and you may see it entering the posterior mediastinum through the aortic opening in the diaphragm. The duct lies on the bodies of the thoracic vertebrae behind the oesophagus, between the aorta and the azygos vein [Fig. 3.46].

When you trace the duct upwards you will see that it crosses the midline obliquely behind the aorta and oeso-phagus, at the level of the intervertebral disc between the fourth and fifth thoracic vertebrae, to enter the superior mediastinum. Afterwards it passes into the neck to enter the beginning of the left brachiocephalic vein. You will only see the terminal part of its course when you dissect the head and neck. The thoracic duct drains the lymph from the whole of the body below the diaphragm, from the left half

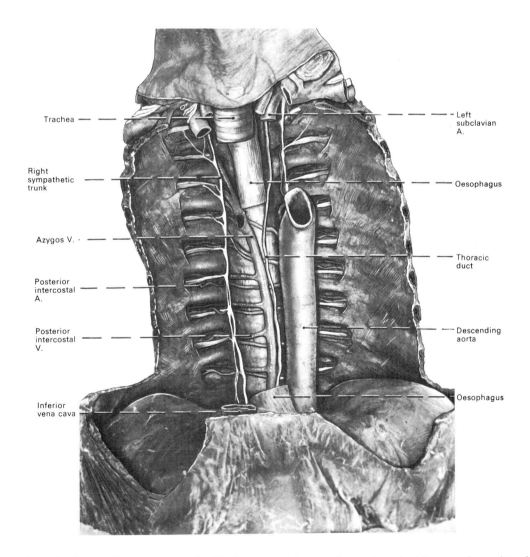

Fig. 3.46 The thoracic duct and the azygos vein. The lower part of the trachea and much of the oesophagus have been excised.

of the head, neck, and thorax, and from the whole of the left upper limb. [See Appendix and Fig. A.3.]

Now turn to the pulmonary trunk and note that, as measured from their origins, the right pulmonary artery is longer than the left, and that it passes behind the aorta and superior vena cava to the hilum of the right lung.

The trachea [Fig. 3.47]

Cut the ligamentum arteriosum, and the azygos vein just before it enters the superior vena cava. Separate the 'stumps' of the pulmonary veins and pulmonary arteries from the underlying main bronchi on both sides and reflect the remains of the pericardium downwards, with the pulmonary trunk and arteries and the remains of the superior vena cava attached to it. Be careful not to destroy the oesophageal plexus as you separate the pericardium from the oesophagus. In separating the fibrous pericardium from its

attachment to the pretracheal layer of the cervical fascia, the connections of the cardiac plexus to the pulmonary plexus will have to be severed. Take care not to damage the main vagal trunks and the left recurrent laryngeal nerve. The reflected structures can be replaced if necessary to see their relations to one another.

The thoracic part of the trachea is now fully exposed, covered by the **pretracheal layer of the cervical fascia.** The trachea is a tube about 10 cm long lying partly in the neck and partly in the thorax. You will see the cardiac plexus lying on it, and probably some lymph nodes will still remain at its bifurcation. These nodes should now be removed. Incise the pretracheal layer of fascia longitudinally in the midline and reflect it to each side, with the cardiac plexus still attached to it, and so clean the trachea. Note that the trachea bifurcates at the level of the plane of the sternal angle [p. 3.7]. Look for the bronchial arteries, which are probably still attached to the cut ends of the bronchi.

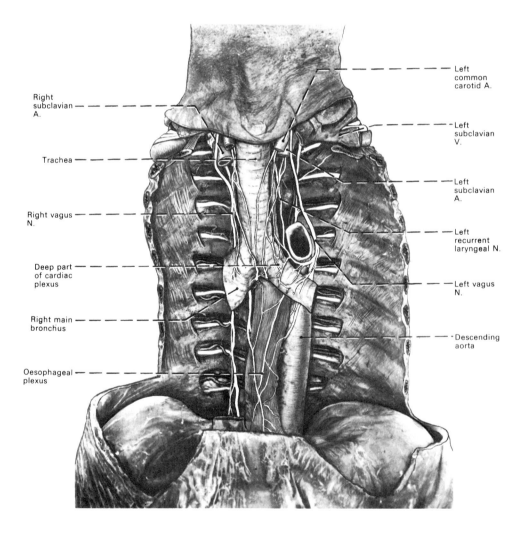

Fig. 3.47 The trachea and the deep part of the cardiac plexus.

The structure of the trachea

The trachea is composed of fibro-elastic tissue reinforced by cartilaginous 'rings', the **tracheal cartilages,** which are deficient posteriorly. Here the wall contains an intrinsic muscle called the **trachealis muscle.** The last cartilage is thick and broad in front, and from its lower border a ridge of cartilage is carried downwards and backwards in the fork between the two bronchi. This ridge of cartilage is called the **carina tracheae.** Note that the aortic arch crosses the trachea, and that the brachiocephalic trunk and left common carotid artery are anterior relations. The oesophagus will be seen to lie behind the trachea throughout its course, with the left recurrent laryngeal nerve in the angular interval between the two. This is an important relation.

The main bronchi [Fig. 3.47]

Examine the **left main bronchus.** Note that it lies more horizontally and that it is longer and narrower than the right.

Trace it as it crosses in front of the descending aorta and the oesophagus to enter the root of the lung, where it divides into two branches, one for the superior and the other for the inferior lobe of the lung. Now examine the **right main bronchus,** which you will see is more in a straight line with the trachea. Note that it passes into the root of the lung behind the pulmonary artery. Note also that on both sides the anterior part of the pulmonary plexus lies in front of the main bronchus, and the posterior part of the pulmonary plexus and bronchial vessels lie behind.

The oesophagus [Fig. 3.48]

Dissect the small bronchial arteries away from the bronchi, and clean away all the lymph nodes you find in the posterior mediastinum. Tease out the oesophageal plexus of autonomic nerves on the surface of the oesophagus. Establish that they are branches of the vagus nerves.

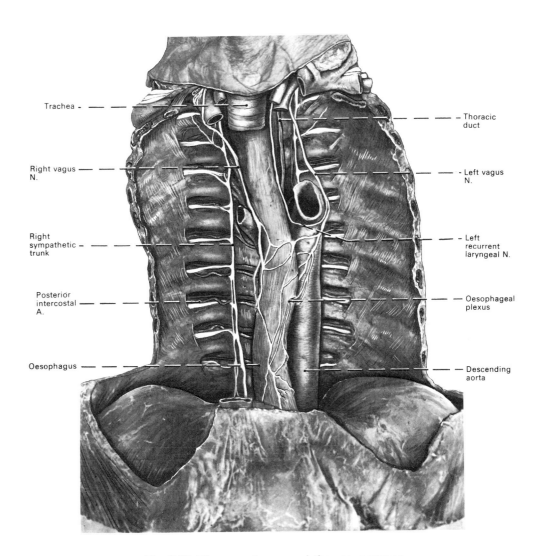

Trachea

Right vagus N.

Right sympathetic trunk

Posterior intercostal A.

Oesophagus

Thoracic duct

Left vagus N.

Left recurrent laryngeal N.

Oesophageal plexus

Descending aorta

Fig. 3.48 The oesophagus and the vagus nerves.

The blood supply of the oesophagus

The thoracic part of the oesophagus is supplied by small branches from the descending aorta and bronchial arteries. With other small arteries which supply its upper and lower parts, these form an essentially longitudinal anastomosis on its surface. In a well-injected cadaver, you may see a few of these arterial branches. Most of the blood from a plexus of veins on the surface of the oesophagus drains into the azygos system of veins. But at the lower end some blood drains into the left gastric vein, which is a tributary of the portal vein of the abdominal cavity. Thus an anastomosis is established between the systemic and portal systems of veins [see p. 4.74]. Make a longitudinal incision in the fascia covering the oesophagus and strip it away from the muscle wall.

The course of the oesophagus [Fig. 3.48]

The oesophagus is about 25 cm long, and lies partly in the neck but mainly in the thorax, a very small part also lying within the abdominal cavity. Note that it has a muscular wall and follow its course through the thorax. Above you will see that it lies behind the trachea and in front of the vertebral column. Trace it downwards, and you will see that it is crossed by the left main bronchus. You will see that in the posterior mediastinum the oesophagus lies behind the pericardium and the left atrium of the heart. Note that the thoracic aorta crosses behind the oesophagus just above the diaphragm. From the level of the plane of the sternal angle the aorta lies on the left side. The oesophagus pierces the diaphragm at the level of the tenth thoracic vertebra.

Visualize that in the undissected body the left lung is in contact with the oesophagus in the superior mediastinum, and that the two are also in contact in the posterior mediastinum just above the diaphragm. Between these two points the oesophagus is in contact with the right lung and pleura.

The descending thoracic aorta [Fig. 3.48]

Lift the oesophagus out of the way and clean the descending thoracic aorta and trace it towards its termination behind the diaphragm at the level of the twelfth thoracic vertebra. Find and clean the origins of two or three of the nine pairs of **posterior intercostal arteries** which pass to the lower nine intercostal spaces from the aorta. If you can, trace the origins of the two left **bronchial arteries** from the descending aorta which, remember again, also gives branches to the pericardium, oesophagus, and diaphragm.

As you dissect in the posterior part of the intercostal spaces, note again that these and the posterior mediastinum are drained by means of the posterior intercostal veins which mostly pass into the azygos system of veins [Fig. 3.46]. These veins also drain the main bronchi, the oesophagus, and the pericardium.

Section 3.6

The joints of the thorax

Before you complete your dissection of the thorax, you should examine the joints of the ribs and costal cartilages. You will not study the joints of the vertebral column until a much later stage of your dissection of the body.

The costovertebral joints

The joints of the heads of the ribs [Fig. 3.49]

You have already seen [p. 3.5] that typically the head of a rib articulates with the body of its numerically-corresponding thoracic vertebra, the body of the vertebra above, and with the intervertebral disc between these two vertebrae.

The joints of the heads of the ribs are synovial joints. Each has an **articular capsule** which is strengthened anteriorly by a ligament which consists of three bands passing to the bodies of the adjacent vertebrae and to the intervening intervertebral disc. This ligament is called the **radiate ligament of the head of the rib** [Fig. 3.49]. There is also an **intra-articular ligament of the head of the rib** which joins the crest of the head of the rib to the intervertebral disc. It divides the joint cavity into two parts, but is absent where the rib articulates with one vertebra only.

To establish these points examine the costovertebral joints of either the fifth or sixth rib. First expose the whole course of an intercostal nerve and look again at its rami communicantes [p. 3.21]. Remove the sympathetic trunk from over the head of the rib, and remove also the adjacent posterior intercostal arteries and veins. If you then clean the head of the rib and the adjacent vertebral bodies, the radiate ligament will be clearly seen. Rock the cut end of a rib to demonstrate its range of movement.

The costotransverse joints [Fig. 3.49]

Refer again to an articulated skeleton and try to visualize how the neck of the rib is fixed by ligaments both to the

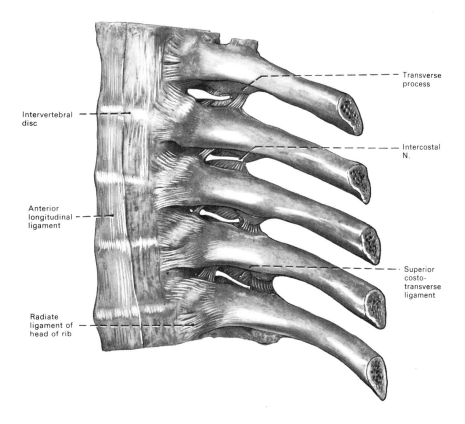

Intervertebral disc

Anterior longitudinal ligament

Radiate ligament of head of rib

Transverse process

Intercostal N.

Superior costo-transverse ligament

Fig. 3.49 The costovertebral joints.

transverse process of the vertebra above and to the transverse process of its corresponding vertebra. The ligaments are the **superior costotransverse ligament** [Fig. 3.49] and the **costotransverse ligament** respectively.

Note, too, that the tubercle of the rib articulates with the transverse process of the numerically-corresponding thoracic vertebra, forming a synovial costotransverse joint. Each joint has a capsule which is reinforced by a strong **lateral costotransverse ligament** [Fig. 3.50]. This ligament extends from the non-articular part of the tubercle to the tip of the transverse process.

Dissection of the costovertebral joints

Turn the body on its side or on its face, press the lateral part of the erector spinae muscle medially, insert the blade of a scalpel between this muscle and the ribs, and divide the attachments of the muscle between the tubercles and the angles of the ribs. When you now press the erector spinae muscle medially, some small flat muscles will come into view. They are the **levatores costarum muscles** [Fig. 3.50]. These are fan-shaped muscles which arise from a transverse process and are inserted into the upper border of the rib below, between the tubercle and the angle.

Remove the remainder of the intercostal muscles and membranes from the spaces above and below the rib you are dissecting. Also remove the levatores costarum muscles. You will then be able to see the lateral costotransverse ligament very clearly. Divide this ligament and the lower part of the articular capsule of the costotransverse joint. If you elevate the rib you will be able to see into the joint. Divide the superior costotransverse ligament by incising it along its attachment to the rib. Next divide the radiate ligament, and then pass the blade of your scalpel between the neck of the rib and the transverse process and so divide the costotransverse ligament. Remove the rib by dividing the posterior part of the capsule of the joint of the head of the rib. Examine the remains of the costotransverse ligament and the intra-articular ligament of the head of the rib. Between the transverse processes of the vertebrae you will see some small muscles called the **rotatores** which pass between the transverse processes and laminae of adjacent vertebrae.

Now study the anterior ends of the ribs. Each has a concavity into which the corresponding costal cartilage fits. The rib and costal cartilage are united by the fusion of the periosteum and perichondrium. You can see the concavity at the end of the ribs by looking at a dried specimen.

The sternocostal joints

Examine the disposition of the sternocostal joints on an articulated skeleton. The cartilages of the true ribs (except the first) articulate with the sternum by synovial joints. Each joint has a capsule which is reinforced anteriorly and posteriorly by **radiate sternocostal ligaments.** An **intra-articular**

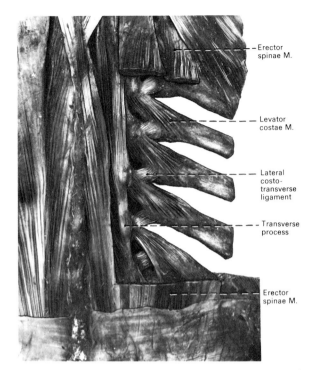

Fig. 3.50 The right levatores costarum muscles. The lateral part of the right erector spinae muscle has been excised.

sternocostal ligament is present in the second sternocostal joint, which thus has two synovial compartments. It is occasionally present in other sternocostal joints. Two small **costoxiphoid ligaments** connect each of the two seventh costal cartilages with the xiphoid process of the sternum. The junction of the first costal cartilage with the sternum is a primary cartilaginous joint which eventually ossifies more or less completely.

The sixth and seventh, the seventh and eighth, and the eighth and ninth costal cartilages articulate at **interchondral joints.** These are synovial joints with an articular capsule. The tenth costal cartilage is usually united to the ninth costal cartilage by fibrous tissue.

The sternocostal and interchondral joints are plane joints capable of gliding movements which take place when the chest wall moves during respiration.

To establish these points on your own dissection, study the sternum and attached ribs which you removed when you opened the thorax. Remove the perichondrium and periosteum from the region of a costochondral junction so that the rib and costal cartilage can be separated and the depression at the end of the rib seen. Then clean a sternocostal joint and note the sternocostal ligaments. Open the joint by incising it in the line of the articular surfaces. Examine the remains of the intra-articular ligament in another joint.

The action of the muscles of respiration

Inspiration of air begins with the contraction of the external intercostal muscles, which raise the ribs. In this action they are aided by those parts of the internal intercostal muscles adjacent to the sternum. As a result the transverse diameter of the thorax is increased. At the same time, owing to the raising of the anterior ends of the ribs, the sternum is pushed forward so that the antero-posterior diameter of the thorax increases. As this movement of the chest wall occurs, the diaphragm contracts and becomes flattened, thereby increasing the vertical diameter of the thorax. The result of this muscular activity is that the intrapleural pressure falls and air is drawn into the lungs.

As the diaphragm flattens it causes an increase in intra-abdominal pressure. This is countered by the relaxation of the muscles of the anterior abdominal wall, causing a bulge to appear in its upper part (the epigastrium). Expiration is due partly to the elastic recoil of the lungs and the relaxation of the diaphragm and the external intercostal muscles. As the latter relax, the main part of the internal intercostal muscles and the transversus abdominis muscles of the abdominal wall contract, as do also the subcostal muscles and the transversus thoracis muscle. All these muscles belong to the same muscle group, and as they depress the ribs, they are muscles of expiration.

At a convenient moment study your own respiratory movements, both when standing and when lying flat on your back. As your thoracic cage expands on inspiration you can see and feel that the ribs and sternum move upwards, and that they move downwards on expiration. Note too how the upper part of your anterior abdominal wall bulges forward on inspiration and flattens on expiration.

Normal respiration is described as being of the thoraco-abdominal type, that is, respiration in which the diaphragm and the intercostal muscles both take part in increasing the size of the thoracic cavity, with the diaphragm playing the major part. The thoracic type of respiration predominates in women in the later months of pregnancy, diaphragmatic movement being restricted by the mass of the uterus in the abdominal cavity.

Chart of contents of the abdomen

Abdominal wall

COMPONENTS	REGIONS		
	Anterior	**Posterior**	**Perineum**
	epigastric hypochondriac umbilical lateral pubic inguinal	lumbar	anal urogenital
Bones	ilium pubis	lumbar vertebrae sacrum ilium	sacrum coccyx ischium pubis
Joints	pubic symphysis	intervertebral sacroiliac	

Muscles	rectus abdominis
	obliques & transverse
	  rectus sheath
	  inguinal ligament
	diaphragm
		spinal extensors
		quadratus lumborum
		iliopsoas
		
		diaphragm
			pelvic diaphragm
			urogenital diaphragm
			  ischiorectal fossa

Nerves	ventral rami of
	  lower thoracic nerves
	  upper lumbar nerves
	branches of lumbosacral plexus
		dorsal rami of
		  lower thoracic nerves
		  lumbar nerves
		lumbosacral plexus
			branches of lumbosacral plexus

Vessels	epigastric intercostal lumbar	lumbar iliolumbar	internal iliac
Organs		spinal medulla cauda equina	anus external genitalia

Abdominopelvic cavity

	REGIONS			
	Abdominal cavity			**Pelvic cavity**
	peritoneal cavity	peritoneal	retroperitoneal	

CONTENTS	peritoneum
	mesenteries
	greater omentum
	lesser omentum
		spleen
		stomach
		liver
		gall-bladder
		transverse colon
		small intestine
		branches of
		  coeliac A.
		  mesenteric As
		tributaries of
		  portal V.
			pancreas
			duodenum
			ascending colon
			descending colon
			suprarenal glands
			kidneys
			ureters
			sympathetic trunks
			abdominal aorta
			inferior vena cava
			common and external
			  iliac vessels
			cisterna chyli
			thoracic duct
				peritoneum
				sigmoid colon
				rectum
				anal canal
				ureters
				urinary bladder
				internal genitalia
				  [except testis
				  and epididymis]
				
				internal iliac vessels

Superior boundary	diaphragm			plane of pelvic inlet
Inferior boundary	plane of pelvic inlet			pelvic diaphragm

Part 4

The abdomen

The abdomen comprises the abdominal and pelvic cavities, and is the part of the trunk that lies below the diaphragm [Fig. 4.1]. It is bounded above by the diaphragm; in front and at the sides by the muscles of the anterior abdominal wall; behind by the lumbar vertebrae and the muscles of the posterior abdominal wall; and below by the pelvic bones and a muscular diaphragm which forms a floor to the pelvic cavity. The smaller pelvic cavity is situated both below and behind the abdominal cavity proper, from which it is separated by the superior aperture of the pelvis (the plane of the pelvic inlet). The rim of the aperture is the linea terminalis, which is formed by the upper border of the pubic symphysis, the pubic crests, the pectens of the pubes, the arcuate lines of the iliac bones and the promontory of the sacrum [Fig. 2.2]. Within the abdominal and pelvic cavities are the stomach, intestines, and rectum; the liver and pancreas; the spleen; the kidneys and suprarenal glands; the ureters and urinary bladder; and most of the reproductive tract. The anal canal, the external genitalia, and in the male the testes, are below the pelvic diaphragm in an area called the perineum.

Your dissection begins with the perineum, which is not an easy region to investigate.

Before you start dissecting, revise and extend the knowledge you already have of the hip-bones, re-reading pages 2.2 to 2.4 before moving to page 4.3.

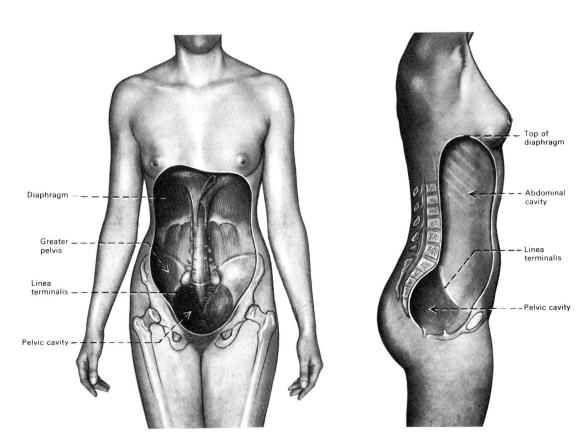

Diaphragm

Greater
pelvis

Linea
terminalis

Pelvic cavity

Top of
diaphragm

Abdominal
cavity

Linea
terminalis

Pelvic cavity

Fig. 4.1 Schematic diagrams of the abdominal cavity.

Section 4.1

The pelvis

Osteology

Examine the pelvis on the articulated skeleton, and note that it is made up of four bones [Fig. 4.2]. The two **hip-bones** bound the pelvic cavity anteriorly and laterally, and the **sacrum** and **coccyx** bound it posteriorly.

The hip-bone [Figs 2.3 and 4.2]

Examine a detached hip-bone. The separate bones from which it is formed—the **ilium**, the **ischium**, and the **pubis**—remain separate throughout childhood, and during this time are united at the **acetabulum** by cartilage only. They fuse together about the time of puberty. Note that the flat portion of the hip-bone which lies above the acetabulum constitutes the ilium. The part that lies below and in front of the acetabulum is the pubis, which consists of the **body of the pubis,** the **superior ramus of the pubis,** and the **inferior ramus of the pubis.** Below and behind the pubis is the ischium. The upper part of the **body of the ischium** forms the lower part of the acetabulum, while the lower part forms the **ischial tuberosity.** The **ramus of the ischium** projects from the front of the tuberosity and is fused with the inferior ramus of the pubis.

The ilium [Fig. 4.2a and b]

Now turn to the ilium and examine the **iliac crest,** which forms the upper border of the large bony plate called the **ala of the ilium.** This crest begins anteriorly at the **anterior superior iliac spine,** which can be located easily both on the skeleton and on the living body. The prominence that limits the notch below the anterior superior iliac spine is the **anterior inferior iliac spine.** About 6 cm behind the anterior superior iliac spine you will see a prominence called the **tubercle of the crest.** This landmark can also be felt on the living body, and marks the highest point of the iliac crest as seen from the front. Tracing the crest backwards you will find that it terminates at the **posterior superior iliac spine,** whose position on the living body is marked by a small dimple above the medial part of the buttock about 4 cm from the midline. Immediately inferior to the posterior superior iliac spine is the **posterior inferior iliac spine.**

The sciatic notches [Fig. 2.1]

Examine the **greater sciatic notch.** It is bounded above by the posterior inferior iliac spine and below by the small

sharp **ischial spine,** which is placed immediately behind the upper end of the body of the ischium. The small notch between the ischial spine and the ischial tuberosity is the **lesser sciatic notch.**

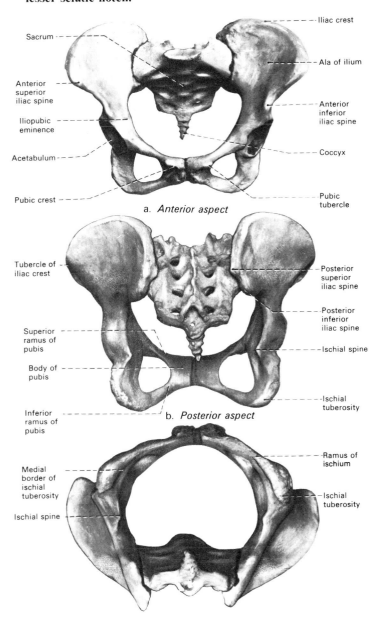

a. *Anterior aspect*

b. *Posterior aspect*

c. *The inferior aperture of the pelvis*

Fig. 4.2 The pelvis.

The pubis [Fig. 4.2a and b]

Follow the anterior border of the ilium downwards and forwards from the anterior inferior iliac spine. Note the **ilio-pubic eminence,** marking the union of the ilium with the pubis. Run your fingers forwards from the eminence along the superior ramus of the pubis, on which is the prominent **pubic tubercle,** and beyond this, the ridge of bone called the **pubic crest,** which forms the upper border of the body of the pubis.

Refer again to the articulated skeleton to see how the pubic bones articulate at the **pubic symphysis** in the midline of the body. Run your fingers downwards along the inferior ramus of the pubis. At its junction with the ramus of the ischium you may find a slight bony thickening.

The sacropelvic surface of the hip-bone [Fig. 2.3a]

Turn to the medial sacropelvic surface of a detached hip-bone. Note the prominent **arcuate line** running backwards from the pubic crest. It forms a large part of the **linea terminalis,** below which lies the **lesser pelvis,** the part of the hip-bone above it forming the walls of the **greater pelvis.** Examine the **auricular surface** at the postero-superior extremity of the arcuate line. It articulates with the sacrum at the sacroiliac joint.

Now examine the pelvic aspect of the ischial tuberosity and note its well-defined medial border. This gives attachment to the falciform process of the sacrotuberous ligament.

The sacrum and coccyx [Fig. 2.7]

Examine the triangular sacrum which is wedged between the two hip-bones. It forms the posterior wall of the pelvic cavity.

The broad upper surface of the bone forms the **base of the sacrum** and projects forwards in the midline as the **promontory** [Fig. 2.7]. The lower end of the bone is called the **apex,** and articulates with the coccyx. The concavity of the anterior or pelvic surface of the sacrum is more uniform in the male than in the female, in which the lower part of the bone is bent forwards, sometimes acutely. The pelvic surface is characterized by four pairs of foramina, the **pelvic sacral foramina,** through which the ventral rami of the sacral nerves emerge. On the dorsal surface you will see the **median sacral crest,** which is formed by the fusion of the spinous processes of the sacral vertebrae. On either side of this crest are the **dorsal sacral foramina,** through which the dorsal rami of the sacral nerves emerge.

The part of the sacrum lateral to the sacral foramina is called the **lateral part of the sacrum.** This is much wider above than below, and on it is the **auricular surface** for articulation with the corresponding surface of the hip-bone.

The coccyx consists of some three to five vestigial tail-vertebrae which are usually fused.

The inferior pelvic aperture [Fig. 4.2c]

Look at the inferior pelvic aperture of an articulated skeleton from below. It is a diamond-shaped space bounded by bony and ligamentous walls. Anteriorly the inferior aperture of the pelvis is limited by the **pubic arch,** which is formed by the conjoined rami of the pubis and ischium of each side. Laterally the inferior pelvic aperture is bounded by the ischial tuberosities, from which the sacrotuberous ligaments pass to the sacrum and coccyx behind [Fig. 2.4].

Surface anatomy

At some convenient time, try to locate on your own body the bony features of the pelvis which can be palpated. First find the anterior superior iliac spine. It lies at the upper and lateral end of the fold of the groin. Then run your fingers backwards along the iliac crest for about 5 cm. The prominent projection you feel is the tubercle of the crest. Continuing backwards along the iliac crest, try to feel the posterior superior iliac spine, remembering that it lies in the floor of a small dimple. In the midline of the body anteriorly, locate the pubic symphysis. Then run your fingers downwards and backwards along the ischiopubic rami, until the prominent ischial tuberosities are felt. In this way you will have demarcated the pubic arch.

Section 4.2

The perineum

The perineum is the small space lying between the upper parts of the thighs and below the muscular diaphragm which forms the pelvic floor, called the pelvic diaphragm.

If one draws a line across the inferior pelvic aperture between the centres of the ischial tuberosities, two triangles are formed. The triangle in front of the line, with the pubic symphysis at its apex, is called the **urogenital region.** It contains the urethra and the external genital organs. The triangle behind the line, with the coccyx at its apex, is called the **anal region.** It contains the anal canal surrounded by its sphincter, and on each side of the canal, an ischiorectal fossa. This is a deep pouch filled with fat which lies between the ischium laterally and the levator ani muscle medially. The upper surface of this muscle forms the floor of the pelvis, and its lower surface forms the roof of the perineum.

Surface anatomy

Begin by examining the male and female external genitalia. In this part of your study you should collaborate with other groups of dissectors, so that when you have finished your dissection of the abdomen you will have studied both a male and a female cadaver.

The male external genitalia

Examine the male external genitalia. The **glans penis** is the swelling at the end of the **penis,** and at its apex is the **external opening of the urethra.** The glans is partly overlapped by a fold of skin called the **prepuce.** Feel the testes in the **scrotum** and note the median **raphe of the scrotum.** Follow the raphe backwards to the anus and forwards to the ventral, or urethral surface of the penis.

The female external genitalia

Next examine a female body. The female external genitalia are collectively known as the **vulva.** The two large folds which bound the vulval or **pudendal cleft** are the **labia majora.** From the embryological point of view they correspond to the scrotum in the male. They are folds of skin, containing fat and connective tissue in which sebaceous and sweat glands are embedded.

Follow these folds anteriorly and you will see that they run into an elevation called the **mons pubis.** This elevation is due to a thickened layer of fat over the pubic symphysis. Follow the folds posteriorly and you will see that they join

to form an indistinct fold called the **posterior commissure of the labia.**

The two smaller folds which come into view when the labia majora are held apart are the **labia minora.** They are folds of skin devoid of fat but richly supplied with blood vessels. Follow these folds forwards and determine that they divide into two parts, one passing over a small organ called the **clitoris,** to form the foreskin or **prepuce of the clitoris,** and the other passing beneath the clitoris to form the **frenulum of the clitoris.** In women who have not borne children the labia minora are joined posteriorly by a fold of skin called the **frenulum of the labia.**

The cleft between the two labia minora is known as the **vestibule of the vagina.** Both the female urethra and the vagina open into this space, as also do some small mucous glands. The **external opening of the urethra** is small and is the more anterior. In the virgin the **opening of the vagina** is partially closed by a thin vascularized membrane of epithelium, perforated centrally, called the **hymen.** You may see the remains of it in the form of small peripheral epithelial tags called the **carunculae hymenales.**

Now examine the opening of the urethra through which the urine passes from the bladder. You will find that it is situated in the midline between the conical projection of the clitoris, which is called the **glans of the clitoris,** and the opening of the vagina.

If the dissection of the cadaver on which you are working has not been taken to the stage at which the lower limbs have been removed from the trunk, the perineum will have to be left until after the completion of the dissection of the abdominal wall and cavity, by which time the dissectors of the lower limb should have completed their work. If the dissection of the lower limbs has not even been begun, the study of the perineum is made very difficult, since it has to be undertaken with the cadaver in the lithotomy position, with the lower limbs abducted and flexed at the hip and knee. When the cadaver is put in this position, there is a danger of the muscles of the lower limbs tearing.

Superficial dissection of the male perineum

With the body in the prone position begin by incising the skin in the midline [Fig. 4.3], starting at the coccyx behind, and skirting the anus as you cut towards the base of the scrotum. Then turn the body over and continue the incision round either side of the neck of the scrotum and then along the urethral (under) surface of the penis, as far as the glans. Remove the skin from the perineum by reflecting it forwards as a flap, and from the penis by reflecting it dorsally. Remove the skin from the pubis but leave the skin over the greater part of the scrotum intact.

The **superficial fascia of the perineum** is now exposed. The superficial fascia of the anal region, which is the posterior

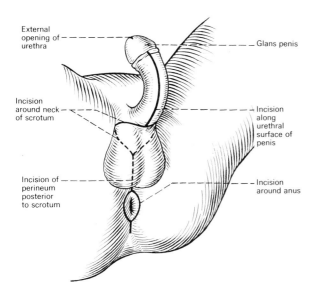

Fig. 4.3 Skin incisions of the male perineum.

part of the perineum behind the line joining the ischial tuberosities, consists of a single layer of connective tissue. The superficial fascia of the urogenital region in front of this line consists of two layers, a superficial **fatty layer** and a deeper **membranous layer.**

Dissect away the fatty layer of the superficial fascia from the perineum. As you trace the fatty layer forwards note that it is continuous with the fascia of the scrotum, penis, and lower abdomen. The area on either side of the anus is the base of a pyramidal fossa called the **ischiorectal fossa.** You can see that the fossa is filled with fat, called the **ischiorectal pad of fat.** In the region of the anus look for small bundles of muscle fibres which connect the wall of the anus to the skin. They are called the **corrugator cutis ani muscle.**

The spermatic cord [Fig. 4.4]

Dissect in the superficial fascia in front of the pubis at the side of the proximal part of the penis above the scrotum, and isolate a firm cord-like structure called the spermatic cord [Fig. 4.4]. If you separate the cord from the fat and trace it upwards and laterally, you will see that it emerges from an opening in the abdominal wall just above the medial part of the inguinal ligament. The opening, which will be dissected later, is called the **superficial inguinal ring.** The right and left rings lie immediately above and lateral to the pubic crests. Having dissected both sides, displace the sper-

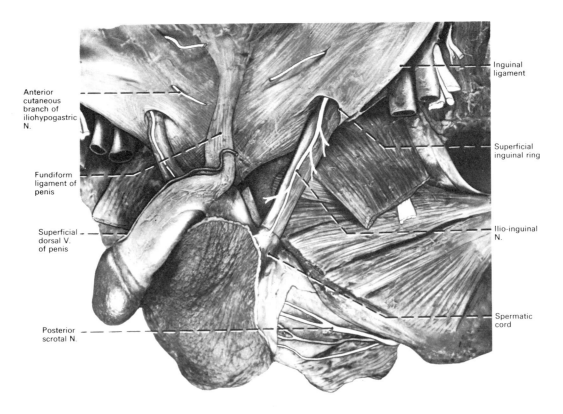

Fig. 4.4 Superficial dissection of the male urogenital region.

matic cords laterally and separate them from the proximal part of the penis. Trace them downwards as they pass into the scrotum.

The cutaneous nerves of the perineum [Fig. 4.6a]

The fascia you will expose when you have removed the superficial fat from the urogenital region is the membranous layer of superficial fascia. Dissect in this fascia at the posterior border of the region and find the **posterior scrotal nerves** [Fig. 4.4], which run close to the lateral margin of the region. Trace them forwards into the scrotum. These nerves are branches of the pudendal nerve, the trunk of which you exposed in your dissection of the gluteal region [p. 2.12]. More laterally on either side you may find one of the **perineal branches of the posterior cutaneous nerve of the thigh** running forwards alongside the posterior scrotal nerves [Fig. 4.6a]. Its cut end will be found crossing the ischiopubic ramus in front of the ischial tuberosity.

Superficial dissection of the female perineum

Incise the skin in the midline from the coccyx to the pubis, skirting both the anus and the labia majora. As in the male cadaver, reflect the skin by turning it forwards as a flap. Dissect away the superficial fatty layer of the superficial fascia. Search in the region where the spermatic cords were picked up in the male cadaver, and try to isolate two small

fibrous bands, one on either side, passing from the sides of the mons pubis into the labia majora. These bands are the **round ligaments of the uterus** [Fig. 4.5]. Like the spermatic cords, they emerge through the superficial inguinal rings. They end by entering the labia majora. Displace them laterally; as you do so, you may pick up the distal ends of the **posterior labial nerves,** which correspond to the posterior scrotal nerves in the male. As in the male cadaver, try to find each cut end of the perineal branches of the posterior cutaneous nerves of the thigh as they pass into the urogenital region over the ischiopubic rami in front of the ischial tuberosities.

The disposition of the pelvic viscera

Before you start to dissect the ischiorectal fossa acquaint yourself with the general arrangement of the pelvic organs [Figs 4.74 and 4.75].

In the midline anteriorly is the **urinary bladder,** whose inferior end is continuous with the **urethra.** In the female the urethra is a small canal a little less than 4 cm in length, which lies in front of the lower end of the vagina. In the male the urethra is continued through, and opens at the end of, the penis.

Posteriorly in the lesser pelvis is the **rectum,** which ends opposite the tip of the coccyx by becoming the **anal canal.** The latter opens externally at the **anus.** In the plane between

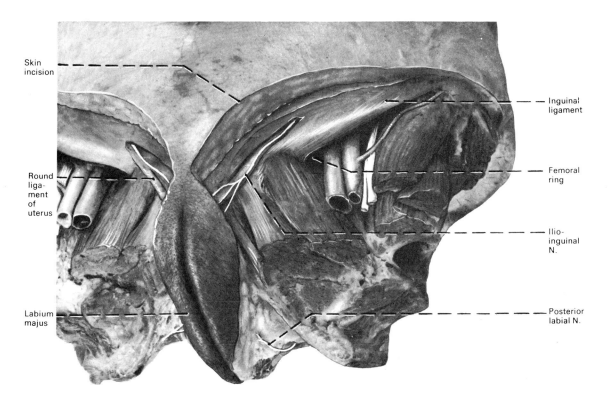

Skin incision

Round ligament of uterus

Labium majus

Inguinal ligament

Femoral ring

Ilio-inguinal N.

Posterior labial N.

Fig. 4.5 Superficial dissection of the female urogenital region.

the bladder and rectum are the reproductive organs. In the male these are the paired glandular structures called **seminal vesicles,** and a single midline structure called the **prostate.** The latter is adherent to the neck of the bladder, and the first part of the urethra passes through it. The seminal vesicles lie on either side of the midline behind the bladder, and their ducts penetrate the prostate to enter the prostatic part of the urethra. The 'essential' reproductive organs in the male are the testes, which are contained in the scrotum.

In the female the reproductive organs are the **uterus** above and the **vagina** below, with the ovaries at the sides of the uterus. The inferior part or cervix of the uterus projects into the upper part of the vagina. The external opening of the vagina is in the perineum between the urethra in front and the anus behind. The 'essential' reproductive organs in the female are the ovaries, which lie on either side of the uterus with which they are connected by two uterine tubes.

The obturator internus muscle [Figs 2.12 and 4.80]

In the living body the side wall of the lesser pelvis, including the obturator foramen, is covered by a flat sheet of muscle fibres which forms the obturator internus muscle. This muscle takes origin from the bone and from the obturator membrane which fills the obturator foramen. The fibres of the muscle converge on, and become continuous with, a series of tendinous bands which pass out of the pelvic cavity through the lesser sciatic notch. You saw the tendon of the muscle in your dissection of the gluteal region, and followed it to its insertion into the anterior part of the medial aspect of the greater trochanter of the femur [p. 2.14].

The pelvic diaphragm [Figs 4.9 and 4.89]

The pelvic organs are partly retained in position by two thin sheets of muscle which pass downwards, backwards, and medially on either side of the pelvis from the back of the pubis and the surface of the two obturator internus muscles. These two sheets of muscle, which are called the **levator ani muscles,** blend together behind and also immediately in front of the rectum. Posteriorly they are also inserted into the coccyx, together with a small muscle called the **coccygeus,** which arises from the ischial spine. Where they are prevented from joining in the midline by the prostate in the male, the vagina in the female, and in both sexes by the lower end of the rectum (or upper part of the anal canal), fibres from the levator ani pass into and blend with these organs as the muscles sweep backwards.

From their disposition it follows that the two levator ani muscles and the smaller coccygeus muscles constitute a muscular sling which pulls the pelvic organs upwards and forwards. These muscles and the layers of fascia covering their upper and lower surfaces form the pelvic diaphragm. The layers of fascia are called, respectively, the **superior fascia** and the **inferior fascia of the pelvic diaphragm.**

The ischiorectal fossa

The ischiorectal fossa is the wedge-shaped region at either side of the anal canal between the obturator internus laterally and the sloping levator ani medially. The apex of the wedge is above, where the two muscles meet, and the base below is formed by the skin and fascia of the anal region of the perineum.

Dissection of the ischiorectal fossa [Fig. 4.6]

Begin your dissection of the fossa by dissecting between the anus and the tip of the coccyx. Remove the fascia and fat on either side of the midline, and expose the **anococcygeal ligament** [Fig. 4.6], which marks the meeting of the two levator ani muscles in the midline between the anus and coccyx. As your dissection becomes deeper, expose and clean the parts of the levator ani and sacrospinous ligament which are attached to the coccyx.

Now work forwards and laterally, carefully removing the fat from the fossa, and leaving behind the deep fascia covering the muscles which bound the fossa. You must take great care not to injure the blood vessels and nerves which lie in the fossa. If you pick up the posterior scrotal (or labial) nerves where you found them in the urogenital region, and trace them backwards, you will find that they pass to the side wall of the fossa. They are useful guides to the main nerves and vessels you have to expose.

As you proceed, try to define the superficial boundaries of the fossa. They are the sacrotuberous ligament posteriorly and a circular muscle called the external anal sphincter, which encircles the anus, medially. Before it was removed during your dissection of the buttock, the gluteus maximus muscle lay superficial to the sacrotuberous ligament, where it also formed the posterior boundary of the fossa.

The anal sphincters [Fig. 4.6]

Dissecting carefully, clean the **external anal sphincter,** which is a cylinder of striated muscle fibres that surrounds the lower part of the anal canal. The sphincter fuses above with the medial fibres of levator ani (which are called the **puborectalis muscle**). Posteriorly some fibres of the sphincter are inserted indirectly into the coccyx by way of the anococcygeal ligament. Anteriorly the external anal sphincter fuses with a part of the perineum which is called the **central tendon of the perineum** (the perineal body). This is a fibromuscular mass between the opening of the vagina and the anus in the female, and between the anus and prostate in the male [Fig. 4.7].

Examine the deep part of the external anal sphincter and note that it cannot be separated from the levator ani muscle. As you will see later, both it and the more superficial part of the external sphincter lie on the outer side of an **internal**

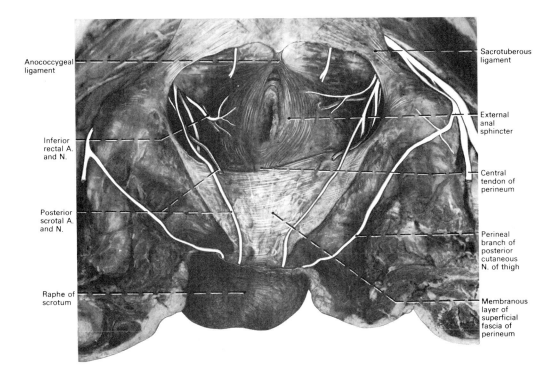

Anococcygeal
ligament

Sacrotuberous
ligament

External
anal
sphincter

Inferior
rectal A.
and N.

Central
tendon of
perineum

Posterior
scrotal A.
and N.

Perineal
branch of
posterior
cutaneous
N. of thigh

Raphe of
scrotum

Membranous
layer of
superficial
fascia of
perineum

a. *Male*

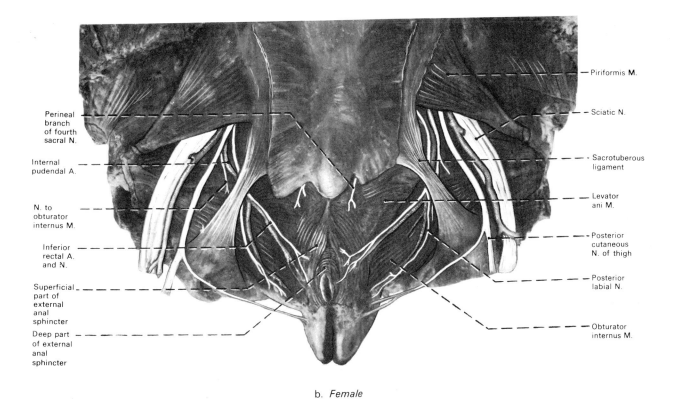

Perineal
branch
of fourth
sacral N.

Piriformis **M.**

Sciatic N.

Internal
pudendal A.

Sacrotuberous
ligament

N. to
obturator
internus M.

Levator
ani M.

Inferior
rectal A.
and N.

Posterior
cutaneous
N. of thigh

Superficial
part of
external
anal
sphincter

Posterior
labial N.

Deep part
of external
anal
sphincter

Obturator
internus M.

b. *Female*

Fig. 4.6 Dissection of the ischiorectal fossa.

anal sphincter, and of the longitudinal layer of the muscular coat of the anal canal.

The nerves and vessels of the ischiorectal fossa [Fig. 4.6]

Having cleaned as much of the fascia covering the levator ani muscle as you can, carefully work your way laterally, continuing to remove the fat in the fossa, and then clean the fascia covering the obturator internus muscle. As you clear the fat, you will find blood vessels and nerves that pass from the lateral wall of the fossa to the anal canal medially, and to the urogenital region of the perineum anteriorly.

As the field of your dissection becomes clearer, trace some of these vessels and nerves into the obturator fascia covering the obturator internus. Their parent trunks (the **pudendal nerve** and the **internal pudendal artery**) lie in a fascial sheath called the **pudendal canal** on the lateral wall of the ischiorectal fossa. You have already dissected them in a more proximal part of their course in the gluteal region [p. 2.12]. Clear away the fascia that forms the pudendal canal, and follow the nerve and vessels both posteriorly and anteriorly as far as possible. In order to expose them, do not hesitate to incise the sacrotuberous ligament posteriorly at its ischial attachment.

Pick up the **posterior scrotal (labial in female) branches of the internal pudendal artery,** and the posterior scrotal (labial) nerves (which you have already followed through the urogenital region) and dissect them posteriorly. You will find that the nerves are branches of a division of the pudendal nerve which is called the **perineal nerve.** The second division, which you will trace later, is the **dorsal nerve of the penis** (or **dorsal nerve of the clitoris**). Your dissection will have defined the **inferior rectal nerves** and the **inferior rectal artery,** which branch from the pudendal nerve and the internal pudendal artery in the posterior part of the pudendal canal.

During your dissection you may have found other small nerves, mostly ending in the subcutaneous tissue behind and to the sides of the anus. They are the cutaneous branches of the second and third sacral nerves, which curl round the lower border of gluteus maximus to supply the skin of the

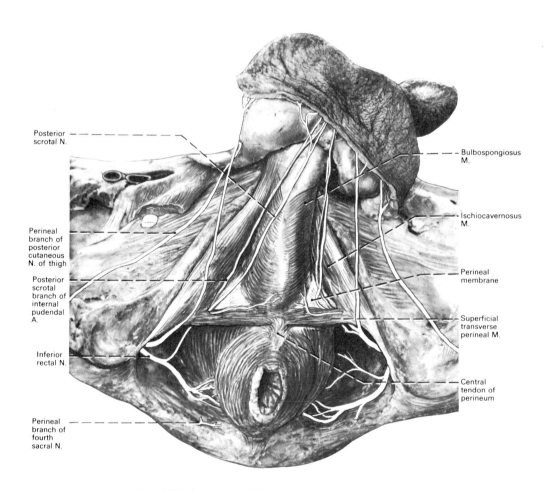

Posterior scrotal N.

Perineal branch of posterior cutaneous N. of thigh

Posterior scrotal branch of internal pudendal A.

Inferior rectal N.

Perineal branch of fourth sacral N.

Bulbospongiosus M.

Ischiocavernosus M.

Perineal membrane

Superficial transverse perineal M.

Central tendon of perineum

Fig. 4.7 The superficial perineal space in the male.

buttock. You may also have seen the perineal branch of the fourth sacral nerve, which runs forwards on the lateral aspect of the coccyx to enter the external anal sphincter.

The fat in the ischiorectal fossa supports the rectum and anal canal. It is poorly supplied with blood, and its powers of resistance to infection are consequently poor. As a result, ischiorectal abscess is a fairly common condition.

With the nerves and arteries identified, you can now complete the removal of the fascia over the levator ani and the obturator internus, and clean both muscles. Search posteriorly near the lesser sciatic foramen and find the **nerve to the obturator internus** as it enters that muscle. You first saw this nerve in the gluteal region below the piriformis muscle and on the medial side of the sciatic nerve. It passed over the ischial spine lateral to the internal pudendal vessels and pudendal nerve, to enter the ischiorectal fossa through the lesser sciatic foramen [p. 2.12].

You will not be able to define the anterior boundary of the ischiorectal fossa until the urogenital region is dissected, but explore a diverticulum which extends backwards above the sacrotuberous ligament. Another recess extends anteriorly deep to the muscles and fascia of the urogenital region. The latter are collectively called the **urogenital diaphragm.** These diverticula are of some importance clinically when abscesses occur in the ischiorectal fossa.

Your next step is the dissection of the urogenital region. Since its disposition is very different in the male and female subject, arrange to follow the dissection on cadavers of both sexes.

Deep dissection of the male perineum

The superficial perineal space [Fig. 4.7]

Examine the membranous layer of superficial fascia [Fig. 4.6] which you exposed when you removed the superficial fat, and note that it is continuous with the fascia of the penis and scrotum. Note also that it is attached laterally to the borders of the pubic arch, and that posteriorly you can trace it as it turns round the posterior border of the **superficial transverse perineal muscles** [Fig. 4.7]. The latter run between the ischial tuberosities and form the posterior boundary of the urogenital region. On the deep surface of these muscles the membranous layer of superficial fascia becomes continuous with a layer of tough fascia called the **perineal membrane** or the **inferior fascia of the urogenital diaphragm.** This membrane is a triangular sheet of fibrous tissue which is attached to the margins of the pubic arch as far posteriorly as the ischial tuberosities. The base of the perineal membrane merges in the midline with the central tendon of the perineum.

Between the membranous layer of the superficial fascia of the perineum and the perineal membrane is the superficial perineal space. In the male it contains the root of the penis, the superficial perineal muscles and also blood vessels, nerves and lymphatics.

The penis [Fig. 4.10]

Before continuing your dissection, note that the penis is composed of three cylindrical columns of erectile tissue which are ensheathed in deep fascia and covered by superficial fascia and skin. Two of these columns form the **corpora cavernosa penis.** They lie on the dorsal aspect of the organ and are fused together in the midline. On their ventral aspect, and lying in the groove between them, is the **corpus spongiosum penis,** which is traversed by the **male urethra.** The corpus spongiosum penis terminates in a conical swelling, the **glans penis,** which forms a cap over the conjoined ends of the two corpora cavernosa penis. Posteriorly the corpus spongiosum penis ends in a bulbous swelling, called the **bulb of the penis,** which is attached to the perineal membrane near its base. Each corpus cavernosum penis ends posteriorly in a **crus** which is attached to the border of the pubic arch and to the adjacent part of the perineal membrane. The crura and bulb are sometimes referred to collectively as the **root of the penis.**

At the base of the glans penis is a ridge called the **corona glandis,** and at its apex is the **external urethral opening.** The junction of the **body of the penis** with the glans is called the **neck of the glans.** On the under-surface of the glans is a fold of skin called the **frenulum of the prepuce,** which carries an artery to the glans. The skin covering the glans is called the **prepuce** or foreskin.

Most of the blood vessels and nerves to the organ lie deeply, but on the dorsum, in the **superficial fascia of the penis,** is the superficial dorsal vein of the penis. The fascia is continuous above with the superficial fascia of the abdominal wall, and below with the superficial fascia of the perineum. The penis is suspended from the linea alba and the pubic symphysis by thickenings of **deep fascia,** called the **fundiform** and **suspensory ligaments of the penis.**

The root of the penis [Fig. 4.7]

Now pull the scrotum forwards and pick up the posterior scrotal vessels and nerves (and, if you find it, a perineal branch of the posterior cutaneous nerve of the thigh), and, using these as a guide as you follow them anteriorly, carefully dissect away the membranous layer of the superficial fascia. As you do so, try to find other branches of the perineal nerve which supply the muscles of the superficial perineal space.

Look for the bulb of the penis in the midline at the base of the perineal membrane. You will see that it is covered by a thin sheet of muscle whose fibres pass forwards around the penis from the central tendon of the perineum and a median raphe on its urethral (under) surface. Clean this muscle, which is the **bulbospongiosus** [Fig. 4.7], and try to isolate the branch of the perineal nerve by which it is supplied. It is inserted not only into the inferior surface of the perineal membrane, but also on to the dorsal surface of the corpus spongiosum, and more anteriorly into the fascia of the dorsum of the penis. On the same plane, but lateral to the bulb of the penis, find the two crura which are attached to the rami of the pubic arch and to the adjacent perineal membrane. Each crus is covered by a thin muscle, called the **ischiocavernosus,** whose fibres pass forwards along the crus. Note that they arise posteriorly from the medial side of the ischial tuberosity and that they are inserted into the crura. The function of these muscles is to compress the root of the penis. There are similar, but much smaller, muscles in the female surrounding the vestibule and the crura of the clitoris respectively.

The transverse muscle fibres which your dissection will have exposed at this stage at the posterior boundary of the urogenital region form the superficial transverse perineal muscles. These feeble muscular slips arise from the ischial tuberosities and pass medially to be inserted into the central tendon of the perineum in the midline [Fig. 4.7].

The dorsal nerves and vessels of the penis [Fig. 4.8]

Now return to the dissection of the pendulous part of the penis. Note, but do not dissect, the **superficial dorsal vein** in the thin, fat-free, superficial fascia of the dorsum. It drains into the right or left external pudendal veins. Make a longitudinal incision in the deep fascia on the dorsum of the penis, and strip away the fascia. In the groove in the midline, which marks the union of the two corpora, dissect out the **dorsal nerves of the penis** [Fig. 4.8], the **dorsal arteries of the penis,** and the **dorsal vein of the penis.** Pulling the organ down from the pubis, define the suspensory ligament, which, as noted already, is a thickening of the deep fascia that is attached to the pubic symphysis, and divide it.

Now trace the dorsal vessels and nerves backwards as far as possible, and establish that the dorsal vein enters the pelvis through a gap immediately below the pubic symphysis. This gap lies between the **arcuate ligament of the pubis** and the **transverse ligament of the perineum.** The former is a ligament on the under-surface of the pubic symphysis, and the latter is the thickened anterior extremity, or apex of the perineal membrane.

Removal of the penis

Divide the dorsal vein and the dorsal arteries and nerves, 3 cm distal to the arcuate ligament of the pubis. Free the scrotum and contents from the under-surface of the root of the penis and pull them upwards over the tip of the penis.

Then separate the crura and bulb of the penis, together with the muscles by which they are covered, from their attachments to the perineal membrane and pubic arch, working from behind forwards. As you do this, you will have to divide the arteries of the bulb of the penis and the nerves which pass into the overlying muscles. You will also

have to divide the urethra where it enters the base (upper surface) of the bulb, and the deep arteries of the penis, which are also branches of the internal pudendal artery. Next remove the superficial transverse perineal muscles. In this way the penis is detached entirely, and the perineal membrane is exposed completely.

Clean the anterior extremity or apex of the membrane, which forms the transverse ligament of the perineum. Observe how the base of the membrane forms one of the boundaries of the ischiorectal fossa. Note, too, that several muscles meet and fuse at the central tendon of the perineum, which is continuous with the midpoint of the base of the membrane. These are the levator ani, the superficial transverse perineal, the bulbospongiosus, and the external anal sphincter muscles. The central tendon of the perineum is much more important in the female than in the male, since it is an indirect support for the pelvic organs, and is liable to be torn during childbirth.

The deep perineal space in the male

The perineal membrane covers another space or stratum of the perineum, called the deep perineal space. This space is a closed pouch, whose superficial surface is the **perineal membrane,** and whose deep surface is the **superior fascia of the urogenital diaphragm.** The latter fills in the gap between the medial margins of the two ischiopubic rami. These two fascial layers fuse anteriorly at the transverse ligament of the perineum (i.e. the apex of the perineal membrane), and posteriorly at the posterior border of the urogenital region. Both layers are attached laterally to the pubic arch. The deep perineal space is occupied by a sheet of muscle. This is formed centrally by the **urethral sphincter muscle,** which surrounds the membranous part of the urethra, and peripherally by the two **deep transverse perineal muscles,** which lie deep to the much smaller superficial transverse perineal muscles at the posterior border of the urogenital region.

The **membranous part of the urethra** is the section of the urethra which lies between the prostate above (this organ lies above the fascia of the urogenital diaphragm) and the bulb of the penis below. The latter is attached to the superficial surface of the perineal membrane. The membranous part of the urethra is little more than 1 cm long, and perforates the perineal membrane about 2.5 cm below and posterior to the pubic symphysis.

In the male the deep perineal space also contains two small glands, called the **bulbo-urethral glands,** the ducts of which pierce the perineal membrane to open into the penile or spongy portion of the urethra. These glands, each the size of a pea, lie between the fibres of the urethral sphincter muscle. They tend to atrophy as age advances, and it is unlikely that you will find them.

In the deep perineal space close to the sides of the pubic arch are the proximal parts of the **dorsal arteries of the penis,** which are terminal branches of the internal pudendal

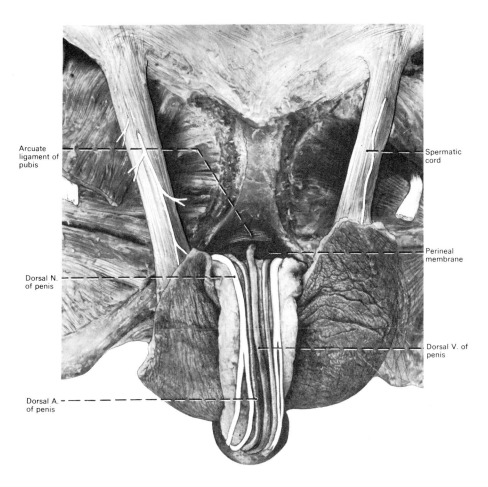

Arcuate
ligament of
pubis

Dorsal N.
of penis

Dorsal A. --
of penis

Spermatic
cord

Perineal
membrane

Dorsal V. of
penis

Fig. 4.8 Dissection of the dorsum of the penis.

arteries. These vessels divide in the deep perineal space into the dorsal and **deep arteries of the penis.** The latter almost immediately penetrate the crura of the penis to supply the corpora cavernosa. Each internal pudendal artery also gives off a branch to the deep transverse perineal muscle and to the bulb of the penis, and so to the corpus spongiosum. Note also the corresponding branches of the perineal nerve.

You can appreciate at this stage that the anterior diverticulum of the ischiorectal fossa extends forwards above the base of the urogenital diaphragm, and above the posterior part of the deep perineal space.

Exposure of the levator ani muscle in the male

Remove the inferior and superior fascias of the urogenital diaphragm and the tissues between them in the 'space' they form (the deep perineal space) by cutting along their attachments to the ischiopubic rami, dividing the urethra transversely as you do so.

Strip the remaining fascia from the under-surface of the levator ani muscles forwards and medially as far as the anterior border of these muscles. Note the gap in the midline

between the two anterior borders. It is filled with fascia, above which lies the prostate [Fig. 4.9].

You should also find the dorsal nerves of the penis. These accompany the dorsal vessels forwards on to the dorsum of the penis.

The blood supply and structure of the penis [Fig. 4.10]

The **dorsal arteries of the penis** supply the skin and fascia and are continued into the glans. Blood leaves the penis by first, a **superficial dorsal vein** which lies in the superficial fascia, and which, as already noted [p. 4.12], drains into the right or left external pudendal veins; and second, a **dorsal vein** which lies beneath the deep fascia and which drains into the prostatic venous plexus around the neck of the bladder.

The penis is innervated by the pudendal nerves and by the pelvic autonomic nerves.

Complete the dissection of the detached penis. Cut through the organ by making a transverse (coronal) incision through the centre of the body [Fig. 4.10]. Note the centrally-situated **deep artery** in each corpus cavernosum, with the **arteries of the bulb** lying below the urethra. Split

4.13

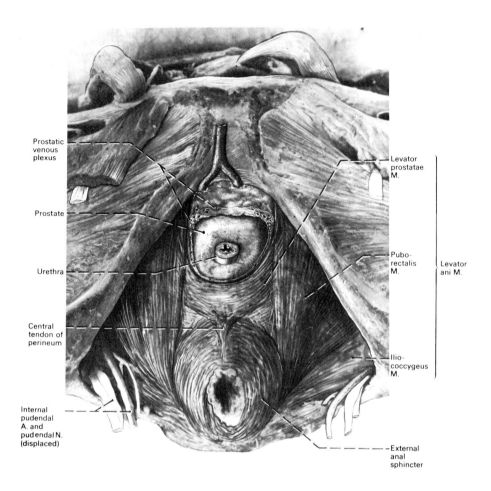

Fig. 4.9 Dissection of the male pelvic diaphragm. The fascia on the under-surface of the levator ani muscles has been removed.

the penis by a longitudinal (sagittal) incision throughout its extent. In the bulb try to find the openings of the bulbo-urethral glands on the ventral wall of the urethra, and at the distal end of the urethra note the **navicular fossa**

of the urethra in the dorsum of the glans penis. You will see small crypts, or **lacunae urethrales,** scattered over the floor of the spongy portion of the urethra.

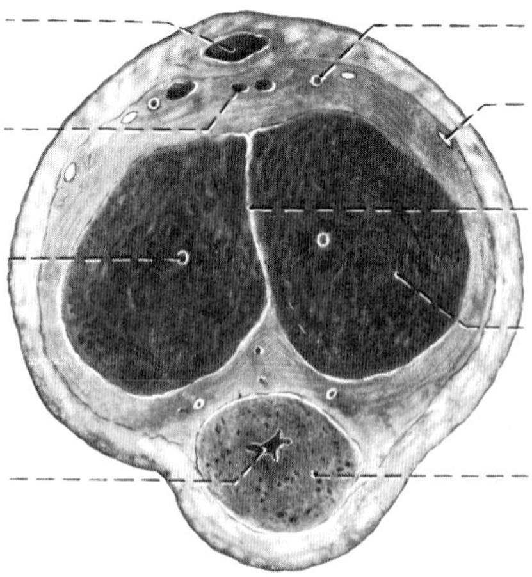

Deep dissection of the female perineum

The superficial perineal space [Fig. 4.11]

The dissection of the female urogenital region proceeds in much the same way as in the male. Begin by picking up the perineal branch of the posterior cutaneous nerve of the thigh in the urogenital region, and more medially the posterior labial nerves [Fig. 4.11]. You should have found the cut end of the former crossing the bone in front of the ischial tuberosity. You have already traced these nerves as far as the insertion of the round ligaments into the labia majora.

Clear away the membranous layer of superficial fascia after its attachments have been noted. Then examine the contents of the superficial perineal space. On each side of the vaginal and urethral openings you will see a mass of erectile tissue called the **bulb of the vestibule.** This tissue is covered by the **bulbospongiosus muscle.** Laterally find the

Fig. 4.10 Cross-section of the penis.

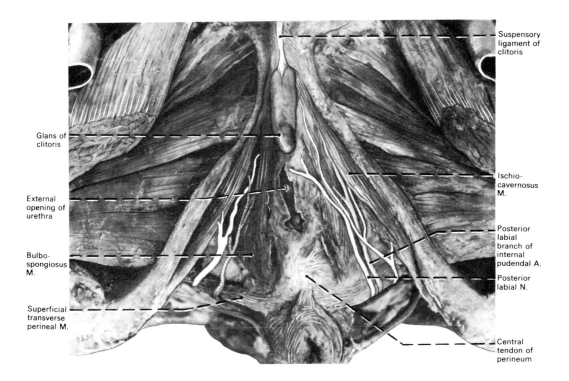

Suspensory ligament of clitoris

Glans of clitoris

External opening of urethra

Bulbo-spongiosus M.

Superficial transverse perineal M.

Ischio-cavernosus M.

Posterior labial branch of internal pudendal A.

Posterior labial N.

Central tendon of perineum

Fig. 4.11 The superficial perineal space in the female.

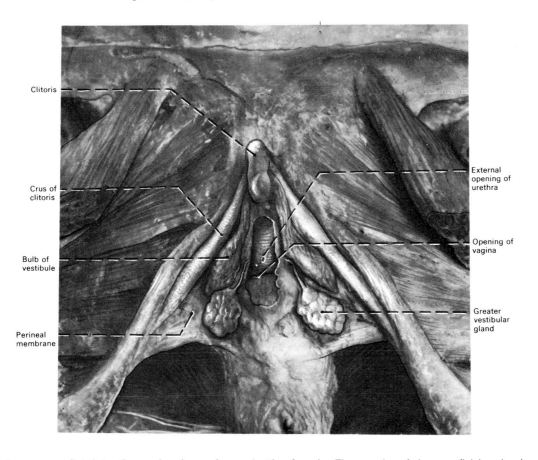

Clitoris

Crus of clitoris

Bulb of vestibule

Perineal membrane

External opening of urethra

Opening of vagina

Greater vestibular gland

Fig. 4.12 Structures superficial to the perineal membrane in the female. The muscles of the superficial perineal space have been removed.

ischiocavernosus muscles covering the **crura of the clitoris,** which are in the same position as the crura of the penis, but very much smaller.

Dissect away the bulbospongiosus muscles on either side, and trace the two bulbs forward to their union on the under-surface of the clitoris in front of the urethra. Try to find the **greater vestibular glands** [Fig. 4.12]. These mucous glands are about the size of a pea in adult life, but are often atrophied in old age and therefore difficult to identify in a dissecting-room cadaver. They lie on either side of the vagina, within the bulbospongiosus muscle, in contact with the posterior part of the bulb of the vestibule. Their ducts, which you may be able to see, open into the vestibule between the labia minora and the remnants of the hymen. Reflect the bulb of the vestibule from the **perineal membrane,** to which it is attached, and turn it medially.

The clitoris [Fig. 4.12]

The clitoris corresponds anatomically to the penis, except that it is not traversed by the urethra. Remove the skin and fascia and try to find the **suspensory ligament of the clitoris** [Fig. 4.11], which is similar to that of the penis. Dissect out the **dorsal arteries of the clitoris** and **dorsal nerves of the clitoris** on the dorsum of the clitoris. Then pull the organ downwards and detach the crura from the perineal mem-brane and pubic arch, beginning anteriorly and working backwards. There is no need to remove the clitoris com-pletely or to examine it further. Branches of the perineal nerve may be seen supplying muscles in the superficial perineal space.

The deep perineal space in the female

As in the male, the deep perineal space in the female encloses the **deep transverse perineal muscles** and the **urethral sphincter muscle,** which surrounds the urethra. The internal pudendal arteries and the proximal parts of the dorsal nerves and arteries of the clitoris lie close to the ischiopubic rami. Part of the vagina also lies within the deep perineal space.

Exposure of the levator ani muscle in the female

Since it is difficult to dissect the deep perineal space, proceed directly to remove the inferior and superior fascias of the urogenital diaphragm, and the muscle fibres and vessels between them, by cutting along their attachments to the ischiopubic rami, dividing the vagina and urethra trans-versely as you do so. Clear away the remaining fascia from the under-surface of the levator ani muscles, stripping it for-wards and medially. You will recall that this layer of fascia is called the inferior fascia of the pelvic diaphragm [p. 4.8]. Note that the vagina passes through the gap between the two levator ani muscles.

Section 4.3

The anterior abdominal wall

Surface anatomy

With a skeleton available for reference, begin the study of the abdomen by examining the surface of the abdominal wall on the cadaver. At a convenient moment revise what you learn on your own body.

The regions of the abdomen [Fig. 4.13]

The abdomen is divided into regions [Fig. 4.13]. With the point of your scalpel lightly draw a line transversely across the body through a point midway between the jugular notch of the sternum and the upper border of the pubic symphysis. This line represents the **transpyloric plane,** which passes through the first lumbar vertebra and, very commonly, through the pylorus, or distal end of the stomach (the pylorus is the junctional zone between the stomach and intestine). Draw a further horizontal line transversely across the body at the level of the tubercles of the iliac crests. This is known as the **transtubercular plane.** Draw a vertical line upwards on each side, commencing from a point midway between the pubic symphysis and the anterior superior iliac spine. In this way the abdomen is divided into nine regions, called from above down:

The right and left **hypochondriac regions,** with the **epigastric region** between them.

The right and left **lateral regions,** with the **umbilical region** between them.

The right and left **inguinal regions,** with the **pubic region** between them.

The transpyloric plane runs between the tip of the ninth costal cartilage and the lower border of the first lumbar vertebra. You will see later that this plane not only marks the position of the pylorus, which lies 1 to 2 cm to the right of the midline, but also the levels of the blind end, or fundus, of the gall-bladder, the hilum of the left kidney, and the lowest limit of the spinal medulla.

In a young healthy adult the navel, or **umbilicus,** lies at the level of the intervertebral disc between the third and fourth lumbar vertebrae. As age advances and fat is deposited, the umbilicus tends to lie below this level.

The rectus abdominis muscle [Fig. 4.14]

On either side of the midline is a straight and flat muscle called the rectus abdominis muscle [Fig. 4.14]. If you cannot identify this on the cadaver, you will easily be able to do so later on your own body. The margins of the muscle can be made to stand out when the muscle is contracted (as it is when you lie on your back and then raise your head and shoulders). You will then see not only the lateral border of the muscle forming the **linea semilunaris,** but also creases which cross the muscle transversely. These creases are produced by **tendinous intersections,** of which there are usually three: one at the level of the umbilicus, another at the lower border of the xiphoid process, and a third midway between these two. The intersections are intramuscular sheets of

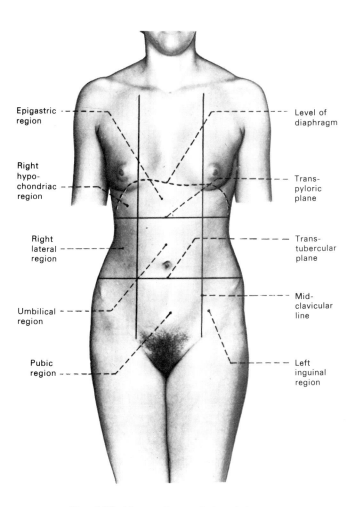

Epigastric region

Level of diaphragm

Right hypo-chondriac region

Trans-pyloric plane

Right lateral region

Trans-tubercular plane

Mid-clavicular line

Umbilical region

Pubic region

Left inguinal region

Fig. 4.13 The regions of the abdomen.

fibrous tissue which subdivide the rectus abdominis muscle and which are continuous with the anterior layer of the rectus sheath.

The vertical crease between the two recti in the midline overlies a band of fibrous tissue called the **linea alba**. The medial borders of the two rectus abdominis muscles are

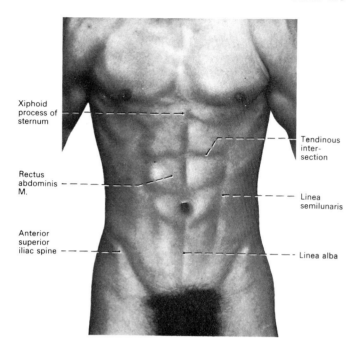

Fig. 4.14 The anterior abdominal wall.

further apart above than below the umbilicus; this, too, can be seen on the living body.

Reflection of the skin and superficial fascia

Begin the dissection of the abdomen by making an incision in the midline, from the transverse incision previously made on the thorax above to the pubic symphysis below, skirting the umbilicus. Reflect the skin in a lateral direction and remove it, exposing the superficial fascia.

The superficial fascia [Fig. 4.15]

Make a horizontal incision through the superficial fascia midway between the umbilicus and the pubic symphysis. Below the level of the umbilicus a **fatty layer** forms the superficial part of the superficial fascia. It is in this layer that fat is deposited in obese people. Beneath this fatty layer is the deep **membranous layer** of superficial fascia. The existence of these two layers is best demonstrated by scraping off the fatty layer, using a scalpel, and so exposing the deeper membranous layer. Remember that the superficial fatty layer is continuous with that of the perineum and thighs, and that it has no bony attachments. In the scrotum the superficial fatty layer is represented by a layer of fascia containing fibres of smooth muscle and called the tunica dartos.

The membranous layer

Now insert your fingers deep to the membranous layer and free it from the underlying deep fascia. The deep fascia of

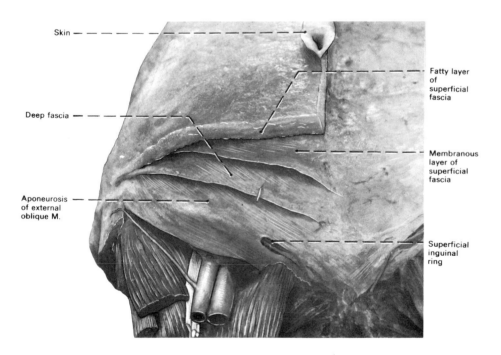

Fig. 4.15 The fascial layers of the anterior abdominal wall.

the abdominal wall is a thin, weak envelope of connective tissue which separates the superficial fascia from the underlying aponeurosis of the external oblique muscle of the abdomen. It is difficult to demonstrate. As you work downwards, separating the membranous layer, note that the latter does not blend with the inguinal ligament. In a cadaver whose lower limbs had not been dissected you would see that the membranous layer joins the **fascia lata** just below the ligament. Medially the membranous layer continues over the external genitalia into the membranous layer of the superficial fascia of the perineum.

Sometimes the proximal portion of the male urethra may be ruptured as a result of falling astride a hard object, resulting in the escape of urine into the superficial perineal space during micturition. The course which the urine then takes is determined by the attachments of the membranous layer of superficial fascia. It cannot pass backwards into the ischiorectal fossa because the membranous layer is attached posteriorly to the perineal membrane. It cannot pass later-

ally because the fascia is attached to the ischiopubic rami. It therefore seeps into the scrotum, and upwards, deep to the membranous layer of superficial fascia of the abdominal wall. It cannot pass downwards into the thighs because of the attachment of the membranous layer of abdominal fascia to the fascia lata just below the inguinal ligament.

The cutaneous vessels and nerves [Figs 4.16 and 4.17]

Your next task is to remove all the superficial fascia of the abdominal wall, and to define some of the vessels and nerves which pass into and through it to the skin. To do this incise the fascia in the midline from the xiphoid process above to the top of the pubic symphysis below, being careful not to cut the fibrous band in the midline called the linea alba. On either side reflect the fascia laterally from the midline, noting the nerves and vessels which you will see penetrating the fibrous aponeurosis which your reflection will expose. Do not spend time cleaning any except the lowest nerves in the series.

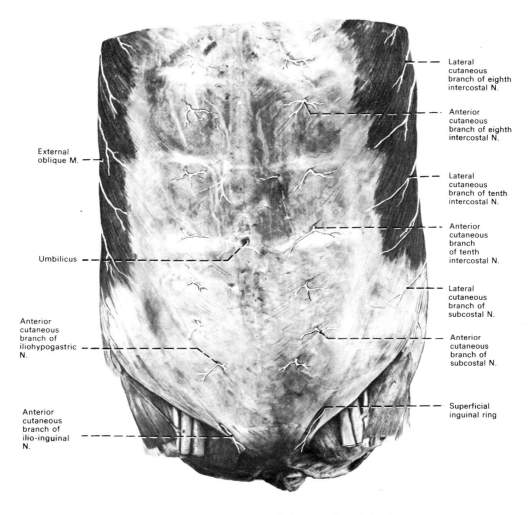

Fig. 4.16 The cutaneous nerves of the anterior abdominal wall.

The cutaneous nerves which emerge in series near the midline are the **anterior cutaneous branches** of the seventh to eleventh **intercostal nerves** and the **subcostal nerve** (the twelfth thoracic nerve) [Fig. 4.16]. Just above the pubic symphysis you should find the anterior cutaneous branch of the **iliohypogastric nerve,** which is a branch of the first lumbar nerve. The nerves which you will find passing into the superficial fascia from the muscles on the lateral aspect of the abdominal wall are the **lateral cutaneous branches** of the lower six thoracic nerves. Search posterior to the anterior superior spine for the vertically-disposed lateral cutaneous branch of the subcostal nerve, as it descends into the thigh over the iliac crest. Immediately behind it you should find the lateral cutaneous branch of the iliohypogastric nerve. No time should be spent on the dissection of the vessels which accompany these nerves. Those in the upper part of the abdominal wall are superficial branches of the two terminal branches of the internal thoracic artery,

the **superior epigastric artery** and **musculophrenic artery,** both of which you will see later. Those in the lower part are mainly branches of the femoral artery, ascending from the upper part of the thigh [p. 2.21]. The arteries in the middle part of the abdominal wall are the terminal branches of the lowest two **posterior intercostal arteries,** the **subcostal artery,** and all the **lumbar arteries.**

The oblique and transverse muscles of the abdominal wall

When you have finished reflecting the superficial fascia and examining the nerves and vessels it contains, study the surface you have exposed. You will see that the whole of the front of the abdominal wall is covered by a white fibrous sheath. To appreciate the nature of this sheath it is necessary to obtain a general idea of the disposition of the muscles of the abdominal wall.

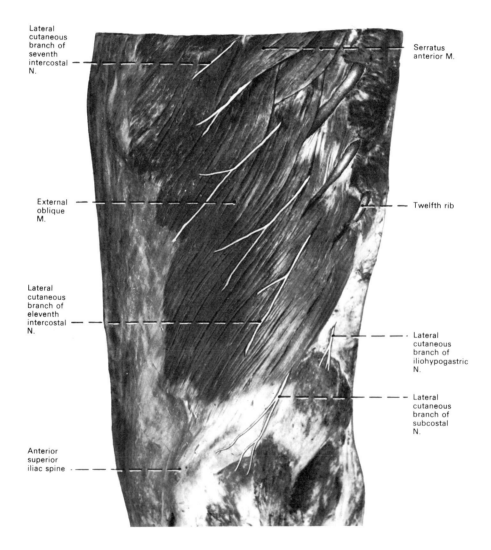

Fig. 4.17 The left external oblique muscle of the abdomen.

As you have already noted, the muscle of the abdominal wall on either side of the midline is the rectus abdominis. This is a flat and long muscle which reaches from the pubic crest below to the cartilages of the fifth, sixth, and seventh ribs above. Its maximum width is about 7.5 cm. Lateral to the rectus abdominis the abdominal wall is made up of three muscular sheets, the external oblique [Fig. 4.17] being the most superficial, the transversus abdominis the deepest, with the internal oblique muscle of the abdomen between the other two. Between the internal oblique and transversus abdominis muscles, which correspond respectively to the internal intercostal and the intercostales intimi muscles of the thorax, will be found segmentally-disposed nerves and blood vessels whose cutaneous branches you have already seen.

The fibres of the **external oblique,** which is the largest of the three muscles, arise from the lower eight ribs and pass downwards and forwards, ending in a fibrous aponeurosis at the lateral side of the rectus abdominis. These aponeurotic fibres are directed downwards and medially over the rectus abdominis. The **internal oblique muscle** arises below from the inguinal ligament and the iliac crest, and passes upwards and medially to be inserted mainly into an aponeurosis which splits at the lateral margin of the rectus muscle, one layer fusing with the aponeurosis of the external oblique muscle in front of the rectus abdominis, the other passing behind. The **transversus abdominis** has an extensive origin along a line which extends from the ribs above, to the iliac crest and inguinal ligament below. Its transversely-disposed muscle fibres end mainly in an aponeurosis which joins the posterior lamina of the aponeurosis of the internal oblique, behind the rectus abdominis.

The aponeuroses on the front and back of the rectus fuse at the medial margin of the muscle to form the fibrous linea alba. In this way each rectus becomes enclosed in a sheath.

The external oblique muscle of the abdomen

With this general picture of the muscles of the abdominal wall in mind, examine the external oblique muscle of the abdomen and its aponeurosis [Fig. 4.17]. Remove all the fascia from its surface and note that its fibres run downwards, forwards, and medially. Turn the cadaver on its side or on to its face, and clean the posterior part of the muscle. You will see that the muscle has a free posterior border, which stretches between the twelfth rib and the iliac crest. The muscle arises by fleshy slips from the lower eight ribs. These slips interdigitate with the slips of origin of the serratus anterior and the latissimus dorsi muscles.

The aponeurosis of the external oblique muscle [Fig. 4.17]
Turn the cadaver on to its back and follow the external oblique muscle to its insertion. You will see that the fleshy fibres which arise from the lower two ribs are inserted into the anterior half of the outer lip of the iliac crest. They form

the posterior part of the muscle. The remainder of the muscle ends in a broad aponeurosis whose lateral margin lies roughly along a line which extends from the ninth costal cartilage above to the anterior superior iliac spine below [Fig. 4.17].

Note how the two aponeuroses run into each other in the midline to help form the **linea alba.** This median raphe extends from the pubic symphysis below to the xiphoid process above. Between the anterior superior iliac spine laterally and the pubic tubercle medially note that the aponeurosis forms the **inguinal ligament.** Try to establish that the lower border of the aponeurosis is rolled back upon itself so that the upper surface of the inguinal ligament is grooved. You may see that some of the lower fibres decussate across the midline and join the opposite inguinal ligament.

Reflection of the external oblique muscle [Fig. 4.18]
Now carefully detach the slips of the external oblique muscle from the ribs and turn the uppermost part of the muscle forwards [Fig. 4.18]. Then turn the subject on its side and completely isolate the posterior free border of the external oblique muscle. With the handle of a scalpel separate it from the underlying internal oblique muscle of the abdomen. Having done this, cut through the insertion of the external oblique into the outer lip of the anterior half of the iliac crest. Turn the body on to its back and divide the aponeurosis of the muscle by incising it horizontally, starting at the level of the anterior superior iliac spine, and continuing as far medially as the lateral border of the rectus abdominis muscle. You should now be able to reflect the upper and bigger part of the external oblique muscle medially and so expose the internal oblique muscle.

The internal oblique muscle of the abdomen

Origin of the internal oblique muscle [Fig. 4.19]
Clear the fascia from the surface of the internal oblique as far backwards as the dense **thoracolumbar fascia** from which part of the muscle arises, turning the cadaver as you do so if it facilitates your dissection. You will also see fibres of the internal oblique arising from the anterior two-thirds of the iliac crest [Fig. 4.19], deep to the part of the insertion of the external oblique muscle, which you have separated from the bone. The most medial fibres of the internal oblique muscle, which arise from the lateral two-thirds of the inguinal ligament, are still covered by the part of the aponeurosis of the external oblique muscle which you have not yet reflected. You will see them later when the inguinal region is dissected [p. 4.26].

The aponeurosis of the internal oblique muscle [Fig. 4.19]
Meanwhile trace those fibres of the internal oblique that arise from the iliac crest. Follow them as they pass upwards and medially until they become aponeurotic at the lateral

4.21

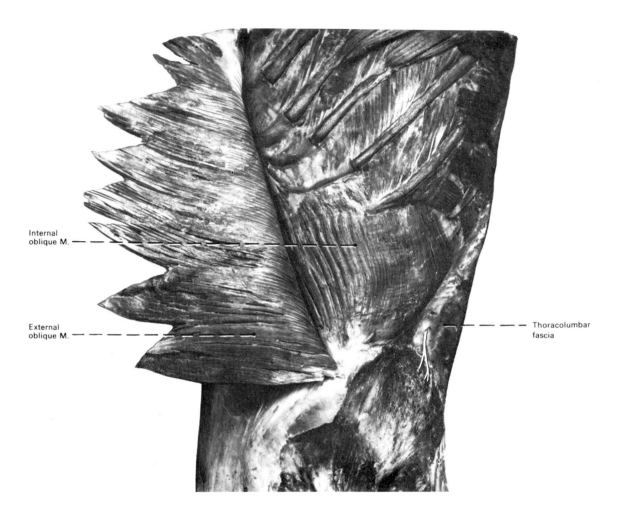

Internal
oblique M.

External
oblique M.

Thoracolumbar
fascia

Fig. 4.18 The reflection of the left external oblique muscle of the abdomen.

border of the rectus abdominis. Here the aponeurosis splits into two lamellae which ensheathe the rectus abdominis as they pass into the linea alba. You can easily see that the anterior lamella fuses with the aponeurosis of the external oblique muscle. Trace the aponeurosis of the internal oblique muscle upwards and note that it is attached to the seventh, eighth, and ninth costal cartilages. Finally, trace the fibres of the internal oblique that arise from the thoraco-lumbar fascia as they pass almost vertically upwards to be inserted, as muscle, into the tenth, eleventh, and twelfth ribs.

About 2 cm medial to the anterior superior iliac spine, find the anterior cutaneous branch of the iliohypogastric nerve piercing the internal oblique muscle. Follow this nerve as far as you can under cover of that part of the external oblique aponeurosis which has not yet been reflected [Fig. 4.19].

Reflection of the internal oblique muscle

You must now separate the internal oblique muscle from its origin from the thoracolumbar fascia and iliac crest, and at the same time detach it from its insertion into the lower ribs. Cut the muscle 1 to 2 cm anterior (lateral) to the thoraco-lumbar fascia in order to separate the muscle from this part of its origin. Great care will be necessary near the iliac crest, for here the internal oblique muscle and the trans-versus abdominis, which lies deep to it, often adhere closely to each other [Fig. 4.20]. The best guide to the plane between the two muscles are two vessels, the **deep circumflex iliac artery,** and its **ascending branch,** which run along the iliac crest between the two muscles. Try to find these vessels. The transverse direction of the fibres of the transversus abdo-minis muscle will act as a further guide to your reflection of the oblique fibres of the internal oblique muscle.

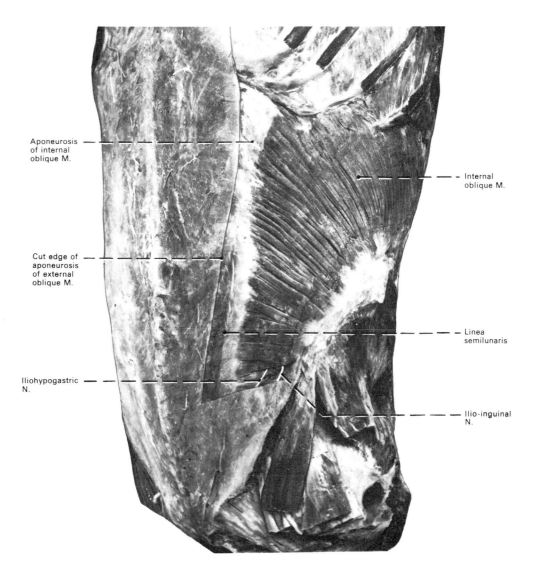

Aponeurosis
of internal
oblique M.

Internal
oblique M.

Cut edge of
aponeurosis
of external
oblique M.

Linea
semilunaris

Iliohypogastric
N.

Ilio-inguinal
N.

Fig. 4.19 The left internal oblique muscle of the abdomen.

As you proceed, note that the main nerves and blood vessels of the abdominal wall pass between the transversus abdominis and internal oblique muscles to their destinations. Look out especially for the iliohypogastric nerve and the ilio-inguinal nerve, both of which are to be seen on the transversus abdominis muscle above the iliac crest [Fig. 4.20].

The transverse abdominis muscle [Fig. 4.20]

When you have turned the internal oblique muscle medially, you can study both the transversus abdominis muscle and the thoracolumbar fascia, which you should first carefully clean. You will see that the muscle arises from the anterior two-thirds of the internal lip of the iliac crest and posteriorly from the thoracolumbar fascia, and also from the deep surfaces of the cartilages of the lower six ribs. Later

you will see that the slips of the muscle which arise from the cartilages interdigitate with the slips of origin of the diaphragm. The lowest fibres of the muscle arise from the lateral third of the inguinal ligament, but these are still covered by the part of the aponeurosis of the external oblique muscle which you have not yet reflected.

The inguinal canal

The superficial inguinal ring [Figs 4.4 and 4.16]

When, earlier on, you identified the spermatic cord in the male and the round ligament of the uterus in the female, you traced them upwards and laterally to the site of their emergence from the abdominal wall [pp. 4.6–4.7]. This is called the superficial inguinal ring, which you should now examine. Note first that it is much smaller in the female

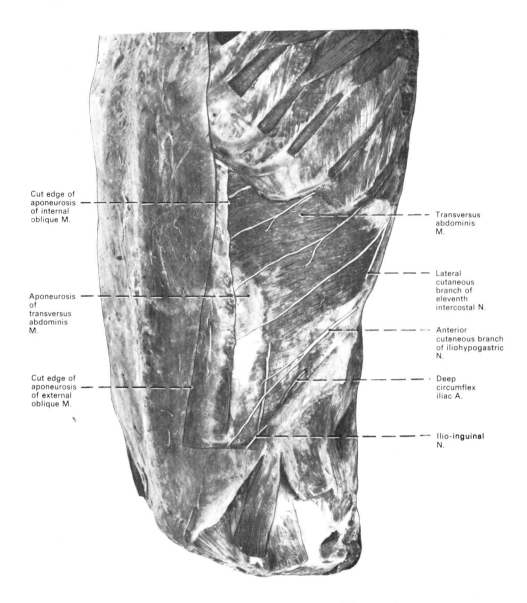

Cut edge of
aponeurosis
of internal
oblique M.

Aponeurosis
of
transversus
abdominis
M.

Cut edge of
aponeurosis
of external
oblique M.

Transversus
abdominis
M.

Lateral
cutaneous
branch of
eleventh
intercostal N.

Anterior
cutaneous branch
of iliohypogastric
N.

Deep
circumflex
iliac A.

Ilio-inguinal
N.

Fig. 4.20 The left transverusus abdominis muscle.

than in the male, and that it is not a ring but a triangle, with its base lying immediately above the pubic crest and with its long axis directed upwards and laterally. Then observe that the ring does not constitute a hole in the aponeurosis of the external oblique, unless one is made artificially. Its edges are prolonged as a thin fascia, called the **external spermatic fascia,** which covers the spermatic cord or round ligament, which have pushed their way from inside the abdomen, across the pubic crest and into the perineal region during embryonic development.

Make an incision through the external spermatic fascia which covers the ring, removing just sufficient to define the margins or crura of the ring [Fig. 4.21]. Note that the inguinal ligament itself forms the **lateral crus** of the ring, and that

the latter is attached to the pubic tubercle. The **medial crus** of the ring is the part of the aponeurosis which is attached to the front of the pubis. You may see some strands passing between the two crura which help to prevent their separation. Normally the ring is just large enough in the male to admit the tip of the little finger. In the female, as already observed, the ring is even smaller. The importance of the ring is that while it transmits the spermatic cord or round ligament, it is also a weakness in the abdominal wall through which gut or associated mesentery can herniate from the abdominal cavity to form an inguinal hernia.

Find a nerve which is adherent to the spermatic cord, and which also emerges from the ring. This is the ilio-inguinal nerve. If you have not already noticed it, try to find it now.

The nerve supplies the skin over the proximal part of the penis in the male, or the mons pubis and adjacent external genitalia in the female [Fig. 4.22].

The lacunar ligament

Now make an oblique incision through the aponeurosis of the external oblique muscle, parallel to and 2 cm above the inguinal ligament, starting 2 cm medial to the anterior superior iliac spine and ending at the apex of the superficial inguinal ring. Turn the two flaps away from each other [Fig. 4.22]. By this means you will have a good view of certain structures which are intimately connected with the anatomy of an inguinal hernia, which is a common surgical condition.

When you look at the inguinal ligament from its inner surface, note that it is grooved, and that it is prolonged along the pecten of the pubis. This prolongation, which is

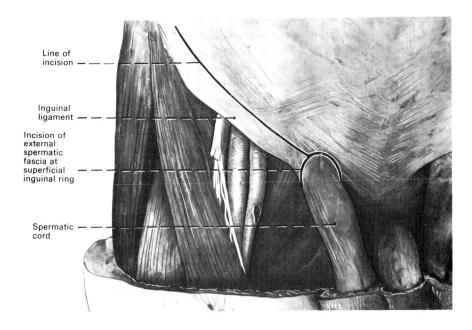

Fig. 4.21 Incision to expose the right inguinal canal.

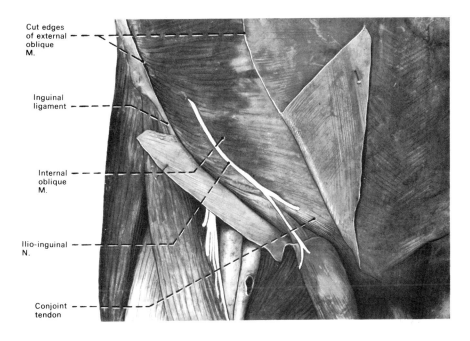

Fig. 4.22 The right inguinal canal. The upper part of the right external oblique muscle of the abdomen has been excised; the lower part has been incised and reflected.

called the lacunar ligament, is particularly important because it forms part of the floor of the inguinal canal as well as the medial border of the femoral ring.

The external spermatic fascia [Fig. 4.21]

In the male, examine the spermatic cord, whose main component is the **ductus deferens.** It is through the latter that the spermatozoa produced in the testis pass into the proximal part of the urethra, which is in the pelvic cavity. Since the testis migrates during the course of its development from within the abdomen through the inguinal canal into the scrotum, it and the attached ductus deferens and associated vessels are recovered by layers of tissue derived from the various layers of the abdominal wall.

The outer layer, the external spermatic fascia [Fig. 4.21], is, as you have seen, a thin sheath of fascia which begins at the superficial inguinal ring, and covers the cord as it passes into the scrotum. In effect, this layer is derived from the aponeurosis of the external oblique muscle of the abdomen.

The cremasteric fascia [Fig. 4.23]

The layer of tissue you can see on the cord on the deep aspect of the aponeurosis of the external oblique, lateral to the superficial inguinal ring, is called the cremasteric fascia [Fig. 4.23]. It is derived from the internal oblique muscle. If you examine this fascia you will see that it contains muscle fibres. These are called the **cremaster muscle,** which consists of fibres reflected from the internal oblique muscle as it arches over the spermatic cord. Trace the fibres of the cre-

master muscle along the cord past the superficial inguinal ring, and on to the testis in the scrotum. Notice that they form loops on the cord and testis. If you clean these loops carefully, you may see that some become attached to the pubic tubercle. When the cremaster muscle contracts, it draws up the testis. Its nerve supply is derived from the genital branch of the genitofemoral nerve. Unless you find this nerve immediately, do not spend time searching for it. The skin over the upper part of the femoral triangle is supplied from the femoral branch of the genitofemoral nerve [Fig. 2.22]. If this area of skin is stroked, the corresponding testis is drawn up; this is known as the cremasteric reflex.

You have already found the ilio-inguinal nerve in front of the spermatic cord [Fig. 4.22]. Trace the nerve laterally and upwards to the point where it pierces the internal oblique muscle, and medially and downwards through the superficial inguinal ring. About 2.5 cm medial to the anterior superior iliac spine search for the anterior cutaneous branch of the iliohypogastric nerve, which you may have seen emerging from the internal oblique muscle. Clean and trace this nerve as it passes medially to the point where it pierces the aponeurosis of the external oblique muscle above the superficial inguinal ring.

The lower part of the internal oblique muscle

You will now be able to see the lowest fibres of the internal oblique muscle arising from the lateral two-thirds of the inguinal ligament [Fig. 4.23]. Clean and trace the uppermost of these fibres and note that they become aponeurotic, and that all run in front of the rectus abdominis muscle to pass

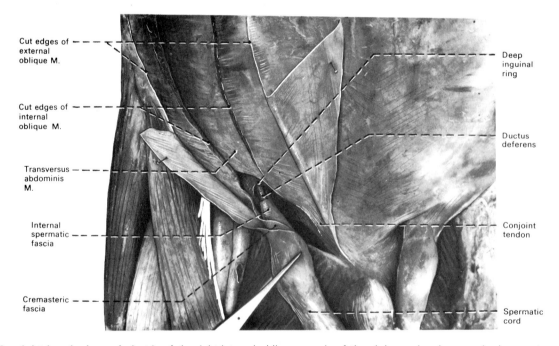

Cut edges of external oblique M.

Cut edges of internal oblique M.

Transversus abdominis M.

Internal spermatic fascia

Cremasteric fascia

Deep inguinal ring

Ductus deferens

Conjoint tendon

Spermatic cord

Fig. 4.23 The right inguinal canal. A strip of the right internal oblique muscle of the abdomen has been excised, so as to expose the right transversus abdominis muscle and the right deep inguinal ring. The edges of this ring have been defined by removing part of the internal spermatic fascia. The spermatic cord has been displaced laterally.

4.26

into the linea alba. Note, too, that the lower (more medial) fibres of the internal oblique muscle become aponeurotic, and that they arch over the spermatic cord (or round ligament of the uterus). The arch forms the lower border of the internal oblique muscle.

Using your scalpel, separate the attachment of the internal oblique muscle from the inguinal ligament and turn the detached part of the muscle upwards and medially. By doing so, you will expose the lowest and most medial fibres of the transversus abdominis muscle as they arise from the lateral third of the inguinal ligament.

The conjoint tendon [Fig. 4.23]

Turn your attention again to the lowest fibres of the internal oblique muscle as they arch over the spermatic cord. Note that they fuse with fibres of the transversus abdominis muscle, so forming what is called the conjoint tendon. Trace the tendon to its insertion into the pubic tubercle and the pubic crest, and also into the medial part of the pecten of the pubis. Observe that the conjoint tendon lies behind the spermatic cord immediately opposite the superficial inguinal ring, thereby strengthening a potentially weak area of the abdominal wall.

The internal spermatic fascia [Fig. 4.23]

Displace the spermatic cord upwards and medially and observe that there are no muscle fibres behind the lateral part of the cord. The glistening membrane you will have exposed is the **transversalis fascia,** which forms the posterior wall of the inguinal canal. You will see that the spermatic cord emerges from this fascia about 1 cm above the midpoint of the inguinal ligament, taking the fascia with it as a diverticulum whose mouth, which faces towards the abdominal cavity, is called the deep inguinal ring. This evaginated fascia, or internal spermatic fascia, ensheaths the cord and testis, deep to the cremasteric fascia.

The deep inguinal ring [Fig. 4.23]

Clear away the internal spermatic fascia so as to define the boundaries of the deep inguinal ring. When you have done so you will see the main and central part of the spermatic cord disappearing into the abdominal cavity. Note that the deep inguinal ring is covered anteriorly by the lowermost fibres of the internal oblique muscle. The inferior epigastric artery can be seen at the medial side of the ring.

The round ligament of the uterus [Fig. 4.5]

In the female the place of the spermatic cord is taken by a fibromuscular strand called the round ligament of the uterus. On each side you should have seen the superficial and distal part of the round ligament emerging from the superficial inguinal ring and passing into the labium majus [p. 4.7]. In the inguinal canal the round ligament is invested by the same sheaths as is the spermatic cord, but it lacks

a cremaster muscle. Like the spermatic cord it leaves the abdominal cavity through the deep inguinal ring.

The scrotum and its contents

Now examine the scrotum, testis, and spermatic cord.

Dissect away the skin of the scrotum, noting the presence of fine muscle fibres, both on its deep surface and in the superficial fascia. These fibres form the **tunica dartos.** When they contract they cause the skin of the scrotum to become rugose.

Incise the superficial fascia at both sides of the scrotum, and remove the testes and spermatic cords with the fascial layers by which they are covered.

You will now see that an incomplete fascial septum divides the scrotum into two compartments, one for each testis. This septum is formed both by fascia and by the fibres of the tunica dartos, which by now will have become more obvious. Follow the distal part of the ilio-inguinal nerve through the subcutaneous tissue as it enters the scrotal region from above, and also the posterior scrotal nerves, branches of the pudendal nerve, which enter the scrotum from below and behind.

The testis [Figs 4.24 and 4.25]

Examine the testis before you remove its fascial coverings. You will see that it is an oval body about 4 cm long. The coiled tube on its posterior border is the epididymis, which you will see merges imperceptibly with the spermatic cord. The ductus deferens, which is the main constituent of the cord, continues into the epididymis, and all three have the same fascial coverings. The testis develops during embryonic life on the posterior abdominal wall, and, as already noted, migrates out of the abdominal cavity, along the inguinal canal, into the scrotum, carrying with it evaginations of the various layers of the abdominal wall [Fig. 4.23]. These are the external spermatic fascia from the external oblique muscle; the cremasteric fascia from the internal oblique muscle; and the internal spermatic fascia from the transversalis fascia.

Make a longitudinal incision on the posterior surface of the spermatic cord, and try to strip each of these three layers of fascia. Do not spend more than a few minutes trying to do this. You will find dissection easier later with the testis and cord in a dish of water. It would be a waste of time, in the female cadaver, to try to demonstrate the three layers around the round ligament.

The tunica vaginalis [Fig. 4.24]

The dull membrane round the testis which is exposed when the three layers of fascia are removed is the tunica vaginalis [Fig. 4.24]. The tunica surrounds the testis on all sides except posteriorly.

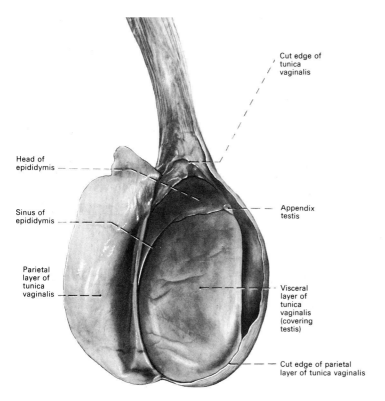

Fig. 4.24 The tunica vaginalis of the right testis. The parietal layer of the tunica vaginalis has been incised and turned laterally.

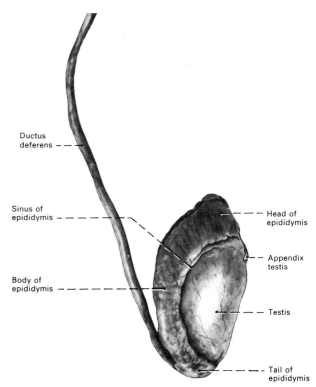

Fig. 4.25 The right testis and epididymis.

The tunica vaginalis is a serous sac which is invaginated by the testis. The inner or **visceral layer** adheres closely to the surface of the testis except posteriorly, where the epididymis and ductus deferens are attached, and where the visceral layer becomes continuous with the outer **parietal layer.** Carefully incise the parietal layer of the tunica. The space between it and the serous layer contains just sufficient exudate to make it possible for the testis to move without friction. Examine the junction of the testis and epididymis from its lateral aspect. You will see that a small recess of the cavity of the tunica vaginalis intervenes between the testis and the body of the epididymis. This is known as the **sinus of the epididymis.**

The epididymis [Fig. 4.25]

Examine the epididymis [Fig. 4.25]. You will see that it consists of an enlarged upper end, or **head**; a central portion, or **body**; and a lower pointed end, or **tail.** On the head of the epididymis, either above or below, and sometimes on the lateral edge of the body, you may note minute tags of tissue, the **appendix testis.** These are vestigial remnants of embryonic structures of no importance to your dissection.

The spermatic cord

Now slit open one of the two spermatic cords along its entire length. You will have no difficulty in picking out the hard

ductus deferens which begins at the lower end and runs up the medial side of the epididymis. The ductus is a muscular tube with a narrow lumen, which connects the epididymis with the seminal vesicles and prostate in the pelvis. Surrounding the ductus deferens you will find a collection of small veins, called the **pampiniform plexus.** These are the most bulky constituents of the spermatic cord. At the deep inguinal rings the veins of each pampiniform plexus unite to form the testicular veins. As you will see later, the right testicular vein drains into the inferior vena cava and the left into the left renal vein.

In a well-injected specimen, you should be able to find in the spermatic cord the **testicular artery,** and sometimes a smaller artery which runs into the ductus deferens. If you can see them, trace these vessels to the testis. The testicular artery arises from the aorta on the upper part of the posterior abdominal wall and passes through the deep inguinal ring to enter the spermatic cord; the **artery of the ductus deferens** is a branch of either the umbilical artery or one of the arteries which supply the bladder. Another small artery, the **cremasteric artery,** supplies the coats of the spermatic cord. It is a branch of the inferior epigastric artery.

The structure of the testis [Fig. 4.26]

Remove one testis by cutting through the cord. Examine it under water by making a transverse incision through it

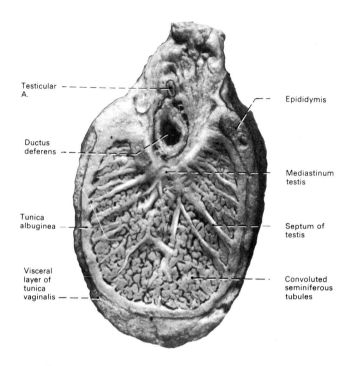

Testicular A.

Ductus deferens

Tunica albuginea

Visceral layer of tunica vaginalis

Epididymis

Mediastinum testis

Septum of testis

Convoluted seminiferous tubules

Fig. 4.26 Transverse section of the left testis.

and the epididymis [Fig. 4.26]. Note its tough outer fibrous covering, called the **tunica albuginea**; it projects into the posterior part of the testis to form the **mediastinum testis**. From the latter you will be able to follow the **septa of the testis,** which divide the organ into the **lobules of the testis.** Some of the **convoluted seminiferous tubules** which occupy the lobules should be teased out. Examine the epididymis and note how greatly coiled it is. When the tunica vaginalis has been removed it may be possible to see the very fine **efferent ducts of the testis** which connect the head of the epididymis with the testis.

The rectus abdominis muscle and the rectus sheath

Now make a vertical incision along the midline of the whole of each rectus sheath, and separate the flaps so formed, at the same time dividing the attachment of the sheaths to the pubes below [Fig. 4.27]. Some difficulty will be experienced where the sheaths adhere to the **tendinous intersections** in the rectus abdominis muscles. Note the anterior cutaneous branches of the intercostal nerves piercing the muscle.

The pyramidalis muscle [Fig. 4.27]

Look for a small triangular muscle, called the pyramidalis muscle, that lies in front of the rectus abdominis [Fig. 4.27].

It is sometimes missing. When present, note its origin from the pubic crest and its insertion into the **linea alba.** A branch of the subcostal nerve enters its deep surface.

The rectus abdominis muscle [Fig. 4.27]

Now examine the rectus abdominis muscle on one side. It is a straight, broad and flat muscle which arises from below by two heads. Clean the lower end of the muscle and note that one head arises from the pubic crest and the other from the anterior ligament of the pubic symphysis.

Follow the muscle upwards to its insertion, by means of muscular slips, into the xiphoid process and the fifth, sixth, and seventh costal cartilages. Separate the upper and lower ends of the muscle from their attachments, and turn the muscle laterally, using the nerves and vessels which enter its deep surface as a hinge [Fig. 4.28]. The nerves are the anterior cutaneous branches of the lower six thoracic nerves. They pierce the posterior layer of the rectus sheath before entering the muscle on its posterior aspect.

The anterior layer of the rectus sheath [Fig. 4.27]

As you will have seen, the anterior layer of the rectus sheath covers the entire muscle [Fig. 4.29a]. It is formed by the aponeurosis of the external oblique muscle, which is reinforced, below the costal margin, by the anterior lamella of the aponeurosis of the internal oblique muscle; and below a line joining the anterior superior iliac spines of the two sides, by the combined aponeuroses of the internal oblique and the transversus abdominis muscles [Fig. 4.29b].

The posterior layer of the rectus sheath [Fig. 4.28]

With the rectus abdominis muscle reflected laterally, you can now examine the posterior layer of the rectus sheath which, you will see, is an unbroken sheet in the area between the costal margin and a line joining the two anterior superior iliac spines. At this level the posterior fibrous layer of the sheath ends in a crescentic margin called the **arcuate line.** Above this line the posterior layer is formed by the fusion of the posterior lamella of the aponeurosis of the internal oblique with the aponeurosis of the transversus abdominis. Below the arcuate line you will see that the aponeuroses of both the internal oblique and transversus abdominis muscles pass in front of the rectus abdominis. In this region the muscle is separated from the peritoneal lining of the abdominal cavity only by the transversalis fascia [Fig. 4.29].

The epigastric vessels [Fig. 4.28]

You will see a prominent and vertically-disposed set of vessels lying behind the lower part of the muscle. These are the **inferior epigastric artery** and **vein** [Fig. 4.28]. The artery is the largest single vessel supplying the abdominal wall. If you trace it downwards, you will see that it arises just above the inguinal ligament from the external iliac artery (which you will examine later), and that it ascends in the extra-

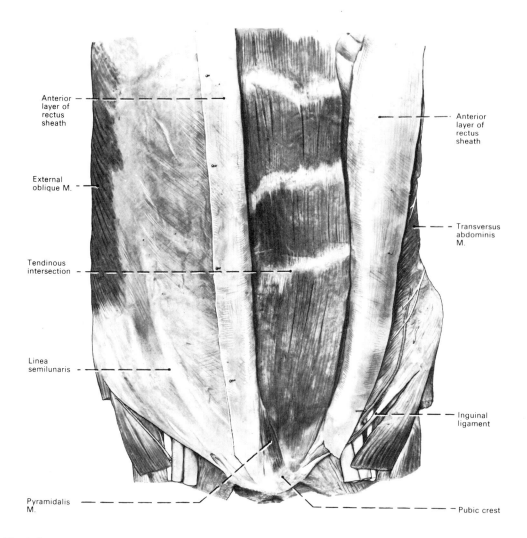

Anterior
layer of
rectus
sheath

External
oblique M.

Tendinous
intersection

Linea
semilunaris

Pyramidalis
M.

Anterior
layer of
rectus
sheath

Transversus
abdominis
M.

Inguinal
ligament

Pubic crest

Fig. 4.27 The left rectus abdominis muscle. The anterior layer of the left rectus sheath has been incised vertically and opened.

peritoneal tissue to the medial side of the deep inguinal ring. The inferior epigastric artery pierces the transversalis fascia before entering the rectus sheath by passing in front of the arcuate line.

Trace the artery upwards until you find it anastomosing with another artery that is descending from the lower end of the sternum. This is the **superior epigastric artery,** one of the two terminal branches of the internal thoracic artery. The other is the **musculophrenic artery** which runs along the costal attachment of the diaphragm, supplying its under-surface and the adjacent musculature.

Now return to the abdominal wall. Detach the trans-versus abdominis muscle from both the inguinal ligament and the anterior part of the iliac crest and turn it upwards. By doing so you reveal more of the transversalis fascia. This fascia becomes very thin superiorly where it blends with the fascia on the under-surface of the diaphragm; but you can

see that it is thick below, where it forms the posterior wall of the inguinal canal.

The thoracolumbar fascia

Turn the cadaver over and examine the thoracolumbar fascia [Fig. 4.30]. Note that the fascia consists of fibrous tissue which covers the deep muscles of the back of the trunk all the way from the base of the neck above to the sacrum below. In the thorax it consists of a single thin layer, but in the lumbar region, where it is thicker, it not only ensheathes and gives origin to muscles, but considerably strengthens the posterior abdominal wall. Here it consists of three layers [Fig. 4.31] called the anterior, middle, and posterior layers, of which the latter, which gives origin to part of the latissimus dorsi muscle, is much the strongest. These three layers pass laterally from the vertebral column

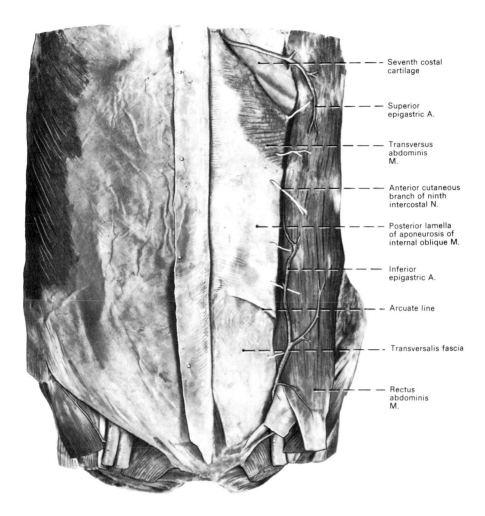

Seventh costal
cartilage

Superior
epigastric A.

Transversus
abdominis
M.

Anterior cutaneous
branch of ninth
intercostal N.

Posterior lamella
of aponeurosis of
internal oblique M.

Inferior
epigastric A.

Arcuate line

Transversalis fascia

Rectus
abdominis
M.

Fig. 4.28 The posterior layer of the rectus sheath. The left rectus abdominis has been reflected laterally.

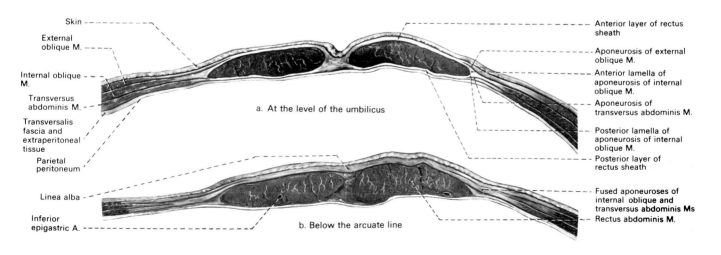

Skin

External
oblique M.

Internal oblique
M.

Transversus
abdominis M.

Transversalis
fascia and
extraperitoneal
tissue

Parietal
peritoneum

Linea alba

Inferior
epigastric A.

Anterior layer of rectus
sheath

Aponeurosis of external
oblique M.

Anterior lamella of
aponeurosis of internal
oblique M.

Aponeurosis of
transversus abdominis M.

Posterior lamella of
aponeurosis of internal
oblique M.

Posterior layer of
rectus sheath

Fused aponeuroses of
internal oblique and
transversus abdominis Ms

Rectus abdominis M.

a. At the level of the umbilicus

b. Below the arcuate line

Fig. 4.29 Horizontal sections of the anterior abdominal wall.

4.31

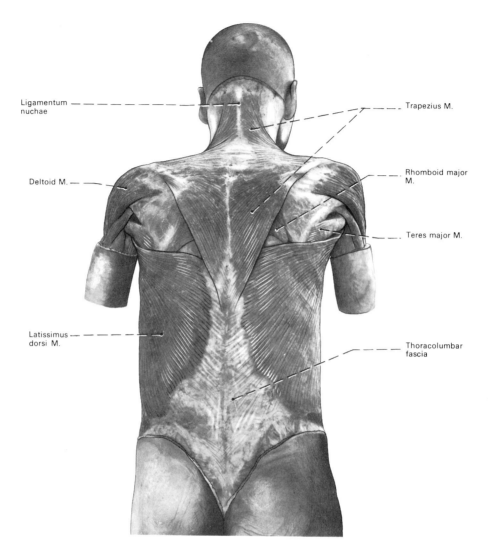

Ligamentum nuchae

Trapezius M.

Deltoid M.

Rhomboid major M.

Teres major M.

Latissimus dorsi M.

Thoracolumbar fascia

Fig. 4.30 The posterior layer of the thoracolumbar fascia.

to enclose the erector spinae and quadratus lumborum muscles, beyond which they fuse, to give origin to the internal oblique and transversus abdominis muscles.

The blood supply of the anterior abdominal wall

Before you complete the study of the abdominal wall, note the following further facts, which you need not confirm by dissection, about its blood and nerve supply.

The largest artery of the abdominal wall is, as already noted, the **inferior epigastric artery** [Fig. 4.32], whose anastomosis with the **superior epigastric artery,** a branch of the internal thoracic artery, you have already seen. You have also seen the branches of the femoral artery to the genitalia and inguinal region [pp. 2.21, 2.24]. Note now the small pubic branch of the inferior epigastric artery, which runs behind the superior ramus of the pubis. This branch is of

some importance since, by its enlargement and anastomosis with an enlarged pubic branch of the obturator artery, it sometimes forms a larger abnormal obturator artery, which replaces the normal obturator artery. You will see the obturator artery when you dissect the pelvis [p. 4.87].

Another branch of the external iliac artery which supplies the anterior abdominal wall is the **deep circumflex iliac artery.** This passes along the iliac crest between the transversus abdominis and internal oblique muscles. You have already seen this vessel [p. 4.22].

The veins of the abdominal wall follow the course of the arteries and require no special mention, except that around the umbilicus there are a number of small veins called the **paraumbilical veins.** These paraumbilical veins drain into the abdominal cavity along the falciform ligament of the liver, and so into the portal vein, which you will study later, and which gathers almost all of the blood of the alimentary canal [p. 4.74]. Obstruction of the portal vein therefore may reveal itself as varicosities around the umbilicus.

The nerve supply of the anterior abdominal wall

Note the following facts about the nerves of the anterior abdominal wall, which you have already seen. The muscles of the wall are supplied by the ventral rami of the lower six or seven thoracic nerves, which are often called the thoraco-abdominal nerves [Fig. 4.16]. The iliohypogastric nerve and ilio-inguinal nerve, which are branches of the first lumbar nerve, also supply the internal oblique muscle and the transversus abdominis muscle. The pyramidalis muscle is supplied by the subcostal nerve.

The lower six **intercostal nerves** descend into the abdominal wall from behind the costal margin, and in this part of their course they run between the transversus abdominis

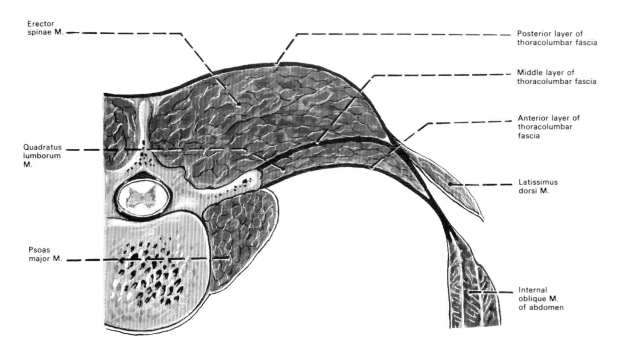

Fig. 4.31 Schematic transverse section of the thoracolumbar fascia.

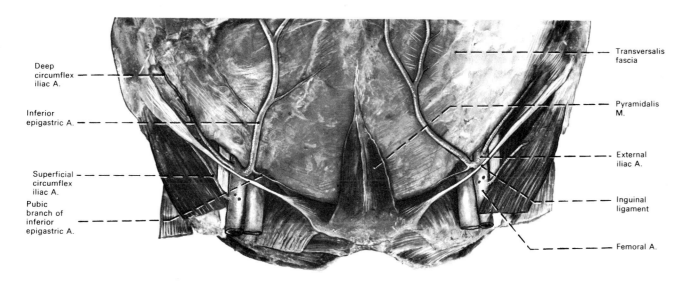

Fig. 4.32 The inferior epigastric arteries. The muscles of the anterior abdominal wall have been excised.

THE ANTERIOR ABDOMINAL WALL

and internal oblique muscles. They give off lateral cutaneous branches which become cutaneous along the lateral surface of the body, and anterior cutaneous branches which pierce the rectus sheath and rectus abdominis muscle, and become cutaneous in series near the midline of the body. The levels innervated by these nerves are indicated by the fact that the seventh thoracic nerve supplies the skin of the epigastrium, the tenth thoracic nerve the skin around the umbilicus, and the twelfth thoracic nerve the skin midway between the umbilicus and the pubis. Remember that the ventral ramus of the twelfth thoracic nerve is known as the subcostal nerve.

The **subcostal nerve** passes across the posterior abdominal wall (on the anterior surface of the quadratus lumborum muscle and behind the kidney), and perforates the transversus abdominis muscle to reach the anterior abdominal wall. It subsequently runs a course similar to the other thoraco-abdominal nerves, except that its lateral cutaneous branch runs downwards over the iliac crest to supply the skin of the thigh in the region of the greater trochanter [see p. 2.9].

The **iliohypogastric** and **ilio-inguinal nerves** also pass between the quadratus lumborum and the kidney, in series with the subcostal nerve, and they run a similar course between the transversus abdominis and internal oblique muscles. The ilio-inguinal nerve is the smaller of these two divisions of the first lumbar nerve and has no lateral cutaneous branch.

The functions of the abdominal muscles

The muscles of the abdominal wall help to keep the viscera in position, and by controlling the intra-abdominal pressure, they materially assist the flow of venous blood and lymph from the lower part of the body into the thorax. When they contract, they increase the intra-abdominal pressure and so force the diaphragm upwards into the chest, thus emptying the lungs of air. This movement is initiated especially by the transversus abdominis muscle, which is therefore a muscle of expiration. Since the contraction of the abdominal muscles increases intra-abdominal pressure, they, in co-operation with the diaphragm and the levator ani, are used in all expulsive efforts (e.g. defaecation and parturition).

When lying flat on your back, the contraction of the rectus abdominis muscle helps lift the upper half of the body. The external and internal oblique muscles of the abdomen are essentially rotators of the trunk, the external oblique muscle of one side acting with the internal oblique muscle of the opposite side. Try these movements on yourself as opportunity allows. Lie on your back and lift your head and shoulders and raise both lower limbs. Note that as they do so your rectus abdominis muscles contract. Next try rotating your trunk when standing upright. You can feel your external and internal oblique abdominal muscles contract as you do so. You will not be able to distinguish their separate actions.

Section 4.4

The peritoneal cavity

Open the abdomen by means of the following cruciate incision. First make a vertical incision through the linea alba (keeping to the left of the midline above the umbilicus), from the xiphoid process above to the pubic symphysis below, and then a transverse incision just below the level of the umbilicus, extending on either side to the lateral margins of the body. Turn aside the four triangular flaps so formed. You will find that the upper right flap cannot be turned back as freely as the others, because a fold, called the falciform ligament [Fig. 4.33], attaches it to the liver.

The peritoneum

Note that the structures which form the walls of the abdominal cavity (above, the diaphragm; in front, the muscles of the anterior abdominal wall; behind, the muscles of the posterior abdominal wall and the lower part of the vertebral column; and below, the muscles of the pelvic diaphragm) are lined on their deep aspect by a continuous layer of serous membrane called the peritoneum. Most of the abdominal and pelvic organs invaginate this serous sac, in the same way as the heart, lungs, and testes invaginate the serous sacs by which they are surrounded.

The peritoneum consists of a **parietal layer** which lines the walls of the abdominal cavity and a **visceral layer** which covers the abdominal organs to a variable extent. A film of fluid between these two layers facilitates the movement of the organs. The potential space between the two layers is called the peritoneal cavity.

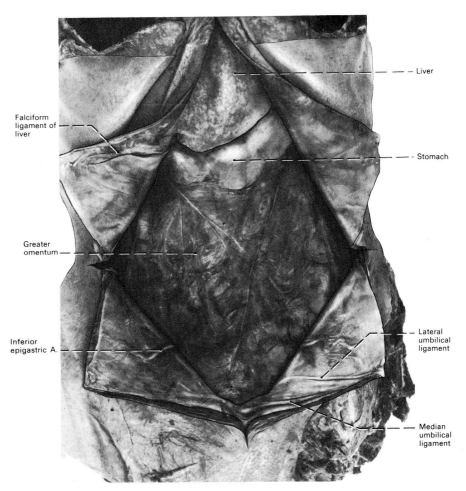

Fig. 4.33 The anterior aspect of the peritoneal cavity.

The ligaments attached to the umbilicus

Look at the **falciform ligament** [Fig. 4.33]. It is a double fold of peritoneum which extends from the umbilicus to the antero-superior surface of the liver. If you examine its free edge you will see that it contains a cord-like structure which passes to the inferior border of the liver. This is the **round ligament of the liver,** which is formed by the remains of the left umbilical vein of the foetus. Between the folds of the falciform ligament are some small veins, already referred to, which connect the portal vein with the paraumbilical veins of the anterior abdominal wall around the umbilicus [see p. 4.32].

Look at the deep surface of the two lower flaps of abdominal wall which you have turned down. Note that there are three cord-like structures which can be seen through the peritoneum, extending upwards on the anterior abdominal wall towards the umbilicus. They are the **median umbilical ligament** and the two **lateral umbilical ligaments.** If you follow the course of the median umbilical ligament you will see that it extends from the apex of the bladder to the umbilicus. It is the remains of the urachus, which is a foetal structure. The lateral umbilical ligaments emerge from the pelvis and are the distal obliterated parts of the umbilical arteries of the foetus [Fig. 4.33].

The disposition of the abdominal viscera

Without disturbing them unduly you should now get a general view of the disposition of the abdominal viscera. You are looking into the main peritoneal cavity.

First examine the **liver.** This large organ lies almost entirely under cover of the ribs and costal cartilages, occupying a large part of the right hypochondriac region and extending across the epigastric region, where it lies directly behind the abdominal wall. Adherent to the right side of the inferior border of the liver, you will see the blind end or fundus of the **gall-bladder.** Below, and to some extent behind the left side of the liver you will find the **stomach,** which is very variable in size [Fig. 4.33].

The apron-like flap of peritoneum suspended from the lower border of the stomach is the **greater omentum.** This flap contains a variable amount of fat and is fairly vascular. If you lift up the greater omentum, coils of **small intestine** will come into view [Fig. 4.34]. If you move these coils from side to side, you will see that they are suspended from the posterior abdominal wall by a double fold of peritoneum, called the **mesentery** [Fig. 4.36].

Now follow the course of the **large intestine,** which you will easily distinguish from the small intestine by the fact that its wall shows three longitudinal bands of muscle, each

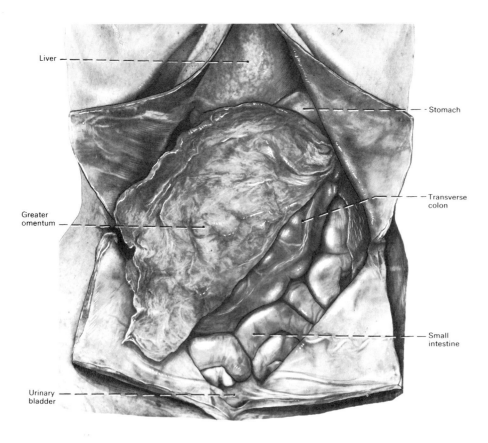

Fig. 4.34 The peritoneal cavity with the greater omentum turned aside.

about 0.5 cm wide; as well as by the fact that the large intestine is usually wider in diameter. Look in the right iliac fossa for a blind pouch of large intestine called the **caecum** [Fig. 4.35]. On the medial side of the caecum, about 4 cm from its blind end, the small intestine runs into the large intestine at the **ileocaecal opening.** Below the opening is a narrow, pencil-like diverticulum of the caecum called the **vermiform appendix.** The appendix is usually about 10 cm long, but may vary from 2 cm to 20 cm.

The upper part of the caecum is continuous with the **ascending colon,** which you should now trace upwards, on the right side of the abdominal cavity. Beneath the liver you will find that the ascending colon bends sharply at the **right colic flexure,** where it becomes continuous with a part of the large intestine called the **transverse colon.** To see the transverse colon clearly you must turn the greater omentum upwards [Fig. 4.34]. As you do so note that this flap of peritoneum is attached to the transverse colon as well as to the lower border of the stomach. You will see that the transverse colon lies somewhat horizontally in the abdominal cavity, between the lower part of the liver on the right and the spleen on the left. Below the spleen the transverse colon becomes continuous with the **descending colon** at the **left**

colic flexure. Follow the descending colon down the left side of the abdominal cavity as far as the linea terminalis of the pelvis [see p. 4.4].

Feel for the pyloric or right extremity of the stomach. It becomes continuous with the small intestine. You should be able to feel that the calibre of the stomach narrows where it joins the small intestine. This part of the stomach is the **pyloric canal.** Distally its wall is thickened to form a **pyloric sphincter.**

The first part of the small intestine is called the **duodenum.** You will not be able to study the duodenum at this stage, since it lies behind the transverse colon under cover of the peritoneum covering the posterior abdominal wall.

With your fingers, feel behind the ribs in the left hypochondriac region. The organ about the size of a fist which lies to the extreme left is the **spleen.** You will see that it is in contact with the colon below, and with the stomach above. Behind the right extremity of the transverse colon you should be able to feel part of the right **kidney,** and behind the left extremity of the colon and the spleen, part of the left kidney.

The disposition of the pelvic viscera

Lift the mass of small intestine out of the pelvis and note the disposition of the pelvic viscera [Fig. 4.36]. In the male cadaver you will find the **urinary bladder** in front, forming a rounded mass covered by peritoneum. Behind, and continuous with the descending colon, is the **sigmoid colon,** suspended by a mesentery from the posterior abdominal wall. It continues as the **rectum,** which it often overhangs. The rectum, which lies under cover of the peritoneum on the posterior wall of the pelvis, leads into the terminal part of the alimentary tract, called the **anal canal.**

In the female cadaver, locate the urinary bladder in front, and in the midline, between it and the rectum posteriorly, the body of the **uterus.** From the upper part of the uterus the **uterine tubes** pass laterally, each in a double fold of peritoneum called the **broad ligament of the uterus** towards the walls of the pelvis. The **ovaries** are attached to the posterior aspect of the broad ligaments at their supero-lateral angles [Fig. 4.40].

Now study the peritoneum. Cut round the umbilicus, leaving the falciform ligament attached to it, and then separate the attachment of the ligament to the anterior abdominal wall on each side with a scalpel or scissors. This will allow you to turn back the right upper flap of the abdominal wall. You will also be able to separate the round ligament of the liver from the free edge of the falciform ligament.

The reflections of the peritoneum

Remember that the peritoneum is an uninterrupted sheet of membrane which is invaginated to varying extents, and

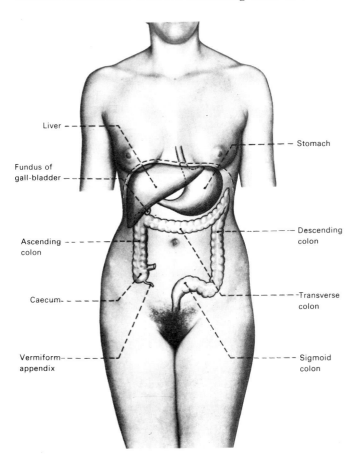

Liver

Fundus of gall-bladder

Ascending colon

Caecum

Vermiform appendix

Stomach

Descending colon

Transverse colon

Sigmoid colon

Fig. 4.35 A surface projection of the liver, stomach, and large intestine.

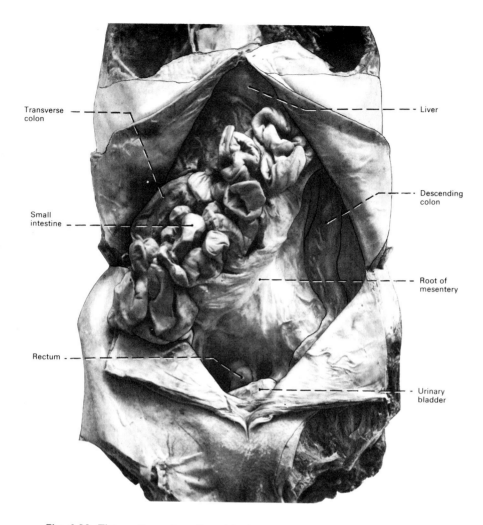

Fig. 4.36 The peritoneal cavity with the small intestine turned upwards.

in different ways, by most of the abdominal viscera. As a result, the abdominal cavity contains a number of complicated peritoneal folds and recesses. The blood vessels, nerves, and lymphatics pass to and from the abdominal viscera between the layers of peritoneum. Refer to Fig. 4.37 which, while schematic, will aid you as you explore the disposition of the peritoneum in your cadaver.

The coronary ligament of the liver

Insert your fingers between the diaphragm and the right lobe of the liver, and gently push your hand backwards. Your fingers will be stopped by a peritoneal fold which connects the diaphragm with the diaphragmatic surface of the liver. This fold of peritoneum is the superior layer of the coronary ligament of the liver, which is reflected from the liver on to the under-surface of the diaphragm.

The visceral peritoneum covering the diaphragmatic surface of the organ is continuous around the sharp inferior border with that on the visceral surface of the liver. The hilum of the liver, or porta hepatis, is on this surface. It is

a transverse cleft behind the neck of the gall-bladder, and through it vessels, nerves, and ducts pass to and from the liver.

The lesser omentum

You will not be able to see the porta hepatis itself, but if you press the liver upwards and pull the stomach down, you should be able to see a fold of peritoneum which is attached to the porta hepatis above, and to the superior or right border of the stomach below. This border is called the lesser curvature of the stomach. The peritoneal fold is the lesser omentum [Fig. 4.38]. It forms the upper part of the anterior wall of a recess of the peritoneal cavity called the **omental bursa** [Fig. 4.37].

The epiploic foramen

If you continue to hold the liver and stomach apart, you will notice that the right border of the lesser omentum is free. At this border the anterior and posterior peritoneal layers of the lesser omentum become continuous with each

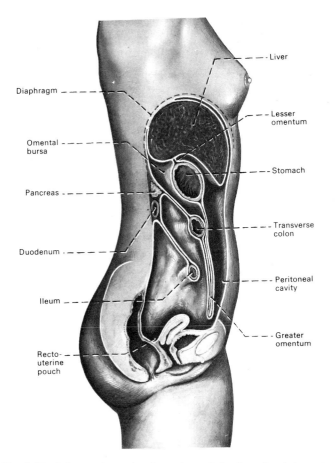

Fig. 4.37 Schematic sagittal section of the female abdomen.

other. If you pass your finger behind the border of the lesser omentum you will enter the omental bursa through an opening called the epiploic foramen [Fig. 4.38]. If you hold the free margin between your finger and thumb you may feel certain structures which you will dissect later. These are the bile-duct, descending from the porta hepatis, and the hepatic artery and portal vein, ascending to the liver. Also running between the two layers of the lesser omentum are the right and left gastric arteries and veins, and branches of the anterior and posterior vagal trunks, which are derived from the vagus nerves, on their way to the stomach. You will dissect these structures later.

The greater omentum [Figs 4.33 and 4.34]

Trace the greater omentum from the inferior and left border or greater curvature of the stomach. The greater omentum varies in shape, size, and in the extent to which it is impregnated with fat. The vessels you can see in it are the right and left gastroepiploic arteries and veins. If you examine Fig. 4.37 you will see that the greater omentum is formed by the continuation downwards of the peritoneum on the anterior and posterior walls of the stomach, and that these two layers of peritoneum are then folded back on themselves. The main part of the greater omentum thus consists of four sheets of peritoneum. The posterior two layers become adherent to the anterior surface of the transverse colon and its mesentery. You may not be able to establish this point in your dissection.

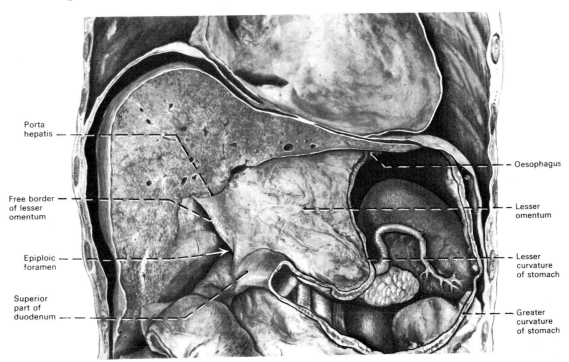

Fig. 4.38 The lesser omentum. A sectioned body from which the walls of the stomach and the peritoneum behind the omental bursa have been excised.

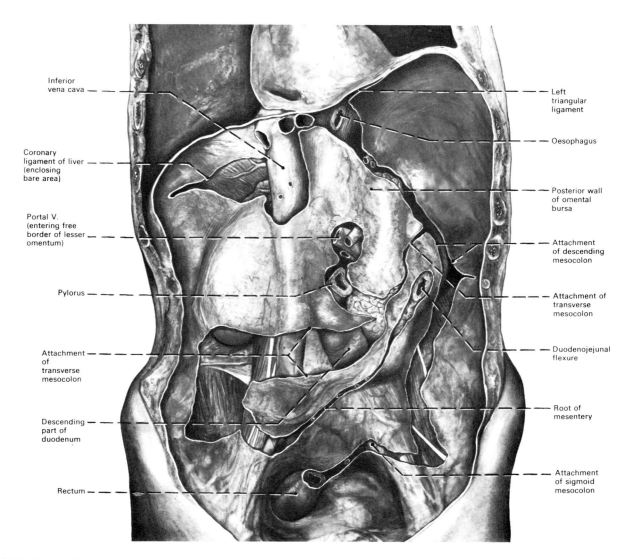

Inferior
vena cava

Coronary
ligament of liver
(enclosing
bare area)

Portal V.
(entering free
border of lesser
omentum)

Pylorus

Attachment
of
transverse
mesocolon

Descending
part of
duodenum

Rectum

Left
triangular
ligament

Oesophagus

Posterior wall
of omental
bursa

Attachment
of descending
mesocolon

Attachment of
transverse
mesocolon

Duodenojejunal
flexure

Root of
mesentery

Attachment
of sigmoid
mesocolon

Fig. 4.39 The peritoneal reflections on the posterior abdominal wall. The liver, spleen, and most of the alimentary tract have been excised. The descending colon had a short mesentery. The left dome of the diaphragm is abnormally high and the duodenum and pancreas lie further to the left than is usual.

The transverse mesocolon [Fig. 4.37]

Trace the peritoneum on the under-surface of the transverse colon to the posterior abdominal wall. It forms a flap called the transverse mesocolon, which is the mesentery or sling of the transverse colon. Since the posterior two layers of the greater omentum are attached to its superior (anterior) surface, the transverse mesocolon theoretically consists of four sheets of peritoneum (you will not be able to establish this on your specimen). This anatomical fact is based on comparative and embryological studies.

The transverse mesocolon is attached to the posterior abdominal wall along the line of the pancreas [Figs 4.37 and 4.39]. This is a retroperitoneal transversely-placed gland about 12 to 15 cm long, whose ducts open into the duodenum. At this stage you cannot see the pancreas, nor can you examine the reflection of the peritoneum of the transverse mesocolon upwards from the gland's anterior surface.

Note, however, that this layer of peritoneum covers the posterior abdominal wall, and also structures which lie on it (e.g. the left kidney), and forms the upper part of the posterior surface of the omental bursa [Fig. 4.39]. To the left the layer is reflected from the surface of the left kidney on to the spleen, and more centrally, it is reflected on to the diaphragm, and from the latter on to the upper border of a part of the visceral surface of the liver called the caudate lobe. The peritoneum adheres to this lobe as far as the porta hepatis, and is then continued from the liver as the posterior layer of the lesser omentum [Fig. 4.37].

To the right the superior layer of the transverse mesocolon passes over the upper part of the duodenum and right kidney on to the diaphragm, and from there on to the lower part of the posterior part of the diaphragmatic surface of the right lobe of the liver, from which it passes forwards to cover the right-hand side of the visceral surface of the liver. The line of reflection on this part of the liver is known as the lower layer of the coronary ligament [Fig. 4.39].

The mesentery

Now trace the inferior layer of peritoneum of the transverse mesocolon downwards from the body of the pancreas, which you may be able to feel. This layer of peritoneum covers the lower part of the duodenum and from here it passes forwards as the superior layer of the mesentery by which the small intestine is suspended from the posterior abdominal wall [Fig. 4.37].

All the 7 m of small intestine, except the duodenum which constitutes the first 25 cm, is suspended by this mesentery (the duodenum, as already observed, is retroperitoneal). The bulk of the small intestine invaginates the peritoneal cavity from behind, the line of invagination being represented by the line of attachment of the **root of the mesentery** to the posterior abdominal wall [Fig. 4.39]. This line runs obliquely across from the left side of the second lumbar vertebra above to the upper part of the right sacroiliac joint below, and is about 15 cm long. Note that the mesentery fans out, and that it becomes pleated as it approaches the gut. You will examine the attachment of the mesentery later, and will also dissect the superior mesenteric artery and vein and their branches and tributaries which pass to and from the small intestine between its two layers (which also contain filaments from the sympathetic and vagus nerves, and a number of lymph nodes and lymphatic vessels, all embedded in fat).

The pelvic peritoneum

Trace the peritoneum from the under-surface of the mesentery as it runs down to the sacrum [Fig. 4.37]. It encloses the sigmoid colon within the **sigmoid mesocolon.**

In the male cadaver trace the peritoneum below the sigmoid mesocolon over the rectum. Note that it is reflected from the latter on to the urinary bladder anteriorly. The peritoneal fossa between the two is called the **rectovesical pouch.** In the female [Fig. 4.40], trace the peritoneum from the rectum to the upper part of the posterior surface of the vagina, and then upwards over the back of the uterus. The peritoneal fossa between the two is called the **recto-uterine pouch.** The peritoneum covers the uterus, from whose vesical surface you will see that it is reflected on to the urinary

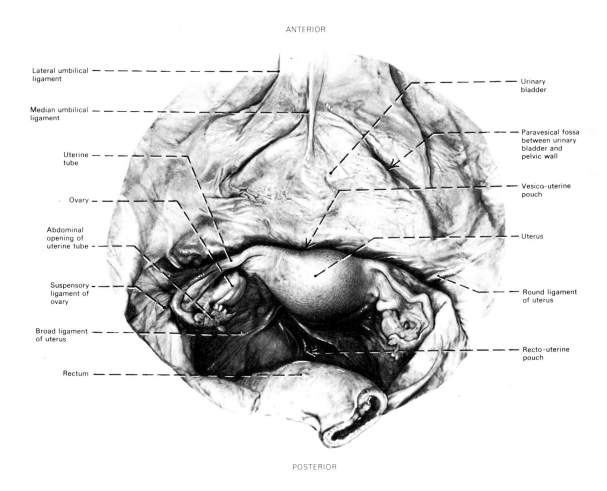

Fig. 4.40 **The female pelvis (viewed from above).**

bladder. The space between the uterus and bladder is called the **vesico-uterine pouch.**

From the superior surface of the bladder, trace the peritoneum on to the anterior abdominal wall, then on to the under-surface of the diaphragm, and then, as the superior layer of the coronary ligament, on to the liver [Fig. 4.37].

The peritoneal reflections in transverse section

Now look at Fig. 4.41, which shows the peritoneal reflections in a transverse section through the abdomen, at the level of the epiploic foramen, and try to verify the features it displays by tracing the peritoneal reflections with your fingers. You will see that at this level the liver is completely surrounded by peritoneum, and that the peritoneum is reflected from the diaphragmatic surface of the liver on to the anterior abdominal wall as the falciform ligament.

The falciform ligament [Figs 4.33 and 4.41]

To understand the falciform ligament it is useful to imagine that originally the peritoneum was reflected in a straight transverse line from the superior part of the diaphragmatic surface of the liver on to the diaphragm, and that it was subsequently pulled down on to the anterior abdominal wall in a midline fold by the round ligament of the liver, which connects the porta hepatis of the liver with the umbilicus.

The lienorenal and gastrosplenic ligaments [Fig. 4.41]

If you trace the peritoneum which forms the left side of the falciform ligament towards the left, it will be seen to line the deep surface of the anterior and left portions of the abdominal wall and, when it reaches the posterior abdominal wall, to cover the left kidney. From here it is reflected on to the spleen as the posterior layer of a peritoneal fold called the **lienorenal ligament.** The peritoneum encloses the spleen completely and is reflected from it on to the anterior surface of the stomach as the anterior layer of another peritoneal fold called the **gastrosplenic ligament.** The layer of peritoneum you are tracing covers the anterior wall of the stomach, from which it passes, at the lesser curvature, to form the anterior layer of the lesser omentum, whose free right border you have already examined. At this stage of your dissection you will not be able to trace the peritoneum any further in the transverse plane, but by reference to Fig. 4.41 try to visualize the following further facts about the reflection of peritoneum at the general level of the epiploic foramen.

The peritoneum of the posterior surface of the lesser omentum is reflected on to the posterior wall of the stomach, and continues from the latter as the posterior layer of the gastrosplenic ligament, whose anterior layer you have already felt. The posterior layer of the ligament is then reflected, as the anterior layer of the lienorenal ligament (whose posterior layer you felt earlier on), on to the left kidney. The peritoneum then passes over the left kidney and the posterior abdominal wall as the posterior wall of the omental bursa.

By now it will be clear to you that the invaginations of the peritoneum form a series of complex folds by which the

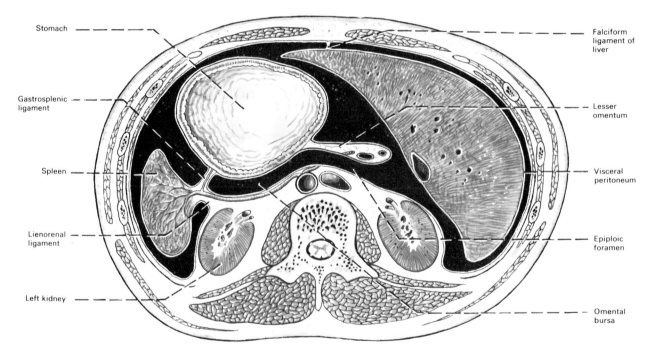

Fig. 4.41 Schematic transverse section of the abdomen at the level of the epiploic foramen (viewed from above).

viscera are slung either to each other or from the posterior abdominal wall. Some of these folds, which may be referred to as omenta, mesenteries, or ligaments, are large and of great importance; others are small and insignificant. They not only suspend the organs but provide pathways along which blood vessels, nerves, and lymphatics can run.

A further point to note at this stage is that in the male the peritoneal cavity is a closed sac. In the female the lateral extremities of the uterine tubes open into the pelvic part of the cavity, which therefore communicates with the exterior by way of the uterine tubes, the uterus, and the vagina.

Section 4.5

The stomach

The stomach *in situ*

Pull the stomach downwards so that it comes more clearly into view. In the cadaver its shape is very variable, and gives little idea of its appearance during life. Usually it is empty, small, and contracted. The larger part lies behind the liver and the diaphragm and is sheltered by the ribs. A smaller part, however, lies directly posterior to the anterior abdominal wall. In the living and full condition, and in the upright posture, the stomach is usually J-shaped, the lowest part of the body extending into the greater pelvis, and the **pylorus** lying at the level of the first lumbar vertebra [Fig. 4.42].

The cardiac part of the stomach

The stomach is a hollow muscular organ lined by a mucous coat, and is almost entirely covered by peritoneum. Slip your fingers upwards under the left costal margin to the posterior side of the left lobe of the liver. Note that here the stomach is fixed by its junction with the part of the oeso-phagus which penetrates the diaphragm. You can also approach the oesophageal part of the stomach by pulling the latter away from the left side of the visceral surface of the liver. This portion of the stomach is known as the cardiac part of the stomach and its opening from the oeso-phagus is called the **cardiac opening.** You will have a far better opportunity of examining it later.

The pyloric part of the stomach

Below and to the right the stomach is fixed at its junction with the duodenum at the **pyloric opening.** Loose connective tissue ties most of the duodenum to the posterior abdominal wall, but the position of the origin of the duodenum at the pyloric end of the stomach, and that of its termination, where it passes into the jejunum, which is the next part of the small intestine, are not absolutely fixed, and depend on the state of distension of the stomach and intestine. In the supine position the pylorus lies in the transpyloric plane, which, as you have already noted [p. 4.17], passes through the lower part of the first lumbar vertebra. In a person standing after a good meal the pylorus may be as low as the third lumbar vertebra. In between its two 'fixed' points the stomach is freely mobile, and its position, shape, and

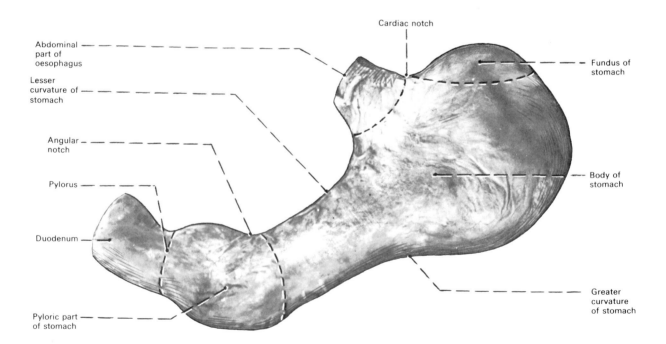

Fig. 4.42 The stomach.

size vary with the state of its distension by air, or food, or both.

The curvatures of the stomach [Fig. 4.42]

Look at the superior border or **lesser curvature** of the stomach. Its concavity faces to the right. Compare it with the much longer inferior border or **greater curvature** of the stomach, which faces to the left and downwards, and which is four to five times as long. Note that the right edge of the terminal part of the oesophagus runs uninterruptedly into the start of the lesser curvature, whereas the junction of the oesophagus with the start of the greater curvature is marked by a notch, since the greater curvature first runs upwards. This notch is called the **cardiac notch.** The part of the stomach which is in contact with the diaphragm above the level of the cardiac notch is called the **fundus.** The part below is called the **body** of the stomach. Try and make out a less conspicuous notch at the lowest point on the lesser curvature. This is called the **angular notch,** and it marks the commencement of the **pyloric antrum,** the beginning of the pyloric part of the stomach [Fig. 4.57].

Removal of the left lobe of the liver

In order to simplify the dissection of the stomach, remove the left lobe of the liver. To do this, pull the left end of the liver from the diaphragm and cut through the fold of peritoneum called the **left triangular ligament** which connects the two. Then make a vertical incision through the liver immediately to the left of the fissure on the visceral surface,

in which the round ligament lies, and to the left of the continuation of this fissure on to the posterior part of the diaphragmatic surface. Detach the incised lobe and preserve it for further study.

Now re-examine the oesophagus, the cardiac part of the stomach, and the lesser curvature. If you forcibly separate the stomach from the remaining part of the liver, the lesser omentum will be well displayed. Before proceeding, you will find it useful to re-read the description of this structure given on pages 4.38 and 4.39.

The blood supply of the stomach

In dissecting the stomach, your first task is to examine its blood supply, and it is useful to obtain a preliminary outline of the arrangement of the vessels before you start [Fig. 4.43].

The coeliac trunk

The main source of blood to the stomach is the coeliac trunk, which is a short wide vessel which springs from the anterior surface of the aorta just below the level where it passes from the thorax into the abdomen. The coeliac trunk almost immediately splits into three branches:

1. The **common hepatic artery,** which mainly supplies the liver through its largest branch, the hepatic artery.
2. The **left gastric artery,** which is distributed almost entirely to the stomach.
3. The **splenic artery,** which supplies the pancreas (as it runs along its superior border), the spleen, and the stomach.

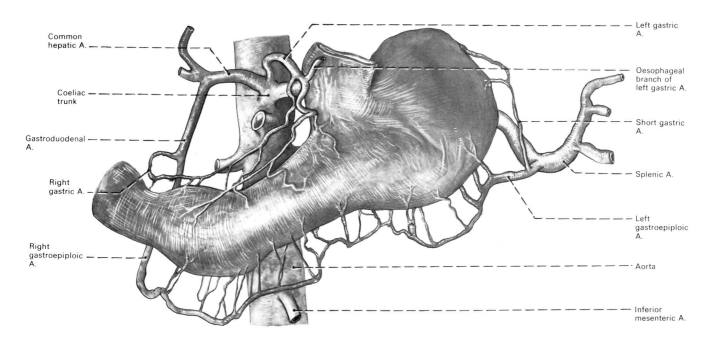

Fig. 4.43 The arteries of the stomach. In this specimen the right gastric artery is a branch of the gastroduodenal artery instead of arising directly from the common hepatic artery.

The arteries of the stomach

The vessels which supply the stomach are [Fig. 4.43]:

1. **The left gastric artery,** which is the smallest branch of the coeliac trunk, and which runs along the lesser curvature from the left end of the latter towards the pylorus.
2. The **right gastric artery,** which is a branch of the common hepatic artery, and which runs from the right along the lesser curvature to anastomose with the left gastric artery.
3. The **short gastric arteries,** which are branches of the splenic artery, and which supply the fundus.
4. The **left gastroepiploic artery,** which is a branch of the splenic artery, and which runs along the greater curvature from the left.
5. The **right gastroepiploic artery,** which is given off by the gastroduodenal artery, and which runs along the greater curvature from the right. The gastroduodenal artery is a branch of the common hepatic artery.

These arteries are accompanied by veins, all of which eventually drain into an important vein called the portal vein, which you will study later.

Cut to one side of the xiphoid process and incise the diaphragm for a few centimetres to allow the margins of the ribs to part. This will allow you better access to the upper part of the abdomen.

The left gastric artery [Fig. 4.43]

Start your dissection of the vessels by dissecting away the lesser omentum from the left end of the lesser curvature of the stomach and find the left gastric artery. Clean this artery, and follow its main trunk as far as possible towards its origin from the coeliac trunk. As you dissect the vessel along the

lesser curvature, you may find that it divides into two parallel branches. Try also to find the **oesophageal branches** which the left gastric artery sends to the terminal part of the oesophagus. Adjacent to the latter you should see a small reflection of peritoneum which passes from the fundus of the stomach to the diaphragm. It is called the gastrophrenic ligament.

Next, clean the anterior surface of the termination of the oesophagus and find the anterior vagal trunk, and trace it on to the anterior wall of the stomach. You may find some small lymph nodes around the cardiac part of the stomach. Remove them if you do.

The common hepatic artery [Fig. 4.43]

The right gastric artery

Now turn to the right end of the lesser curvature, and clear away the lesser omentum so as to expose the right gastric artery. In cleaning this vessel, try to define its anastomosis with the left gastric artery and also trace it to its origin from the common hepatic artery.

The hepatic artery

Now look at the right free border of the lesser omentum, which is very variable in appearance, sometimes being a taut, dense membrane, and at other times a slack, occasionally fenestrated sheet of peritoneum. By dissecting away the peritoneum define in its right free border three vertically-disposed structures [Fig. 4.44]:

1. The bile-duct on the right.
2. The hepatic artery (the terminal branch of the common hepatic artery) on the left.
3. The portal vein behind and between the two.

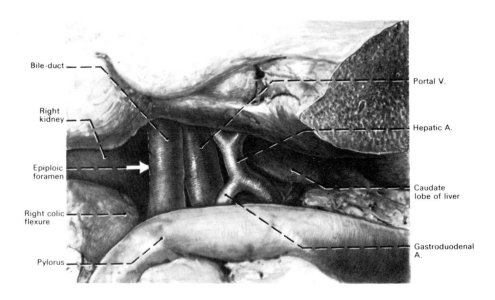

Fig. 4.44 Structures in the free border of the lesser omentum.

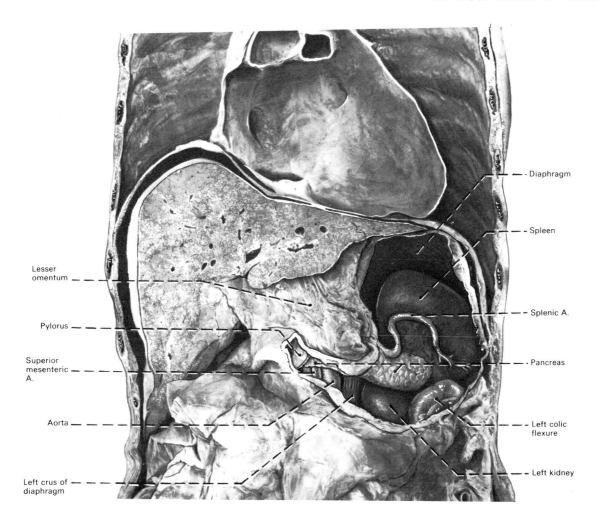

Lesser omentum

Pylorus

Superior mesenteric A.

Aorta

Left crus of diaphragm

Diaphragm

Spleen

Splenic A.

Pancreas

Left colic flexure

Left kidney

Fig. 4.45 The stomach bed. A sectioned body from which the walls of the stomach and the peritoneum covering the stomach bed have been excised.

Clean and isolate these structures as far as possible. As you trace the bile-duct towards the liver, you may find the cystic duct, which joins the neck of the gall-bladder to the common hepatic duct to form the bile-duct; and also the **cystic artery** passing to the gall-bladder, and which arises from the hepatic artery or from one of its branches. Later, when the liver is removed, you will have a better opportunity of examining these structures. Note now that both the bile-duct and the portal vein disappear behind the pancreas and the superior part of the duodenum. Clean them as far as this point.

When the bile-duct, hepatic artery, and portal vein have been cleaned, use your finger to hook them out of the way towards the midline. Now see if you can recognize behind them, and under cover of the peritoneum, the large inferior vena cava, whose termination in the thorax you have already seen [p. 3.26], and to its medial side a long triangular slip of muscle called the right crus of the diaphragm. These two structures form the posterior boundary of the epiploic foramen. You will see both of them more clearly later.

The gastroduodenal artery

Before leaving this part of the dissection, find the gastroduodenal artery, which branches off the common hepatic artery above the start of the duodenum, and descends behind the superior part of the duodenum. Pull the transverse colon away from the stomach. If you dissect further into the peritoneum you will see that the gastroduodenal artery breaks up on the head of the pancreas into the **superior pancreatico-duodenal artery,** which runs along the medial side of the duodenum, and the **right gastroepiploic artery.** Follow the latter for a short distance into the greater omentum, at its attachment to the greater curvature of the stomach.

The left gastroepiploic artery [Fig. 4.43]

Next, pull the fundus of the stomach downwards and to the right, and define the fold of peritoneum which is reflected from the greater curvature of the stomach near the fundus, and which continues into the greater omentum on the one hand, and on to the hilum of the spleen on the other. The latter reflection forms the gastrosplenic ligament [Fig. 4.41].

4.47

It encloses the left gastroepiploic artery, which passes along the greater curvature of the stomach, and the **short gastric arteries,** which pass to the fundus of the stomach, all of these vessels being branches of the splenic artery [Fig. 4.43].

Clean away the peritoneum on the anterior surface of the gastrosplenic ligament, and expose the vessels within the ligament. Clean and follow the left gastroepiploic artery as it passes to the right along the greater curvature, between the two layers of the greater omentum. Occasionally you may find that the left gastroepiploic artery anastomoses with the right gastroepiploic artery, which you should now clean completely as you trace it, towards the right, to its origin from the gastroduodenal artery.

Now tease away the anterior layers of the greater omentum immediately distal to the main vessels that run along the greater curvature of the stomach. Do this over the whole length of the stomach. This will free the stomach, which you can then turn upwards, so that you can look into the omental bursa which lies behind the stomach. The full extent of the transverse mesocolon will also now be apparent.

The stomach bed

The stomach bed [Fig. 4.45] is the name given to the structures on which the stomach lies, and which are in contact with its postero-inferior surface. Confirm, as far as the present stage of the dissection will allow, that the stomach bed is made up of the body of the pancreas, the left crus of the diaphragm, the left kidney and the left suprarenal gland, the spleen, and part of the transverse mesocolon. You will have another opportunity of examining the stomach bed at a later stage, when you complete the dissection of the stomach.

Having done this, dissect away the peritoneum which covers the body of the pancreas on the posterior wall of the omental bursa. You will now see the **splenic artery** running a tortuous horizontal course along the superior border of the pancreas. Clean this vessel and follow it as it passes with the tail of the pancreas between the two layers of the lienorenal ligament to the spleen. Note again that this ligament is a double fold of peritoneum which extends between the kidney and the spleen, and that the continuation of its anterior layer into the posterior layer of the gastrosplenic ligament forms the left lateral wall of the omental bursa at the level of the transpyloric plane. Now clean and trace the splenic vessels into the hilum of the spleen, and note again that the upper part of the visceral surface of the spleen at which you are looking forms part of the stomach bed.

Section 4.6

The small intestine

The next part of the dissection is the removal of the small intestine, but before doing this the following facts should be noted.

The duodenum

The duodenum [Fig. 4.46], into which the stomach opens, is 25 cm long, C-shaped, and begins at the pyloric opening. It is almost entirely retroperitoneal, and is the most fixed part of the small intestine. It is also the widest part. All that you can do at this stage of your dissection is to discern its general shape. The duodenum is described as having four parts:

1. The short first, or **superior part,** runs upwards and backwards, and is the part between the pylorus and the neck of the gall-bladder above.
2. The second, or **descending part,** lies in front of the medial part of the right kidney, and descends as far as the right side of the third lumbar vertebra. It is crossed by the transverse colon.
3. The third, or **horizontal part,** runs transversely across the inferior vena cava and abdominal aorta on the posterior abdominal wall.
4. The fourth, or **ascending part,** runs upwards to its termination at the **duodenojejunal flexure,** which you will have no difficulty in finding.

The jejunum and the ileum

The remainder of the small intestine is composed of the jejunum and the ileum, and is slung from the posterior abdominal wall by the mesentery, and is thus extremely mobile. The jejunum is about 2.5 m long and passes imperceptibly into the ileum, which is about 4 m long. Note again that this part of the small intestine occupies a central position in the abdominal cavity, below the liver and the stomach, and behind the transverse mesocolon, the transverse colon, and the greater omentum. The lowest coils of the intestine lie in the pelvic cavity [Fig. 4.47].

Start your dissection by lifting up the small intestine, and you will see that the **mesentery** consists of a thick double fold of peritoneum filled with fat and blood vessels. As already observed, the mesentery is fan-shaped, and its root, about 15 cm long, runs obliquely across the posterior abdominal wall from the left side of the second lumbar vertebra to the right sacroiliac joint. Note that there is less fat in the mesentery which supports the jejunum than in that supporting the ileum.

The blood supply of the small intestine

The vessels which supply the small intestine are derived from a large artery, the **superior mesenteric artery** [Fig. 4.47], which arises from the abdominal aorta, below the coeliac

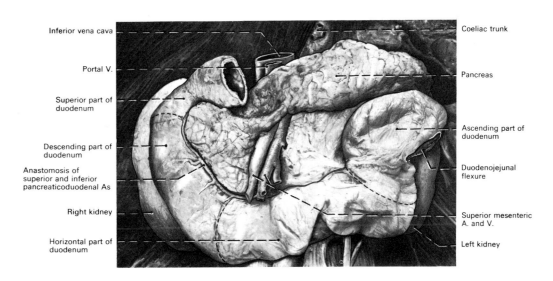

Fig. 4.46 The duodenum and the pancreas.

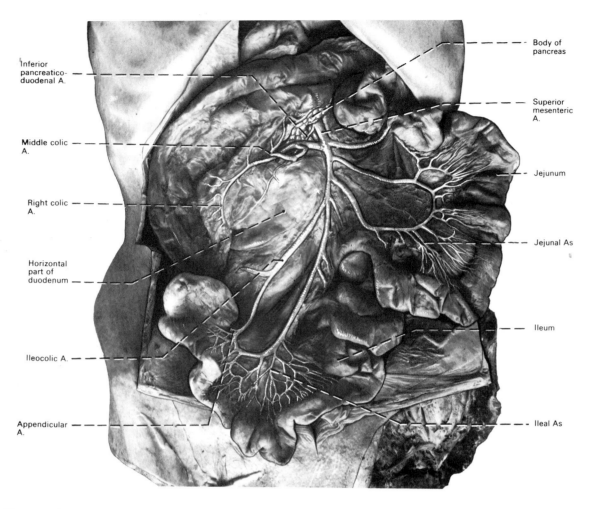

Inferior
pancreatico-
duodenal A.

Middle colic
A.

Right colic
A.

Horizontal
part of
duodenum

Ileocolic A.

Appendicular
A.

Body of
pancreas

Superior
mesenteric
A.

Jejunum

Jejunal As

Ileum

Ileal As

Fig. 4.47 The superior mesenteric artery. The transverse colon has been lifted upwards, and the small intestine displaced downwards and to the left.

trunk and behind the pancreas, and which crosses the horizontal part of the duodenum before it enters the mesentery. As you will see in a moment, the superior mesenteric artery runs obliquely downwards in the mesentery (with a concavity to the right), giving off from its left side a series of **jejunal** and **ileal arteries** to the small intestine. It ends in the right iliac fossa by anastomosing with one of its own branches. The superior mesenteric artery also gives off:

1. The **inferior pancreaticoduodenal artery,** which lies on the head of the pancreas, supplying it together with the duodenum. This vessel anastomoses with the superior pancreaticoduodenal artery, a branch of the gastroduodenal artery [see p. 4.47].

2. The **middle colic artery,** which enters the transverse mesocolon and is distributed to the transverse colon.

3. The **right colic artery,** which passes behind the peritoneum to the right to supply the ascending colon.

4. The **ileocolic artery,** which passes behind the peritoneum to the right, and gives off an ascending branch to the ascending colon and a descending branch to the caecum and vermiform appendix. The descending branch ends by anastomosing with the distal end of the superior mesenteric artery.

The arterial arcades [Fig. 4.47]

It will be seen shortly that the jejunal and ileal arteries divide, subdivide, and anastomose, forming a series of arterial arcades, before giving off their straight terminal branches to the small intestine. Those to the jejunum are characteristically longer than those to the ileum. In the jejunum the mesentery between these arcades appears as semi-translucent windows, while that to the ileum is made opaque by fat. Throughout its course the superior mesenteric artery is closely related to the superior mesenteric vein and its tributaries.

4.50

With this picture of the blood supply of the small intestine in mind, start cleaning the superior mesenteric vessels. Remove the peritoneum from the front of the mesentery and trace the branches of the artery to the small intestine, noting the arterial arcades. Identify and trace the ileocolic artery, which is the lowest branch that springs from the right side of the superior mesenteric artery. If necessary, remove a little peritoneum of the posterior abdominal wall in order to see this vessel more clearly. Above the ileocolic artery, find the origins of the right and middle colic arteries, but do not trace them for the moment; nor should you try to find the inferior pancreaticoduodenal artery at this stage. During the dissection of the mesentery you will see some of the **mesenteric lymph nodes.** These should be removed as they are encountered.

Dissection of the jejunum and ileum

With scissors cut through the mesentery near its attachment to the small intestine. This is best done with an assistant holding the gut. Tie two strong ligatures about 2.5 cm apart close to the duodenojejunal flexure and divide the gut between them. Do the same on the proximal side of the ileo-caecal opening. Remove the small intestine and place it in a sink.

First compare the external appearance of the jejunum and ileum. You can see that the jejunum is wider, thicker, and more vascular than the ileum. In the living body, therefore, it is redder.

The interior of the jejunum and ileum [Fig. 4.48]

Remove the string ligatures at either end of the small intestine and open the gut with scissors along its whole length, and wash it thoroughly under running water. You will see that its mucous coat is thrown into a series of **circular folds** [Fig. 4.48], by which the surface area is increased. The folds also delay the passage of food, thus facilitating digestion and absorption. With the aid of a handlens you will see that finger-like processes called **intestinal villi** project from the mucosa. When you come to study the intestine in your histology class, you will see that each villus contains a central lymphatic vessel, or lacteal, through which most of the digested fat is absorbed into the lymph stream; and also a network of blood vessels by which the remaining products of digestion are absorbed into the portal system of veins.

Notice particularly that as the jejunum passes into the ileum the circular folds and villi become less numerous, so that the mucous coat of the ileum is comparatively un-wrinkled. In this part of the gut you may see with the naked eye pale patches of varying shape in the mucosa. These are islands of lymphoid tissue called **aggregated lymphatic fol-**

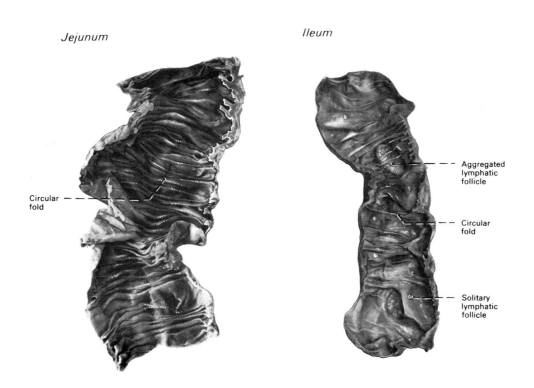

Fig. 4.48 The interior of the small intestine.

licles. They are numerous and obvious in young individuals, but tend to disappear in the aged.

Examine the ileum carefully. In 2 per cent of persons a small blind pouch known as the **diverticulum ilei** [Fig 4.49] will be found within a metre from the termination of the ileum at the ileocaecal opening. This is a vestigial structure (the proximal part of the vitellointestinal duct), but is of some clinical importance.

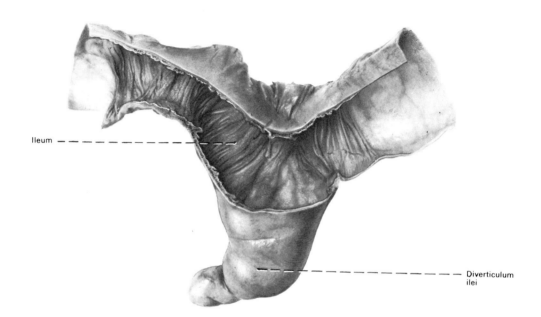

Ileum

Diverticulum ilei

Fig. 4.49 The diverticulum ilei.

Section 4.7

The liver and gall-bladder

Now begin the dissection of the liver, which is the largest gland in the body. It normally weighs about 1.5 kg. First replace the detached left lobe of the liver in its original position. Note again that the liver lies chiefly in the right hypochondriac region beneath the diaphragm and behind the ribs; that a small part crosses the midline; and that here the liver is covered only by the upper part of the anterior abdominal wall. Since the thorax has been dissected, you can now see that the left extremity of the liver is separated from the apex of the heart by only the central tendon of the diaphragm. You may also be able to determine that anteriorly the superior part of the **diaphragmatic surface** of the liver lies at the level of the fifth rib, and posteriorly about 1 cm below the inferior angle of the right scapula. Another important observation, and one easy to confirm at this stage, is that the sharp **inferior border** of the liver, which separates the anterior part of the diaphragmatic surface from the **visceral surface**, does not normally extend below the right costal margin. If you find that it does on your cadaver, the liver was enlarged during life.

Removal of the liver

Now remove the whole liver from the body. First remove the detached part of the left lobe, and then cut through the bile-duct and portal vein in the right free border of the lesser omentum, just above the duodenum. Divide the hepatic artery just beyond the point of origin of the gastroduodenal and right gastric arteries, which you will thus leave in the body. Continue to cut through what is left of the lesser omentum, moving from right to left, until you reach the diaphragm behind the liver. Then re-identify the **inferior vena cava** where it forms the posterior boundary of what was the epiploic foramen, and remove the peritoneum from its surface. Trace the inferior vena cava upwards and cut it transversely where it is anchored to the substance of the liver by its tributaries. Forcibly lift the liver upwards and forwards. Behind, on the right side, find the fold of peritoneum which forms the inferior layer of the coronary ligament of the liver, and which constitutes the line of reflection of peritoneum from the liver on to the diaphragm (or occasionally on to the right kidney). This peritoneal fold lies adjacent to the point where the inferior vena cava enters the liver. Divide it, and continue your cut towards the right along the lower edge of the posterior part of the diaphragmatic surface of the right lobe of the liver.

Now, on the extreme right, divide the right triangular ligament [Fig. 4.50], which is a fold of peritoneum that is formed by the merging of the superior and inferior layers of the coronary ligament. Then, working towards the left, cut through the peritoneal fold which forms the superior layer of the coronary ligament, noting as you do so that it marks the reflection of peritoneum from the upper posterior part of the diaphragmatic surface of the right lobe on to the diaphragm. Having done this, gently pull the liver from the diaphragm, and define the upper limit of the abdominal portion of the inferior vena cava. Divide the latter as it pierces the diaphragm. The liver is now attached to the diaphragm only by the falciform ligament. This connection can be cut through without difficulty. Then remove the liver from the body.

The peritoneal attachments of the liver

The falciform ligament [Fig. 4.50]

The falciform ligament, by which the liver is arbitrarily divided into a small left lobe and a large right lobe, will be easily seen on the superior and anterior parts of the diaphragmatic surface of the liver. You may sometimes see a shallow concavity on the superior part of the liver at the junction of the right and left lobes. This is where the heart rested, with the central tendon of the diaphragm intervening.

The bare area of the liver [Fig. 4.51]

Beginning from the falciform ligament on the sharp inferior border in front [Fig. 4.50], trace the cut edge of the peritoneum backwards on the diaphragmatic surface of the liver, first on its anterior part, and then across its superior part. Then follow the peritoneum to the left towards the apex of the left lobe, where it forms the **left triangular ligament.** Beginning from the same point on the inferior border of the liver in front, trace the right side of the falciform ligament posteriorly and then to the right. Here it becomes the superior layer of the **coronary ligament,** which in turn passes into the **right triangular ligament.** The posterior layer of the triangular ligament is formed by the right extremity of the inferior layer of the coronary ligament [Fig. 4.51]. Between the reflections of the superior and inferior layers of the coronary ligament from the liver, identify the **bare area** which is devoid of peritoneum. This bare area of liver is tri-

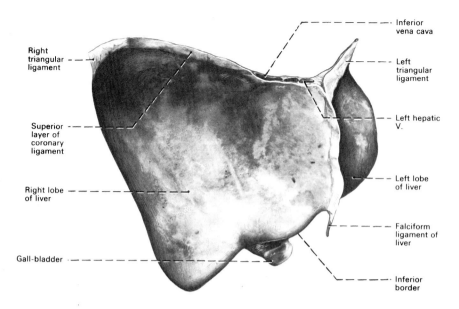

Fig. 4.50 Anterior view of the diaphragmatic surface of the liver.

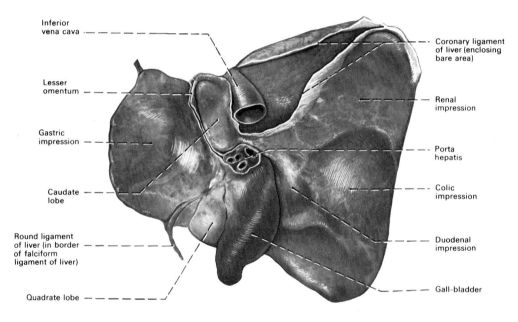

Fig. 4.51 The visceral surface of the liver.

angular in shape, with its base, formed by the inferior vena cava, near the midline. You will almost always find that the inferior vena cava is partially embedded in the liver substance. The other two sides of the triangular bare area are formed by the superior and inferior layers of the coronary ligament, which fuse together at the apex of the triangle to form the right triangular ligament.

The lesser omentum [Figs 4.38 and 4.51]

Examine the attachment of the lesser omentum to the **porta hepatis** on the visceral surface of the liver, where the com-

mon hepatic duct leaves and the hepatic artery and the portal vein enter the organ. From the left extremity of the porta hepatis trace the anterior and posterior layers of the lesser omentum upwards and backwards along the margins of a fissure which forms the right-hand border of the posterior part of the diaphragmatic surface of the left lobe. This is the **fissure for the ligamentum venosum,** a remnant of an embryological structure. Between this fissure and the inferior vena cava you will see the small **caudate lobe** of the liver. To the left of this lobe and fissure is a small swelling, called the **tuber omentale.**

4.54

Although you may find this difficult to understand, all the reflections of peritoneum you have now traced on the liver are part of a continuous peritoneal sheet.

The visceral surface of the liver

Impressions on the liver [Fig. 4.51]

Near the upper end of the fissure for the ligamentum venosum, on the posterior part of the diaphragmatic surface of the left lobe, look for a well-marked notch. Before you removed the liver, the oesophagus rested in it. The concavity on the visceral surface of the left lobe below and to the left of the **oesophageal impression** is called the **gastric impression,** because in the undisturbed abdomen it accommodates part of the fundus and body of the stomach.

If you trace the visceral surface of the left lobe to the right in front of the porta hepatis, you will encounter the **fissure for the round ligament.** To the right of this fissure and between it and the gall-bladder is the **quadrate lobe,** which in the living body is in contact with the superior part of the duodenum. The descending part of the duodenum is in contact with an impression to the right of the gall-bladder. This, the **duodenal impression,** extends behind the right-hand side of the porta hepatis. A **renal impression,** for the right kidney, can normally be seen on the posterior part of the visceral surface of the right lobe. In close relation with the inferior vena cava, and jutting into the bare area, is the **suprarenal impression** for the right suprarenal gland, a small organ which caps the kidney. On the anterior part of the visceral surface of the right lobe you may see the **colic impression** caused by the right colic flexure and the adjacent part of the transverse colon.

The porta hepatis [Fig. 4.51]

Now clean the porta hepatis and define its contents carefully. It separates the caudate lobe behind from the quadrate lobe in front, and transmits the **hepatic artery,** the **portal vein,** and the **right** and **left hepatic ducts,** which unite to form the common hepatic duct. It also contains some lymph nodes. In most cases the hepatic ducts are centrally situated, with the artery lying anteriorly and the vein posteriorly.

The gall-bladder

The bile-duct [Fig. 4.52]

Find the bile-duct at the point where you divided it when you removed the liver, and from it trace and clean the **cystic duct,** which leads to the neck of the gall-bladder [Fig. 4.52]. Beyond the point where the cystic duct joins the bile-duct is the **common hepatic duct,** leading into the porta hepatis.

The cystic artery [Fig. 4.52]

Clean and define the hepatic artery and the portal vein, removing the lymph nodes around them. Next trace the vein, artery, and duct into the liver as far as their division into right and left branches. Find and clean the small but important cystic artery, which usually arises from the right branch of the hepatic artery. It passes down behind the cystic duct and divides into anterior and posterior branches which are distributed to the wall of the gall-bladder. When dissecting the right branch of the portal vein look for the **cystic vein** which drains into it.

Dissection of the gall-bladder [Fig. 4.52]

Next examine the gall-bladder. Note that it lies in a fossa on the lower part of the visceral surface of the liver [Fig.

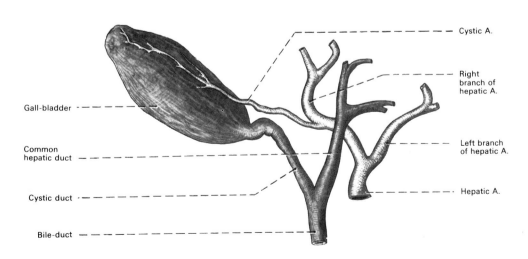

Fig. 4.52 The biliary tract and the hepatic artery.

Gall-bladder

Common hepatic duct

Cystic duct

Bile-duct

Cystic A.

Right branch of hepatic A.

Left branch of hepatic A.

Hepatic A.

4.51]. You will see that it is a pear-shaped sac, which just projects beyond the inferior border of the liver. The gall-bladder consists of a blind end called the **fundus,** a **body,** and a **neck.** The fundus is the most dependent part, and when full of bile can occasionally be palpated in the angle between the ninth costal cartilage and the lateral border of the right rectus abdominis muscle. The neck is continuous with the cystic duct.

Replace the liver in the abdomen and try to visualize that the body of the gall-bladder rests on the transverse colon, while the neck lies on the junction of the superior and descending parts of the duodenum.

Again remove the liver and clean the gall-bladder so as to free it from the liver. In so doing, note that peritoneum, continued from the visceral surface of the liver, covers the gall-bladder on all but its upper surface, which is in direct contact with the liver substance.

The gall-bladder and cystic duct should now be opened. Within the cystic duct you may see the **spiral fold** of the mucous coat.

The round ligament of the liver

Now pick up the round ligament of the liver [Fig. 4.51], in the free edge of what remains of the falciform ligament, and trace it into its fissure on the visceral surface of the liver. Its significance is entirely embryological. It is the remnant of the **left umbilical vein** of the foetus by which oxygenated blood was conveyed from the placenta, through the left branch of the portal vein, to a vessel called the **ductus venosus** behind the liver, from which it passed directly to the upper part of the inferior vena cava. In this way blood from the placenta by-passed the liver on its way to the heart. By removing the remains of the left lobe of the liver, try to follow the round ligament into the left branch of the portal vein. After birth the ductus venosus is reduced to a fibrous cord called the **ligamentum venosum,** which you should try to trace in its fissure to the left of the caudate lobe on the posterior part of the diaphragmatic surface of the liver.

The structure of the liver

Cut a section of liver and note its granular appearance. You will see that inward prolongations of fibrous tissue from the fibrous outer capsule form a fibrous perivascular capsule around the sectioned branches of the hepatic ducts, portal vein and hepatic arteries. Contrast these aggregations with the larger, more solitary and thin-walled hepatic veins.

Section 4.8

The large intestine

The large intestine *in situ*

You must now study the large intestine as far as the start of the sigmoid colon, before examining the duodenum, pancreas, and spleen. First note that the large gut is pouched or sacculated, and that three bands of longitudinal muscle fibres called **taeniae coli,** each about 5 mm wide, run the length of the gut from the caecum as far as the rectum. You will see tags of peritoneum filled with fat, called the **appendices epiploicae,** scattered over the free surface of the colon. The sacculations (called **haustra coli),** bands, and appendices are characteristic features of the large intestine, and distinguish it from the small intestine.

Follow the taenia coli on the anterior surface of the caecum, and you will see that all the taeniae lead to the base of the vermiform appendix [Fig. 4.53]. Surgeons find this a useful way of locating the appendix at operation. A mesentery of varying size, called the mesoappendix, connects the appendix to the mesentery of the small intestine.

Peritoneal recesses

Now consider the peritoneal relations of the ascending and descending colon. These two parts of the large intestine are for the most part retroperitoneal, since the peritoneum covers them only in front and partially at the sides. Look for a fossa behind the caecum (the **retrocaecal recess**), and if one is present, pass a finger into it. Occasionally it is so deep that you will be able to feel the inferior end of the right kidney.

The caecum [Fig. 4.53]

Now examine the caecum. It is about 6 cm long, and is a blind cul-de-sac of the large intestine which lies in the right iliac fossa below the ileocaecal opening. Note its position above the lateral part of the inguinal ligament, and note also that it is usually completely ensheathed by peritoneum. The caecum lies immediately behind the anterior abdominal wall and the greater omentum, and is sometimes also covered by coils of small intestine. It lies on the muscles of the posterior abdominal wall (the psoas major and iliacus muscles). These are at present covered with fascia and will be seen more clearly at a later stage of the dissection. After you have lifted the caecum from the posterior abdominal wall, note that in addition to the taenia coli on its anterior surface, there is a second taenia on its postero-medial, and a third on its postero-lateral aspect.

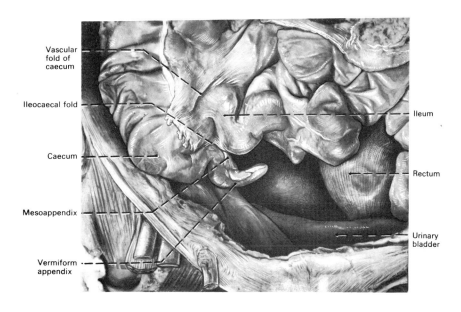

Fig. 4.53 The caecum and the vermiform appendix.

The vermiform appendix [Fig. 4.53]

Examine the vermiform appendix, which communicates with the caecum about 2 cm behind and below the ileocaecal opening, and on whose surface the three taeniae of the caecum converge. As already noted, it is very variable in length, and averages about 10 cm. Find its triangular **mesoappendix,** which encloses the **appendicular artery,** and which is an extension of the distal part of the mesentery of the small intestine.

Remember that the position of the appendix is variable. It sometimes turns up behind the caecum to lie in the retrocaecal recess ('retrocaecal appendix'), or it may extend downwards and to the left, either behind the small intestine or over the linea terminalis of the pelvis ('pelvic appendix').

Dissection of the colon

Remove the peritoneum on the posterior abdominal wall between the root of the mesentery and the ascending colon, and clean and trace the blood vessels to the ascending colon and right colic flexure. The arteries which you display are branches of the right colic and ileocolic arteries, which you will see arising from the concavity of the trunk of the superior mesenteric artery [Fig. 4.54].

Now incise the peritoneum on the posterior abdominal wall, immediately to the lateral side of the caecum and ascending colon, and push and turn these structures aside. Note that the ascending colon lies immediately under the lateral part of the anterior abdominal wall, and on the muscles of the posterior abdominal wall. These muscles will be dissected later. Replace the liver in the abdomen for a moment, and again observe the relationship of the right colic flexure to the liver and to the inferior end of the right kidney.

The blood supply of the transverse colon [Fig. 4.54]

Now re-examine the transverse colon and the transverse mesocolon [p. 4.40]. Again trace the latter to the anterior border of the pancreas, and note how the peritoneum diverges at this border. Place the stomach in the position it occupied originally, and note that the **transverse mesocolon** makes a large contribution to the stomach bed. By teasing and dissecting the peritoneum which makes up the mesocolon, clean the vessels to this part of the transverse colon and trace them to their origin from the **middle colic artery.** Clean the latter vessel, and trace it to its origin from the concavity of the superior mesenteric artery. You will be able to demonstrate that branches of the middle colic artery anastomose not only with branches of the **right colic artery** but also with those of the **left colic artery,** which springs from another branch of the aorta called the inferior mesenteric artery, which you will dissect later.

Relations of the transverse colon

Now examine the relations of the transverse colon and the left colic flexure. The position of the transverse colon varies with that of the body, and with the amount of digested food it contains, but in the formalin-injected cadaver its most dependent portion usually lies at the level of the umbilicus. Note how the transverse colon ascends as it passes to the left, for the left colic flexure lies at a higher level than the right colic flexure. Confirm the anterior relations of the transverse colon. It is covered by the anterior abdominal wall, the part of the greater omentum immediately below the greater curvature of the stomach, and the most inferior part of the omental bursa, which may extend in front of the transverse colon. Sometimes the transverse colon lies on the stomach.

Sever the attachments of the transverse mesocolon and greater omentum close to the transverse colon, and verify the latter's posterior relations. Confirm that the transverse colon lies, from right to left, on the descending part of the duodenum, the head of the pancreas, the root of the mesentery, the duodenojejunal flexure, and on coils of small intestine (now removed), and finally on the spleen, where at the left colic flexure it bends to become the descending colon. It is important to remember that the fundus of the gall-bladder lies on the transverse colon near the right colic flexure.

Find a fold or reflection of peritoneum which passes from the left colic flexure to the diaphragm. It is called the **phrenicocolic ligament.** Note that the spleen rests on it.

The descending colon

Now examine the descending colon. It is covered by peritoneum in the same way as is the ascending colon, and you will see that its anterior relations are the anterior abdominal wall, and sometimes also the greater omentum and coils of small intestine. The posterior relations of the descending colon cannot yet be seen; it lies on the muscles of the posterior abdominal wall, and descends into the greater pelvis. Remove the peritoneum from the posterior abdominal wall on the medial aspect of the descending colon, and expose and clean the blood vessels which pass to it from that direction. They are branches of the left colic artery [Fig. 4.54], which springs from the inferior mesenteric artery, and they anastomose above with branches of the middle colic artery (a branch of the superior mesenteric artery), and below with the sigmoid arteries (branches of the inferior mesenteric artery).

The inferior mesenteric artery [Fig. 4.54]

The inferior mesenteric artery, whose dissection you will complete later, is a branch of the abdominal aorta, and arises about 3 cm below the superior mesenteric artery. It gives off:

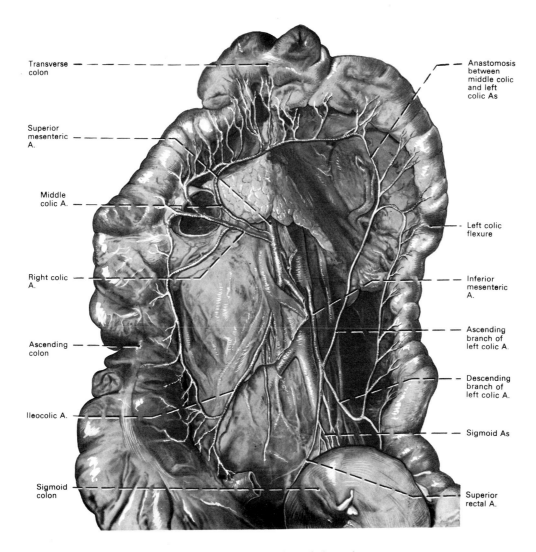

Transverse colon

Superior mesenteric A.

Middle colic A.

Right colic A.

Ascending colon

Ileocolic A.

Sigmoid colon

Anastomosis between middle colic and left colic As

Left colic flexure

Inferior mesenteric A.

Ascending branch of left colic A.

Descending branch of left colic A.

Sigmoid As

Superior rectal A.

Fig. 4.54 The arteries of the colon.

1. The **left colic artery,** which supplies the descending colon, left colic flexure, and the adjacent part of the transverse colon.
2. Two or three **sigmoid arteries,** which descend in the sigmoid mesocolon to supply the sigmoid colon.
3. The **superior rectal artery,** which descends in the sigmoid mesocolon to supply the sigmoid colon, rectum, and anal canal.

These vessels are accompanied by tributaries of the inferior mesenteric vein, which eventually joins the splenic vein behind the pancreas.

Trace and clean the inferior mesenteric artery and its left colic and sigmoid branches as far as the linea terminalis of the pelvis below. Also clean the inferior mesenteric vein from the linea terminalis below to the inferior border of the pancreas above.

Removal of the colon

Incise the peritoneum along the lateral border of the descending colon, and turn the gut medially from the posterior abdominal wall. Then cut the vessels away from the mesenteric border of the whole colon, starting with the ascending colon and working your way along the transverse colon and descending colon, freeing the right and left colic flexures. Tie a ligature around the lower end of the descending colon and then divide the colon above the ligature. Then remove all of the large intestine except the sigmoid colon and rectum from the body.

The interior of the colon

Take the detached colon to a sink and wash out its contents. Note the course of the three taeniae coli from the caecum to the end of the descending colon. Open the colon through-

4.59

out its extent, and note that the mucous coat is thrown into a series of crescentic folds quite different from the circular folds of the jejunum. Note, too, that there are no villi. Look especially at the junction of the ileum with the caecum [Fig. 4.55]. The junction is a horizontal slit-like opening with upper and lower lips caused by the muscular coat of the small intestine invaginating the wall of the large intestine.

These form the **ileocaecal valve.** Look for two ridges of mucosa which extend for some distance round the wall of the gut from each end of the slit. These constitute the **frenula of the ileocaecal valve.**

About 2 cm below and behind this valve look for the **opening of the vermiform appendix.** You will see that it is also guarded by a small, mucosal valve.

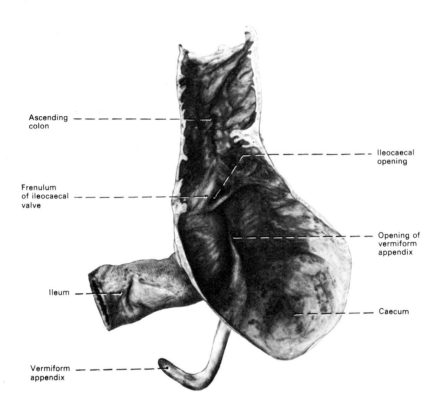

Fig. 4.55 The interior of the caecum (posterior view).

Section 4.9

The duodenum, pancreas, and spleen

Now examine the duodenum, pancreas, and spleen, displacing the stomach, as necessary, in order to facilitate your dissection.

Exposure of the pancreas

As you have seen, the pancreas lies behind the peritoneum, its anterior border forming the line along which the superior and inferior layers of the transverse mesocolon are reflected.

Parts of the pancreas [Fig. 4.56]

Dissect all the remaining peritoneum from the anterior surface of the pancreas and the duodenum. Note, as already described, that the latter is a C-shaped piece of gut, with its concavity facing to the left. The part of the pancreas that lies in the concavity of the duodenum is called the **head.** The main horizontal part which extends across the midline is the **body.** The **tail,** as you can see, rests on the spleen. Note that the pancreas consists of a tightly-packed mass of lobules which, as you dissect, will be seen to be held together by fine areolar tissue.

Clean the superior mesenteric vessels, and you will see that they run posterior to the body of the pancreas but anterior to a hook-shaped extension from the head, called the **uncinate process.** Clean the blood vessels which lie in the concavity of the duodenum between the latter and the head of the pancreas. They form an anastomosis of the superior and inferior pancreaticoduodenal vessels [Fig. 4.46]. To the right of the superior mesenteric artery is the prominent superior mesenteric vein, which you will later see uniting behind the pancreas with the splenic vein to form the portal vein.

The part of the pancreas anterior to the union of the two veins is called the **neck** of the pancreas. The body of the pancreas runs from the neck to the left across the posterior abdominal wall in a slightly upward direction.

The anterior surface of the pancreas [Fig. 4.56]

The part of the pancreas which faces you is called the anterior surface. This surface is limited below by the anterior border, which separates it from the inferior surface of the pancreas. The root of the transverse mesocolon is attached to the anterior border, and from it peritoneum is reflected over the anterior surface in an upward direction to form the posterior wall of the omental bursa.

The anterior surface of the pancreas is limited above by the superior border of the organ. Clean this border and display the splenic artery running along it to the left. Follow

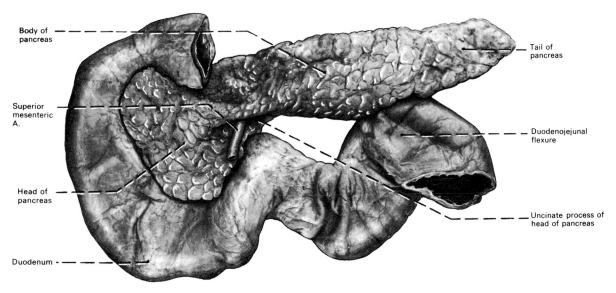

Fig. 4.56 Anterior view of the duodenum and pancreas.

Body of pancreas

Superior mesenteric A.

Head of pancreas

Duodenum

Tail of pancreas

Duodenojejunal flexure

Uncinate process of head of pancreas

the tail of the pancreas to the visceral surface of the spleen in front of the hilum. Before you cleared away the peritoneum, the tail passed between the two folds which formed the lienorenal ligament [Fig 4.41].

Place the stomach as near to its original position as possible, and observe that it rests on the anterior surface of the pancreas. Note, too, that in the undissected abdomen the left half of the inferior surface of the pancreas would be related to the duodenojejunal flexure and the left colic flexure, with coils of small intestine intervening between the two.

The duodenum *in situ*

Now replace the liver and again look at the duodenum as it lies *in situ*, noting how these two organs are related to each other, and remembering the large duodenal impression on the visceral surface of the liver to the right of the gall-bladder, extending behind the porta hepatis [p. 4.55]. Having done this, remove the liver.

Parts of the duodenum [Fig. 4.46]

For descriptive purposes the duodenum is divided into four parts [Figs 4.46 and 4.56]. The first or **superior part** is about 5 cm long, and is the most movable part of the duodenum. It runs from the pylorus upwards and backwards to the neck of the gall-bladder, where it turns downwards into the **descending part.** The latter is about 8 cm long, and runs vertically downwards to the right of the first, second, and third lumbar vertebrae, where it turns obliquely upwards,

forwards, and to the left to become the **horizontal part.** This is about 10 cm long and runs obliquely across the midline in front of the inferior vena cava and aorta. The horizontal part is followed by a short **ascending part** (2.5 cm long) which ascends on the left side of the aorta, and which at the level of the upper border of the second lumbar vertebra turns forwards into the duodenojejunal flexure.

Relations of the duodenum

In the centre of the descending part of the duodenum is an area which is not covered by peritoneum. Here the transverse colon is a direct relation. Above this area you will see that the body of the gall-bladder lies on the duodenum, with the neck of the gall-bladder on the line of demarcation between the superior and descending parts. Lift the right (lateral) margin of the duodenum, cutting the peritoneum in order to do so, and note that the duodenum lies on the medial half of the right kidney and on the right renal vessels. Remove just enough of the connective tissue between the two to display this relationship. Observe the way the superior mesenteric vessels cross in front of the horizontal part of the duodenum to enter the root of the mesentery [Fig. 4.46].

Removal of the stomach

Now return to the stomach [Fig. 4.57] and study those parts of the organ which were inaccessible in your earlier dissection. Examine the cardiac notch at the junction of the fundus with the oesophagus. Look at the fundus and note

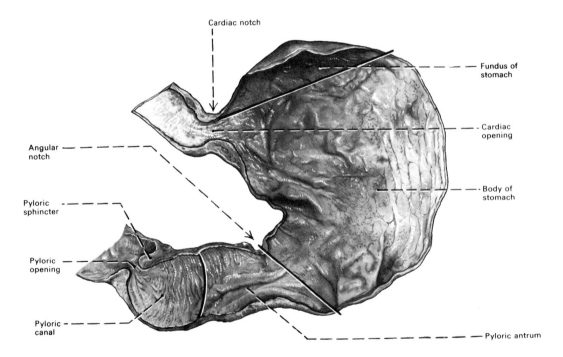

Fig. 4.57 The interior of the stomach.

that it lies on the anterior part of the visceral surface of the spleen. Once more follow the left gastric artery along the lesser curvature of the stomach to its origin from the coeliac trunk. If you did not find it before, try now to identify the branch which the left gastric artery sends to the oesophagus [p. 4.46]. Also re-identify the **gastrosplenic ligament,** which connects the body of the stomach to the spleen. Remember that the vessels in it are the left gastroepiploic and short gastric arteries, which are branches of the splenic artery. Then divide the ligament and its contained vessels close to the stomach.

The upper end of the gastrosplenic ligament is continuous with a reflection of peritoneum which passes between the diaphragm and the fundus of the stomach. This is the **gastrophrenic ligament.** Next re-identify the **anterior vagal trunk** as it descends from the anterior surface of the oesophagus on to the anterior wall of the stomach. Turn the stomach upwards and trace a branch of the **posterior vagal trunk,** which passes from the posterior surface of the oesophagus

on to the posterior wall of the stomach. If you have any difficulty in finding the vagal trunks in the abdomen, you will pick them up easily on the thoracic part of the oesophagus [see Fig. 3.48]. You can then trace them through the diaphragm.

In order to remove the stomach, divide the right and left gastric arteries where they make contact with the lesser curvature, and the right gastroepiploic artery on the greater curvature near the pylorus. In each case leave the distal part of the artery attached to the stomach. Cut through the abdominal part of the oesophagus and the superior part of the duodenum. You will now be able to remove the stomach from the abdominal cavity and examine its structure, in so far as this can be done with the naked eye or a handlens.

The structure of the stomach

First strip the peritoneum and follow the terminal branches of some of the gastric arteries over the surface of the stomach. Then look for the **longitudinal layer of the**

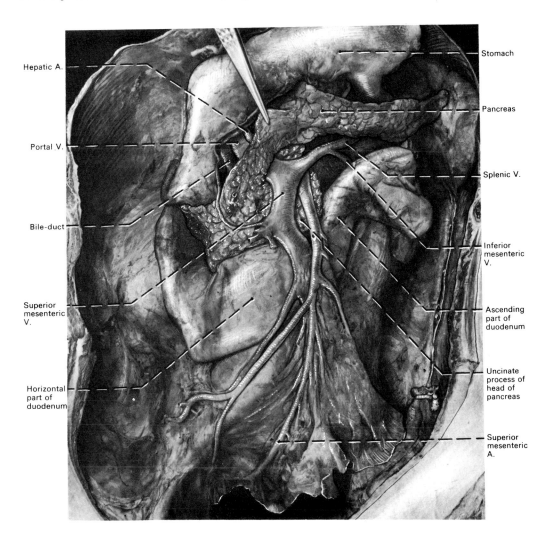

Fig. 4.58 The formation of the portal vein. The stomach and the pancreas have been turned upwards.

4.63

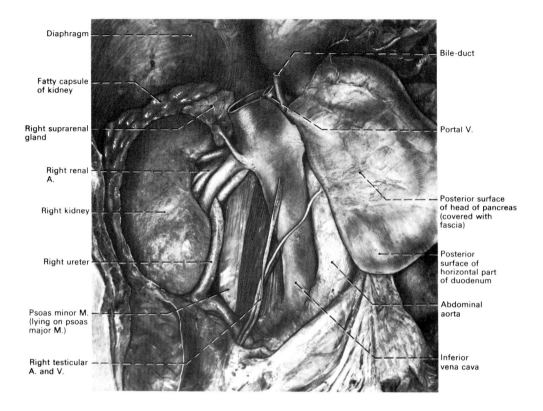

Fig. 4.59 The structures behind the duodenum and head of the pancreas. The duodenum and head of the pancreas have been turned to the left.

muscle coat which you will find is often incomplete. Beneath this you will probably be able to define the complete **circular layer of the muscle coat** which is more conspicuous than the incomplete muscle coat of **oblique fibres** that lies deep to it. Cut the **pyloric sphincter** longitudinally and note the thickening of the circular muscle in this region. Then open the stomach along the lesser curvature and clean its mucosa at the sink.

The gastric mucosa is thrown into a series of folds when the stomach is empty.

Removal of the duodenum, pancreas, and spleen

Structures behind the duodenum and pancreas

Separate the body of the pancreas from the posterior abdominal wall, turning it upwards so as to expose its posterior surface. Clean and display the union of the splenic and superior mesenteric veins where they form the **portal vein** [Fig. 4.58]. About 3 cm to the left of this union note the inferior mesenteric vein entering the splenic vein, and then divide it.

Now lift up the descending part of the duodenum and head of the pancreas, and turn them together to the left, revealing several anatomical structures of great importance [Fig. 4.59]. First, there is the **bile-duct** (which sometimes lies in the substance of the pancreas), together with the com-

mencement of the portal vein. You should trace the duct downwards to the point where it enters the medial side of the descending part of the duodenum. You severed the upper part of the duct and also the portal vein when you removed the liver. Behind these structures, on the posterior abdominal wall, you will see the **inferior vena cava,** with the **abdominal aorta** to its left. Clean the fascia off the inferior vena cava and also off the psoas major muscle on which the vessel lies, but do not disturb any fascia lateral to the medial border of the right kidney.

Branches of the abdominal aorta [Fig. 4.66]

Before completing the removal of the pancreas, continue the cleaning and identification of the branches of the abdominal aorta which you have already exposed, being careful as you approach the aorta not to clear away the matted nerve fibres and ganglia by which it and the commencement of its branches are surrounded, and which you will dissect later. At this stage these plexuses look like part of the retroperitoneal fascia.

Identify the right and left **inferior phrenic arteries** which arise from each side of the abdominal aorta and pass upwards to the under-surface of the diaphragm. Then immediately below, define the origin of the **coeliac trunk** [Fig. 4.60], noting that it is a large unpaired vessel which arises from the anterior surface of the aorta, about 1 cm above

4.64

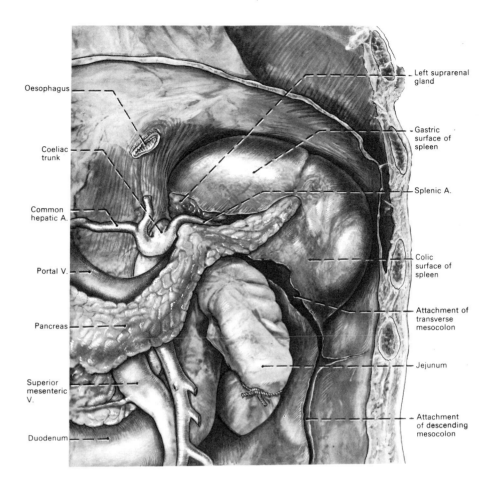

Fig. 4.60 The spleen and the pancreas.

the origin of the **superior mesenteric artery.** Note that the left renal vein, a big vessel, passes in front of the aorta below the origin of the superior mesenteric artery. As you dissect between the coeliac trunk and the superior mesenteric artery, be careful not to cut the small **middle suprarenal arteries** which arise between them from each side of the aorta. Now divide the superior mesenteric artery 1 cm from its origin, and the coeliac trunk a little closer to its origin.

Then continue to shell the pancreas off the fascia of the posterior abdominal wall. As you approach the spleen, re-identify the remains of the lienorenal ligament between the spleen and the kidney. It contains the splenic vessels and the tail of the pancreas.

The spleen [Figs 4.60 and 4.61]

The spleen should now be examined *in situ* [Fig. 4.60]. Observe that it lies obliquely, with its long axis in line with the tenth rib, and that its anterior end does not extend forwards beyond the axillary line. Note, too, that its convex **diaphragmatic surface** is in contact with the diaphragm. On its concave **visceral surface** find the **hilum** of the spleen, with the splenic vessels running to and from it between what is left of the two layers of the lienorenal ligament. In front

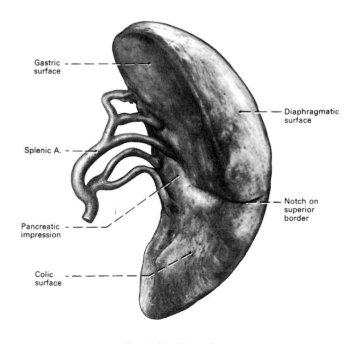

Fig. 4.61 The spleen.

of the hilum is a large concave surface which is in contact with the stomach, and behind it a (usually) smaller surface which is in contact with the left kidney and left suprarenal gland. Inferior to both of these is an impression which is made by the left colic flexure.

The **gastrosplenic ligament** has already been cut. Now free the spleen from the **lienorenal ligament** and divide the anastomosis between the middle colic artery and the ascending branch of the left colic artery. Remove the spleen from the abdominal cavity together with the duodenum, the pancreas, the superior mesenteric vessels (enclosed in the remains of their mesentery), and the splenic vessels.

Both the size and form of the spleen vary greatly between different cadavers. In the living body its size is dependent on the volume of blood it contains, while its form varies with the state of distension of the stomach and colon. Its position also varies slightly with the respiratory excursions of the diaphragm.

The diaphragmatic surface [Fig. 4.61] is evenly convex and easily recognizable when the organ is removed from the body. Anteriorly it is separated from the visceral surface by a superior border, which usually shows two or three notches at its anterior end. The visceral surface is formed, in part, by the concave **gastric surface** and the less concave and narrower **renal surface** behind the hilum, with the lower part of which the tail of the pancreas makes contact. The lower part of the visceral surface is flat, and before the abdomen was disturbed, was in contact with the left colic flexure.

Dissection of the pancreas and duodenum

The pancreas [Fig. 4.56]

Examine the pancreas, and note again how the uncinate process of the head projects upwards behind the body, from which it is separated by the superior mesenteric artery and the origin of the portal vein [Fig. 4.56]. Note that the body of the pancreas is triangular in cross-section, with an anterior surface which faces slightly upwards, separated by an anterior border from an inferior surface. Remember again that the transverse mesocolon was reflected along the line of the anterior border, and that the anterior surface was covered by the peritoneum which formed the posterior wall of the omental bursa. Examine the posterior surface, and note that its most important relations from right to left are the inferior vena cava, the abdominal aorta (and the superior mesenteric vessels and portal vein), the left kidney (and suprarenal gland on its upper end), and the spleen [Figs 4.59 and 4.60]. Confirm, too, that the splenic artery runs along the superior border of the pancreas, with the splenic vein below it, behind the body of the pancreas, and that the bile-duct is closely related to the posterior surface of the head of the pancreas, which lies in the concavity of the duodenum [Fig. 4.62].

The pancreatic ducts [Fig. 4.62]

Make a horizontal cut in the posterior surface of the pancreas to find the **pancreatic duct.** It runs fairly close to the posterior surface and looks like a thin white-walled vein. It receives numerous small tributaries, and can be traced into, and then through the head of the pancreas, where it comes to lie close to the end of the bile-duct.

Now open the duodenum along its posterior surface. Wash its mucous coat under running water, and note that it, too, is thrown into a series of circular folds, beginning about 2 cm from the pylorus. Look for a small swelling, called the **greater duodenal papilla,** on the postero-medial wall about 10 cm from the pylorus, hidden to some extent by a fold of mucosa. A longitudinal fold of the mucous coat,

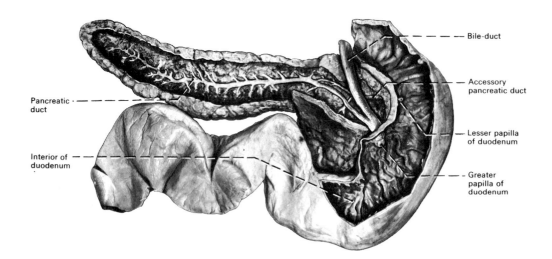

Fig. 4.62 Posterior view of the pancreas and duodenum. The posterior surface of the pancreas and part of the duodenal wall have been excised.

called the **longitudinal fold of the duodenum,** often provides a good guide to the papilla, which lies at its distal end. Dissect this small swelling carefully, and you will see that it is formed by the junction in the duodenal wall of the bile-duct with the pancreatic duct. Try to pass a fine probe or bristle into these two ducts. Their common lumen is called the hepatopancreatic ampulla. Also try to find another small opening into the duodenum about 2 cm above the greater duodenal papilla. It is the **lesser duodenal papilla,** where the small **accessory pancreatic duct** opens. This duct drains the lower part of the head and crosses the pancreatic duct, with which it may communicate.

Section 4.10

The posterior abdominal wall

Now that you have examined most of the alimentary tract, as well as the liver, pancreas, and spleen, you can start dissecting the posterior abdominal wall and the structures which lie on it. Before you begin, try to get an impression of their general arrangement.

In the midline are the bodies of the lumbar vertebrae, and in the angle between them and their transverse processes is a vertically-disposed muscle, called the psoas major [Fig. 4.63], which passes down, at the side of the linea terminalis of the pelvis, behind the inguinal ligament, to become attached to the lesser trochanter of the femur. This part of

the muscle was examined when you dissected the thigh [p. 2.23].

Above the level of the iliac crest to the lateral side of the psoas major, is the quadratus lumborum muscle, and lateral to this the posterior part of the transversus abdominis muscle. Below the iliac crest the iliacus muscle lies lateral to the psoas major muscle.

In the midline below the promontory of the sacrum is the pelvic surface of the sacrum, covered by the belly of the piriformis muscle, whose insertion you studied when you dissected the buttock [p. 2.11].

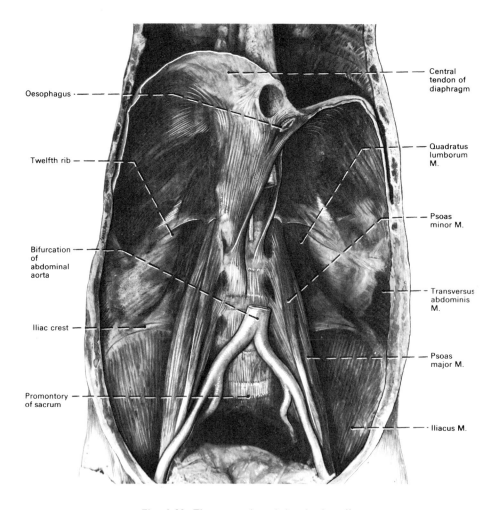

Fig. 4.63 The posterior abdominal wall.

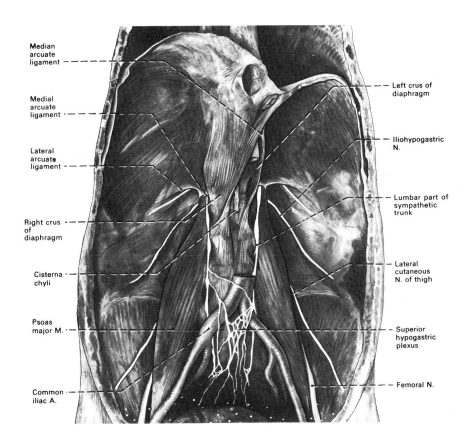

Median arcuate ligament

Medial arcuate ligament

Lateral arcuate ligament

Right crus of diaphragm

Cisterna chyli

Psoas major M.

Common iliac A.

Left crus of diaphragm

Iliohypogastric N.

Lumbar part of sympathetic trunk

Lateral cutaneous N. of thigh

Superior hypogastric plexus

Femoral N.

Fig. 4.64 The lumbar parts of the sympathetic trunks and the crura of the diaphragm.

Lying on the bodies of the lumbar vertebrae is the abdominal aorta, with the inferior vena cava to its right side. The aorta bifurcates into two common iliac arteries at the level of the fourth lumbar vertebra (approximately that of the umbilicus), and these pass downwards and laterally.

The kidneys, with the suprarenal glands on their superior ends, lie on the upper part of the posterior wall of the abdomen, mainly on the diaphragm and the quadratus lumborum muscles. The hilum of each kidney faces anteromedially, and into it passes the renal artery, and from it the renal vein and ureter emerge. The ureters pass down the posterior abdominal wall into the pelvis, where they enter the urinary bladder.

Now return to the cadaver in order to clean the abdominal aorta and its branches, the inferior vena cava and its tributaries, and the autonomic nerve plexuses by which they are surrounded. It is best to start the dissection of the latter first, lest they are destroyed as the vessels are cleaned. Before you begin, it is useful to get a general idea of the disposition of the abdominal autonomic nerves.

The autonomic nerve plexuses of the abdomen

These plexuses are formed by the three **splanchnic nerves,** branches of the thoracic parts of each sympathetic trunk,

and by **lumbar splanchnic nerves,** branches of the lumbar parts of the sympathetic trunks [Fig. 4.64]. The sympathetic trunks pass behind the diaphragm as they leave the thorax to enter the abdomen. The lumbar parts of the sympathetic trunks lie on each side of the bodies of the lumbar vertebrae, to the side of and behind the aorta and inferior vena cava. They pass into the pelvis and end by fusing together in front of the coccyx. You will not find it easy to dissect the trunks themselves until you have completed the dissection of the aorta and inferior vena cava.

The abdominal autonomic plexuses receive contributions from the **vagus nerves,** which constitute the main parasympathetic nerve trunks of the body, and from parasympathetic fibres that emerge with the second and third (sometimes third and fourth) sacral nerves (**pelvic splanchnic nerves**), and which are distributed along the blood vessels to the organs they supply. The vagal fibres, which are part of the parasympathetic outflow from the brain stem, are responsible for the parasympathetic innervation of the abdominal viscera as far distally as the region of the left colic flexure. The pelvic parasympathetic fibres supply the distal part of the alimentary canal and all the pelvic organs.

There is one further general point to note before you start dissecting. Both the sympathetic and parasympathetic autonomic nerves begin as preganglionic fibres which

4.69

synapse on terminal neurons whence the pathways of stimulation are continued along postganglionic fibres. Most of the neurons with which the preganglionic sympathetic fibres synapse are concentrated either in the ganglia of the sympathetic trunk itself or in ganglia of very variable size which lie on or close to the aorta. From these ganglia postganglionic fibres are distributed to the viscera and blood vessels by the perivascular plexuses. There is an important exception to this rule, since the cells of the medulla of the suprarenal gland themselves serve as a sympathetic ganglion.

Almost without exception the parasympathetic fibres remain preganglionic until they reach the organ or tissue which they innervate, and in which are the terminal neurons with which they synapse.

Dissection of the coeliac ganglia

When you start dissecting the fascia that covers the front and the sides of the upper part of the abdominal aorta you will have to be careful not to damage the two inferior phrenic arteries which pass from the aorta to each side of the diaphragm, and also the origins of the coeliac trunk and superior mesenteric artery, and in between them, on either side, the small middle suprarenal arteries. In the upper part of your dissection you will not be impeded by the inferior vena cava, since you excised the upper segment of this big vessel when you removed the liver; lower down you will have to isolate the inferior vena cava from the aorta.

The crura of the diaphragm

Carefully clear away the fascia from the posterior abdominal wall on either side of the upper part of the abdominal aorta, in order to expose the two crura of the diaphragm [Fig. 4.64]. As you will see more clearly later, the crura are two powerful slips of muscle by means of which the diaphragm takes origin from the vertebral column. You will find that the **right crus** is attached to the upper three lumbar vertebrae and the intervening intervertebral discs, while the smaller **left crus** arises only from the upper two lumbar vertebrae and the disc between them. Uniting the two crura you will see a thin, sometimes indistinct, tendinous band, called the **median arcuate ligament,** behind which the aorta passes as it lies on the bodies of the twelfth thoracic vertebra and first lumbar vertebra.

Clean the crura and the median arcuate ligament carefully. As you clean each crus note that it is perforated by one or more of the thoracic splanchnic nerves. Continue cleaning the fascia on the lateral side of each crus, and expose the upper and rounded part of each psoas major muscle. As you clean the surface of the psoas in an upward direction, be careful not to damage the lumbar part of the sympathetic trunk, which you will find entering the abdominal cavity from behind a tendinous arch which marks the posterior border of the diaphragm over the psoas major

muscle. This arch is called the **medial arcuate ligament** [Fig. 4.64].

The coeliac ganglia

If you follow the splanchnic nerves from the surface of the crura of the diaphragm, you will find that they end in two, large, irregularly-shaped ganglia, not unlike lymph nodes in appearance, which lie on the crura of the diaphragm. These are the coeliac ganglia [Fig. 4.65]. The right coeliac ganglion lies behind the inferior vena cava, and the left, to the left of the aorta, behind the splenic vessels. Lateral to the coeliac ganglia are the suprarenal glands.

The coeliac plexus

As you dissect the front of the aorta, you will see that the two coeliac ganglia are connected by a coeliac plexus of nerves. This important plexus surrounds the coeliac trunk and the root of the superior mesenteric artery, and is composed of a dense network of nerve fibres. The plexus and ganglia receive the **greater** and **lesser splanchnic nerves,** and also a large number of branches from the **posterior vagal trunk.** They send preganglionic branches to the medulla of the suprarenal glands, and give off numerous secondary plexuses along the arteries which are distributed to the viscera.

The abdominal aortic plexus

As you clean the abdominal aorta and separate it from the inferior vena cava, be careful not to damage the lumbar splanchnic nerves which spring from the sympathetic trunk and pass into the abdominal aortic plexus [Fig. 4.65]. On the right side they pass between the aorta and the inferior vena cava. On the left side they are obvious as they pass across the abdominal aorta. Also be careful as you dissect not to destroy the two renal veins. The left renal vein crosses the front of the aorta just below the origin of the superior mesenteric artery.

The abdominal aorta

Having defined and dissected the start of the autonomic nerve plexuses of the abdominal cavity, try to avoid cutting nerves as you continue with the dissection of the branches of the aorta, on which you should now focus your attention.

You have seen that the abdominal aorta [Fig. 4.66], which is a continuation of the thoracic aorta, begins at the **aortic opening** in the midline of the posterior border of the diaphragm at the level of the twelfth thoracic vertebra. It ends, as already observed, and as your dissection will show, at the level of the fourth lumbar vertebra by dividing into two common iliac arteries. It lies in front of the vertebral column, and you have already removed from its anterior surface, from above downwards, the posterior layer of peritoneum of the omental bursa, the pancreas, the horizontal part of the duodenum, the root of the mesentery and coils

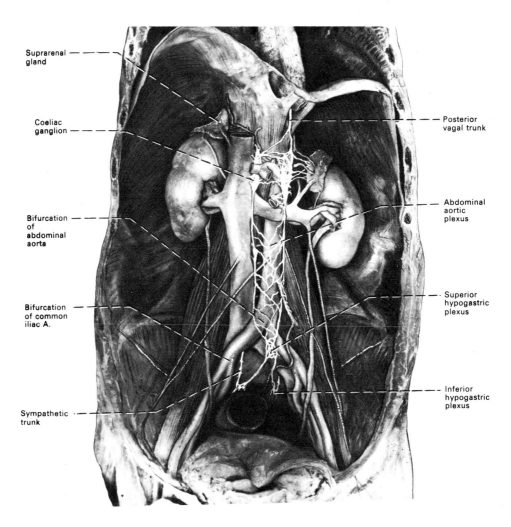

Fig. 4.65 The abdominal aortic plexus. The right kidney is higher than usual.

Labels (clockwise): Suprarenal gland — Coeliac ganglion — Bifurcation of abdominal aorta — Bifurcation of common iliac A. — Sympathetic trunk — Posterior vagal trunk — Abdominal aortic plexus — Superior hypogastric plexus — Inferior hypogastric plexus

of small intestine. As you have seen, the abdominal aorta is enmeshed in a plexus of sympathetic nerves, while lymph nodes, which you should remove as you dissect, lie both in front of it and at the sides.

The branches of the abdominal aorta

The branches of the abdominal aorta, paired unless otherwise stated, come off in the following order:

1. The **inferior phrenic arteries** [Fig. 4.66]. These, as you have seen, are distributed to the under-surface of the diaphragm, and each gives off a **superior suprarenal artery** to the suprarenal gland. Clean these vessels.

2. The **coeliac trunk** [Figs 4.43 and 4.66]. Note again that this unpaired artery springs from the front of the abdominal aorta, just below the aortic opening behind the diaphragm, and that in the undissected body it lies on the superior border of the pancreas behind the omental bursa. It is surrounded by the coeliac nerve plexus, and on either side of it are the two large coeliac ganglia. The

artery is just over 1 cm long, and terminates by dividing into the three large branches which you have already dissected. Refresh your memory about:

i. The **left gastric artery** [Fig. 4.43], which runs along the lesser curvature of the stomach, to supply not only the stomach but also the termination of the oesophagus [see p. 4.46].

ii. The **splenic artery** [Fig. 4.43], passing along the superior border of the pancreas, and then between the two layers of the lienorenal ligament, to the spleen. Remember that this vessel gives off **splenic** and **pancreatic branches, short gastric arteries,** and also the **left gastroepiploic artery.** The latter runs, at first, with the short gastric arteries, between the two layers of the gastrosplenic ligament, and then enters the greater omentum to pass along the greater curvature of the stomach [see p. 4.47].

iii. The **common hepatic artery** [Fig. 4.43], which, after passing to the right along the body of the pancreas

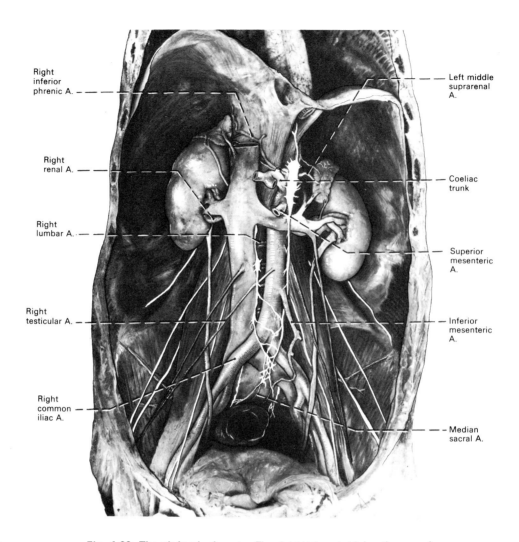

Right inferior phrenic A.

Right renal A.

Right lumbar A.

Right testicular A.

Right common iliac A.

Left middle suprarenal A.

Coeliac trunk

Superior mesenteric A.

Inferior mesenteric A.

Median sacral A.

Fig. 4.66 The abdominal aorta. The right kidney is higher than usual.

and the superior part of the duodenum, continues as the **hepatic artery,** and ascends to the porta hepatis. The hepatic artery lies in the right free border of the lesser omentum, where it divides into right and left branches which pass into the interior of the liver. Remember that the right branch usually gives off the important **cystic artery** to the gall-bladder, and that the common hepatic artery, before continuing as the hepatic artery, gives off the **right gastric artery** (which runs along the lesser curvature of the stomach to anastomose with the left gastric artery), and the **gastroduodenal artery,** which almost immediately divides into:

a. the **superior pancreaticoduodenal artery,** which descends on the head of the pancreas, which it supplies together with the duodenum [p. 4.47];

b. the **right gastroepiploic artery,** which runs between the two layers of the greater omentum along the

greater curvature of the stomach, and occasionally anastomoses with the left gastroepiploic branch of the splenic artery [see p. 4.48].

Remember that all the arteries supplying the stomach and intestines anastomose freely with each other.

3. The **middle suprarenal arteries** [Fig. 4.69]. These arise on either side of the superior mesenteric artery and pass to the suprarenal glands, which you will dissect later. At present do not disturb the fatty fascia in which the kidneys and suprarenal glands lie.

4. The **superior mesenteric artery** [Fig. 4.47], which springs from the front of the aorta just below the coeliac trunk. Remember that this unpaired vessel passes down behind the neck and in front of the uncinate process of the head of the pancreas, and that it supplies practically all the small intestine, as well as the caecum, and the ascending and transverse colons. Remember, too, that in its course

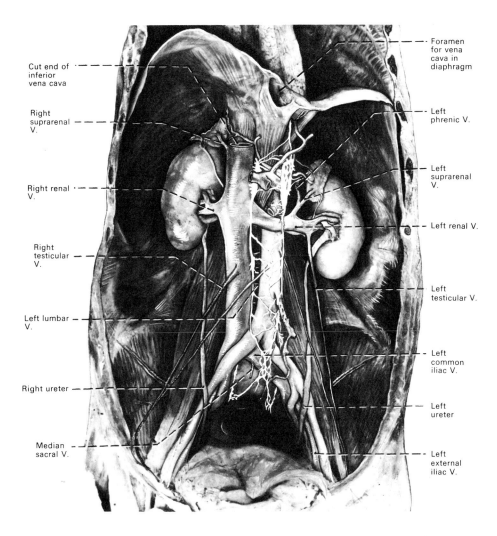

Cut end of inferior vena cava

Right suprarenal V.

Right renal V.

Right testicular V.

Left lumbar V.

Right ureter

Median sacral V.

Foramen for vena cava in diaphragm

Left phrenic V.

Left suprarenal V.

Left renal V.

Left testicular V.

Left common iliac V.

Left ureter

Left external iliac V.

Fig. 4.67 The inferior vena cava. The right kidney is higher than usual.

in the root of the mesentery, the superior mesenteric artery forms an arch with its concavity to the right, and that the **middle colic artery,** the **right colic artery,** and the **ileocolic artery** spring from this side [see p. 4.50].

5. The **renal arteries** [Fig. 4.66], which are two large vessels that run almost horizontally to the hilum of each kidney. The right artery passes behind the inferior vena cava and the right renal vein, and the left artery lies posterior to the left renal vein which, as you have seen, crosses the aorta just below the origin of the superior mesenteric artery. Each artery gives an **inferior suprarenal artery** to the suprarenal gland.

6. The **testicular arteries** [Fig. 4.66], which arise just below the renal arteries, descend obliquely across the posterior abdominal wall to enter the spermatic cords at the deep inguinal rings. If you were careful when you cleaned the left renal vein, you will have seen that it receives the left testicular vein, the left suprarenal vein, and the phrenic

veins of the left side [Fig. 4.67]. In the female, the place of the testicular arteries is taken by the **ovarian arteries,** which pass to the ovaries in the pelvis. Do not trace these vessels further than the linea terminalis of the pelvis [p. 4.4].

7. The **lumbar arteries** (four pairs), which arise from the back of the aorta and pass to the lateral part of the abdominal wall [Fig. 4.66].

8. The **inferior mesenteric artery** [Fig. 4.66], an unpaired vessel which arises from the front of the aorta, about 4 cm above its bifurcation, and supplies that part of the large intestine which is not supplied by the superior mesenteric artery.

9. The **median sacral artery,** a small unpaired vessel which arises at the bifurcation of the aorta, and which descends on the front of the sacrum [Fig. 4.91].

10. The **common iliac arteries** [Fig. 4.66], which you will study later.

4.73

The inferior vena cava

Now study the inferior vena cava [Fig. 4.67], the upper part of which was removed with the liver, while the remainder should by now have been thoroughly cleaned.

You will see that it commences in front of the body of the fifth lumbar vertebra by the union of the two **common iliac veins,** and that it ascends on the vertebral column to the right of the aorta. It passes through the liver, pierces the central tendon of the diaphragm at the level of the eighth thoracic vertebra, and almost immediately enters the right atrium of the heart. You can see that because it lies on the right of the midline the inferior vena cava overlies the right sympathetic trunk, part of the right suprarenal gland and the right coeliac ganglion.

Running into the inferior vena cava (starting from below), you should have found the third and fourth **lumbar veins,** the **right testicular** (or **ovarian) vein,** the **renal veins,** and the **right suprarenal vein.** The inferior vena cava also receives the **right phrenic vein** and the **hepatic veins.** You will already have noted that the left testicular (or ovarian) vein, the left suprarenal vein, and the left phrenic vein join the left renal vein [Fig. 4.67].

The portal vein

Before you proceed with your dissection of the posterior abdominal wall, recall that the blood from the stomach, small and large intestines, pancreas, and spleen does not drain into the inferior vena cava but into the portal vein [Fig. 4.68], which enters the liver at the porta hepatis, having passed upwards in the free edge of the lesser omentum behind the bile-duct and the hepatic artery. Recall, too, that the portal vein is formed behind the neck of the pancreas by the union of the **splenic vein** and the **superior mesenteric vein,** and that it drains the stomach through the **right gastric vein** and the **left gastric vein,** and the spleen and pancreas via the splenic and superior mesenteric veins, which also drain part of the stomach. The alimentary canal is drained by the superior and inferior mesenteric veins and by the **pancreatico-duodenal veins.** The gall-bladder is drained by the **cystic vein,** which joins the right branch of the portal vein. The portal vein also drains a small part of the anterior abdominal wall near the umbilicus, through **paraumbilical veins** which pass up in the falciform ligament of the liver [p. 4.32].

The tributaries of the portal vein commence as capillaries, the most important being those in the villi of the small in-

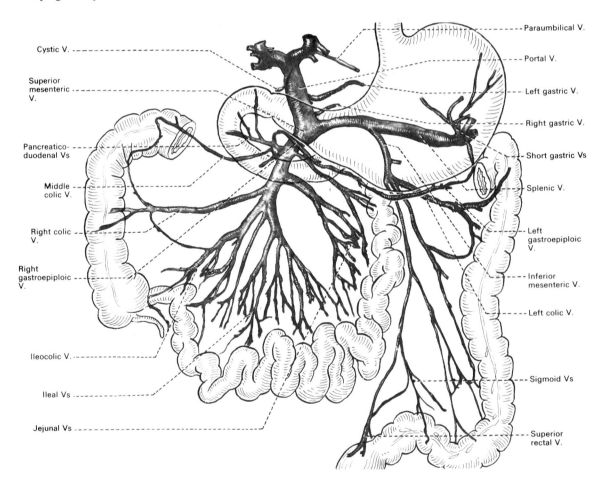

Fig. 4.68 Tributaries of the portal vein.

testine. Within the liver, the branches of the portal vein again break up into other minute vessels, called sinusoids, which are common to the portal vein and hepatic artery. Thus the portal vein, which transports the major part of the products of digestion, begins and ends as a series of capillaries. The circulation of the blood in the vessel is largely, but not entirely, controlled by variations in the intra-abdominal pressure.

At the lower end of the anal canal, at the lower end of the oesophagus and around the umbilicus, capillaries of the portal system anastomose with capillaries of the systemic venous system. Varicosities are liable to occur in these regions.

The cisterna chyli

The upper part of the abdominal aorta and inferior vena cava should have been sufficiently freed as they were cleaned for you to turn them aside to look for a narrow white sac, some 5 to 7 cm long, which is usually collapsed like an empty vein. This is the **cisterna chyli** [Fig. 4.64]. If you do not find it behind the aorta, separate the fibres of the right crus of the diaphragm and look for it on the bodies of the first and second lumbar vertebrae. The upper end of the cisterna chyli is continuous with the **thoracic duct** [Fig. 3.46]. You can confirm this fact by finding the thoracic duct in the thorax and by tracing it, with the aorta, behind the median arcuate ligament into the abdomen. Do not spend any time searching for them, but note that three main lymph trunks usually pass into the cisterna chyli: an **intestinal trunk** from the small intestine, and paired **lumbar trunks** which drain the lower limbs and the lower half of the trunk. In addition, small paired **posterior intercostal trunks** often descend from the thorax. The veins which you will see as you dissect behind the aorta join together to form the azygos vein [Fig. 3.46]. Do not spend any time on their dissection.

The lumbar part of the sympathetic trunk

You should now follow the course of the lumbar parts of the sympathetic trunks as far as you can towards the promontory of the sacrum [Fig. 4.64]. Observe again that each sympathetic trunk enters the abdomen by passing behind the medial arcuate ligament. Note that it runs downwards in front of the vertebral column, along the medial border of the psoas major muscle. Later you will see that after passing behind the common iliac artery, each trunk lies in front of the sacrum medial to the pelvic sacral foramina [Fig. 4.64]. As already noted [p. 4.69], the two trunks unite in front of the coccyx in a small ganglion, called the **ganglion impar** [Fig. 4.91]. Observe that the right lumbar trunk lies behind the inferior vena cava, and that the left trunk lies behind the left renal vessels and the inferior mesenteric artery.

Usually there are four ganglia on the lumbar part of each trunk, and either four or five on the pelvic portion. Try now to define the four **lumbar ganglia. Grey rami communicantes** pass from the ganglia to the neighbouring spinal nerves. The upper two (or three) lumbar nerves, but not the lower three (or two), send **white rami communicantes** to their corresponding ganglia. Normally the second lumbar nerves mark the caudal limit for the outflow of preganglionic fibres to the sympathetic trunks.

Secondary autonomic plexuses

Branches from the lumbar parts of the sympathetic trunks join the abdominal aortic plexus, and form **iliac plexuses** around each iliac artery. You have already seen that the coeliac and abdominal aortic plexuses form secondary plexuses of nerves and nerve cells along the branches of the abdominal aorta. In addition, it is sufficient to note, without trying to confirm by dissection, the following:

1. The **hepatic plexus** is the largest of the secondary plexuses, and receives branches from both vagus nerves.
2. The **suprarenal plexus,** accompanying the middle suprarenal artery, in addition to receiving branches from the coeliac plexus and ganglia, also receives branches directly from the phrenic nerve and the greater splanchnic nerve.
3. The **renal plexus** is joined by the lowest splanchnic nerve and also by branches from the vagus nerve.
4. The **superior mesenteric plexus** is a direct continuation of the lower part of the coeliac plexus, and receives a branch from the posterior vagal trunk.
5. The **abdominal aortic plexus** [Fig. 4.65] receives filaments from all the lumbar sympathetic ganglia, and branches from it are distributed to the **testicular** (or **ovarian**) **plexuses, the inferior mesenteric plexus**, the **iliac plexuses**, and the **superior hypogastric plexus.**
6. The **inferior mesenteric plexus** receives the majority of its branches from the abdominal aortic plexus.

The iliac arteries

Return to the aorta, and carefully clean the region where it bifurcates into the **common iliac arteries** [Figs 4.63 to 4.67] on the left side of the fourth lumbar vertebra. As you clean the latter vessels, follow them for 4 to 5 cm downwards and laterally, and note that each common iliac artery divides at the level of the promontory of the sacrum, in front of the sacroiliac joint, into a larger **external iliac artery** and a smaller **internal iliac artery** which passes into the lesser pelvis. Clean and follow the external iliac artery as far as the inguinal ligament, where it becomes the **femoral artery,** and note that the external iliac artery gives off the **inferior epigastric artery** [Fig. 4.32] and **deep circumflex iliac artery** [Fig. 4.20] to the abdominal wall. You have already dissected both these vessels [pp. 4.22, 4.29]. You should remember that the inferior epigastric artery ascends on the posterior aspect of the anterior abdominal wall close to the medial margin of the deep inguinal ring. It supplies the neighbouring muscles and enters the rectus sheath at the arcuate line, to anastomose with the superior epigastric artery. The inferior epigastric artery gives off the cremasteric artery to supply the coverings of the spermatic cord, and a pubic branch [Fig. 4.32] which passes to the back of the pubic symphysis. The deep circumflex iliac artery runs towards and then along the iliac crest, between the transversus abdominis muscle and internal oblique muscle, to supply these and adjacent muscles.

The hypogastric plexuses [Fig. 4.65]

As you clean the bifurcation of the aorta and the common iliac arteries, note the fibres from the lumbar part of the sympathetic trunk which join the terminal part of the abdominal aortic plexus. If you dissect in the triangle between the two common iliac vessels, you will find a rich plexus of nerves called the **superior hypogastric plexus**. This lies mainly in front of the left common iliac artery, the fifth lumbar vertebra and the promontory of the sacrum, and

between the common iliac arteries. It is formed by the union of numerous branches from the abdominal aortic plexus, by branches from the lumbar ganglia and by parasympathetic fibres from the second and third sacral nerves. Below it divides into right and left **inferior hypogastric plexuses** [Fig. 4.65].

Dissection of the kidneys and suprarenal glands

The kidneys

By this stage of your dissection the general position of the kidneys [Fig. 4.69] will be obvious. They lie behind the peritoneum on the posterior abdominal wall, surrounded by fat and fascia. Each kidney is about 12 cm long and is closely invested by a **fibrous capsule,** which is separated by a **fatty capsule** from the **renal fascia.** Behind the renal fascia is a large pad of fat, sometimes called the **paranephric body.**

Incise the renal fascia in the midline of the anterior surface of each kidney, and remove the fat from the surface of the organ. Note that the renal fascia and its contained fat enclose both the kidney and the suprarenal gland. The latter lies on the superior end of the kidney. Clean all the

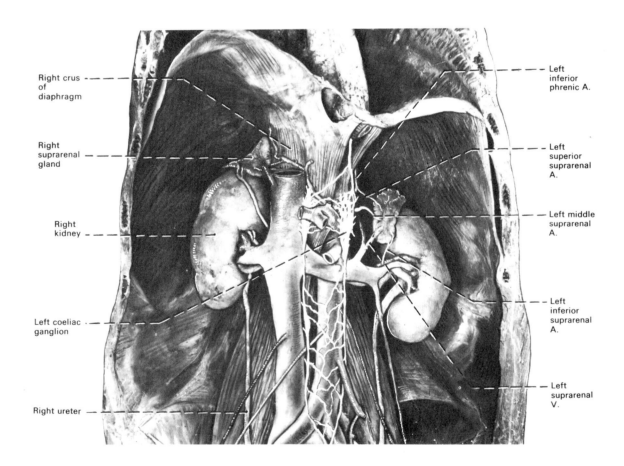

Fig. 4.69 The kidneys and the suprarenal glands. The right kidney is higher than usual.

Right crus of diaphragm

Right suprarenal gland

Right kidney

Left coeliac ganglion

Right ureter

Left inferior phrenic A.

Left superior suprarenal A.

Left middle suprarenal A.

Left inferior suprarenal A.

Left suprarenal V.

fat away on both sides, so that the shapes of the two kidneys and suprarenal glands are properly defined. Continue your dissection until you have cleaned the artery entering, and the vein and ureter leaving, each **renal hilum.**

The suprarenal glands

Now examine the suprarenal glands [Fig. 4.69]. You will see that the right gland is pyramidal in shape, while the left is semilunar, and that each lies on the medial border of the superior end of the corresponding kidney, and on the adjacent crus of the diaphragm. Note that the right gland lies behind the inferior vena cava and the liver, while the left lies behind the pancreas, stomach, and spleen. Confirm that the medial sides of both glands are closely related to the coeliac ganglia and plexus. Identify the solitary vein which drains each gland, and which emerges from a point on the anterior surface, called the **hilum.** If the veins are still intact in the whole of their course, note that the shorter right one drains directly into the inferior vena cava, and the longer left vein into the left renal vein.

The suprarenal gland is supplied by three small variable arteries, none of which enters the hilum. The superior suprarenal artery is a branch of the inferior phrenic artery; the middle suprarenal artery a branch of the aorta; and the inferior suprarenal artery a branch of the renal artery. Numerous nerves from the coeliac plexus will be seen entering the medulla of both glands. Remove the right gland and cut it in coronal section, when its pale **cortex** will stand out in striking contrast with the darker central **medulla.**

Anterior relations of the kidney

Turn your attention to the kidneys, and by replacing the organs you have removed, try to verify their anterior relations. You will see that the anterior surface of the right kidney [Figs 4.46 and 4.69] is in contact with the right suprarenal gland above and medially; the liver laterally; the duodenum medially; and the right colic flexure and coils of small intestine inferiorly. Try to appreciate that the anterior surface of the left kidney [Figs 4.45, 4.46, and 4.69] is in contact with the left suprarenal gland above and medially; the spleen laterally; the stomach and pancreas medially; and the left colic flexure and coils of small intestine inferiorly.

Note that the right kidney usually lies a little lower than the left, whose hilum lies in the transpyloric plane.

The ureter [Fig. 4.67]

Next, trace each ureter from the hilum of the kidney downwards over the posterior abdominal wall as far as the linea terminalis of the pelvis, noting the structures with which it is related [Figs 4.67 and 4.69]. Note that each ureter begins at the lower end of a funnel-shaped sac called the **renal pelvis** [Fig. 4.71]. The ureters lie behind the peritoneum on the psoas major muscle. The right ureter lies lateral to the in-

ferior vena cava and is crossed by the testicular (or ovarian) vessels and the vessels of the alimentary canal. The renal pelvis lies behind the descending part of the duodenum. The left ureter is crossed by the testicular (or ovarian) vessels and by branches of the left colic and sigmoid vessels.

Posterior relations of the kidney [Fig. 4.70]

Lift each kidney, and clean away any fat that remains on its posterior surface and on the adjacent abdominal wall. By so doing you will remove the paranephric body. If the kidney is then turned towards the midline, its posterior relations can be studied [Fig. 4.70]. They will be seen to be much the same on the two sides. The upper part of each kidney is in contact with the diaphragm. This separates the left kidney from the pleura and the eleventh and twelfth ribs; and the right kidney, which is normally slightly lower than the left, from the pleura and twelfth rib only.

You will see that below the diaphragm the kidneys lie medially on the psoas major muscle, centrally on the quadratus lumborum muscle, and laterally on the transversus abdominis muscle.

Identify the subcostal nerve, the iliohypogastric nerve and the ilio-inguinal nerve, which emerge in series. The subcostal nerve appears below the lateral arcuate ligament; the iliohypogastric and ilio-inguinal nerves emerge between the psoas major and quadratus lumborum muscles [pp. 4.79–4.80]. The lateral arcuate ligament is a band of fibrous tissue which stretches over the quadratus lumborum muscle, from the transverse process of the first lumbar vertebra to the twelfth rib. In the same way the medial arcuate ligament passes over the psoas major muscle from the front of the transverse process to the body of the same vertebra. Both arches give origin to fibres of the diaphragm [Fig. 4.72].

Note that as the blood vessels and ureter enter or leave the kidney at the renal hilum, the ureter lies behind the vessels.

The structure of the kidney [Fig. 4.71]

Make a vertical incision in the anterior surface of the right kidney just deeply enough to cut its fibrous capsule. The blade of your scalpel should not go in more deeply than a millimetre or two. Strip the capsule from the surface of the kidney and note that it is entirely independent of the renal fascia.

Using a knife with a long blade, slit the right kidney into anterior and posterior halves by cutting vertically through the convex lateral margin until you reach the renal pelvis [Fig. 4.71]. When the organ is sectioned in this way it will be seen to be composed of a **cortex** peripherally and a **medulla** centrally. In the medulla you will see a number of conical **renal pyramids,** with **renal columns** between them. The apex of each pyramid forms a **renal papilla,** and a hand-lens will help you to see a number of small openings which are the terminations of the papillary ducts. These ducts open

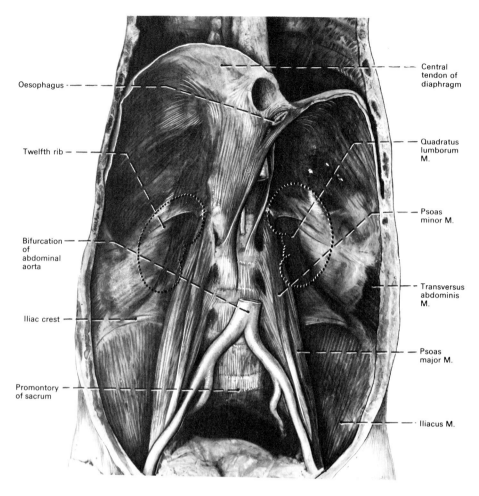

Oesophagus

Twelfth rib

Bifurcation of abdominal aorta

Iliac crest

Promontory of sacrum

Central tendon of diaphragm

Quadratus lumborum M.

Psoas minor M.

Transversus abdominis M.

Psoas major M.

Iliacus M.

Fig. 4.70 **The posterior relations of the kidneys.** The position of the kidneys is marked by the dotted outlines.

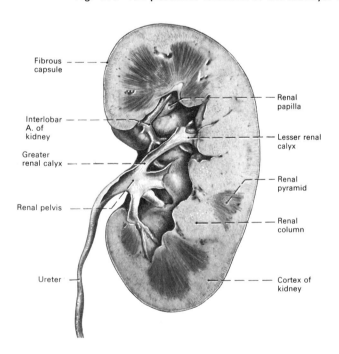

Fibrous capsule

Interlobar A. of kidney

Greater renal calyx

Renal pelvis

Ureter

Renal papilla

Lesser renal calyx

Renal pyramid

Renal column

Cortex of kidney

Fig. 4.71 **Coronal section of the kidney.**

into small channels called the **lesser renal calyces,** which in turn open into two larger channels called the **greater renal calyces.** These join to form the **renal pelvis.** Remove any fat which may be present in the **renal sinus,** in order to get a better view of the renal pelvis which lies within it.

The diaphragm

Examine the diaphragm [Fig. 4.72], which is a large dome-shaped muscle separating the thoracic and abdominal cavities. Strip the peritoneum and fascia from its under-surface in the direction of its fibres. You will see that the diaphragm arises from the posterior aspect of the xiphoid process and from the inner surfaces of the lower six costal cartilages, where it interdigitates with the slips of origin of the transversus abdominis muscle. The diaphragm also arises by means of the **left** and **right crura,** which you have already seen, attached to the upper lumbar vertebrae [p. 4.70]. In addition, its posterior fibres arise on each side of the midline from the medial and lateral arcuate ligaments.

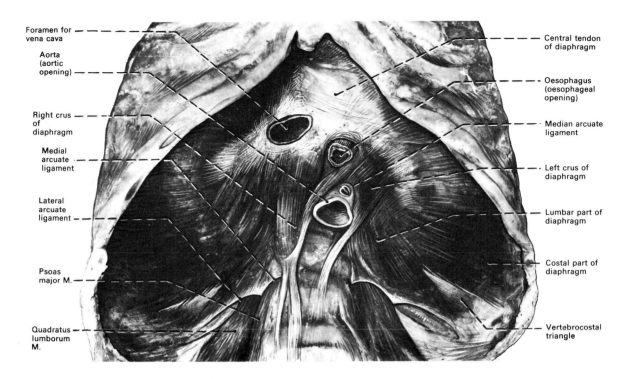

Foramen for vena cava

Aorta (aortic opening)

Right crus of diaphragm

Medial arcuate ligament

Lateral arcuate ligament

Psoas major M.

Quadratus lumborum M.

Central tendon of diaphragm

Oesophagus (oesophageal opening)

Median arcuate ligament

Left crus of diaphragm

Lumbar part of diaphragm

Costal part of diaphragm

Vertebrocostal triangle

Fig. 4.72 The diaphragm.

Note that the central part of the diaphragm is a tri-lobed tendon which lies in front, and on either side, of the vertebral column. This is the tendon of insertion of the muscle fibres of the diaphragm. When they contract, they pull on the tendon and flatten the whole diaphragm.

Openings in the diaphragm [Fig. 4.72]

Note that the **foramen for the vena cava** (through which the right phrenic nerve also passes) lies in the tendon at the level of the eighth thoracic vertebra. The fact that this big vein passes through the tendon, and not the muscle, means that the flow of blood through it is not interrupted when the diaphragm contracts. Look for the left phrenic nerve, which pierces the diaphragm independently, lateral to the pericardium.

Then find the **oesophageal opening** at the level of the tenth thoracic vertebra, just behind the central part of the tendon. The oesophagus passes obliquely through the muscle so that the diaphragm helps to fix the cardiac opening which controls the flow of food and fluid into the stomach. Also re-identify the anterior and posterior vagal trunks in the oesophageal opening.

Now re-examine the **crura,** and note that both have a tendinous origin, and that the right one is larger and more powerful than the left. If they are still there, note again the greater and lesser splanchnic nerves which perforate the crura. Look again at the oesophageal opening, and note that it is formed by a splitting of the fibres of the right crus.

Now look at the so-called **aortic opening** at the level of the twelfth thoracic vertebra. You will see that it lies behind the muscle, and that it is not a true opening in the diaphragm. Confirm that it is bounded in front by the fibrous band called the **median arcuate ligament,** which joins the two crura, and behind by the body of the twelfth thoracic vertebra. Define not only the aorta as it passes through the opening, but also the azygos vein and the thoracic duct. Again define the **medial** and **lateral arcuate ligaments** and, as you do so, find the sympathetic trunks passing into the abdomen behind the medial, and the subcostal artery and nerve passing behind the lateral ligament. Examine the diaphragm carefully for evidence of defects in the musculature, especially in the region of the arcuate ligaments. Such defects, covered only by fibrous tissue, may allow some of the abdominal contents to pass into the thorax, producing a diaphragmatic hernia.

The diaphragm is the chief muscle of respiration and helps to control intra-abdominal pressure. It is innervated by the phrenic nerves. The lower six thoracic nerves also convey sensory nerve fibres from the periphery of the muscle.

The muscles of the posterior abdominal wall

The quadratus lumborum muscle [Fig. 4.70]

Now turn your attention to the quadratus lumborum muscle, and clean the fascia from its anterior surface. You will see that it arises below from the iliac crest and the **ilio-lumbar ligament** [Fig. 4.79], which connects the crest to the transverse process of the fifth lumbar vertebra, and that it is inserted above into the transverse processes of the upper lumbar vertebrae and into the last rib. It is innervated by the upper four lumbar nerves. The main action of the muscle is to steady the twelfth rib as a base for the contraction of the diaphragm. The quadratus lumborum also flexes the vertebral column laterally.

The psoas muscles [Fig. 4.70]

Remove what fascia remains on the **psoas major muscle** [Fig. 4.70], being careful not to damage the thin genitofemoral nerve which emerges from its substance and runs downwards on its surface. Note that the fascia which encloses the muscle forms a fibrous sheath, the thickened upper margin of which is the medial arcuate ligament. Note that the muscle arises from the bodies and transverse processes of all the lumbar vertebrae. It also arises from their intervertebral discs (including that between the twelfth thoracic and first lumbar vertebrae), and from the aponeurotic arches which cover the lumbar vessels. The psoas major is the main flexor of the hip joint, and also flexes the vertebral column. You studied its insertion and action when you dissected the thigh [p. 2.23].

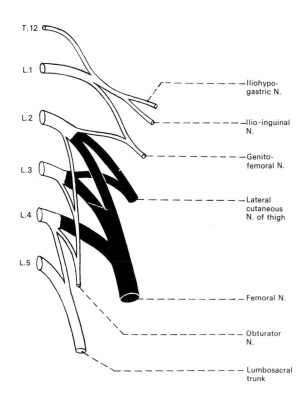

Fig. 4.73 Schema of the left lumbar plexus. The posterior divisions of the ventral rami of the spinal nerves concerned and their derivatives are shown black; the corresponding anterior divisions are shown in outline.

Lying on the psoas major muscle you may find another smaller muscle called the **psoas minor** [Fig. 4.70]. It has a very small belly and a long tendon which passes into the sheath of the psoas major and the pecten of the pubis. It is present in about 60 per cent of bodies and arises from the twelfth thoracic and first lumbar vertebrae.

The lumbar plexus

The iliohypogastric and ilio-inguinal nerves

In your study of the lumbar plexus [Fig. 4.73], begin by searching at the upper and lateral side of the psoas major muscle, to isolate the iliohypogastric and ilio-inguinal nerves (both branches of the first lumbar nerve) as they emerge from the muscle. You have already dissected these nerves as they lie between the kidney and the quadratus lumborum muscles [p. 4.77]. Both emerge from the lateral side of the psoas major, and pass obliquely down on the quadratus lumborum muscle. They pierce the transversus abdominis muscle shortly after they leave the lateral border of the quadratus lumborum. You have also dissected these nerves in the distal part of their course [pp. 2.20, 4.20, 4.24–4.25]. Both nerves send motor fibres to most of the muscles of the abdominal wall, before innervating the skin of the lower part of the abdominal wall and the external genitalia (as well as a small area of the buttocks and the part of the thigh adjacent to the genitalia).

The genitofemoral nerve

Now identify the genitofemoral nerve, which is formed by branches of the first and second lumbar nerves, and which emerges about halfway down the muscle on its anterior surface. It is crossed by the ureter as it runs down on the psoas major muscle to the region of the inguinal ligament. The nerve divides into two branches, the division sometimes taking place high up, and sometimes near the inguinal ligament. One of its two branches is the **genital branch,** which enters the inguinal canal at the deep inguinal ring, to supply the cremaster muscle, and emerges at the superficial inguinal ring to supply the skin of the external genitalia. The second branch is the **femoral branch,** which descends on the lateral aspect of the external iliac and femoral vessels, and supplies a small area of skin over the femoral triangle [p. 2.20].

The lateral cutaneous nerve of the thigh [Fig. 4.64]

Look for the lateral cutaneous nerve of the thigh, which emerges at the lateral side of the psoas major muscle, and runs obliquely over the iliacus muscle to the anterior superior iliac spine. It passes behind the inguinal ligament to supply a large area of skin on the antero-lateral aspect of the thigh [p. 2.20].

The obturator nerve [Fig. 4.89]

Search also for the obturator nerve, where it emerges from

the medial border of the psoas major muscle at the linea terminalis of the pelvis. It passes behind the common iliac vessels and then runs along the lateral wall of the lesser pelvis to the upper part of the obturator foramen, within which the nerve divides into an **anterior branch** and a **posterior branch,** both of which pass into the thigh to supply the adductor group of muscles [pp. 2.28–2.29]. An **accessory obturator nerve** [p. 2.29] is present in about one in ten bodies. When present, it runs over the medial surface of the psoas major muscle to enter the thigh by passing over the superior ramus of the pubis. It supplies the pectineus muscle and the hip joint.

The femoral nerve

Now look for the femoral nerve [Fig. 4.64], which is a large branch that emerges at the lateral border of the psoas major muscle, below the lateral cutaneous nerve of the thigh. It passes down between the psoas major and the iliacus muscles to enter the thigh behind the inguinal ligament. It supplies the quadriceps femoris and sartorius muscles as well as the skin over the front of the thigh and the medial side of the lower limb [pp. 2.22–2.23].

The formation of the lumbar plexus

All these nerves are branches of the lumbar plexus, which you must now expose. Before doing this, it will help you to note that the lumbar plexus [Fig. 4.73], which lies in the substance of the posterior part of the psoas major muscle, is formed by the ventral rami of the upper four lumbar nerves, augmented by a small branch of the twelfth thoracic nerve.

The first lumbar nerve divides into iliohypogastric and ilio-inguinal nerves;

branches from the first and second lumbar nerves unite to form the genitofemoral nerve;

branches from the second and third lumbar nerves form the lateral cutaneous nerve of the thigh;

branches from the second, third, and fourth lumbar nerves form the obturator and femoral nerves;

branches from the third and fourth lumbar nerves occasionally form the accessory obturator nerve;

branches from the fourth and fifth lumbar nerves join to form the **lumbosacral trunk,** which descends on the pelvic surface of the sacrum, where it joins the ventral ramus of the first sacral nerve to help form the sacral plexus.

Exposure of the lumbar plexus

To expose the plexus you must use forceps, and if necessary the blade of a scalpel. Pick away the fibres of the left psoas muscles so as to remove them entirely above the linea terminalis. As already observed, the psoas major arises from the sides of the bodies of the lumbar vertebrae and their transverse processes. Begin by lifting the iliohypogastric and ilio-inguinal nerves, and by tracing them into the substance of the psoas major muscle, nibbling away the muscle fibres by which they are surrounded. Trace these two nerves to their connection with the ventral ramus of the first lumbar nerve, where the latter emerges from the intervertebral foramen. When you have done this, continue the removal of the muscle fibres in a downward direction until you have exposed the whole lumbar plexus. As you dissect, it will help you if you follow into the muscle all the nerves you have found emerging from it.

The lumbosacral trunk is easy to find. Note that it passes almost vertically down into the pelvis to the medial side of the upper end of the sacroiliac joint.

Section 4.11

The pelvic cavity

The final stage of your dissection of the abdomen comprises the study of the contents of the pelvis. You should study not only the cadaver you yourself are dissecting, but also one of the opposite sex. Therefore arrange, as conveniently as is possible, to work on two cadavers.

Dissection of the male pelvis

Begin by identifying the **sigmoid colon** and **rectum** posteriorly, and the **urinary bladder** anteriorly, with the **rectovesical pouch** in the midline between them [Fig. 4.74]. The

peritoneum passes to the side walls of the pelvis from the superior surface of the bladder.

Note the shape and direction of the sigmoid colon, which is the final reservoir for the faeces. Its long axis is directed transversely. Examine the **sigmoid mesocolon** by which it is suspended, and note that the mesocolon is attached both to the lateral pelvic wall and to the sacrum. Its line of attachment is shaped like an inverted V, with the apex lying near the bifurcation of the left common iliac artery and in front of the left sacroiliac joint. Dissect away the peritoneum from the superior side of the mesocolon and ex-

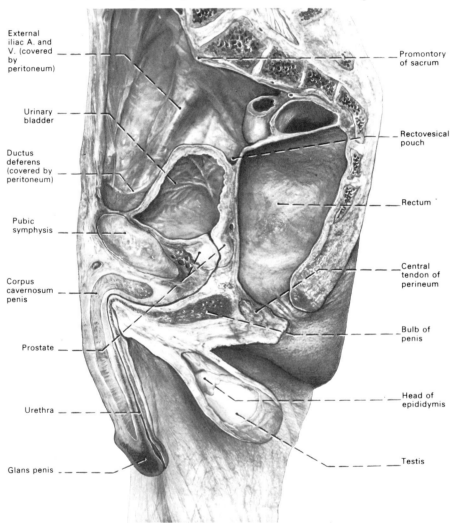

Fig. 4.74 Median section of the male pelvis. The abnormal distension of the rectum was produced *post mortem* during the preparation of the body.

amine its contents. The arteries you will find are the **sigmoid arteries** and the **superior rectal artery,** branches of the inferior mesenteric artery. The superior rectal artery is the terminal branch, and you should trace it as far distally as this stage of the dissection will allow.

Dissection of the female pelvis

As in the male pelvis, the sigmoid colon and rectum lie posteriorly and the urinary bladder anteriorly [Fig. 4.75]. Between the two, however, are the **uterus** and **vagina.** Follow the peritoneum over the uterus, on to the superior surface of the bladder. Between the two is the shallow **vesico-uterine pouch.** Follow the peritoneum down the intestinal surface of the uterus. Note that it dips down far more deeply on this than on the vesical surface of the uterus. Inferiorly it passes to the upper third of the vagina, from which it is reflected on to the anterior surface of the rectum. The deep peritoneal fossa which is formed in this way behind the

uterus is called the **recto-uterine pouch.** It can be reached through the upper and posterior third of the vagina and is, therefore, of surgical importance. Its lateral boundaries are formed by peritoneum which is reflected over two condensations of fibromuscular tissue that stretch over the pelvic diaphragm from the uterus to the rectum and sacrum. The peritoneal reflections over these bands are known as the **recto-uterine folds**; the fibromuscular strands are called the **recto-uterine muscle.** The sigmoid colon and coils of small intestine may lie in the recto-uterine pouch.

Now examine the sigmoid colon and mesocolon, as in the male cadaver.

The uterus *in situ* [Fig. 4.75]

Having done so, turn to the uterus. You will see that the peritoneum is reflected from the lateral borders of this organ on to the lateral pelvic wall in the form of two thin folds. These are the **broad ligaments of the uterus** [Fig. 4.76]. You can see that they divide the pelvic cavity into two com-

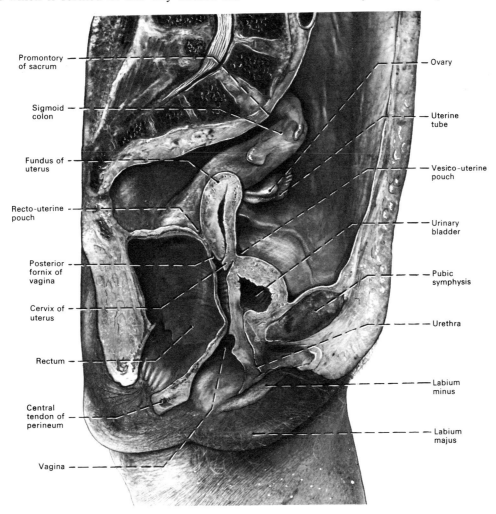

Fig. 4.75 Median section of the female pelvis. The abnormal distension of the rectum and lower part of the vagina was produced *post mortem* during the preparation of the body. Consequently the peritoneum of the recto-uterine pouch does not extend on to the vagina. The uterus is less anteflexed than is usual.

4.83

partments. Hold the upper margin of each broad ligament between the finger and thumb. You will be able to feel the **uterine tube** [Fig. 4.75], which you can follow medially to the upper part of the uterus. Follow the tube laterally, and it will lead to the **ovary,** which you may find lying in a small fossa on the lateral pelvic wall. At the lateral extremity of the tube you will see a circular fringe formed by the **fimbriae of the tube** [Fig. 4.76]. Within it is a small opening called the **abdominal opening of the uterine tube,** which opens into the pelvic cavity. The fimbriae are extensions of the mucous coat, covered by loose fibromuscular tissue and peritoneum.

The ovary [Fig. 4.76]

Now examine the ovary. The ovaries correspond to the testes in the male. You will see that each is oval in shape, grey in colour, and that its surface is irregular and scarred. Each is about 2.5 cm long, 2 cm broad, and 1.2 cm thick. The older the cadaver you are dissecting, the smaller will be the ovary. In women who have not borne children the ovary lies with its long axis more in the vertical than in the horizontal plane.

During pregnancy the ovary rises with the uterus into the abdominal cavity, and it may never regain its former position. In women who have borne several children you may find the ovaries lying transversely in the recto-uterine pouch. Closely examine the place where the ovary normally lies.

You will see that it is situated immediately below the bifurcation of the common iliac artery, with the ureter immediately behind it.

The attachments of the ovary [Fig. 4.76]

Examine the anterior aspect of the ovary. You will see that it is attached to the posterior layer of the broad ligament by a short fold of peritoneum. This is called the **mesovarium.** Examine the **tubal end** of the ovary. You will see that it is attached to the lateral pelvic wall by a peritoneal fold, called the **suspensory ligament of the ovary.** Find the **uterine end** of the ovary. You will see that this is attached to the lateral border of the uterus by a rounded cord called the **ligament of the ovary,** which you should follow as it runs within the broad ligament [see Fig. 4.76].

If you examine the fimbriae of the uterine tube, you will find that they are more closely related to the medial than to the lateral surface of the ovary. Look at the lateral surface of the ovary, and you will see that it is in contact with the lateral pelvic wall. When the vermiform appendix extends into the pelvis, it is likely to be in direct contact with the right ovary and tube.

The blood supply of the ovary [Fig. 4.86]

The ovary receives its blood supply from a long, slender branch of the abdominal aorta called the **ovarian artery,** and

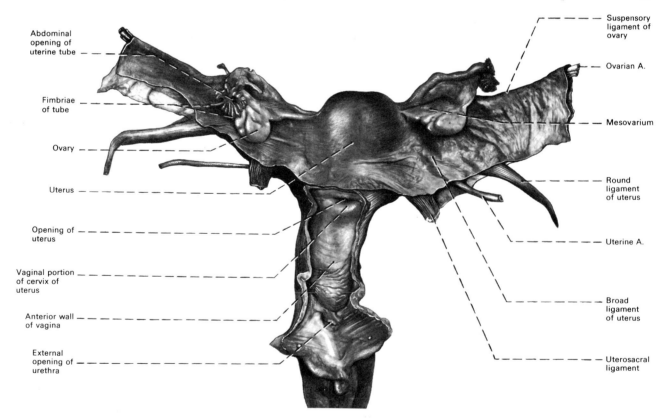

Fig. 4.76 Posterior view of the female genital organs. The posterior wall of the vagina has been excised.

4.84

also from branches of the **uterine artery** which pass to it through the broad ligament. You have seen that the ovarian artery arises from the aorta immediately below the renal artery. This intra-abdominal origin of the vessel reflects the fact that the ovary develops from cells which originate high up on the posterior abdominal wall. Remember that the **right ovarian vein** drains into the inferior vena cava and the **left ovarian vein** into the left renal vein. The ovary is also drained by the **uterine venous plexus.**

Carefully dissect the suspensory ligament of the ovary, and find the ovarian vessels between its two layers [Fig. 4.76]. Trace the ovarian artery towards its proximal part, which you have already dissected. Now trace the distal part into the broad ligament and follow it into the mesovarium, and so into the **hilum of the ovary.** In a well-injected subject it may be possible to see that branches of the ovarian artery also pass to the uterine tube [Fig. 4.86].

The round ligament of the uterus [Fig. 4.76]

On the antero-lateral surface of the uterus, in front of the uterine attachment of the ovarian ligament, you will find the medial end of the round ligament of the uterus. Dissect away the peritoneum of the anterior surface of the broad ligament to expose this ligament, and trace it as far as the abdominal wall. You will find that it hooks round the inferior epigastric artery at the deep inguinal ring, and enters the inguinal canal. From here it has already been traced through the inguinal canal into the labium majus [Fig. 4.5]. The round ligament is a fibromuscular cord, and with its fellow of the opposite side, it keeps the uterus tilted forwards.

Dissect away the peritoneum from the vesico-uterine and recto-uterine pouches and from the side walls of the pelvis.

The cervix of the uterus [Figs 4.75 and 4.76]

In order to get a clear idea of the way the cervix of the uterus is held in the pelvic diaphragm, it is helpful to pass a finger into the vagina and to feel at its upper end for the **vaginal portion** of the neck, or cervix, of the uterus. At the same time, with your other hand hold the lower part of the uterus within the pelvis. The cervix projects as a knob into the vagina. On the rounded end of the cervix you may be able to feel a small, depressed aperture of irregular shape. This is the **opening of the uterus,** through which the cavity of the uterus communicates with the vagina.

The fornix of the vagina [Fig. 4.75]

The circular recess at the upper end of the vagina, between its walls and the vaginal portion of the cervix, is called the fornix of the vagina. For descriptive purposes the fornix is usually divided into anterior, posterior, and lateral fornices. Pass your finger in front of the cervix and explore the anterior vaginal fornix [Fig. 4.75]. Your finger will be lying behind the bladder and the commencement of the urethra.

Now move your finger into the lateral fornix at the side of the cervix. By pushing laterally you may just be able to feel the ureter. Finally, explore the posterior vaginal fornix behind the cervix. This is the largest of the fornices. If you push your finger backwards it will come into contact with the recto-uterine pouch of peritoneum, the sigmoid colon, and behind the latter the rectum and sacrum.

Dissection of the iliac fossae

You have already removed the abdominal part of the left psoas major muscle from the cadaver. Now clear away any fascia that may remain on the right psoas major and clean the iliacus muscle on both sides, noting that it arises from most of the pelvic surface of the ala of the ilium [Fig. 4.77]. On the undissected side note again that the femoral nerve lies in the angle between the psoas major and iliacus muscles, medial to the lateral cutaneous nerve of the thigh.

Clean the external iliac vessels, removing any lymph nodes which lie on either side of them, and trace these vessels as far as the inguinal ligament, below which they descend into the thigh as the femoral vessels.

Dissection of the ureter in the male [Fig. 4.77]

Identify the ureter in the abdomen, and as you trace it downwards and forwards, note that it lies, deep to the peritoneum, on the bifurcation of the common iliac artery and anterior to the internal iliac artery. Strip away any peritoneum and fascia by which it may still be covered, and trace the ureter as it descends in front of the internal iliac artery. Clean the latter vessel, but do not follow its branches at this stage. You will see that the ureter turns medially when it reaches the pelvic diaphragm. Follow it forwards, and you will find that it terminates by joining the lateral angle of the fundus of the bladder.

The ductus deferens and the seminal vesicle

Isolate the ductus deferens at the deep inguinal ring, and trace it as it crosses the anterior aspect of the lateral pelvic wall. Clean and follow it to the posterior aspect of the bladder, on the medial side of a slightly lobulated structure called the seminal vesicle [Fig. 4.83]. This organ varies in size, but is usually about 4 to 5 cm long and about 1 cm wide.

Dissection of the ureter and uterine artery in the female

The ureter

Identify and dissect the ureter in the same way as in the male cadaver. You will find that the ureter lies immediately behind the ovary, within the bifurcation of the common iliac artery, and anterior to the internal iliac artery. Follow the ureter through the pelvic extraperitoneal tissue, clearing

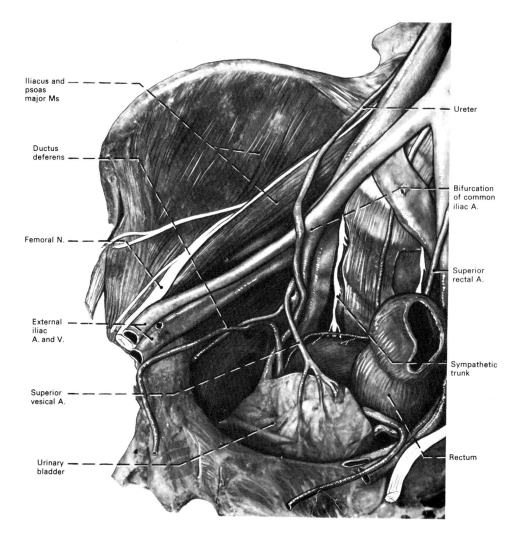

Iliacus and
psoas
major Ms

Ductus
deferens

Femoral N.

External
iliac
A. and V.

Superior
vesical A.

Urinary
bladder

Ureter

Bifurcation
of common
iliac A.

Superior
rectal A.

Sympathetic
trunk

Rectum

Fig. 4.77 The contents of the pelvis in the male.

away the latter as necessary, and note that at the level of
the ischial spine the ureter passes beneath the base of the
broad ligament. Dissect carefully at this point, and clean
an artery which you will find passing above the ureter, where
it lies close to the lateral vaginal fornix. This is the uterine
artery. Next trace the ureter forwards into the bladder, and
note that in this part of its course one or both ureters, more
frequently the left, may come to lie in front of the upper
part of the vagina.

The uterine artery [Fig. 4.86]

Now trace the uterine artery to its origin, which varies from
body to body. As you dissect it towards the pelvic wall, you
will find that it arises either directly from the internal iliac
artery, or from a common trunk, together with other pelvic
branches of the artery. Remove enough of the broad ligament on one side to enable you to trace the artery to its
termination. You will find that the uterine artery passes
vertically upwards along the lateral margin of the uterus to-

wards the medial end of the uterine tube. If your cadaver
is well injected, you may also find that some of its branches
anastomose with branches of the ovarian artery. Notice that
the uterine artery is very tortuous.

The internal iliac artery

Return to the internal iliac artery [Fig. 4.78] on the right
side of the pelvis, and clean as many of its branches as you
can as they pass forwards on the lateral pelvic wall, removing the accompanying veins as you do so. From above
downwards on the lateral wall of the pelvis you should see:

1. The obliterated part of the **umbilical artery** which, as the
   lateral umbilical ligament, passes obliquely upwards
   across the linea terminalis of the pelvis into the medial
   umbilical fold of peritoneum, and towards the umbilicus.
   Branches from the proximal and patent part of the
   umbilical artery, called the **superior vesical arteries,** may
   be found passing to the bladder.

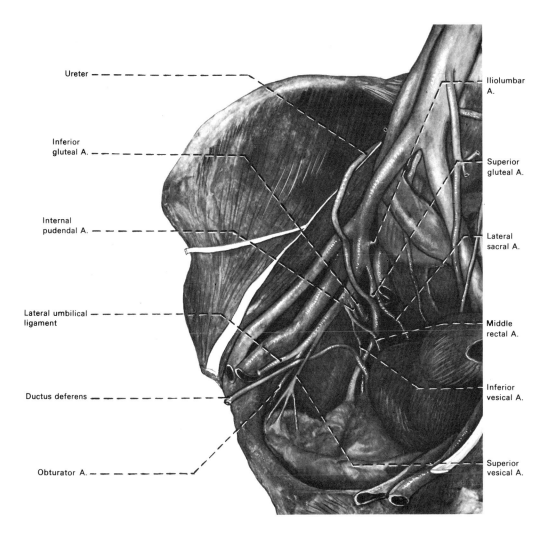

Ureter

Inferior gluteal A.

Internal pudendal A.

Lateral umbilical ligament

Ductus deferens

Obturator A.

Iliolumbar A.

Superior gluteal A.

Lateral sacral A.

Middle rectal A.

Inferior vesical A.

Superior vesical A.

Fig. 4.78 The right internal iliac artery. The bladder and rectum have been displaced to the left.

2. The obturator nerve and the **obturator artery** and vein. These follow a horizontal course, closely applied to the pelvic wall, and pass through the obturator foramen. To refresh your memory, follow the nerve upwards, out of the pelvis, to its origin from the lumbar plexus.
3. In the male, the **inferior vesical artery** to the bladder, or in the female, the **vaginal artery.**
4. In the female, the **uterine artery.**
5. The **middle rectal artery.**

Trace these vessels as far as possible to their terminations on the pelvic organs which they supply. If this proves difficult do not persist, as the vessels can be followed more easily after the right hip-bone has been removed.

Note again that the origin of all these vessels varies greatly from cadaver to cadaver. Both the uterine artery, from which the vaginal artery often arises, and the inferior vesical artery, may originate from almost any other of these branches of the internal iliac artery. Frequently all of them arise from a common stem, called the **anterior division** of

the internal iliac artery. The two terminal branches of this division of the internal iliac artery are the **inferior gluteal artery** and the **internal pudendal artery,** both of which you have already seen as they left the pelvis through the lower part of the greater sciatic foramen [p. 2.11]. Their course in the pelvis will be more easily seen when the hip-bone is removed.

When an anterior division of the internal iliac artery is clearly defined, there will also be a short **posterior division,** closely applied to the pelvic wall. Clean this division and trace its branches (which otherwise arise in variable fashion). They are:

1. The **iliolumbar artery,** which runs obliquely upwards deep to the psoas major muscle to enter the iliacus muscle, which it supplies.
2. The **lateral sacral arteries,** which pass to the pelvic sacral foramina.
3. The **superior gluteal artery,** the largest branch of the posterior division, which passes above the piriformis muscle

through the greater sciatic foramen into the buttock [p. 2.11].

The superior surface of the pelvic diaphragm

Lining the lateral pelvic wall deep to (i.e. lateral to) the branches of the internal iliac artery, is the obturator internus muscle, covered by a pelvic fascia. Clean the fascia but do not remove it.

You will be able to see only as much of the superior part of the obturator internus muscle as is not covered by the levator ani muscle and the fascia on its superior surface (the **superior fascia of the pelvic diaphragm**). If you pull the pelvic organs away from the pelvic wall, and so stretch the levator ani muscle, you will be able to see that its lateral attachment is curved and often prolonged upwards on to the side wall of the pelvis by a thin aponeurosis which joins the fascia covering the obturator internus.

When the aponeurosis is only slightly developed, its upper border is called the **tendinous arch of the levator ani,** from which the fibres of the muscle pass medially, downwards, and posteriorly to form a major part of the pelvic diaphragm [Fig. 4.89].

The fascia covering the aponeurosis and muscle fibres of the levator ani is, as previously noted, the superior fascia of the pelvic diaphragm. This fascia is thickened along a line which passes from the pubic bone to the ischial spine and is called the **tendinous arch of the pelvic fascia.** Since the superior limit reached by the muscle fibres of the levator ani varies in different individuals, it is difficult to be precise about the level of the tendinous arch of the levator ani relative to that of the pelvic fascia.

Removal of the right hip-bone

When you have dissected the structures on the right lateral wall of the pelvis, you should remove the right hip-bone so as to make subsequent dissection easier.

Begin by pushing the bladder backwards from the pubes, and thus expose the **retropubic space** filled with fat, lying between the bladder and the anterior wall of the pelvis. Next examine the **pubic symphysis.** The opposed surfaces of the pubic bones are connected by the **interpubic disc.** Above, the two bones are joined by the **superior pubic ligament,** and below by the **arcuate ligament of the pubis** [Fig. 4.8]. Cut through the interpubic disc with your scalpel. Then divide:

1. The right external iliac vessels midway between their origins and the inguinal ligament.
2. The right ductus deferens and the right testicular artery (or, in the female, the round ligament of the uterus) at the deep inguinal ring.
3. The right obturator nerve and vessels at the obturator canal.

4. The right psoas major and minor muscles, as well as the femoral nerve, the lateral cutaneous nerve of the thigh, and the genitofemoral nerve, near the linea terminalis.

On the right side incise the pelvic fascia along the linea terminalis, and posteriorly along the inferior margin of the greater sciatic notch. Push the pelvic contents and the right levator ani muscle away from the right pelvic wall, towards the midline of the pelvis. Using a scalpel, separate the most anterior fibres of the levator ani muscle from the back of the right pubic bone (close to the bone). The obturator internus muscle is now completely exposed on the right side. You can already see that it arises from the medial surface of the inferior ramus of the pubis, from the ramus of the ischium, from the obturator membrane, and from the bone above, behind and in front of the obturator foramen [Fig. 4.80].

The sacroiliac joint [Figs 4.79 and 4.80]

You should now examine the vertebropelvic ligaments and the right sacroiliac joint, which belongs to the category of plane synovial joints. Feel for the transverse process of the fifth lumbar vertebra and the adjacent part of the iliac crest. Clean this region and examine the **iliolumbar ligament** which spans this gap, and which gives origin to part of the quadratus lumborum muscle. Next clean the anterior part of the sacroiliac region and note the **ventral sacroiliac ligaments** which cover the anterior and inferior surfaces of the joint. Now lift the upper cut ends of the right psoas

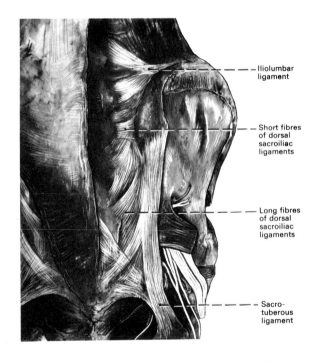

Fig. 4.79 The posterior aspect of the right sacroiliac joint.

Iliolumbar ligament

Short fibres of dorsal sacroiliac ligaments

Long fibres of dorsal sacroiliac ligaments

Sacro-tuberous ligament

muscle(s) and pull the medial part of the iliacus muscle later-ally in order to expose this region. You will also find certain ligamentous fibres, from the iliolumbar ligament, passing downwards from the lower border of the fifth lumbar trans-verse process to blend with the ventral sacroiliac ligaments.

Turn the body over on to its face. Then clean and define the **sacrotuberous ligament** [Fig. 4.79]. Note that below and laterally it is attached to the medial margin of the ischial tuberosity. Above and medially it is attached, from above downwards, to the posterior iliac spines, to the adjacent sur-face of the sacrum, and to the lateral margin of the lower part of the sacrum and the upper part of the coccyx. Remove the ligament from its lateral attachment and reflect it medi-ally, taking care not to damage the underlying structures. Now examine the **sacrospinous ligament,** and note that later-ally it is attached to the ischial spine and medially to the lateral margins of the sacrum and coccyx. In front it blends with the coccygeus muscle. Cut the ligament and the muscle from their spinous attachments.

With the handle of your scalpel, make sure that the right piriformis muscle, the right sciatic nerve, the right superior and inferior gluteal vessels and the right pudendal nerve and internal pudendal vessels are no longer attached by fascia, either to the hip-bone or to neighbouring muscles. Now free the thoracolumbar fascia and the muscles from the posterior aspect of the sacroiliac region and pull them medially. Next identify the **dorsal sacroiliac ligaments,** which pass from the lateral part of the sacrum to the posterior superior iliac spine. The lower fibres are long, and the upper ones short.

Deep to the dorsal sacroiliac ligaments are the **interosseous sacroiliac ligaments.** These are the main bond between the sacrum and ilium. The ligaments are some of the strongest in the body, and lie in a depression behind and above the joint cavity. Cut the dorsal and interosseous sacroiliac liga-ments along a vertical line and as deeply as possible.

Turn the body on to its back and sever the ventral sacro-iliac ligaments. Cut the iliolumbar ligament together with the lower fibres of the quadratus lumborum muscle from the iliac crest. Now try to wrench the hip-bone from the sacrum. In elderly people the sacroiliac joint is usually fused (ankylosed), and it may be necessary to cut through it with a saw. If you have been able to wrench the two bones apart, look at the **auricular surfaces** of the sacrum and ilium [Fig. 4.80]. These contain irregularities that fit into one another and so make the joint more stable.

The downward, inward, and rotatory pressure to which the sacrum is subjected by the weight of the body is offset by the mechanical arrangement of the ligaments and the set-ting of the two sacroiliac joints.

Take the opportunity to examine the obturator internus muscle and the obturator canal on the separated hip-bone, and the right levator ani muscle on the body. On the left side of the cadaver clean and examine the internal iliac artery and its branches. Re-identify the main structures which you can see, now that the right hip-bone has been removed [Fig. 4.81].

Dissection of the urogenital organs in the male

You must now remove, in one piece, the urinary bladder, the seminal vesicles, the two ductus deferens, the prostate, the ureters, and the kidneys [Fig. 4.82]. Before starting, note the following. At the neck of the bladder, where it is applied to the pelvic diaphragm, is a firm pyramidal organ, with its base applied to the neck of the bladder and its apex to the pelvic diaphragm. This is called the **prostate** [Fig. 4.74]. You saw its apex when you were dissecting the perineum [Fig. 4.9]. Connected with this organ and passing upwards behind the bladder and beneath the peritoneum are the two **seminal vesicles** [Fig. 4.83].

In order to remove these structures from the pelvic and abdominal cavities, divide the blood vessels to the bladder close to their origins from both internal iliac arteries, noting as you do so that the superior vesical arteries supply the upper part of the bladder, and that the inferior vesical arteries are distributed to the fundus and neck of the bladder and the proximal part of the urethra [Fig. 4.78]. As you have already seen, both these vessels arise from the anterior division of the internal iliac artery, when the artery divides into two divisions [p. 4.87]. Now cut the peritoneal reflection between the rectum and bladder. Divide the left ductus deferens at the deep inguinal ring, and also the renal vessels.

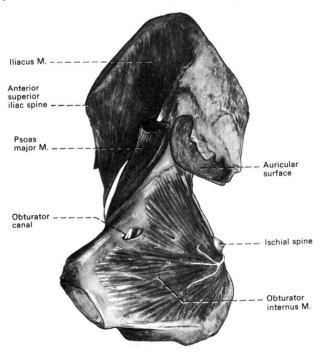

Fig. 4.80 Medial aspect of the right hip-bone (as seen when removed from the cadaver).

Iliacus M.

Anterior superior iliac spine

Psoas major M.

Auricular surface

Obturator canal

Ischial spine

Obturator internus M.

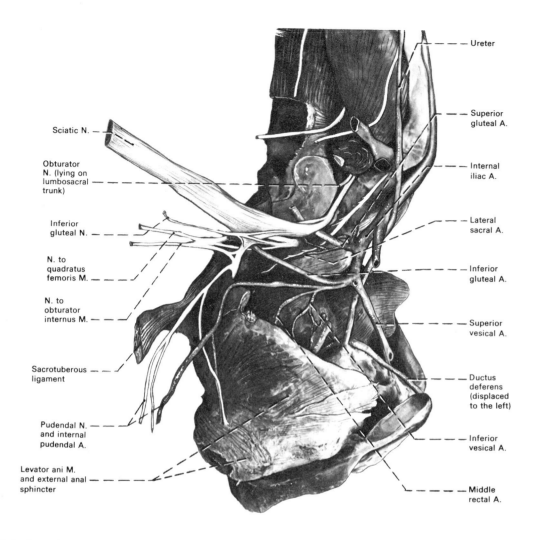

Sciatic N.

Obturator
N. (lying on
lumbosacral
trunk)

Inferior
gluteal N.

N. to
quadratus
femoris M.

N. to
obturator
internus M.

Sacrotuberous
ligament

Pudendal N.
and internal
pudendal A.

Levator ani M.
and external anal
sphincter

Ureter

Superior
gluteal A.

Internal
iliac A.

Lateral
sacral A.

Inferior
gluteal A.

Superior
vesical A.

Ductus
deferens
(displaced
to the left)

Inferior
vesical A.

Middle
rectal A.

Fig. 4.81 The right lateral aspect of the male pelvis after removal of the right hip-bone. The sciatic nerve and some other branches of the sacral plexus are displaced upwards.

The pelvic connective tissue

Before removing the prostate and bladder from the pelvic diaphragm, try to obtain a general picture of the **pelvic fascia** and connective tissue, which extends down to the pelvic diaphragm, and which is continuous with the extraperitoneal tissue, that lies deep to the peritoneum of the abdomen. The pelvic connective tissue surrounds and serves as a padding for all the organs in the pelvic cavity, at the same time as it blends with the fascia which covers the obturator internus muscles laterally, the piriformis muscles on the posterior pelvic wall, and the two levator ani muscles and the smaller coccygeus muscles, which together form the pelvic diaphragm below.

The fascia on these muscles is called the **parietal pelvic fascia,** and that which covers the pelvic organs the **visceral pelvic fascia.**

At certain places condensations of the pelvic connective tissue and pelvic fascia, reinforced by smooth muscle fibres,

form the 'ligaments' of the pelvic diaphragm. These are better marked in the female than male body.

To verify some of these points, push the left side of the bladder off the fascia covering the pelvic diaphragm. Do this with your fingers. You will find that the prostate is enclosed in a strong capsule of fibrous tissue. This capsule blends with condensations of the pelvic connective tissue which form weak ligaments that hold the prostate and neck of the bladder to the pubic bones in front, and to the pelvic walls at the sides. Try to define the left **puboprostatic ligament** connecting the prostatic capsule with the pubis, and the left lateral ligament of the bladder passing laterally. (In the female the puboprostatic ligament is represented by a corresponding **pubovesical ligament.**) Having defined the ligaments, divide both close to the prostate. Then push and lift the bladder off the pelvic diaphragm, working on both sides, and with your fingers shell the prostate out of the dense **fascial sheath of the prostate.** The urethra, which traverses the gland, was divided on the external surface of the pelvic diaphragm during the dissection of the perineum. The prostate comes away cleanly, but its fascial sheath is left behind.

When you have completed this operation and removed the organs from the pelvis and abdominal cavity, you can start examining each in turn [Fig. 4.82]. Begin by cleaning the fascia from the bladder wall, and particularly from the point where the latter is entered by the ureters. Note the

plexus of veins that lies between the neck of the bladder and the prostate. Trace the vesical arteries into the bladder wall and then clean the seminal vesicles and the terminal parts of the two ductus deferens which lie between the vesicles.

The seminal vesicle [Fig. 4.83]

You will see that each seminal vesicle is a nodular body about 5 cm long which lies behind the fundus of the bladder and between it and the rectum. Remove the tough fascial capsule by which it is surrounded. You will see that the seminal vesicle consists of a coiled tube which gives off several diverticula. Later you will find that its duct unites with the ductus deferens to form a common duct, called the **ejaculatory duct,** which passes through the posterior wall of the prostate to open within the prostatic part of the urethra.

The urinary bladder [Figs 4.74, 4.82, and 4.83]

Now examine the urinary bladder, which is a hollow muscular organ lined by a mucous coat. The muscle wall is composed of plain muscle fibres, separated by very loose submucous tissue from the mucous coat, which is thrown into a series of folds when the bladder is empty, except over the trigone of the bladder.

Replace the bladder in the pelvis and note its relations [Fig. 4.74]. It lies immediately in front of the rectum, and when empty, behind the pubic bones. As it fills it rises above the linea terminalis, in the space between the transversalis fascia and the peritoneum.

Remove the bladder from the pelvis, and note that it is shaped rather like an inverted pyramid. Look at the anterior limit or **apex** of its superior surface [Fig. 4.82], to which there may still be attached the remains of the **median umbilical ligament** (the vestige of the foetal **urachus).** Note that

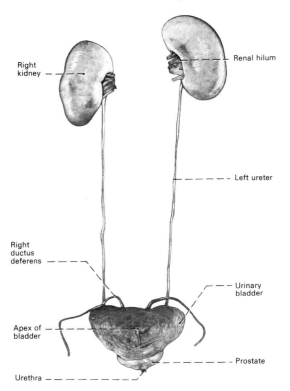

Right kidney

Renal hilum

Left ureter

Right ductus deferens

Urinary bladder

Apex of bladder

Prostate

Urethra

Fig. 4.82 The male urinary organs.

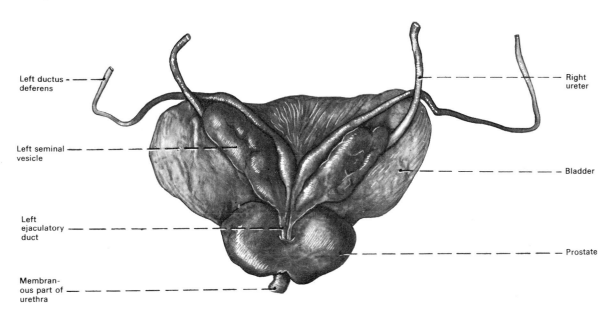

Left ductus deferens

Right ureter

Left seminal vesicle

Bladder

Left ejaculatory duct

Prostate

Membranous part of urethra

Fig. 4.83 The seminal vesicles and the prostate.

the **fundus** of the bladder, which is directed backwards and slightly downwards, is separated from the rectum by the two ductus deferens and the two seminal vesicles [Fig. 4.83]. The inferior part of the bladder, called the **neck,** is continuous with the urethra and rests upon the prostate.

Look again at the superior surface of the bladder. It is flat or concave when the bladder is empty, but becomes rounded or convex as the organ fills. You have already noted [p. 4.82] that the superior surface of the bladder is covered by peritoneum and that it is often in contact with coils of the small intestine. Look at the two infero-lateral surfaces, below the superior surface and in front of the fundus. Again replacing the bladder in the pelvis, you will see that these surfaces are in contact anteriorly with the fat which lies in the retropubic space. As you have seen, this potential space lies between the pubes and the bladder and is filled in by fatty extraperitoneal tissue. You can see that the bladder rests on the pelvic diaphragm, and that the obliterated parts of the umbilical arteries pass forwards on its lateral aspects on their way to the umbilicus, as the lateral umbilical ligaments [Fig. 4.78]. An important point which you should note now is that in the child the bladder lies mainly above the pubic symphysis and in contact with the anterior abdominal wall.

The interior of the urinary bladder [Fig. 4.84]

Now make a wide opening in the bladder, using a cruciate incision with its centre at the apex of the bladder. You will see that in the empty state the mucosa of the bladder is wrinkled, except for a smooth triangular area at the fundus, known as the **trigone of the bladder** [Fig. 4.84]. Here the mucous coat is tense and adherent to the muscle wall. In life the mucosa is pink in colour, due to the presence of many blood vessels.

Look at the angles of the trigone. Each of the upper angles is formed by the **opening of the ureter,** and the apex below is formed by the **internal opening of the urethra.** Immediately above the urethral opening you may see an elevation called the **uvula vesicae** caused by the middle lobe of the prostate.

The ureters pass through the bladder wall obliquely, and in so doing make a ridge in the mucous coat for a short distance on the lateral side of each ureteric opening. As the pressure rises in the bladder with the accumulation of urine, the distal ends of the ureters in the bladder wall are compressed, and in this way urine is prevented from flowing back up the ureters towards the kidney.

It is possible that you may see another ridge joining the two ureteric orifices. This ridge, which is called the **inter-ureteric fold,** is formed by a band of plain muscle fibres. Sometimes the lateral boundaries of the trigone, between the ureteric openings and the urethra, are demarcated by yet another line of muscle fibres which continue through the urethral orifice to merge with the longitudinal muscle fibres of the posterior wall of the urethra. Both the neck of the

bladder and the beginning of the urethra have a sphincter, the **vesical sphincter.** This is formed by a reduplication of the circular muscle fibres of the bladder wall around the internal urethral opening.

The prostate [Fig. 4.83]

Now examine the prostate, which, like the seminal vesicles, is present only in the male. In a normal healthy adult it is chestnut-shaped and has smooth surfaces. It varies greatly in size, but on average its **base** measures about 3×2 cm, and its length from the base to the **apex** 2 cm. In old men it may be much larger and nodular. The base is applied to the neck of the bladder [Fig. 4.83]. In its original position in the body the apex projected through the interval between the medial margins of the two levator ani muscles on to the fascia covering the superior surface of the muscles within the deep perineal space [Fig. 4.9].

Look at the posterior surface of the prostate. You will see that the upper part of this surface is perforated by the ejaculatory ducts, each of which is formed by the union of the duct which emerges from the apex of the seminal vesicle with the corresponding ductus deferens. The ejaculatory ducts traverse the prostate and open into the prostatic part of the urethra.

The smooth anterior part of the prostate is divided by a rounded anterior border into two infero-lateral surfaces.

The prostatic part of the urethra

Now open the prostatic part of the urethra by a median incision through the rounded anterior border of the gland.

Examine the central ridge on the posterior wall of the urethra. It is known as the **urethral crest.** On this crest you will see an elevation called the **colliculus seminalis** [Fig. 4.84]. In the centre you will find a small opening, into which you should try to insert a fine probe. You will find that it enters a blind diverticulum about 5 mm long, known as the **prostatic utricle.** This corresponds embryologically to the uterus and vagina in the female.

At the sides of the mouth of the prostatic utricle, on the urethral crest, you will find the slit-like openings of the ejaculatory ducts. On either side of the crest itself you will see a depression known as the **prostatic sinus** [Fig. 4.84]. Into it open the mouths of the glands which ramify in the fibro-muscular tissue that makes up the matrix of the prostate.

The part of the prostate which lies above the openings of the ejaculatory ducts is called the **middle lobe,** and, as you may have seen, forms the uvula vesicae.

The capsules of the prostate

The prostate has two capsules. You have already seen the outer one, which is called the **fascial sheath of the prostate** (or 'false capsule'), and which is formed by the pelvic fascia. It was left in the pelvis when you removed the organ. The inner **capsule of the prostate** is formed by a condensation

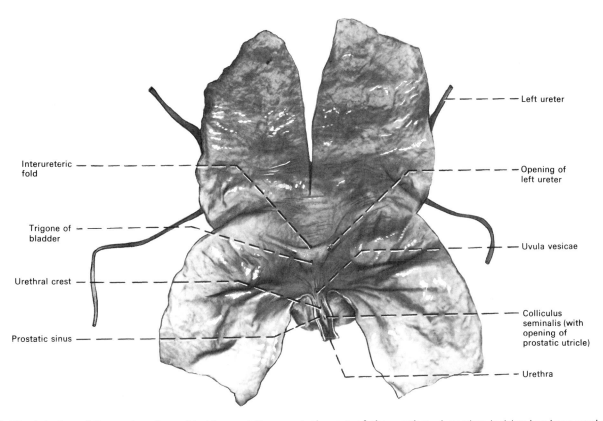

Left ureter

Interureteric fold

Opening of left ureter

Trigone of bladder

Uvula vesicae

Urethral crest

Colliculus seminalis (with opening of prostatic utricle)

Prostatic sinus

Urethra

Fig. 4.84 The interior of the male urinary bladder and the prostatic part of the urethra. A cruciate incision has been used to open the bladder, which is viewed from the front.

of fibrous tissue on the surface of the prostate itself. Try to establish its presence.

The space between the capsule and the sheath is filled by the **prostatic venous plexus** which, in addition to draining the prostate, also drains the external genitalia. The anterior fibres of the levator ani muscles are closely applied to the fascial sheath of the prostate, and so help support the gland.

The ductus deferens [Fig. 4.83]

Now examine the structures on the posterior aspect of the bladder and prostate, and note that in this position the ureter crosses behind the ductus deferens, as the ductus deferens descends on the medial aspect of the seminal vesicle [Fig. 4.83]. Note that near its termination the ductus deferens is dilated. The dilatation is called the **ampulla of the ductus deferens.** Using scissors, open the seminal vesicles and note their lobulated appearance.

Dissection of the urogenital organs in the female

You have already dissected away the peritoneum of the recto-uterine pouch [Figs 4.40 and 4.75]. By blunt dissection separate the rectum from the vagina, and note the plane in which the long axis of the vagina lies. Separate the bladder from the pelvic diaphragm with your fingers. Then, pulling the bladder away from the pelvic diaphragm, divide the urethra. Next divide the vagina, also close to the pelvic dia-

phragm. Having refreshed your memory about the origin of the uterine, vesical, vaginal, and ovarian arteries [pp. 4.84–4.87], divide them close to their origins. Clean and follow the vaginal artery as it runs forward on the pelvic diaphragm to supply the vagina. You will see that it sends branches both to the lower part of the bladder and to the rectum.

Completely strip the suspensory ligament of the ovary from the lateral wall of the pelvis [Fig. 4.85]. By pushing downwards gently with your fingers, separate the lateral attachments of the broad ligaments from the walls of the pelvis until you come to the pelvic diaphragm. Using scissors, completely separate the ligaments from the pelvic wall. When you reach the pelvic diaphragm, continue to strip the peritoneum in a medial direction, if necessary incising the base of the broad ligament so as to free it completely from the pelvic diaphragm. Be careful not to damage the ureters as they pass beneath the ligament to the side of the lateral fornices of the vagina on their way to the bladder.

The ligaments of the uterus [Fig. 4.85]

As you do this dissection, note an important series of condensations of fibrous tissue and muscle fibres in the parietal and visceral pelvic fascia which radiate from the cervix of the uterus and the vault of the vagina as 'ligaments' which support and fix the cervix of the uterus. They are:

1. The **pubocervical ligaments.** Parts of this condensation of fibrous tissue, which pass forwards to the pubes, are

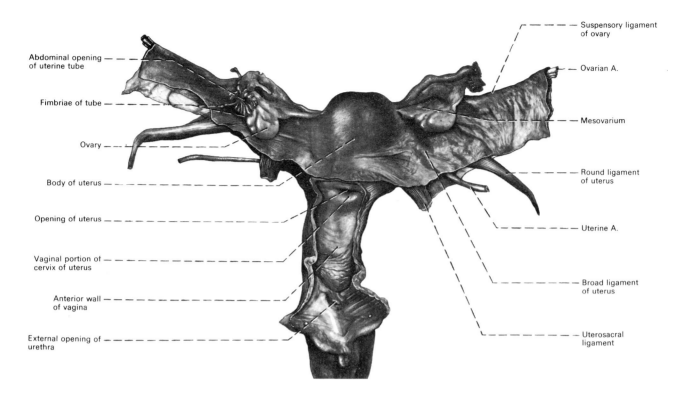

Abdominal opening
of uterine tube

Fimbriae of tube

Ovary

Body of uterus

Opening of uterus

Vaginal portion of
cervix of uterus

Anterior wall
of vagina

External opening of
urethra

Suspensory ligament
of ovary

Ovarian A.

Mesovarium

Round ligament
of uterus

Uterine A.

Broad ligament
of uterus

Uterosacral
ligament

Fig. 4.85 Posterior view of the female genital organs. The posterior wall of the vagina has been excised.

attached to the neck of the bladder and constitute the **pubovesical ligaments** [see p. 4.90].

2. The **transverse ligaments of the cervix,** which pass laterally to the lateral pelvic walls (usually two or three strands).

3. The **uterosacral ligaments** [Fig. 4.85], which pass posteriorly to the rectum and lateral border of the sacrum, sometimes reaching as high as the promontory. Their muscle fibres are called the **recto-uterine muscles,** and they are covered by the **recto-uterine folds** of the peritoneum.

These folds form the upper lateral boundaries of the recto-uterine pouch. The main lymph vessels which drain the cervix of the uterus pass along the ligaments, and beneath the folds, to the internal iliac lymph nodes which lie alongside the internal iliac artery.

Divide the left round ligament of the uterus at the deep inguinal ring, and also the renal vessels. You can now remove the bladder, the uterus, the uterine tubes, the ovaries, the kidneys, and the ureters.

The broad ligaments

First examine what is left of the two broad ligaments of the uterus [Fig. 4.85]. Each consists of a double fold of peritoneum which is reflected as a flap from the lateral border of the uterus to the pelvic wall. The supero-lateral corner of the ligament forms the **suspensory ligament of the ovary,** through which, as you have seen, the ovarian vessels pass to the ovary. At the base of the broad ligament, where the two layers of peritoneum by which it is formed are reflected

anteriorly and posteriorly on to the pelvic diaphragm, extra-peritoneal tissue enters the ligament to form the **para-metrium.** Again study the way the ovary is attached to the posterior layer of the broad ligament by the **mesovarium.** The part of the broad ligament which lies above the meso-varium, and containing the uterine tube, is called the **meso-salpinx.** The part below it is called the **mesometrium.** You will see that the uterine tube lies within the broad ligament, as also do the **round ligament of the uterus,** the **ligament of the ovary,** and the uterine and ovarian vessels, nerves, and lymphatics.

Now clean the distal ends of the ureters as they enter the bladder. Then complete the cleaning of the vesical, the uterine, the vaginal and the ovarian arteries, tracing each to its destination.

The vagina [Fig. 4.85]

Now examine the vagina [Fig. 4.85]. It is a fibromuscular canal lined by a mucous coat, which extends from the **vesti-bule of the vagina** (the cleft between the labia minora) to the uterus. It is about 8 cm long. When you divided it above the pelvic diaphragm you left its lower part in the remains of the perineum.

Open the upper part of the vagina by cutting along one of its lateral borders with scissors, and note that its **anterior** and **posterior walls,** which are normally in apposition, are ridged in the midline, and that transverse folds pass later-ally, forming **rugae.** In transverse section the vagina forms an H-shaped cleft. The posterior wall is longer than the anterior wall. The two levator ani muscles blend with the lateral walls, which are therefore fixed. You can see this if you examine the pelvic diaphragm. Note that the part of the vagina that is still left in the body is adherent to the pelvic diaphragm.

Note, too, that the axis of the vagina passes obliquely upwards and backwards.

The vaginal wall is covered externally by pelvic fascia, and contains a rich venous plexus.

Relations of the vagina

Note the relationship of the upper third of the vagina to the fundus of the bladder, from which it is separated by loose connective tissue [Fig. 4.75]. The lower two-thirds of the vagina are closely applied to the urethra, which you should now dissect from the anterior vaginal wall.

Note how the cervix of the uterus projects into the upper part of the anterior vaginal wall, and that here the two organs are closely bound together by connective tissue. Examine the vaginal portion of the cervix, which is convex in shape. Note the opening of the uterus [Fig. 4.85].

As already observed [p. 4.85], the vaginal portion of the cervix is separated from the upper part of the vaginal wall by the fornix of the vagina. You can now see that the anterior fornix is in contact with the fundus of the bladder and the termination of the ureters, especially the left ureter, and that the lateral fornices are in fairly close relation with the uterine arteries and the ureters. If you consider the relations of the posterior vaginal fornix, you will again be able

to realize that this is in direct relationship with the recto-uterine pouch.

The uterus [Figs 4.85 and 4.86]

Now study the uterus, which in the normal position lies in the pelvis between the bladder and the rectum [Figs 4.40 and 4.75]. It is a pear-shaped organ consisting of four parts. The upper part is called the **fundus** of the uterus [Fig. 4.86], and lies above each uterine opening of the tube. The main part, or **body** of the uterus, lies below the fundus and above an ill-defined **isthmus** of the uterus. The narrow terminal cylindrical part below the isthmus is called the **cervix** of the uterus. In a mature non-pregnant woman, the uterus is about 7.5 cm long, 5 cm wide at the fundus, and its walls are about 2 cm thick. After the menopause the uterus shrinks in size, and as most dissecting-room subjects are elderly people, the cadaver you are dissecting is likely to have a small uterus. The cylindrical cervix, as you have already noted, perforates the upper part of the anterior vaginal wall. The part of the cervix lying above the vagina is called the **supravaginal portion of the cervix,** and the part lying within the vagina is called the **vaginal portion of the cervix.** This ends at the opening of the uterus, which is round in women who have not borne children, but is transverse and often fissured in those who have.

The position of the uterus

The uterus as a whole is tilted forward over the bladder, in a position called anteversion. The body of the uterus itself is normally bent forward at the isthmus. This position is

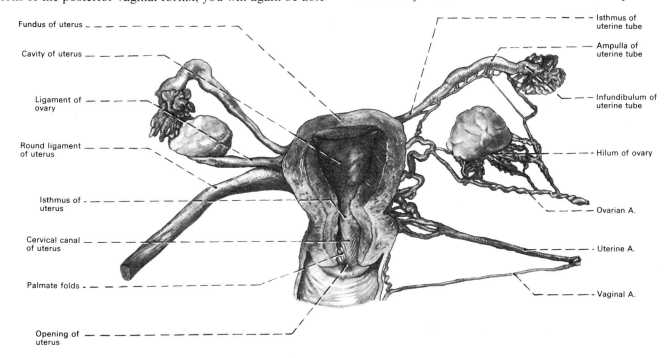

Fundus of uterus

Cavity of uterus

Ligament of ovary

Round ligament of uterus

Isthmus of uterus

Cervical canal of uterus

Palmate folds

Opening of uterus

Isthmus of uterine tube

Ampulla of uterine tube

Infundibulum of uterine tube

Hilum of ovary

Ovarian A.

Uterine A.

Vaginal A.

Fig. 4.86 The interior of the uterus. Part of the posterior walls of the uterus and vagina have been excised. The uterine cavity is much larger than usual.

called anteflexion. You can appreciate, however, that the uterus is movable except at the cervix, where it is fixed in the upper part of the vagina, and that its position will vary with the degree of distension of the adjacent viscera, especially of the bladder on which the uterus lies. The uterus does not usually lie in the midline, but inclines to the right.

Try to realize again that in the undissected body the intestinal (posterior) surface of the uterus, which is more convex than the vesical (anterior) surface, is in relationship with the rectum, from which it may be separated by the sigmoid colon and coils of small intestine lying in the recto-uterine pouch. You have already seen that each lateral border of the uterus is in direct relationship with the uterine vessels, the medial border of the broad ligament, and the parametrium within the ligament [Fig. 4.85].

The interior of the uterus

Now cut the uterus in the coronal plane from the fundus downwards, and note the thickness of the fibromuscular walls [Fig. 4.86].

You will see that the **cavity of the uterus** is triangular, with its base above and its apex below. The cavity is extremely small when compared with the external size of the organ. The apex of the cavity of the body is continuous with the **cervical canal of the uterus** at the level of the isthmus. The cervical canal is fusiform (spindle-shaped), and opens into the vagina at the opening of the uterus. You may see the minute **palmate folds** in its mucous coat.

The uterine tubes [Fig. 4.86]

Now examine the uterine tubes [Fig. 4.86]. Each tube is about 10 cm long, and about 5 mm in diameter. At one end it opens into the cavity of the uterus and at the other into the peritoneal cavity, through the **abdominal opening.** Note again that in the female there is, therefore, a direct communication between the peritoneal cavity and the exterior via the uterine tubes, uterus, and vagina. (Remember that in the male the peritoneal cavity is a closed sac.)

Each uterine tube lies between the two layers of the broad ligament near its superior border [Fig. 4.85]. The tube passes laterally and posteriorly, and its lateral half usually lies in direct contact with the medial surface of its corresponding ovary.

Open the uterine tube throughout its extent, and you will see that its mucous coat is thrown into longitudinal folds which almost obliterate the lumen. Note the fringe of **fimbriae** around the abdominal opening. You may find that one fimbria, larger than the rest, is adherent to the medial surface of the ovary. This is known as the **ovarian fimbria.**

Each uterine tube consists of four parts [Fig. 4.86]. A narrow portion, called the **uterine part,** passes from the uterine cavity into the wall of the uterus. This leads to a straight part called the **isthmus,** which in turn leads to a conspicuously tortuous part called the **ampulla.** The uterine tube fin-

ally ends in the dilated **infundibulum,** which opens at the abdominal opening. The diameter of the lumen of the tube varies from 1 mm in the uterine part to 6 mm in the ampulla and infundibulum.

The urinary bladder [Fig. 4.75]

Examine the urinary bladder. It is a hollow muscular organ lined by a mucous coat. The wall is composed of plain muscle fibres, separated by very loose submucous tissue from the mucous coat, which is drawn into a series of folds when the bladder is empty [Fig. 4.87]. Try to visualize the position which the bladder normally occupies in the pelvis [Fig. 4.75]. It lies immediately in front of the uterus and the upper part of the vagina, and when empty, behind the pubic bones. As it fills it rises above the linea terminalis of the pelvis, between the transversalis fascia and the peritoneum.

Note the shape of the bladder. It is roughly like an inverted pyramid. Look at the anterior limit (or **apex**) of the superior surface, to which there may still be attached the remains of the **median umbilical ligament** [Fig. 4.40] (which is the vestige of the foetal **urachus).** Note that the **fundus** of the bladder is directed backwards and slightly downwards. The inferior part of the bladder, called the **neck,** is continuous with the urethra and rests on the fascia covering the muscles of the deep perineal space.

Look again at the superior surface of the bladder. It is flat or concave when the bladder is empty, but becomes rounded or convex as the organ fills. You have already noted [p. 4.83] that this surface is covered by peritoneum, and that it is often in contact with coils of the small intestine. Look at the two infero-lateral surfaces, below the superior surface and in front of the fundus. If you replace the bladder in the body you will see that these surfaces are in contact anteriorly with the fat which lies in the retropubic space. As you have noted, this potential space lies between the pubes and the bladder. You can see that the bladder rests on the pelvic diaphragm, and that the obliterated parts of the umbilical arteries pass forwards on its lateral aspects to the umbilicus as the lateral umbilical ligaments. Note that in the child the bladder lies mainly above the pubic symphysis, and that it is in contact with the anterior abdominal wall.

The interior of the urinary bladder [Fig. 4.87]

Now open the bladder widely, using a cruciate incision with its centre at the apex of the bladder. You will see that in the empty state the mucosa of the bladder is wrinkled, except for a smooth triangular area at the fundus, which is known as the **trigone of the bladder** [Fig. 4.87]. Here the mucous coat is adherent to the muscle wall. In life the mucous coat is pink in colour, due to the presence of many blood vessels.

Look at the angles of the trigone. Each of the upper angles is formed by the **opening of the ureter,** while the apex below

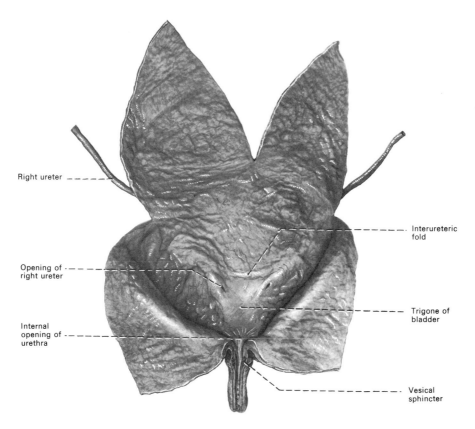

Right ureter

Opening of
right ureter

Internal
opening of
urethra

Interureteric
fold

Trigone of
bladder

Vesical
sphincter

Fig. 4.87 The interior of the female urinary bladder and urethra. A cruciate incision has been used to open the bladder, which is viewed from the front.

is formed by the **internal opening of the urethra.** The ureters pass through the bladder wall obliquely, and in so doing make a ridge in the mucous coat for a short distance on the lateral side of each ureteric opening. As the pressure rises when the bladder fills with urine, the distal ends of the ureters within the bladder wall become compressed, and in this way urine is prevented from passing backwards up the ureter to the kidney.

It is possible that you may see a transverse ridge joining the two ureteric openings. This ridge, which is called the **interureteric fold,** is formed by a band of plain muscle fibres.

Sometimes the lateral boundaries of the trigone are demarcated by yet another line of muscle fibres which join the ureteric openings and the opening of the urethra, and which are continued through the urethral opening, where they merge with the longitudinal muscle fibres of the posterior wall of the urethra.

Both the neck of the bladder and the beginning of the urethra have a sphincter, the **vesical sphincter.** This is formed by a reduplication of the circular muscle fibres of the bladder wall around the internal opening of the urethra.

Before returning to the dissection of the remaining structures of the pelvis, open the part of the female urethra which you have already freed from the anterior vaginal wall.

Its mucous coat is markedly ridged, an indication of the fact that during life the female urethra is very dilatable.

The sigmoid colon and rectum

Dissection of the sigmoid colon

Follow the sigmoid colon [Fig. 4.88], which is the continuation of the descending colon, from its commencement on the medial border of the left psoas major muscle. You will see that it descends on the lateral pelvic wall, then turns to the right across the pelvic cavity. If you visualize the position of the organs you have already removed, you will be able to realize that the sigmoid colon lies between the bladder and rectum in the male, and either on the uterus and the bladder, or between the uterus and rectum in the female. The sigmoid colon may reach as far as the right lateral pelvic wall before sweeping backwards in front of the sacrum, where at the level of the third sacral vertebra it becomes the rectum. Sometimes it forms an ascending loop of variable length. Like all other parts of the large intestine, except the rectum, the sigmoid colon is characterized by **appendices epiploicae** and **taeniae coli.**

You have already dissected the sigmoid mesocolon and its contents [p. 4.82]. Now trace the **superior rectal artery** (the continuation of the inferior mesenteric artery) in the distal part of its course, removing the **superior rectal vein** as you

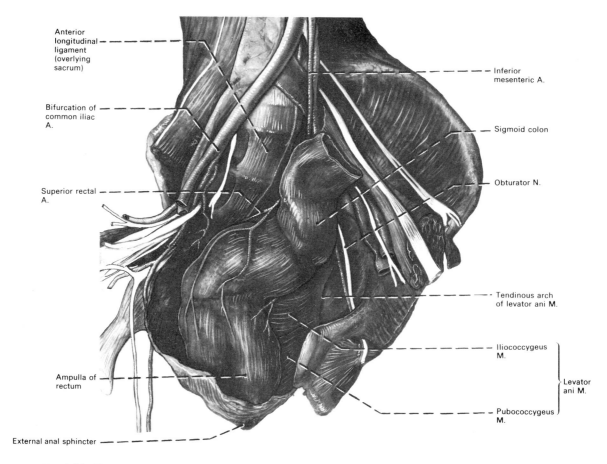

Anterior
longitudinal
ligament
(overlying
sacrum)

Bifurcation of
common iliac
A.

Superior rectal
A.

Ampulla of
rectum

External anal sphincter

Inferior
mesenteric A.

Sigmoid colon

Obturator N.

Tendinous arch
of levator ani M.

Iliococcygeus
M.

Levator
ani M.

Pubococcygeus
M.

Fig. 4.88 The rectum and sigmoid colon. The right hip-bone and the urinary bladder have been removed.

do so. To do this you will have to separate the rectum from the posterior wall of the pelvis. You will see that the vessels pass down on the posterior aspect of the rectum before sinking into the wall of the gut.

Dissection of the rectum

Now examine the rectum [Fig. 4.88] and note its relations. The rectum is about 15 cm long, and begins anterior to the third sacral vertebra as a continuation of the sigmoid colon. You will see that it is devoid of taeniae coli and appendices epiploicae. As the rectum descends in front of the sacrum and coccyx, you will notice that it fits the concavity of these bones, and that just below the tip of the coccyx it bends sharply backwards at the **perineal flexure,** where it becomes the anal canal. You will also see that the lower half of the rectum is ballooned to form the **ampulla of the rectum.** Note that in its upper third the rectum is covered by peritoneum in front and at the sides; that in its middle third it is covered only in front; and that its lower third is devoid of peritoneum. In the male the rectum forms the posterior wall of the rectovesical pouch, and in the female the posterior wall of the recto-uterine pouch [Figs 4.74 and 4.75].

The rectum is not a reservoir for faeces, and is normally empty. Notice that its long axis is curved in the transverse

plane. It first sweeps to the right, then to the left, and finally to the right again. These lateral flexures are of no importance in themselves, but correspond with the three semi-lunar **transverse folds of the rectum** in the rectal wall [Fig. 4.90]. These consist of muscle fibres covered by a mucous coat, and they are not effaced when the rectum is distended. They play a part in controlling the descent of the faeces.

The anal canal

At the tip of the coccyx the rectum runs into the anal canal, which is about 2.5 cm long, and which is directed downwards and backwards to end at the **anus.** The anal canal is guarded by three sphincters; the **internal anal sphincter,** which is a reduplication of circular muscle fibres; the **puborectalis muscle** (part of the levator ani); and the **external anal sphincter,** which you have already dissected [p. 4.8, Figs 4.6 and 4.9]. These three sphincters blend around the lower half of the anal canal.

The blood supply of the sigmoid colon and rectum

Now divide the inferior mesenteric artery [Fig 4.88] near its origin from the aorta, divide the middle rectal artery on either side, and then cut through the rectum or anal canal close to the pelvic diaphragm and as near to the anus as possible. Place the sigmoid colon and rectum in a sink and wash them out. Then incise them down the midline and examine their structure. The transverse folds of the rectum will be obvious either in the detached portion of the gut or in the small part that remains *in situ*. The latter, however, should not be opened until the pelvic diaphragm has been examined.

The blood supply to the lower part of the alimentary canal is derived from the **sigmoid arteries** and the **superior rectal artery** (both of which are branches of the inferior mesenteric artery), the **middle rectal arteries** (branches of the internal iliac arteries), and the **inferior rectal arteries** (branches of the internal pudendal arteries).

The venous drainage is partly by way of the **superior rectal vein** and partly by the **middle rectal veins** and the **inferior rectal veins,** which pass into the systemic system via the internal iliac veins. The superior rectal vein is continued as the inferior mesenteric vein. The latter becomes a tributary of the splenic vein, which drains into the portal vein. The lower end of the anal canal is the most dependent point at which the portal and systemic venous systems meet.

The pelvic diaphragm and anal canal

Dissect away the fascia from the pelvic diaphragm to expose the fibres of the levator ani and coccygeus muscles [Fig. 4.89].

The pelvic diaphragm, as you have already learnt [p. 4.8], is a muscular diaphragm, concave superiorly, which separates the pelvic cavity above from the perineum below. It is formed by the levator ani and coccygeus muscles, and by the pelvic fascia which covers them. At the anterior part of this muscular shelf is a gap that is filled in by the pelvic fascia which lies above the deep perineal space. In the male, as you have already seen, the urethra, when it emerges from the apex of the prostate, passes through this gap into the perineum. In the female the urethra and vagina pass through the fascia which fills the gap.

The levator ani muscle [Fig. 4.89]

Examine the levator ani muscle, which forms the anterior two-thirds of the pelvic diaphragm, and whose inferior surface you dissected when you studied the perineum [pp. 4.8, 4.13, 4.16]. It consists of pubic and iliac parts. Note that the anterior or **pubic part** constantly arises from the pelvic surface of the body of the pubis, and from a linear attachment extending laterally to the obturator canal. This anterior origin is both fleshy and tendinous. The posterior or **iliac part** of the muscle is more variable. Usually it is attached to the lower margin of the obturator canal, the ilium just below the linea terminalis, the inferior margin of the greater sciatic notch and the ischial spine. This iliac part of the muscle is often aponeurotic and poorly developed, or even deficient. In that case you will find that the aponeurotic origin has

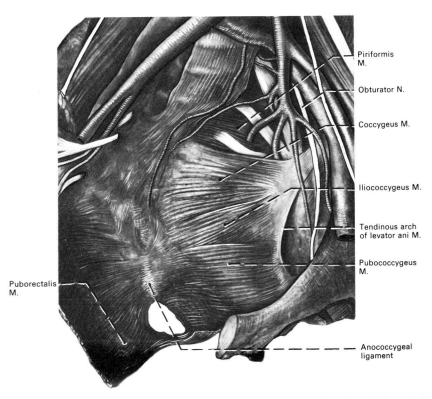

Fig. 4.89 The pelvic diaphragm (as seen when looking towards the left side of the pelvic cavity).
The right hip-bone has been removed.

shrunk to a tendinous band, called the **tendinous arch of the levator ani muscle,** which runs from the pubic part of the muscle to the ischial spine, and which gives rise to a thin layer of muscle fibres [see p. 4.88].

The pubic part of the levator ani muscle is composed of three sets of muscle fibres that run backwards, downwards, and medially: a medial set, called the **levator prostatae muscle** in the male and the **pubovaginalis muscle** in the female; an intermediate set, the **puborectalis muscle;** and a lateral set, the **pubococcygeus muscle** [Fig. 4.89].

If the pelvic viscera were still in place, you would be able to see that in the male the levator prostatae muscle is inserted into the prostate and into the central tendon of the perineum. In the female the pubovaginalis muscle crosses the side of the vagina to reach the central tendon of the perineum. Some of its fibres actually blend with the vaginal wall, and together with fibres from the contralateral muscle form a sphincter for that organ. The puborectalis muscle passes across the side of the rectum to loop around the anorectal junction by joining with its fellow of the opposite side. Some of the fibres of the puborectalis become continuous with the deeper part of the external anal sphincter [Fig. 4.9] and the longitudinal coat of the rectum. The pubococcygeus muscle is inserted into the coccyx and lowest part of the sacrum.

The iliac part of the levator ani muscle is called the **iliococcygeus muscle.** Its fibres pass downwards and medially

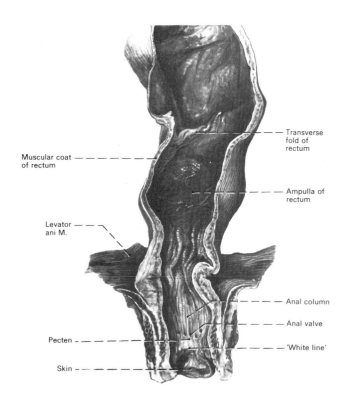

Fig. 4.90 The interior of the rectum and the anal canal.

Transverse fold of rectum

Muscular coat of rectum

Ampulla of rectum

Levator ani M.

Anal column

Anal valve

Pecten

'White line'

Skin

and become inserted into the coccyx. They interweave with those of the iliococcygeus of the opposite side, thus forming the **anococcygeal ligament** in the midline.

The levator ani muscle is innervated by branches of the third and fourth sacral nerves and by the inferior rectal nerves.

Its main functions are to help hold the pelvic viscera in place and increase intra-abdominal pressure.

The coccygeus muscle [Fig. 4.89]

You will see that the posterior part of the pelvic diaphragm is a fan-shaped muscle, called the coccygeus. Its deep posterior surface blends with the sacrospinous ligament. The muscle arises from the pelvic aspect of the ischial spine and is inserted into the lower part of the lateral border of the sacrum and the first piece of the coccyx. It is innervated by the third and fourth sacral nerves.

As you have already noted [p. 4.8], the pelvic diaphragm supports the pelvic organs, and acts as an auxiliary sphincter for the anal canal. It also helps to regulate intra-abdominal pressure.

In a female subject make a vertical incision in the lower part of the urethra, which is still in the body. Do the same with the lower part of the vagina. You may be able to see the rugae and the remains of the hymen.

The anal canal [Fig. 4.90]

In both sexes open the part of the rectum and the anal canal which are still *in situ*, by making a vertical incision in the midline anteriorly.

The anal canal [Fig. 4.90] is lined in its upper part by a mucous coat identical with that of the rectum, and in its lower part by stratified squamous epithelium. At the anus the latter is replaced by pigmented skin containing hairs, sebaceous glands, and sweat glands.

In the mucosa lining the upper half of the anal canal you will find a series of vertical folds called the **anal columns.** The folds contain the terminal branches of the superior rectal arteries and the commencement of the corresponding veins. Look at the bases of these columns, and you will see that they are linked together by semilunar **anal valves,** each of which bounds a cavity called an **anal sinus.** The anal valves also mark the lowermost extent of the part of the anal canal which is lined by columnar epithelium. About 1.5 cm below the anal valves lies the **'white line'** which marks the uppermost limit of that part of the anal canal which is lined by stratified squamous epithelium. The middle part of the anal canal, which lies between the anal valves and the 'white line', is a transitional zone known as the **pecten.** It is lined by stratified columnar epithelium. The upper part of the anal canal above the 'white line' is developed as part of the gut from the endoderm of the embryo; the lower part is derived as an ingrowth from the ectoderm of the surface of the embryo.

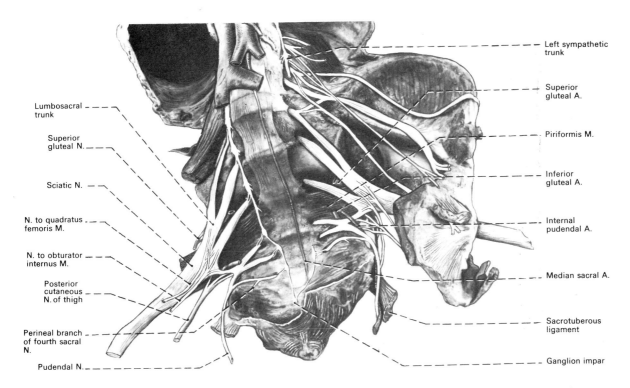

Lumbosacral trunk

Superior gluteal N.

Sciatic N.

N. to quadratus femoris M.

N. to obturator internus M.

Posterior cutaneous N. of thigh

Perineal branch of fourth sacral N.

Pudendal N.

Left sympathetic trunk

Superior gluteal A.

Piriformis M.

Inferior gluteal A.

Internal pudendal A.

Median sacral A.

Sacrotuberous ligament

Ganglion impar

Fig. 4.91 The sacral plexus. The greater portion of the sacral part of the left sympathetic trunk has been excised. The left hip-bone has been displaced laterally after dislocating the left sacroiliac joint. The fifth lumbar vertebra is fused with the sacrum.

After stripping off the mucous coat from the region of the anorectal junction, you should try and define the deep part of the external anal sphincter and the internal anal sphincter, together with the levator ani muscles as they blend with these.

The pelvic nerves

Complete your dissection of the pelvic cavity by examining the pelvic autonomic nerves and the sacral plexus.

The pelvic autonomic nerves

Return to the most inferior part of the abdominal aortic plexus [Fig. 4.65], and try to find further branches from the lumbar parts of the sympathetic trunks crossing in front of the common iliac arteries, and uniting to form the **superior hypogastric plexus** of nerves in the angle between the two vessels. Remember that the plexus sometimes appears as a dense and matted network of fibres.

Follow the superior hypogastric plexus as it descends over the promontory of the sacrum. Also clean the termination of the sympathetic trunks as they descend in front of the sacrum. Note that the superior hypogastric plexus is continued into the pelvis as the two **inferior hypogastric plexuses.** These lie on the sides of the rectum in the male, and on the sides of the rectum and vagina in the female. They receive sympathetic branches from the upper ganglia of the sacral continuation of the sympathetic trunks, and para-

sympathetic branches from the **pelvic splanchnic nerves.** These last arise from the ventral rami of the second, third (and sometimes the fourth) sacral nerves, and contain parasympathetic nerve fibres which are distributed to the pelvic viscera; some of these parasympathetic fibres ascend to be distributed to the descending colon.

The efferent branches of the inferior hypogastric plexuses are distributed to all the pelvic viscera. They accompany the branches of the internal iliac artery, around which they form secondary plexuses. All these secondary plexuses contain both sympathetic and parasympathetic (preganglionic) nerve fibres. The largest and most important are the **vesical plexuses,** the **prostatic plexus,** and the **uterovaginal plexus.**

The sacral plexus [Figs 2.32 and 4.91]

Follow each **lumbosacral trunk** [Fig. 4.91] (formed by the union of a big branch of the fourth lumbar with the whole of the fifth lumbar nerve) as it descends in front of the sacrum. As you clean the lumbosacral trunk you will find that it ends by joining the first sacral nerve soon after this emerges from the first pelvic sacral foramen, just above the upper border of the piriformis muscle.

Having isolated the first sacral nerve, continue dissecting on the surface of the piriformis and define the second and third sacral nerves. You will find that these nerves converge, in the form of a large flat nerve, towards the lower border of the piriformis muscle at the lower part of the greater sciatic foramen. This nerve continues into the gluteal region

4.101

as the **sciatic nerve,** and from it arise the various muscular and cutaneous nerves which you saw when you dissected that region.

Clean and define the origin of the piriformis muscle. You will see that it arises from the pelvic surface of the middle three pieces of the sacrum. Re-examine the branches of the internal iliac artery and especially those of the posterior division (the iliolumbar artery, the lateral sacral arteries, and the superior gluteal artery), and those branches of the anterior division which have not been divided within the pelvis (the internal pudendal artery and the inferior gluteal artery) [pp. 4.86–4.87]. Trace the median sacral artery from the aorta. It is a small vessel which descends over the lower lumbar vertebrae and the middle of the sacrum.

Chart of contents of the head and neck

COMPONENTS	REGIONS		
	Neck	**Face**	**Head**
	anterior lateral posterior	zygomatic · infraorbital · nasal infratemporal · · orbital buccal · oral · mental	frontal parietal temporal occipital
Bones	cervical vertebrae atlas axis hyoid	zygomatic · palatine maxilla mandible	cranial vault cranial base auditory ossicles
Joints	atlanto-occipital atlantoaxial intervertebral of larynx	temporomandibular	cranial sutures of auditory ossicles
Muscles	suboccipital, erector spinae transversospinalis, dorsal [of upper limb] sternocleidomastoid, scalene supra- and infrahyoid pharyngeal, laryngeal	masticatory · of eyeball facial palatal, pharyngeal lingual	of auditory ossicles facial
Nerves	vagus accessory sympathetic trunk cervical plexus brachial plexus	trigeminal · oculomotor facial · trochlear glossopharyngeal · abducent hypoglossal	olfactory optic vestibulocochlear origins of cranial Ns
Arteries	common carotid, subclavian, vertebral	external carotid · ophthalmic	internal carotid vertebral
Veins	external jugular internal jugular subclavian brachiocephalic vertebral venous plexuses	facial · ophthalmic retromandibular	cerebral dural venous sinuses emissary internal jugular
Lymph nodes *superficial* *deep*	anterior and lateral cervical anterior and lateral cervical	parotid facial, submandibular, submental retropharyngeal	occipital, mastoid
Organs	spinal medulla laryngeal pharynx oesophagus larynx trachea thyroid gland parathyroid glands	mouth, teeth, tongue · nose salivary glands · paranasal sinuses nasal pharynx · eye oral pharynx · lacrimal apparatus tonsils	brain ear pituitary gland pineal gland

Part 5

The head and neck

The head and neck are studied together, but because of the arrangement of the bones and soft parts, the dissection cannot follow as orderly a sequence as is possible in other regions of the body. The dissection begins with the back and side of the neck. It then proceeds to the anterior part of the neck, but the face has to be dissected before the deeper cervical structures are exposed, since these cannot be seen until the mandible is removed. The head and neck has, therefore, to be studied in a series of stages which do not necessarily form a logical sequence.

The brain, the eyeball, and the auditory apparatus are examined separately, on specimens which will be provided for the purpose.

The back of the neck

The back of the neck consists of muscles which pass up from the trunk to be inserted either into the cervical vertebrae or into the external surface of the base of the skull (the inferior surface of the skull) behind and at the sides of the foramen magnum, which is the large foramen in the base of the skull [Fig. 5.1]. These muscles are part of a group of extensors and rotators of the vertebral column, which are collectively known as the deep muscles of the back. The bulk of those that are found in the neck arise from the upper six thoracic vertebrae and lower four cervical vertebrae. In addition, there are four, small, deeply-placed muscles at the very base of the skull, which are attached to different parts of the first two cervical vertebrae and to the base of the skull. On each side, these muscles enclose a triangle in which is found the vertebral artery. The latter is a branch of the

subclavian artery, and passes up the neck within the foramina transversaria in the transverse processes of the cervical vertebrae [see p. 5.3]. The vertebral artery ends by traversing the foramen magnum of the skull, and supplying a large part of the brain.

The main interest of the dissection of the back of the neck lies in the fact that the muscles which it displays control the movements of the head and neck.

Osteology

Forward and backward bending of the head on the neck occurs in the joints between the first cervical vertebra and the condyles of the occipital bone at the side of the foramen magnum. Side to side or rotatory movements of the head

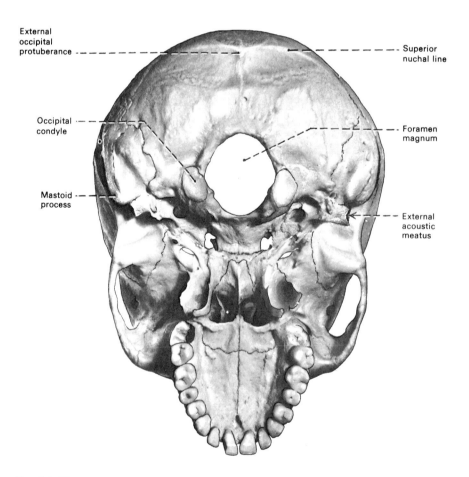

Fig. 5.1 The external surface of the base of the skull. The inferior surface of the skull.

occur between the first and second cervical vertebrae. These two vertebrae articulate both by means of the apposition of lateral articular surfaces, and by way of a median, upwardly-projecting process of the body of the second vertebra, which is held to the anterior arch of the first vertebra by ligaments. The tip of this process is also connected by additional ligaments to the anterior border of the foramen magnum. The dissection of the back of the neck will not be carried far enough to see these joints at this stage, but will expose the muscles which control their movements.

The occipital bone

The skull articulates with the first cervical vertebra, or atlas, by means of a pair of oval convex condyles. These, the **occipital condyles,** lie on either side of the anterior part of the **foramen magnum,** which is within the occipital bone. Note that the part of the bone immediately behind and to the sides of the foramen magnum is on a more horizontally-directed plane than the part above, the two being separated by a ridge called the **superior nuchal line,** which passes from each side of a midline protuberance called the **external occipital protuberance** [Fig. 5.1]. Behind the **external acoustic meatus,** which is the channel leading medially from the external opening of the ear, is the downwardly-projecting **mastoid process.** Note that the superior nuchal line extends on to the posterior part of this process.

The cervical vertebrae

Turn your attention now to the cervical vertebrae. As you saw before [p. 3.3], these are characterized by the presence of a foramen in the transverse process. The facets of articulation between adjacent cervical vertebrae are on a pillar of bone which lies immediately behind the **foramen transversarium.** The first two vertebrae, the atlas and axis, require more detailed examination.

The atlas [Fig. 5.2a]

The atlas consists of a thick bony ring which is formed by an **anterior arch** and a **posterior arch.** These join two bulky **lateral masses** which bear large facets for articulation with

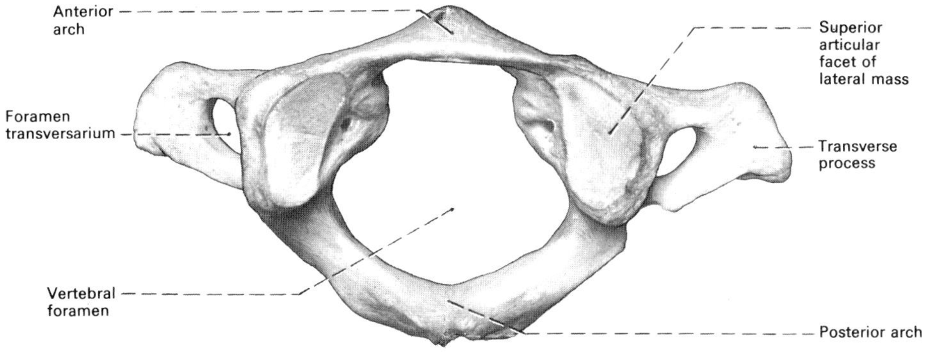

a. *Atlas (from above)*

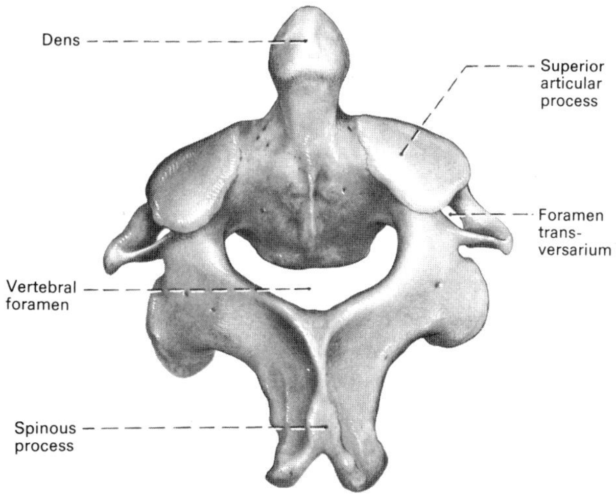

b. *Axis (from above and behind)*

Fig. 5.2 The atlas and the axis.

the occipital bone above and the axis below. The transverse processes are relatively long.

The axis [Fig. 5.2b]

In the articulated skeleton you will see the stout **dens** of the axis lying behind the anterior arch of the atlas. The other special feature of the axis is a pair of large facets for articulation with the facets on the under-surface of the atlas.

Flexion and extension of the skull on the vertebral column occur at the atlanto-occipital joint. Rotation of the skull and atlas around the dens of the axis takes place at the atlantoaxial joint.

Surface anatomy

Now look at the back of your partner's neck and also feel your own. On either side, immediately behind the auricles of the ears, are the mastoid processes [Fig. 5.3]. There is a faint depression in the midline at the base of the skull. A ridge of muscle can sometimes be seen on either side of the midline of the neck, running upwards, obliquely, and medially, and fading out above the area of the small centre-line depression. This ridge is formed by the semispinalis capitis, one of the deep muscles of the neck, on the surface of which lies the thin upper part of the trapezius muscle. The upper margin of the line of attachment of muscles to the skull is easily felt on the living subject. The external occipital protuberance can usually be felt in the centre of this line of attachment. At the base of the neck you can feel and see the spinous processes of two vertebrae. The upper

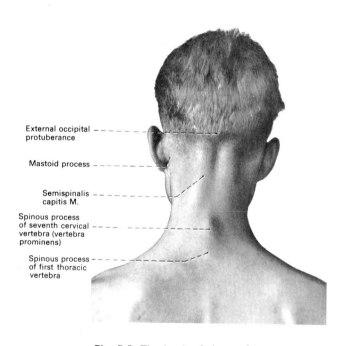

External occipital
protuberance -- -- -- -- --

Mastoid process -- -- -- -- -- --

Semispinalis -- -- -- -- --
capitis M.

Spinous process
of seventh cervical -- -- -- --
vertebra (vertebra
prominens)

Spinous process -- -- -- --
of first thoracic
vertebra

Fig. 5.3 The back of the neck.

is the seventh cervical vertebra, known as the **vertebra prominens,** and the lower that of the first thoracic vertebra.

The superficial muscles of the back of the neck

Early in your dissection of the upper limb [p. 1.7] you exposed the **trapezius muscle** and the **greater occipital nerve,** which pierces the muscle near the superior nuchal line [Fig. 5.4]. You divided the trapezius horizontally at the root of the neck (as in Fig. 1.9) after you had isolated the accessory nerve on its deep surface. You detached the **rhomboid major muscle** and the **rhomboid minor muscle** from the spinous processes of the vertebrae [p. 1.11]. You also separated the **accessory nerve** from the lower half of the trapezius, which was left attached to the scapula when you removed the upper limb. At the same time you detached the **levator scapulae** from the scapula [p. 1.23]. Identify what remains of these muscles and find the accessory nerve on the deep surface of the upper part of the trapezius, whose dissection you must now complete on both sides.

The trapezius muscle [Fig. 5.4]

Place the body face down and slip the handle of your scalpel under the cut lower margin of the cervical part of the trapezius to ease the muscle off the underlying layer of muscles. Then separate the trapezius from its vertebral origin, reflecting the muscle in an upward direction until you reach the external occipital protuberance. Note that between the spinous process of the seventh cervical vertebra and the external occipital protuberance the muscle takes origin from a vertically-disposed fascial band called the **ligamentum nuchae.** Now separate the muscle from the medial part of its origin from the superior nuchal line (leaving it still attached laterally so as not to cut the greater occipital nerve), and turn it to the side.

Lymph nodes will be encountered during the course of the dissection of the neck. Their arrangement is important, but they cannot be properly demonstrated in the cadaver. A brief account of their anatomy is, therefore, given in the Appendix [p. App. 8], and should be referred to from time to time during the course of your dissection.

Of the muscles that were revealed when the trapezius and rhomboids were removed, you have already studied the serratus posterior superior [p. 3.8], which should now be detached from the ribs and spinous processes of the vertebrae and removed.

The deep muscles of the back of the neck

The splenius muscles [Fig. 5.5]

The next layer of muscles which arise from the spinous processes of the vertebrae, and which run upwards and laterally, is now completely exposed. The upper fibres form a

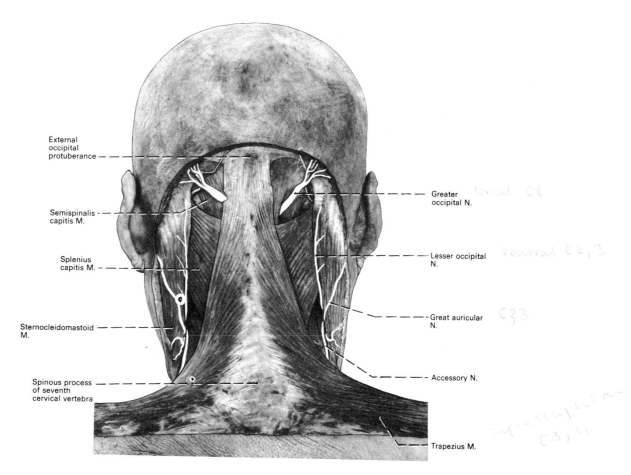

Fig. 5.4 The superficial muscles of the back of the neck.

flat band of muscle, called the **splenius capitis** [Fig. 5.5], which is inserted just below the lateral part of the superior nuchal line. The lower fibres constitute the **splenius cervicis**, and are attached to the transverse processes of the upper cervical vertebrae.

Detach the two splenius muscles from the spinous processes of the vertebrae, and turn them as far laterally as you can, to reveal the deepest of the three groups of muscles on the back of the neck. In the course of this dissection do not spend time on branches of the dorsal rami of the cervical nerves which you will encounter, and which supply all these muscles. Some of their terminal branches become cutaneous.

The semispinalis muscles [Fig. 5.5]

The muscles of the third layer run more or less longitudinally from the transverse processes of the upper thoracic and lower cervical vertebrae to the spinous processes of the cervical vertebrae and to the skull. They form the semispinalis group of muscles. The most superficial is a thick muscle, the **semispinalis capitis**, which is inserted towards the middle of the occipital bone, just below the superior

nuchal line, and which lies immediately deep to the trapezius at this level.

Starting in the lower part of the neck, insert the handle of a scalpel, or the points of your forceps, under the medial margin of this muscle and lift it off the structures deep to it. Continue this separation upwards as far as you are able without separating the muscle from the part of the trapezius muscle which overlies it.

The greater occipital nerve [Figs 5.4 to 5.6]

You identified the greater occipital nerve piercing the trapezius near the superior nuchal line when you cleaned the muscle at the beginning of the dissection of the upper limb. You can now see it running transversely across the deep surface of the semispinalis capitis, which it pierces near the midline, about 4 cm below the external occipital protuberance. The greater occipital nerve supplies the scalp as far forwards as the vertex of the skull.

The occipital artery [Figs 5.5 and 5.6]

Lateral to the point at which the greater occipital nerve pierces the trapezius you may see the occipital artery. This

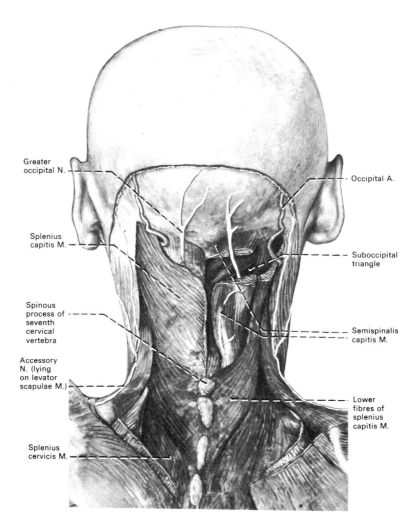

Fig. 5.5 The muscles of the back of the neck. Both trapezius muscles have been reflected and parts of the splenius capitis and semispinalis capitis muscles have been excised on the right side.

is a branch of the external carotid artery, one of the main arterial trunks of the anterior part of the neck. The occipital artery crosses the upper end of the semispinalis capitis, pierces the trapezius muscle, and accompanies the greater occipital nerve upwards into the scalp. If you find the artery preserve it. Its origin in the anterior part of the neck will be seen later.

The suboccipital muscles [Fig. 5.6]

Free the greater occipital nerve from the semispinalis muscle by cutting the fibres medial to the point where the nerve pierces the muscle. Now, starting at the medial edge, a little lower down, cut transversely across the muscle, watching the under-surface of the muscle so that none of the structures deep to it are damaged. You may have difficulty in deciding whether your incision has reached the lateral margin of the muscle. Reflect the lower part of the muscle downwards and then make a second incision in the upper part of the muscle close to the skull. Remove the isolated portion of the muscle [Fig. 5.5].

The small suboccipital muscles lie in the area that is now exposed. They are covered by dense fascia which has to be removed. To do this, first follow the greater occipital nerve to the point where it enters the present field of dissection. Immediately above this point is the **obliquus capitis inferior muscle** [Fig. 5.6]. Its fibres run laterally and slightly upwards from the spinous process of the axis to the transverse process of the atlas. Use your scalpel to clear the fascia from the muscle. The muscle is finely fasciculated and its dissection is made easier by rotating the head of the cadaver so as to stretch the fibres. It may also be necessary to pull the splenius capitis laterally in order to cut through the fascia overlying the lateral end of the obliquus capitis inferior.

A network of veins that lies in the fascia of the suboccipital region should be removed as the dissection proceeds.

Feel for the transverse process of the atlas. Now expose the **obliquus capitis superior muscle.** This muscle arises from the transverse process of the atlas and, passing backwards but only slightly upwards, it is inserted into the occipital bone lateral to the insertion of the semispinalis capitis. The

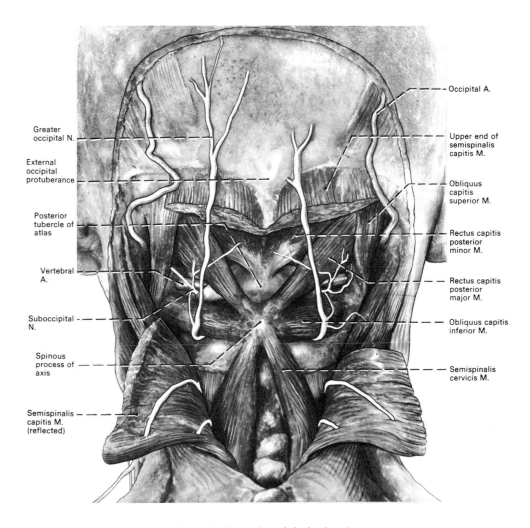

Greater
occipital N.

External
occipital
protuberance

Posterior
tubercle of
atlas

Vertebral
A.

Suboccipital
N.

Spinous
process of
axis

Semispinalis
capitis M.
(reflected)

Occipital A.

Upper end of
semispinalis
capitis M.

Obliquus
capitis
superior M.

Rectus capitis
posterior
minor M.

Rectus capitis
posterior
major M.

Obliquus capitis
inferior M.

Semispinalis
cervicis M.

Fig. 5.6 The suboccipital triangles.

obliquus capitis superior muscle is covered by a thin sheet of tough fascia which should be carefully removed.

Return to the spinous process of the axis and clean the muscle which runs upwards and slightly laterally to the occipital bone. This is the **rectus capitis posterior major.** Near its insertion it may be overlapped by the obliquus capitis superior.

Displace the rectus capitis posterior major laterally, detaching it from the spinous process of the axis if necessary and, using forceps and scalpel, clear away the connective tissue to reveal the **rectus capitis posterior minor muscle.** This muscle extends from the posterior tubercle of the atlas to the occipital bone, medial to the insertion of the rectus capitis posterior major.

Now define the muscle which is inserted on each side into the spinous process of the axis from below. This is the upper part of the **semispinalis cervicis muscle.** You will see that six muscles radiate, three on each side, from the spinous process of the axis [Fig. 5.6].

The suboccipital triangles [Fig. 5.6]

The two suboccipital triangles are defined as the areas on either side of the midline that are bounded by the two obliquus capitis muscles and the rectus capitis posterior major. Place a finger in either of the two triangles and feel for a transverse bar of bone. This is the **posterior arch of the atlas.** The fascia and veins by which it is covered should now be removed. Once the arch has been seen, continue removing fascia and veins in the space immediately above the arch. By this means you should soon uncover the **vertebral artery,** which will be found running horizontally as it winds round the back of the lateral mass of the atlas [Fig. 5.6]. If it is poorly injected, the artery will not be easily identified and may be accidentally damaged. You will study the full course of this vessel at a later stage.

Deep in the suboccipital triangle, between the vertebral artery and the posterior arch of the atlas, the dorsal ramus of the first cervical nerve, called the **suboccipital nerve,** may be found. It supplies the suboccipital muscles but has no cutaneous branch. Do not spend unnecessary time on its dissection.

The actions of the suboccipital muscles

The actions of the suboccipital muscles are easily appreciated, provided you bear in mind that the spinous process of the axis and the transverse process of the atlas are on a deeper plane than the part of the occipital bone into which the muscles are inserted. The neck muscles which are inserted into the vertebrae extend and fix the cervical part of the vertebral column, and those which become attached to the occipital bone, such as the splenius and semispinalis capitis, extend and to a certain extent rotate the head on the neck.

Before proceeding with the next part of the dissection, note again the vertebral artery as it emerges from the foramen transversarium of the atlas and passes medially. Note, too, the course of the greater occipital nerve from the point of its emergence below the obliquus capitis inferior to that of its disappearance under the skin at the superior boundary of the field of dissection.

Section 5.2

The posterior triangle of the neck

The anatomy of the side of the neck is the anatomy of what is called the posterior triangle. This triangle has its apex above, immediately behind the mastoid process, and its base on the clavicle below. The **anterior border** of the triangle is formed by the posterior margin of the sterno-cleidomastoid muscle; the **posterior border** by the lateral margin of the cervical part of the trapezius muscle; and the **base** by the middle part of the clavicle [Fig. 5.7]. As you saw when you dissected the arm [p. 1.17], the sternocleido-mastoid muscle arises below from the anterior surface of the manubrium of the sternum by a tendon, and from the medial third of the clavicle by muscle fibres. Above, the muscle is attached to the mastoid process and the contiguous part of the superior nuchal line of the skull. Refer again to this part of the skull. The insertion of the sterno-cleidomastoid is along a narrow line which passes from the lateral surface of the mastoid process on to the superior

nuchal line. Immediately deep to it is the line along which the splenius capitis is inserted.

Within the confines of the posterior triangle lie muscles most of whose fibres run in much the same general direction—downwards and backwards. The more superiorly-situated of these muscles (the semispinalis capitis, which may just appear at the apex of the triangle, the splenius capitis just below it, and the levator scapulae) have already been seen.

The triangle is covered by skin, and by superficial and deep fascia, the latter forming a fascial roof to the triangle. A thin sheet of muscle fibres, called the **platysma muscle,** runs downwards and laterally in the superficial fascia over the lower part of the triangle. The platysma is a downward extension of a set of subcutaneous facial muscles which, through the pull they exercise on the skin, control facial expression.

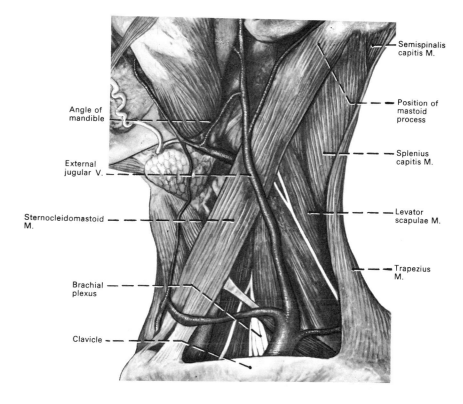

Fig. 5.7 **The left posterior triangle of the neck.**

Angle of mandible

External jugular V.

Sternocleidomastoid M.

Brachial plexus

Clavicle

Semispinalis capitis M.

Position of mastoid process

Splenius capitis M.

Levator scapulae M.

Trapezius M.

Among the non-muscular structures on which the student should spend time while dissecting the posterior triangle are the ventral rami of the cervical nerves. The union of the ventral rami of the first, second, third, and fourth cervical nerves is called the **cervical plexus,** and the union of those of the fifth, sixth, seventh, and eighth cervical nerves and part of that of the first thoracic nerve, the **brachial plexus.** Another nerve of great importance which is encountered in the posterior triangle is the accessory nerve, part of which has already been dissected [p. 1.9].

Other important anatomical structures to be found during this stage of dissection are the subclavian artery and vein, which arch over the first rib, and the external jugular vein. The latter descends, deep to the platysma muscle but superficial to the deep fascia, from behind the angle of the mandible to just above the midpoint of the clavicle.

Surface anatomy

The borders of the posterior triangle can be easily seen and felt in the living subject, especially when the muscles are made to contract [Fig. 5.8]. Examine your own neck or that of a fellow student. Make the tendinous sternal head and the fleshy clavicular head of the sternocleidomastoid muscle stand out by trying to rotate your head against resistance. The muscle that stands out is the one on the side opposite to that to which you are turning your face.

Feel the mastoid process. Now, recalling your dissection of the suboccipital region, and visualizing the way the skull articulates with the vertebral column, try to locate the transverse process of the atlas. Its surface marking is a point midway between the mastoid process and the angle of the mandible; and its position illustrates how much of the bulk of the neck is made up of the vertebral column and the muscles

by which it is surrounded.

Two further features of the side of the neck may be seen on the surface. If you increase the hydrostatic pressure of the blood in the veins of the head by lying down, or by attempting to breathe out when at the same time you prevent the air from being expelled (by contracting the upper part of your throat), the external jugular vein can be seen as a vertical ridge descending from just behind the angle of the mandible to the middle of the clavicle.

The subcutaneous platysma muscle can be seen when it contracts. Contracting it forcibly usually leads to a grimace with the mandible protruded, the angles of the mouth pulled downwards and laterally, and the lips everted [Fig. 5.9]. You will feel the skin on your chest move as you do this, and, if you look in a mirror, you should be able to see strands of muscle fibres standing out under the skin of the neck.

Reflection of the skin

Continue the skin incision which you made from the external occipital protuberance to the mastoid process, as far as the attachment of the lobe of the ear (anatomically, the lobule of the auricle). Pick up the large flap of skin which originally covered the back of the neck, and reflect it forwards as far as the anterior border of the sternocleidomastoid muscle, turning the body over on to its back as you complete the reflection of the skin. If you have reflected the skin carefully, you will be able to see fibres of the **platysma muscle** running downwards and laterally in the superficial fascia [Fig. 5.10]. If the platysma is removed with the flap, do not dissect it off the deep surface of the latter, but try to avoid cutting cutaneous nerves or the external jugular vein.

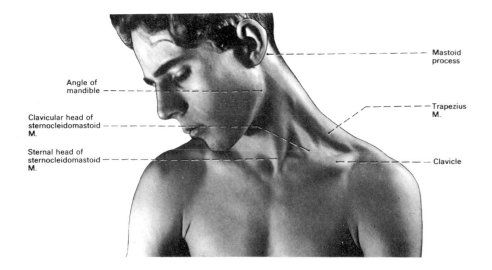

Fig. 5.8 The left side of the neck.

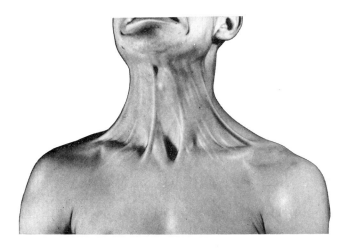

Fig. 5.9 The platysma muscle when contracted.

Dissection of the posterior triangle

The external jugular vein [Fig. 5.11]

If the layer of platysma has not been removed, reflect it in the same direction as you have the skin, taking care not to cut the cutaneous nerves which you may find lying on or close to the sternocleidomastoid muscle. In spite of the fact that it is sometimes very small, you will usually have no difficulty in identifying the external jugular vein which lies immediately deep to the platysma [Fig. 5.11]. It begins at the junction of two veins just below the lobule of the auricle, and you will see it disappearing into the fascia which forms the roof of the posterior triangle, some 4 cm above the first rib. Using blunt dissection, and treating the vein very gently, since it may be easily torn, free it from the surrounding fascia, starting at its upper end, and avoid damaging the cutaneous nerves you may encounter. Follow the vein

downwards through the fascia to the point where it ends by entering the **subclavian vein.** Now divide the vein twice, 1 cm from its start and 1 cm from its termination. Remove the intermediate portion, together with the tributaries which enter it.

If the external jugular vein is very small in the body you are dissecting, look at some other dissection.

The accessory nerve [Fig. 5.11]

Return to the accessory nerve, which you will find lying on the levator scapulae muscle [Fig. 5.11]. By means of blunt dissection, trace it upwards through the fibrous connective tissue towards the posterior border of the sternocleidomastoid muscle. The nerve will stand a fair amount of stretching and pulling, but it may be accidentally cut. You will usually find branches from the second and third cervical nerves running with and joining it. These branches also emerge from under cover of the posterior border of the sternocleidomastoid.

The course of the accessory nerve can be marked on the surface of the neck as a line drawn downwards and backwards from the transverse process of the atlas, across the sternocleidomastoid muscle and posterior triangle, to a point on the anterior border of the trapezius, 5 cm above the clavicle.

The cervical plexus [Fig. 5.12]

Just below the point where the accessory nerve emerges from under the sternocleidomastoid muscle, find three cutaneous branches of the cervical plexus which appear from beneath the muscle and wind round its posterior border [Fig. 5.12]. One of them, the **lesser occipital nerve,** runs upwards and backwards along the posterior border of the sternocleidomastoid muscle. Another, the **great auricu-**

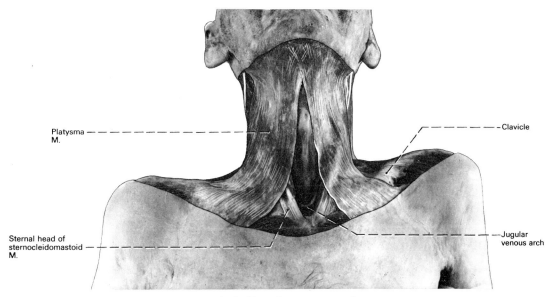

Fig. 5.10 The platysma muscle.

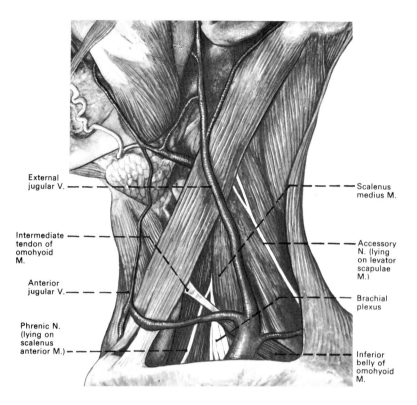

External jugular V. —

Intermediate tendon of omohyoid M. — — —

Anterior jugular V. — —

Phrenic N. (lying on scalenus anterior M.) — —

Scalenus medius M.

Accessory N. (lying on levator scapulae M.)

Brachial plexus

Inferior belly of omohyoid M.

Fig. 5.11 The left posterior triangle. In this body the anterior jugular vein crosses the sternocleidomastoid muscle superficially.

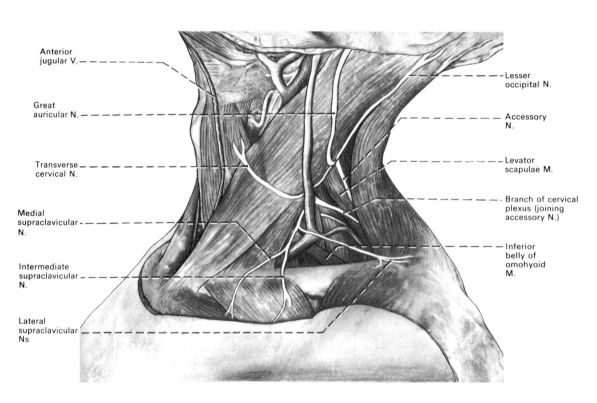

Anterior jugular V. — — —

Great auricular N. — — — —

Transverse cervical N. — — —

Medial supraclavicular N. — — —

Intermediate supraclavicular N. — — —

Lateral supraclavicular Ns — — —

Lesser occipital N.

Accessory N.

Levator scapulae M.

Branch of cervical plexus (joining accessory N.)

Inferior belly of omohyoid M.

Fig. 5.12 The contents of the left posterior triangle.

lar nerve, ascends vertically, crossing the sternocleidomastoid obliquely. The third, the **transverse cervical nerve,** runs horizontally forwards across the sternocleidomastoid muscle. These three nerves are composed of fibres of the second and third cervical nerves, and supply the skin in the areas towards which you find them running. The great auricular nerve supplies the skin overlying the angle of the mandible, much of the skin of the auricle, and the skin covering the mastoid process. Do not trace these nerves further than the skin reflection allows.

A little below these three nerves, three other cutaneous branches of the cervical plexus emerge from behind the sternocleidomastoid muscle. They are the **supraclavicular nerves** which you may have seen already in your dissection of the subcutaneous tissue overlying the pectoralis major muscle [p. 1.11]. They descend in the deep fascia that is attached to the posterior border of the sternocleidomastoid, and after piercing the fascia, cross the clavicle. They supply the skin over the lower part of the neck, the skin over the shoulder, and the skin over the front of the chest as far down as the second rib.

Although these nerves consist of fibres from the third and fourth cervical nerves, the part of the chest wall they supply abuts mainly on the area innervated by the second thoracic nerve. This is because the intervening ventral rami of the spinal nerves, which form the brachial plexus, supply the upper limb. A small part of the first thoracic nerve supplies the skin of the first intercostal space.

Using a finger, or the handle of a scalpel, separate the posterior border and the clavicular head of the sternocleidomastoid from the underlying fascia, and by blunt dissection trace the supraclavicular nerves in this plane of fascia. You will find that they come from the cervical nerves as these emerge from the interval between the upper slips of a flat strap-like muscle, the scalenus anterior, in front, and a thicker muscle, the scalenus medius, behind [Fig. 5.13].

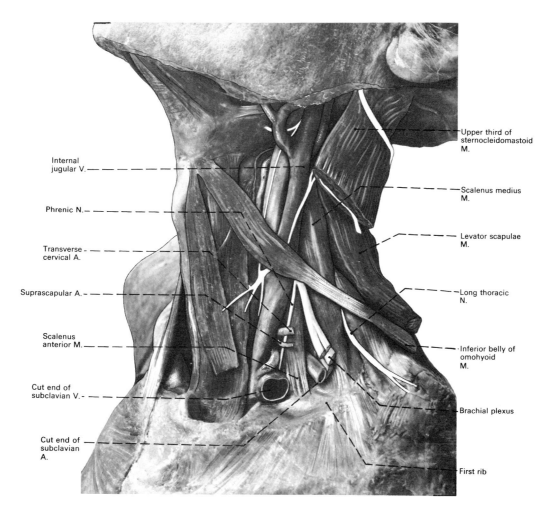

Fig. 5.13 The root of the left side of the neck.

The phrenic nerve

Try now to find the phrenic nerve [Fig. 5.13], which springs from the cervical plexus just below the common trunk of the supraclavicular nerves, or perhaps arises from it, and descends vertically. The phrenic nerve is formed by branches of the third, fourth, and fifth cervical nerves (mainly the fourth). You have already examined the thoracic course of the phrenic nerve on its way to the diaphragm. If you do not find the nerve near the origin of the supraclavicular nerves, you will do so by dissecting the fascia on the anterior surface of the scalenus anterior. Be careful, when you search, not to cut deeply at the lateral border of the muscle, or you will divide one or more of the roots of the nerve. At present you will not be able to see the whole of the cervical course of the phrenic nerve, but you can confirm its presence on the scalenus anterior by pulling gently on the nerve in the thorax, when you will see that the part of the nerve you have exposed in the neck moves.

The transverse cervical and suprascapular arteries

Starting at the apex of the posterior triangle, clear away the fascia in order to identify the muscles which cross the posterior triangle. Preserve the nerves you have already isolated. In the posterior triangle all the branches of the cervical plexus lie inferior to the accessory nerve. Do not try to preserve any small motor nerves you may find supplying the muscles in the triangle.

Towards the base of the triangle you will encounter two horizontally-disposed arteries. Both usually arise under cover of the sternocleidomastoid muscle, from the **thyrocervical trunk,** a branch of the subclavian artery. Trace the arteries laterally. The upper artery is the **transverse cervical artery** [Fig. 5.13] which divides, one branch running deep to the levator scapulae, and then along the medial border of the scapula, the other passing on to the deep surface of the trapezius where it was severed when the upper limb was removed. The lower horizontally-disposed artery is the **suprascapular artery,** which runs laterally, downwards, and backwards to the scapular notch of the scapula. It, too, was divided when the upper limb was removed [p. 1.23].

Muscles of the posterior triangle [Figs 5.11 and 5.13]

The upper end of the **semispinalis capitis** sometimes appears at the apex of the posterior triangle. You have already seen the **splenius capitis** and **levator scapulae muscles.** Note once again that the accessory nerve runs on the surface of the levator scapulae. The **inferior belly of the omohyoid** [Fig. 5.13] is a narrow muscular band which runs almost horizontally across the lower end of the triangle in the fascial layer attached to the sternocleidomastoid. You saw the attachment of this muscle to the scapula before this was removed with the upper limb [p. 1.23]. The three scalene muscles take origin from the cervical transverse processes,

and descend to be inserted into one or both of the first two ribs.

Clean the part of the brachial plexus which was left on the trunk when the upper limb was removed. You will find that above the first rib, the brachial plexus, like the cervical plexus with which it is continuous, lies between the **scalenus anterior** in front and the **scalenus medius** behind. Behind the scalenus medius lies the **scalenus posterior,** which is usually overlapped by the levator scapulae. You may be able to identify the long thoracic nerve [see p. 1.23] whose upper two roots pierce the scalenus medius and appear on its lateral surface. Note once more that the phrenic nerve descends on the anterior surface of the scalenus anterior.

Relations of the scalenus anterior muscle [Fig. 5.13]

With the handle of the scalpel, now define the borders of the scalenus anterior and scalenus medius more clearly. You will see that the scalenus anterior is attached to the first rib between the subclavian artery and vein, the vein lying anterior. The subclavian arteries arise differently on the two sides: the right from the brachiocephalic trunk, the left from the arch of the aorta. Except for those parts of the arteries medial to the scalenus anterior, they take the same course on each side.

Each **subclavian artery** arches over the corresponding first rib behind the scalenus anterior and in front of the brachial plexus. The **inferior trunk of the brachial plexus,** or that part of the first thoracic nerve which contributes to it, lies on the rib inferior to the artery. At the outer border of the rib the subclavian artery becomes the axillary artery, while the axillary vein continues as the **subclavian vein** medial to this border of the rib. The vein passes in front of the scalenus anterior and ends at its medial border by joining the principal vein of the neck, the internal jugular vein, to form the brachiocephalic vein.

The first rib [Fig. 5.14]

You should be able to identify on the first rib of your specimen the subclavian vein, the scalenus anterior muscle, the

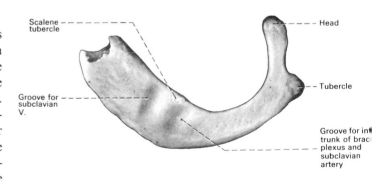

Fig. 5.14 The superior surface of the left first rib.

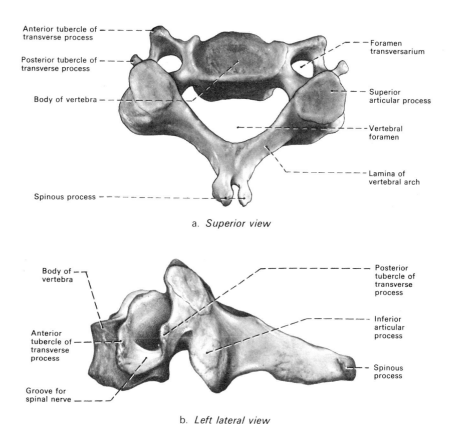

a. *Superior view*

b. *Left lateral view*

Fig. 5.15 The fifth cervical vertebra.

subclavian artery, the inferior trunk of the brachial plexus (formed by the first thoracic and the eighth cervical nerves) and the scalenus medius muscle, in that order from before backwards.

Now look at the first rib on a skeleton. On its upper surface you will see the **scalene tubercle** into which the scalenus anterior muscle is inserted [Fig. 5.14]. On each side of the tubercle, you should be able to make out a faint groove. The one in front is for the subclavian vein; the one behind is for the inferior trunk of the brachial plexus. In spite of this anatomical relationship, the posterior groove is conventionally known as the **groove for the subclavian artery.**

The vertebral origins of the scalene muscles

Now again examine the transverse processes of the third, fourth, fifth, and sixth cervical vertebrae. The bar of bone which forms the lateral boundary of the foramen transversarium is bent downwards to form a transversely-running **groove for the spinal nerve** [Fig. 5.15b]. The ventral ramus of the corresponding spinal nerve lies on this groove. The scalenus anterior muscle is attached to the part of the transverse process anterior to the groove, and the scalenus medius to the part of the process below and posterior to the groove. The two tips which the cervical transverse process acquires as a result of this grooving are called the **anterior** and **posterior tubercles of the transverse process.**

The dome of the pleura

Return to the cadaver, and put your hand in the thorax, placing a finger on the deep surface of the fascia which extends above the first rib. This fascia was lined by the dome of the pleura before the latter was removed. Press gently upwards and you will see that your finger is immediately underneath the fascia that lies medial to the inner border of the first rib behind the subclavian artery.

The posterior triangle in general

Before proceeding with the next part of the dissection, once more examine the course of the accessory nerve, and observe again that the roots of the cervical and brachial plexuses emerge between the scalenus anterior and scalenus medius muscles, and that the nerves increase in thickness from above downwards. Check, too, the course of the phrenic nerve over the lower part of the former muscle. Attempt, also, to determine the actions of the muscles you have dissected, paying particular attention to the sternocleidomastoid muscle. You will recall that to make the sternocleidomastoid of one side stand out in the living body, you rotate the face to the opposite side against resistance. As well as rotating the head, the sternocleidomastoid muscle flexes the neck laterally, to the same side, and forwards.

Section 5.3

The front of the neck

The only important non-muscular structures which you have so far found in the neck are the ventral and dorsal rami of the spinal nerves, one cranial nerve (the accessory nerve), part of the subclavian vessels, and the upper part of the vertebral artery.

The front of the neck is very different. In the midline one finds the **larynx** and **trachea** [Fig. 5.16], and behind them the **oesophagus**; and on either side, the common carotid artery, and the external and internal carotid arteries into which it divides, as well as four important cranial nerves. Closely applied to the trachea and larynx is the thyroid gland. Above the upper border of the larynx, and connected to it by a ligament, is a U-shaped bone called the hyoid bone, to which various muscles of the floor of the mouth and the tongue are attached. The front of the neck also contains the cervical part of the sympathetic trunk, and the internal jugular vein and its tributaries.

The larynx and oesophagus open from, and are continuous with, the lower part of the **pharynx,** the space behind the cavity of the nose and the mouth [Fig. 5.17].

Before you begin to dissect in this region, it is useful to look at a skull. The roof of the **cavity of the mouth** is formed by the palate, and the floor by the muscles which fill the space between the two halves of the body of the mandible and by the tongue lying above them. The side walls of the **cavity of the mouth proper** are formed by the gums and teeth, the space between them and the cheeks being called the **vestibule of the mouth.** The cheeks are attached behind to the muscular walls of the pharynx. The latter reach up to the base of the skull in front of the foramen magnum. The upper part of the pharynx is called the nasal part of the pharynx and is continuous with the nasal cavity [Fig. 5.17].

The next point to appreciate before you continue dissecting is that the structures in the front of the neck are covered by a series of elongated muscles, of which the most important is the sternocleidomastoid.

Surface anatomy

First follow, from below upwards, the midline structures on your own neck. Place your finger in the **jugular notch** on the upper border of the manubrium of the sternum between the sternal attachments of the sternocleidomastoid muscles, and press gently backwards [Fig. 5.18]. You will feel the ridged anterior surface of the trachea. As you follow this upwards, you will feel first the cricoid cartilage and then the larger thyroid cartilage of the larynx. As you will see later, the cricoid cartilage is shaped like a signet ring, with the signet behind. Above it you will be able to feel the cricothyroid ligament by which it is connected to the thyroid cartilage. The thyroid cartilage consists of two large plates or laminae of cartilage applied to the sides of the larynx. They meet anteriorly to form the **laryngeal prominence,** or Adam's apple, which is much more prominent in men than in women.

If you press firmly above the thyroid cartilage you will be able to feel the anterior part of the hyoid bone. Above and in front of it is the floor of the mouth, of which the tongue can be regarded as forming a mobile part.

The thyroid gland consists of two large lateral lobes that are connected in front of the trachea by a narrow band of glandular tissue, called the isthmus of the thyroid gland. The latter is hardly ever palpable, but the lobes of the thyroid gland can sometimes be felt or seen as prominences in the lower part of the neck.

If you press your fingers underneath the anterior border of the sternocleidomastoid muscle, you will feel the pulsation of the carotid arteries, especially when you bend your head forwards slightly.

Reflection of the skin

Make an incision through the skin in the midline from the jugular notch to the point of the chin [Fig. 5.19]. The skin

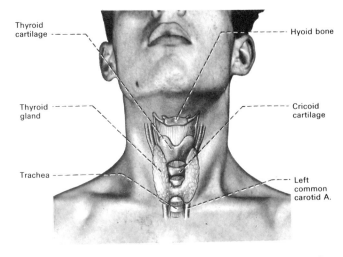

Fig. 5.16 Outline of structures in the front of the neck.

Thyroid cartilage

Hyoid bone

Thyroid gland

Cricoid cartilage

Trachea

Left common carotid A.

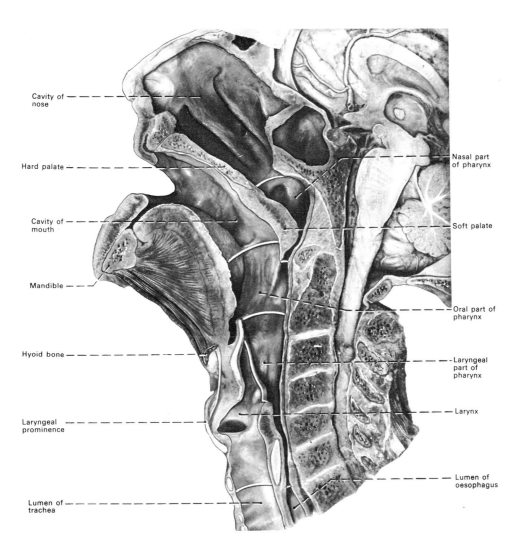

Cavity of nose

Hard palate

Cavity of mouth

Mandible

Hyoid bone

Laryngeal prominence

Lumen of trachea

Nasal part of pharynx

Soft palate

Oral part of pharynx

Laryngeal part of pharynx

Larynx

Lumen of oesophagus

Fig. 5.17 **Median section of the head and neck.** The boundaries of the parts of the pharynx are outlined in white.

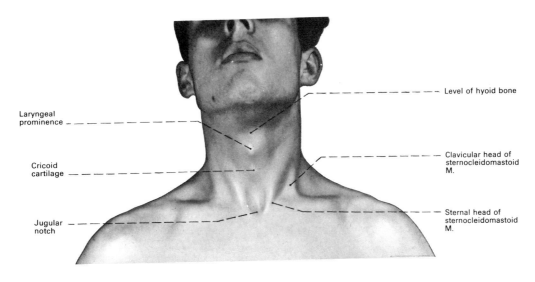

Laryngeal prominence

Cricoid cartilage

Jugular notch

Level of hyoid bone

Clavicular head of sternocleidomastoid M.

Sternal head of sternocleidomastoid M.

Fig. 5.18 **The front of the neck.**

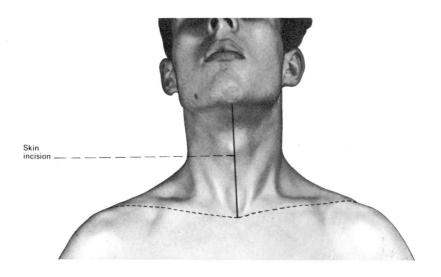

Fig. 5.19 Skin incision of the front of the neck.

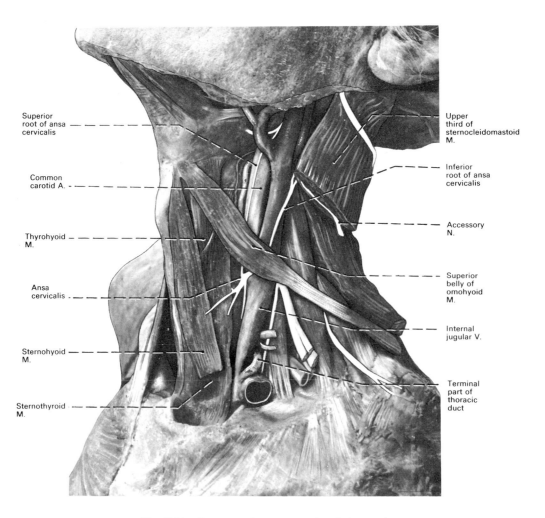

Superior
root of ansa
cervicalis

Common
carotid A.

Thyrohyoid
M.

Ansa
cervicalis

Sternohyoid
M.

Sternothyroid
M.

Upper
third of
sternocleidomastoid
M.

Inferior
root of ansa
cervicalis

Accessory
N.

Superior
belly of
omohyoid
M.

Internal
jugular V.

Terminal
part of
thoracic
duct

Fig. 5.20 The root of the left side of the neck.

5.18

of the neck is thin, so do not cut deeply. Take the large flap of skin which has been dissected off the back and side of the neck, and reflect it towards the lower border or base of the mandible. Then pick up the sheet of platysma just above the jugular notch, and divide it vertically in the midline. Using the handle of a scalpel, separate this layer from the underlying structures by dissecting it upwards from below, and laterally from the midline. Then cut it along the base of the mandible for about 6 cm from the mid-point of the chin, and turn the platysma laterally, leaving it attached to the angle of the mandible. The transverse cervical nerve, which you dissected in the posterior triangle, will be seen running into it, but need not be traced further.

Dissection of the front of the neck

Lying on either side of the midline between the two sterno-cleidomastoid muscles, and covered by deep fascia, are four thin strap-like muscles which are collectively named the **in-frahyoid muscles.** They are crossed by a pair of veins which pass down the neck, one on either side of the midline. These are the **anterior jugular veins** [Fig. 5.12], each of which turns laterally at the lower end of the neck and passes deep to the sternocleidomastoid muscle to join the external jugular vein. Just above the jugular notch the anterior jugular veins are usually united by a large vein, the **jugular venous arch** [Fig. 5.10]. Once you have identified them, do not attempt to preserve these veins.

With forceps pick up the deep fascia covering the in-frahyoid muscles just above the jugular notch and, by means of blunt dissection with scissors, lift it off the underlying **sternohyoid muscle** [Fig. 5.20]. Follow the latter muscle to the hyoid bone.

Now lift off the fascia lateral to the sternohyoid to reveal the **superior belly of the omohyoid,** but do not reflect the fascia beyond the lateral border of the omohyoid.

Removal of the lower part of the sternocleidomastoid muscle

The tendon by which the sternocleidomastoid muscle takes origin from the manubrium of the sternum, as well as its muscular origin from the clavicle, were divided in the course of your dissection of the upper limb [p. 1.17]. The next step in your present dissection is to remove the lower two-thirds of the muscle. Before doing so, the accessory nerve should be followed through, and isolated from, the muscle. Sometimes the nerve does not pierce the muscle, but lies close to its deep surface. The branches of the nerve to the muscle should be divided so as to free the nerve completely.

Separate the sternocleidomastoid muscle from the under-lying omohyoid with the handle of your scalpel. Then reflect the lower end of the muscle upwards, until you reach the point where it is traversed by the accessory nerve. Now divide the muscle along the line of the accessory nerve and completely remove its lower two-thirds.

You can now see a thin tendon which joins the superior and inferior bellies of the omohyoid (the latter you dissected in the posterior triangle [p. 5.14]). By blunt dissection free the whole extent of the omohyoid from underlying structures.

Structures lateral to the larynx and trachea

The internal jugular vein [Fig. 5.20]

You will have no difficulty in making out the large longitu-dinally-disposed internal jugular vein in the fascia deep to the sternocleidomastoid [Fig. 5.20]. When the omohyoid, whose intermediate tendon crosses the vein, is turned aside, you can clear away the fascia by which the vein is sur-rounded, taking care not to damage a fine nerve, the **ansa cervicalis,** which runs obliquely across the vein. This fascia is part of the **carotid sheath.** First pick up the **subclavian vein** and trace it medially to the point where it joins the **internal jugular vein** to form the **brachiocephalic vein.** Then follow the internal jugular vein upwards, dissecting the fascia off its anterior and lateral aspects, as far as the level of the lower border of the thyroid cartilage.

The ansa cervicalis [Fig. 5.20]

As you dissect the fascia off the internal jugular vein, you may encounter, in the fascial sheath of the vein, a fine nerve which crosses the vein obliquely in a downwards and medial direction. Trace this nerve upwards. You will find that it springs, like the cutaneous nerves of the neck that you have already isolated, from the cervical plexus on the front of the scalenus medius muscle. Now trace the nerve down-wards, and note that it is joined by another longitudinally-disposed nerve to form a loop which is called the ansa cervi-calis. The nerve which descends from the cervical plexus is called the **inferior root of the ansa cervicalis;** the other descending nerve is the **superior root of the ansa cervicalis,** which springs from the hypoglossal nerve [see p. 5.63]. Branches of the ansa cervicalis supply the sternohyoid and another strap-like muscle, the sternothyroid, which lies deep to it [Fig. 5.21], as well as the omohyoid. You may see these branches of supply as you dissect, but time should not be spent looking for them especially.

The common carotid artery

Bound by fascia to the medial side of the internal jugular vein, and hidden from view, is the common carotid artery [Fig. 5.21]. Use the handle of a scalpel to separate and retract the vein from the artery. Clear away the connective tissue surrounding the artery as far down as the superior aperture of the thorax, and as far up as the lower border of the thyroid cartilage. The common carotid artery divides

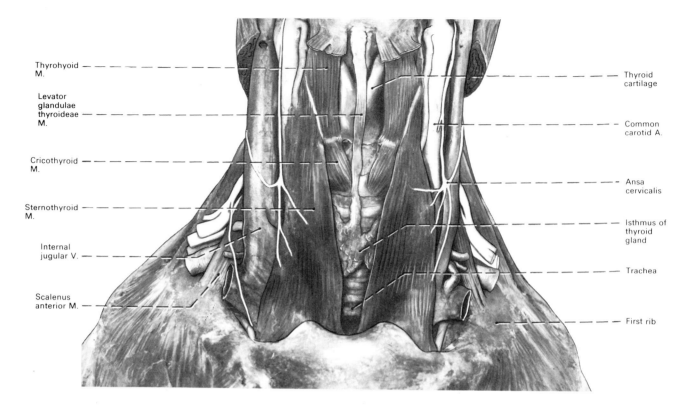

Thyrohyoid M.

Levator glandulae thyroideae M.

Cricothyroid M.

Sternothyroid M.

Internal jugular V.

Scalenus anterior M.

Thyroid cartilage

Common carotid A.

Ansa cervicalis

Isthmus of thyroid gland

Trachea

First rib

Fig. 5.21 Dissection of the front of the neck. The sternocleidomastoid, sternohyoid, and omohyoid muscles have been removed.

into the **internal** and **external carotid arteries.** These cannot be studied at this stage, but note now that the internal carotid is the main artery of the brain, and that it enters the skull through a passage called the carotid canal in the base of the skull. It gives off no branches in the neck. The external carotid artery is the main artery of the face and gives off a number of branches which supply the skin and the deeper structures of the neck and face.

The vagus nerve

By careful dissection, find the vagus nerve [Fig. 5.22] which lies deeply between the artery and the vein. It will be bound by fascia to the artery. Confirm that what you have found is the vagus nerve by pulling gently on the vagus in the thorax and watching for movement of the nerve in the neck.

The carotid sheath

The name carotid sheath is given to the thick fascia which binds together the common carotid artery, the internal jugular vein and the vagus nerve, and which separates them from adjacent structures. Deep, and somewhat medial to the sheath is the cervical part of the **sympathetic trunk.** This trunk should not be dissected at this stage, but note that its course is parallel to that of the vagus nerve. Their mutual relationship is bound to be disturbed by your subsequent dissection.

Structures anterior to the larynx and trachea

The infrahyoid muscles [Figs 5.20 and 5.21]

The **sternohyoid** and **omohyoid muscles** have already been identified. Now carefully separate the sternohyoid muscle from the underlying muscles as far up as the hyoid bone. Free the borders of the sternohyoid and then cut across the muscle horizontally, halfway between the hyoid bone and the jugular notch. Turn back the two ends of the muscle so as to expose the whole of the **sternothyroid muscle,** which is attached to the thyroid cartilage, and its upward extension, the **thyrohyoid muscle,** which runs from the cartilage to the hyoid bone [Fig. 5.21].

Between the medial borders of the sternothyroid and thyrohyoid muscles of the two sides of the neck, identify the following structures which are, in order, starting from below:

1. The trachea.
2. The isthmus of the thyroid gland, which crosses the trachea. You will see veins descending from the isthmus. These are the inferior thyroid veins.
3. The cricoid cartilage covered by two muscles, the cricothyroid muscles, whose fibres fan upwards and backwards.
4. The fused anterior borders of the laminae of the thyroid cartilage.

5.20

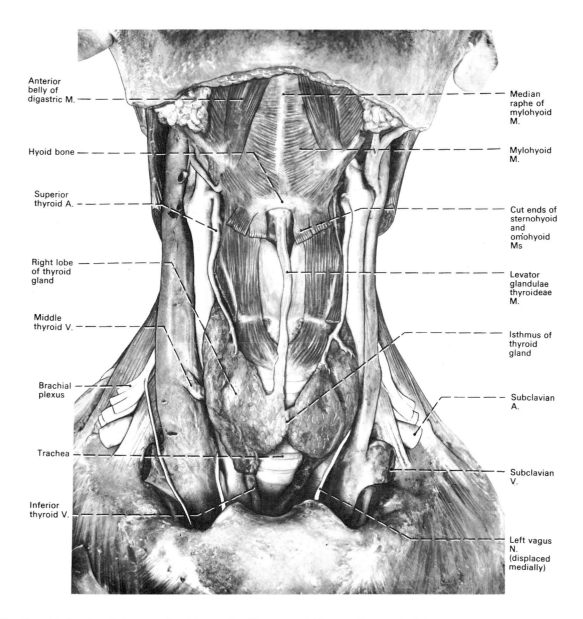

Anterior belly of digastric M.

Hyoid bone

Superior thyroid A.

Right lobe of thyroid gland

Middle thyroid V.

Brachial plexus

Trachea

Inferior thyroid V.

Median raphe of mylohyoid M.

Mylohyoid M.

Cut ends of sternohyoid and omohyoid Ms

Levator glandulae thyroideae M.

Isthmus of thyroid gland

Subclavian A.

Subclavian V.

Left vagus N. (displaced medially)

Fig. 5.22 The thyroid gland and the suprahyoid muscles. The sternocleidomastoid, sternohyoid, omohyoid, and sternothyroid muscles have been removed.

5. The upper borders of the thyroid cartilages, with a membrane, the thyrohyoid membrane, attaching them to the hyoid bone above.

Separate the sternothyroid muscle from the thyroid gland with the handle of your scalpel, and divide the muscle, with scissors, horizontally at the same level as you did the sternohyoid. Reflect both ends of the muscle, using a scalpel or scissors to free its lateral border.

The thyroid gland [Fig. 5.22]

The two **lobes** of the thyroid gland, one on each side of the trachea and the lower part of the larynx, and the **isthmus** connecting them across the front of the trachea, are now

completely exposed [Fig. 5.22]. The lines of insertion of the sternothyroid muscles define the upper limits of the lobes. Note that the thyroid gland overlaps the common carotid arteries but is separated from them by fascia. Occasionally the isthmus is connected to the hyoid bone by a narrow muscular band, the **levator glandulae thyroideae** [Fig. 5.22]. You will examine the thyroid gland again at a later stage.

The suprahyoid muscles [Fig. 5.22]

Now turn your attention to the area in the midline of the neck above the hyoid bone. Carefully pick up the deep fascia and dissect it off the underlying muscle. On either side of the midline you will find a muscle, the **anterior belly of the digastric muscle.** The two anterior bellies converge towards

5.21

the point of the chin. At this stage merely identify their medial borders. The muscles lying on a deeper plane between them are the **mylohyoid muscles.** The two mylo-hyoid muscles meet in a median raphe, so forming the floor of the mouth.

The cervical fascia [Fig. 5.23]

When exposing and tracing structures in the neck you may at times run into difficulties because of the condensations of connective tissue that form various layers of the deep cervical fascia. What is called the **superficial layer** of deep cervical fascia lies immediately deep to the platysma muscle and the subcutaneous nerves and veins of the neck. From its posterior attachment to the ligamentum nuchae this layer encircles the neck, splitting to ensheathe the trapezius and

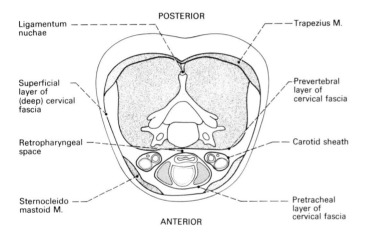

Fig. 5.23 The deep cervical fascia (schematic transverse section).

sternocleidomastoid muscles, between which it forms the fascial roof to the posterior triangle [p. 5.11]. Inferiorly the superficial layer is bound down to the periosteum of the sub-cutaneous parts of the clavicle, scapula, and sternum. Superiorly the principal attachments of the superficial layer are to the hyoid bone, the lower border of the mandible, the mastoid process and the superior nuchal line. You will come across this superficial layer of deep fascia again when you dissect the parotid and submandibular glands [pp. 5.43 and 5.63], which are both encapsulated by it.

In addition to the superficial layer, three deeper layers of deep cervical fascia are generally distinguished. You have already seen the **carotid sheath** which binds together the components of the neurovascular bundle that lies on each side of the midline visceral structures of the neck. The latter, which comprise the larynx, trachea, laryngeal pharynx, and oesophagus, are themselves enclosed by a sleeve of fascia, the **pretracheal layer.** The pretracheal fascia splits to encapsulate the thyroid gland which is thus firmly bound to the trachea. Finally there is a **prevertebral layer** of fascia that covers the scalene and other muscles in the floor of the posterior triangle. You have already removed some of this fascia when you cleaned these muscles and traced the phrenic nerve and brachial plexus [pp. 5.14 to 5.15]. The prevertebral fascia gets its name because it also covers the muscles that clothe the anterior surface of the vertebral column. You will examine these muscles at a much later stage of dissection [p. 5.96].

Although four parts of the deep cervical fascia are defined, they blend with each other in certain places so that partial boundaries are formed to the potential spaces between them. The latter are filled by loose connective tissue. One such space, which you will see later, is the **retro-pharyngeal space** [p. 5.79] between the pharynx and the pre-vertebral fascia.

Section 5.4

Bisection of the head

The exposure of the deep cervical structures would come next in logical sequence, but before this can be done, it is necessary to remove the angle of the mandible, and structures on the side of the face which would otherwise be destroyed must first be examined. At this stage, too, the head is bisected into right and left halves.

If desired, the bisection of the head may be deferred until the face and temporal region, the infratemporal region, and the upper part of the neck have been dissected. If this order is followed the student should now turn to page 5.35 and continue until page 5.70 before turning back to this page The order of dissection then becomes:

Another variation in the sequence of dissection may be adopted before bisecting the head, to enable you to examine the spinal medulla before you study the brain *in situ*. If this procedure is advised by your teacher, then turn to page 5.120 and follow the instructions for the dissection of the deep muscles of the back and the exposure of the spinal medulla; but do not open up the vertebral canal beyond the second thoracic vertebra above, or the fifth lumbar vertebra below. When you have examined the spinal medulla, do not embark on the study of the joints and ligaments of the vertebral column on page 5.124 but return to the task of bisecting the head according to the following instructions.

The advantage of bisection at an earlier stage is that it permits the structures which form the walls of the mouth and pharynx to be dissected from both their medial and lateral aspects. Dissectors of one side of the head are able to work without being inconvenienced by those of the other side, and they can dissect the same structure from its medial aspect while the others approach it from the lateral side. But this dissection has the disadvantage that the contents of the skull will dry out unless special precautions are taken.

The following instruments should be used at this stage:
A frame-saw, a small amputation-saw, bone-cutting forceps [see Fig. 0.1], and a wooden block with a semicircular notch to support the head.

1. Lay the body supine, with the neck in the notch of the block. In order to avoid debris falling on the floor make quite sure that the head does not overlap the edge of the table.
2. Stand at the head of the body.
3. The nose, which is often bent to one side, should be pushed back into the midline, and divided in the midline with a scalpel as deeply as you can.
4. Insert the blade of the frame-saw into this incision and, keeping your saw as nearly as possible in the median plane, start sawing through the mandible and the bone of the forehead [Fig. 5.24a].

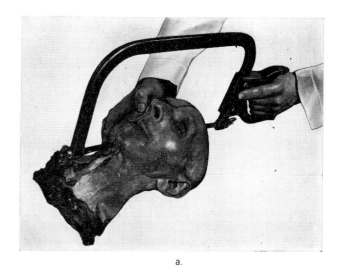

a.

Fig. 5.24 Bisection of the head.

5. When you have divided the mandible, use a scalpel to continue the cut through the soft tissues of the floor of the mouth and upper part of the neck in the same plane. Divide the hyoid bone with bone-cutting forceps at its midpoint, and continue dividing the soft tissues of the neck, with a scalpel, in the median plane, until you reach the midline of the cervical part of the vertebral column.

At this point start sawing again, with someone helping you by holding the head and neck and guarding the divided soft tissues from the saw.

6. Deepen the saw-cut as far as possible, until the handle of the saw meets the table on which the body is lying.

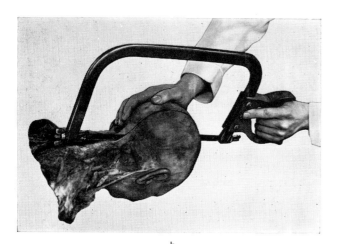

b.

Fig. 5.24

7. Turn the body over, and incise the skin over the occiput with a scalpel, in line with the saw-cut. The soft tissues overlying the spinous processes should then be incised with a scalpel until you reach the bone. Having done so, insert the saw in the incision, and saw forwards in the median plane as deeply as possible [Fig. 5.24b]. The sawcut should be extended into the spinous processes.

8. Turn the body on its side so that the right side is uppermost. Transect all the soft tissues with a scalpel just above the line of the right first rib. The incision should pass between the subclavian vessels below and the lower

end of the thyroid gland above. Use a saw to carry the section through the vertebral column as far as the midline [Fig. 5.24c].

9. Complete the median section of the bone of the skull, where necessary, with the small amputation-saw, until you can separate the two halves. The left half of the head remains attached to the trunk.

The skull is hardly ever bisected exactly in the median plane. While the larynx and pharynx are usually satisfactorily divided, the oesophagus, which lies behind the trachea, often slips to one or other side of the cut. For this and other reasons it is essential that the dissectors of one half of the head should co-operate in their work with those of the other.

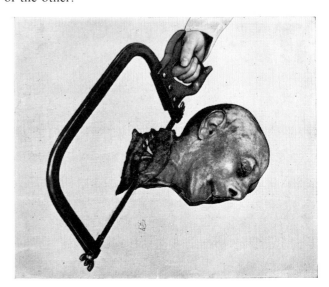

c.

Section 5.5

The contents of the skull

Because the contents of the skull would dry out if the dissection of more superficial structures were continued at this stage, they are examined now. You will continue the dissection of the neck and face after the brain has been removed.

Osteology

With a skull available for reference, examine the medial surfaces of the halves of the head you have divided. First identify the following structures: the **cervical vertebrae** and

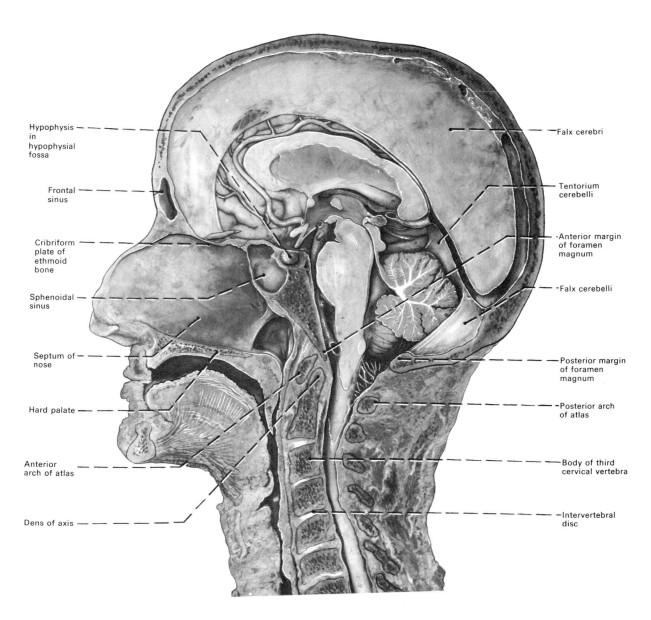

Hypophysis in hypophysial fossa

Frontal sinus

Cribriform plate of ethmoid bone

Sphenoidal sinus

Septum of nose

Hard palate

Anterior arch of atlas

Dens of axis

Falx cerebri

Tentorium cerebelli

Anterior margin of foramen magnum

Falx cerebelli

Posterior margin of foramen magnum

Posterior arch of atlas

Body of third cervical vertebra

Intervertebral disc

Fig. 5.25 Median section of the head and neck.

the **intervertebral discs**; the anterior and the posterior arches of the **atlas**; the dens of the **axis**, extending upwards from the body of the axis, behind the anterior arch of the atlas [Fig. 5.25]. Note especially that the axis lies at the level of the cavity of the mouth, immediately behind the posterior wall of the pharynx.

Now identify the **foramen magnum** on the cadaver, and starting at its posterior margin, follow the sectioned skull over the **calvaria** or skull-cap, to the face in front, and all the way round to the anterior margin of the foramen. As you do so, identify the **occipital bone**, the **parietal bone**, and the **frontal bone**. In the cadaver you will see a large air-filled space, the **frontal sinus**, just above the root of the nose. In the median plane behind the frontal sinus is a crest of bone, the **crista galli of the ethmoid bone** [Fig. 5.26]. Identify this in the skull, since it may have been destroyed when you divided the head. On each side of the crista galli is a small area of perforated bone called the **cribriform plate** of the ethmoid bone [Figs 5.25 and 5.26].

Behind the cribriform plate is the **sphenoid bone**, which lies in front of the foramen magnum. On the upper surface of the sphenoid bone is a deep depression, the **sella turcica**, which is bounded posteriorly by the **dorsum sellae**. The deepest part of the sella turcica is called the **hypophysial fossa**. In the **body of the sphenoid bone**, below the hypophysial fossa, you will see an air-filled space, the **sphenoidal sinus** [Fig. 5.25].

The posterior surface of the body of the sphenoid bone slopes downwards and backwards towards the anterior margin of the foramen magnum. Halfway down, the sphenoid bone meets the **basilar part of the occipital bone**, which forms the anterior margin of the foramen. Below the cribriform plate and the sphenoid bone is one half of the **nasal cavity**, which is bounded inferiorly by the **hard palate**. The median **septum of the nose** between the two halves of the nasal cavity will either be entirely on one half of the divided head, or parts of the septum will be present on both sides.

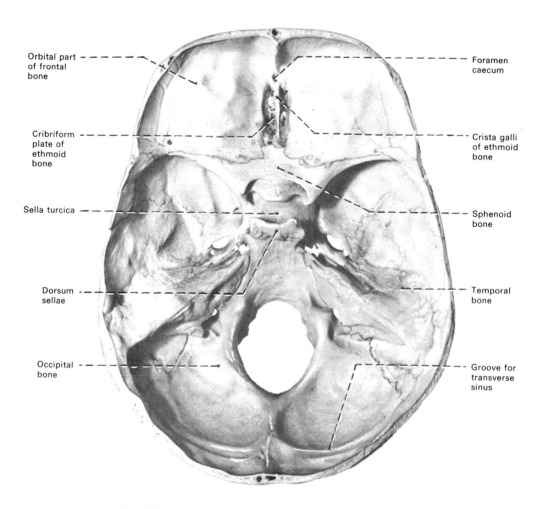

Orbital part
of frontal
bone

Cribriform
plate of
ethmoid
bone

Sella turcica

Dorsum
sellae

Occipital
bone

Foramen
caecum

Crista galli
of ethmoid
bone

Sphenoid
bone

Temporal
bone

Groove for
transverse
sinus

Fig. 5.26 The internal surface of the base of the skull.

The meninges and the brain

The brain lies within the skull, and the spinal medulla lies in the vertebral canal of the vertebral column. Both are separated from the bone by three membranes or meninges, called, from without in, the **dura mater,** the **arachnoid,** and the **pia mater.**

The dura mater

The outermost membrane, or dura mater, is thick, and is easily identified in the vertebral canal and on the inner surface of the occipital bone. The dura mater forms the periosteum of the internal surface of the whole skull, and has a second inner layer which forms median and horizontal folds or septa that help divide the interior of the skull into compartments. Some of the folds may have been damaged when the head was sawn in two, but their normal arrangement can be realized by looking at the two halves of the head together.

A large partition that is disposed vertically in the median plane is the **falx cerebri** [Fig. 5.25]. Its upper border is attached to the under-surface of the calvaria, while its free and lower border arches from the crista galli in front, to a point some 5 cm in front of the occipital bone behind. Here the lower border of the falx cerebri is attached to the upper surface of a horizontal diaphragm of dura mater, the cut edge of which can be clearly seen, especially on the half of the head that lacks the falx cerebri. This horizontal diaphragm is known as the **tentorium cerebelli.** Its lateral border is attached to the inner surface of the skull, and its free, medial border encircles the part of the brain that lies behind the dorsum sellae. You will not be able to see the whole extent of the tentorium cerebelli until the brain has been removed. Below the tentorium you will see a low sagittal partition, the **falx cerebelli,** which is attached to the inner surface of the occipital bone in the midline. At the foramen magnum, the outer layer of the dura mater is continuous with the periosteum on the external surface of the cranium, while the inner layer continues down the vertebral canal to surround the spinal medulla.

The brain

The major subdivisions of the brain [Figs 5.27 and 5.28]

Now identify the three major subdivisions of the brain:

1. The **forebrain** lies above the tentorium cerebelli, and comprises the right and left cerebral hemispheres and the diencephalon, which lies between the two hemispheres [Fig. 5.27].
2. The **midbrain** is the part of the brain lying in the opening in the tentorium cerebelli.
3. The **hindbrain** comprises the pons, medulla oblongata, and the cerebellum, and lies below the tentorium cerebelli.

The cerebral hemispheres [Fig. 5.28]

Each cerebral hemisphere is divided into four lobes, named according to their relation to the four main bones that form the calvaria (the frontal, parietal, occipital, and temporal bones). The anterior convexity of the hemisphere forms most of the **frontal lobe,** and its most anterior or rostral part is the **frontal pole** [Fig. 5.28]. The posterior part of the hemisphere is the **occipital lobe,** which lies on the upper surface of the tentorium cerebelli. Its most posterior part is the **occipital pole.** The **parietal lobe** lies between the frontal and occipital lobes, from which it is demarcated by somewhat arbitrary boundaries. The **temporal lobe** is best seen when the brain has been removed. It lies on the lateral aspect of the brain, in front of the occipital lobe, projecting forwards below the parietal and frontal lobes, but falling well short of the frontal pole.

The hypophysis [Fig. 5.29]

Now examine the **hypophysial fossa.** It is occupied by a small endocrine gland called the **hypophysis,** also known as the **pituitary gland,** which is connected by a stalk, the **infundibulum,** to the part of the brain immediately above it [Fig. 5.29]. The infundibulum may still be visible even if it has been severed or otherwise damaged when the head was divided. If you look at it closely, you will see that the surface of the infundibulum is marked by longitudinal venous channels. The part of the forebrain to which the hypophysis is attached, between the two cerebral hemispheres, is the **diencephalon.** Posteriorly, the diencephalon is continuous with the midbrain, which joins the forebrain to the hindbrain.

The brain stem [Figs 5.27 and 5.28]

The bulge on the anterior surface of the brain immediately behind the dorsum sellae and below the midbrain is the pons. Below the pons is the medulla oblongata, which extends through the foramen magnum to continue into the spinal medulla. The **midbrain, pons,** and **medulla oblongata,** are often collectively referred to as the brain stem.

The cerebellum [Figs 5.27 and 5.28]

The cerebellum lies behind the pons and medulla oblongata. It is roofed over by the tentorium cerebelli. The cerebellum comprises right and left **cerebellar hemispheres** joined by a midline portion, the **vermis.** The falx cerebelli is interposed between the hemispheres.

The arachnoid and the pia mater

The middle layer of the meninges, or arachnoid, lines the inner surface of the dura mater. The innermost layer of the meninges, the pia mater, adheres closely to the brain and spinal medulla. The space between it and the arachnoid is known as the **subarachnoid space.** This space is criss-crossed by fine strands of connective tissue that pass from the arachnoid to the pia mater. In the living body it is filled with **cerebrospinal fluid,** but during the preparation of the cadaver for dissection, the cerebrospinal fluid disappears, and the arachnoid usually collapses on to the pia mater, especially over the cerebral hemispheres. One of the parts of the subarachnoid space that usually persists is just in front of the posterior margin of the foramen magnum, where the space is enlarged and forms a cistern for the cerebrospinal fluid. It is here that the arachnoid itself is most easily identified. There are a number of such cisterns, but the only important one, called the **cerebellomedullary cistern,** is the one lying in the foramen magnum [Fig. 5.27]. In sagittal section, it appears as a triangular space bounded by the dura mater posteriorly, the medulla oblongata anteriorly and the cerebellum superiorly.

Intracranial vessels

The basilar artery [Fig. 5.27]

The arteries and veins of the brain and spinal medulla also lie in the subarachnoid space. This fact can be best appreciated by examining the anterior surface of the pons and medulla oblongata, behind the dorsum sellae. The vessel you will see close to the midline is the basilar artery, which is formed by the junction of the two **vertebral arteries** [see p. 6.3]. These enter the skull through the foramen magnum.

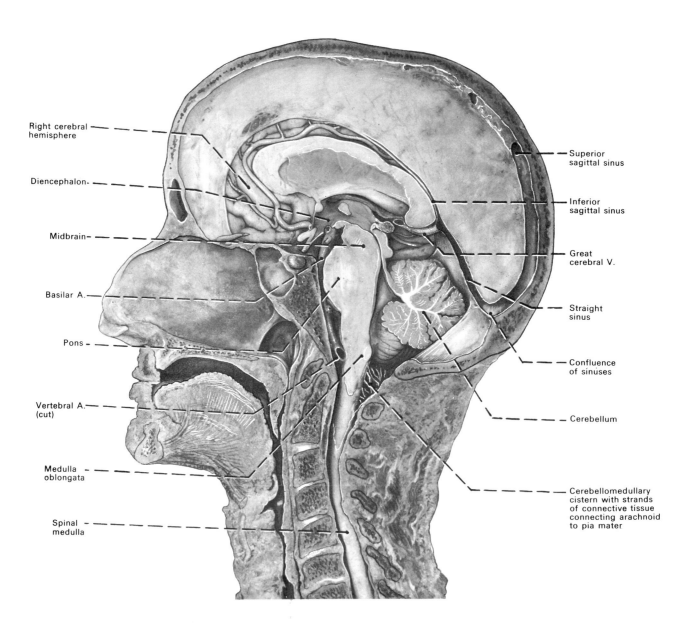

Right cerebral hemisphere

Diencephalon

Midbrain

Basilar A.

Pons

Vertebral A. (cut)

Medulla oblongata

Spinal medulla

Superior sagittal sinus

Inferior sagittal sinus

Great cerebral V.

Straight sinus

Confluence of sinuses

Cerebellum

Cerebellomedullary cistern with strands of connective tissue connecting arachnoid to pia mater

Fig. 5.27 **Median section of the head and neck.**

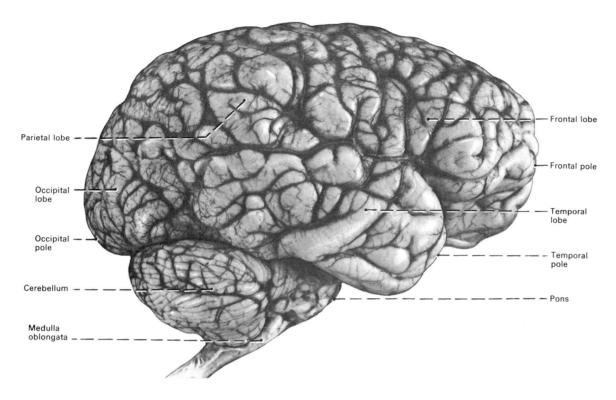

Parietal lobe

Occipital lobe

Occipital pole

Cerebellum

Medulla oblongata

Frontal lobe

Frontal pole

Temporal lobe

Temporal pole

Pons

Fig. 5.28 The right side of the brain. The midbrain is hidden from view.

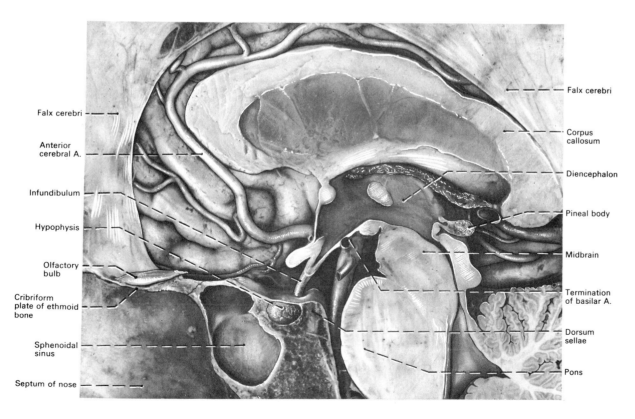

Falx cerebri

Anterior cerebral A.

Infundibulum

Hypophysis

Olfactory bulb

Cribriform plate of ethmoid bone

Sphenoidal sinus

Septum of nose

Falx cerebri

Corpus callosum

Diencephalon

Pineal body

Midbrain

Termination of basilar A.

Dorsum sellae

Pons

Fig. 5.29 Median section of the head. Enlargement of part of Fig. 5.27.

The basilar artery, which breaks up into branches behind the sella turcica, may have been damaged when the head was divided, but you should be able to confirm that it lies within the subarachnoid space [Fig. 5.29].

Sinuses of the dura mater [Figs 5.27 and 5.108]

The veins of the brain drain into venous sinuses which lie between the two layers of the dura mater. These are collectively referred to as sinuses of the dura mater. One, the **superior sagittal sinus,** lies between the layers of the dura mater in the attached border of the falx cerebri, as it arches backwards over the brain. It begins at a small foramen, the **foramen caecum,** just in front of the crista galli [Fig. 5.26]. Open up the superior sagittal sinus, using scissors if necessary, and clean it out so as to see the openings of **cerebral veins** in its walls. If you look carefully you may see a number of small granular elevations on the walls of the superior sagittal sinus, either singly or in clusters. These are the **arachnoid granulations** through which cerebrospinal fluid is absorbed into the blood stream.

At the posterior end of the falx cerebri, the superior sagittal sinus drains into one or both of two **transverse sinuses** which run laterally, one on each side of the head, in the attached border of the tentorium cerebelli. You cannot yet see the course of these sinuses, but at least one of them will have been cut across when the head was divided. Determine into which transverse sinus the superior sagittal sinus drains. It is more commonly the right one.

You will find a sinus, the **straight sinus,** lying along the line of the attachment of the falx cerebri to the tentorium cerebelli [Fig. 5.27]. Unless the posterior part of the skull was cut exactly in the midline, more of the straight sinus will appear on one of the halves of the head than on the other. At its posterior end this sinus joins the superior sagittal sinus and the two transverse sinuses at a junction called the **confluence of the sinuses.**

Open the straight sinus with scissors, cutting forwards from the confluence. At its anterior end the sinus receives the **great cerebral vein,** which is a large vessel that emerges from a point just above and behind the midbrain [Fig. 5.27]. Also draining into the anterior end of the straight sinus is the small **inferior sagittal sinus** which lies in the free border of the falx cerebri.

Look at the interior of a skull and identify the grooves which correspond to the superior sagittal and transverse sinuses.

Removal of the brain

The brain has now to be removed. At a later stage of your dissection, properly prepared specimens of other brains should be provided for study, but the opportunity ought to be taken now to see some of the blood vessels and nerves which run to and from the brain.

If there is any falx cerebri on the half of the head you are dissecting, cut along its attached border just below the superior sagittal sinus, as far back as the posterior end of the straight sinus.

Transect the brain stem at the level of the foramen magnum, taking care not to damage any of the surrounding structures. Very gently bend the lower end of the brain stem backwards and medially, and with a sharp scalpel or fine scissors, divide all the fine nerves and vessels which you find attached to it, cutting close to the surface. Most of the nerves and vessels are attached to the anterior and lateral surfaces of the brain stem. As you section the nerves and vessels, turn the brain stem upwards, at the same time lifting the cerebellum out of the skull. On the postero-lateral surface of the midbrain you will see a fine nerve (the trochlear nerve) which must also be divided.

Now divide the infundibulum [p. 5.27], the nerve close to it (the optic nerve), and the large artery which lies below and lateral to the nerve (the internal carotid artery). Starting anteriorly, lift the cerebral hemisphere out of the skull, and as you do so cut the veins which enter the superior sagittal sinus. Note that the larger of these veins, and posteriorly, the smaller ones as well, are directed obliquely forwards. Blood flows in these vessels against the current in the superior sagittal sinus, which is from before backwards.

You should now be able to remove the brain completely; but be careful not to tear the cranial nerves, otherwise you may not see where they pierce the dura mater. When you have completed the removal of the brain identify the temporal lobe on its lateral surface.

The interior of the skull

The anterior cranial fossa [Fig. 5.31]

Examine the base of the skull from within [Fig. 5.30]. The frontal lobe of the brain lodges in the anterior cranial fossa immediately over the orbit. Most of the floor of this fossa is formed by part of the frontal bone, but if you examine a skull you will see that its sharp posterior margin is part of a lateral process of the sphenoid bone, called the **lesser wing of the sphenoid.** The backwardly-projecting process at the medial end of the posterior border of the lesser wing is called the **anterior clinoid process.** Immediately below the lesser wing is the **superior orbital fissure,** leading into the orbit. In your specimen this fissure is covered over by dura mater.

The middle cranial fossa [Fig. 5.31]

Behind and below the anterior cranial fossa is the middle cranial fossa, which was occupied by the temporal lobe of the brain. Study this fossa in a skull, and you will see that its floor is formed anteriorly by the upper surface of another lateral projection of the sphenoid bone, called the **greater wing of the sphenoid** [Fig. 5.30]. The posterior two-thirds of

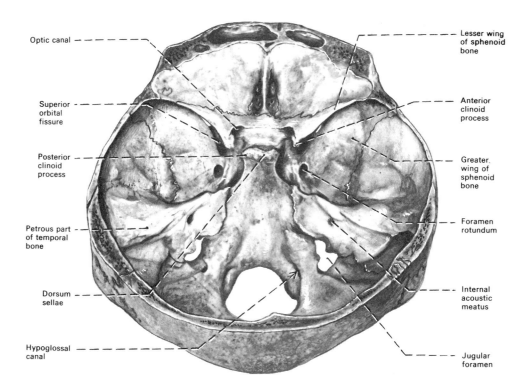

Optic canal

Superior orbital fissure

Posterior clinoid process

Petrous part of temporal bone

Dorsum sellae

Hypoglossal canal

Lesser wing of sphenoid bone

Anterior clinoid process

Greater wing of sphenoid bone

Foramen rotundum

Internal acoustic meatus

Jugular foramen

Fig. 5.30 The internal surface of the base of the skull (from above and behind).

the floor and its postero-medial margin are parts of a large bony mass, called the **petrous part of the temporal bone.** In the cadaver you will find that the floor of the middle cranial fossa is continuous posteriorly with the upper surface of the tentorium cerebelli.

The tentorium cerebelli

Examine the peripheral or attached border of the tentorium cerebelli. Posteriorly it is fixed to the occipital bone along the margins of the **groove for the transverse sinus** [Fig. 5.26]; but laterally you will find that it is attached to the temporal bone where this bone forms the postero-medial margin of the middle cranial fossa. Anteriorly, the attachment of this border extends on to the sphenoid bone, ending on a tubercle, the **posterior clinoid process,** at the lateral end of the superior border of the dorsum sellae [Fig. 5.30]. Identify this process on a skull. Now follow the medial or free border of the tentorium cerebelli forwards. Anteriorly it crosses above the attached border, and is fixed to the anterior clinoid process.

The posterior cranial fossa [Fig. 5.31]

Below the tentorium cerebelli is the posterior cranial fossa, in which the hindbrain lies. Its floor and posterior wall are formed by the occipital bone; its antero-lateral wall by the temporal bone. It is bounded anteriorly by the basilar part of the occipital bone and by the posterior surface of the body of the sphenoid bone.

Arteries to the brain

The brain is supplied by the terminal parts of the internal carotid and vertebral arteries. You will be able to identify the **internal carotid artery** piercing the dura mater medial to the anterior clinoid process, and the **vertebral artery** ascending through the foramen magnum [Fig. 5.31]. The **basilar artery,** which, as you have seen, is formed by the union of the two vertebral arteries, is likely to be intact on one half of the head. It ascends to the superior border of the dorsum sellae where it terminates by dividing into branches. In the region of the hypophysis the internal carotid and basilar arteries and their branches form an anastomosis called the **cerebral arterial circle.** This will be studied later, when the brain is dissected [see p. 6.4].

The cranial nerves

The brain and spinal medulla are connected by nerves to the sense receptors and muscles of the body. There is a pair of spinal nerves attached to each segment of the spinal medulla, and there are twelve pairs of cranial nerves.

The first cranial nerve

The **olfactory nerves** comprise the first cranial nerve, and form leashes of fibres that traverse the perforations in the cribriform plate of the ethmoid bone on either side of the crista galli [see Fig. 5.115]. This small area of bone is inter-

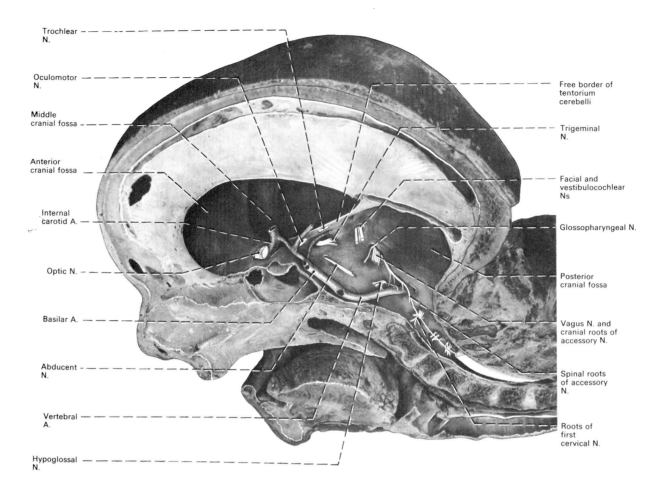

Trochlear N.

Oculomotor N.

Middle cranial fossa

Anterior cranial fossa

Internal carotid A.

Optic N.

Basilar A.

Abducent N.

Vertebral A.

Hypoglossal N.

Free border of tentorium cerebelli

Trigeminal N.

Facial and vestibulocochlear Ns

Glossopharyngeal N.

Posterior cranial fossa

Vagus N. and cranial roots of accessory N.

Spinal roots of accessory N.

Roots of first cervical N.

Fig. 5.31 Oblique view of the right half of the head after removal of the brain.

posed between the anterior cranial fossa above and the mucous coat of the nose in the uppermost part of the nasal cavity below. On one or other half of the head you should be able to confirm that the nasal cavity and anterior cranial fossa lie very close to each other in this region, but it is unlikely that you will see any of the nerves which run from the nasal mucosa to the **olfactory bulb,** which is a small mass of nervous tissue that immediately overlies the cribriform plate [Fig. 5.29]. It is probable that the olfactory bulb has been removed with the brain.

The second cranial nerve

Find the **optic canal** in a skull. It lies at the root of the lesser wing of the sphenoid bone, medial to the anterior clinoid process [Fig. 5.30]. It is traversed by the second cranial or **optic nerve** and the ophthalmic artery, which is a branch of the internal carotid artery. Identify the optic canal on your dissection. The optic nerve is the thick stump of nerve emerging from the canal and lying antero-medial to, and above, the internal carotid artery [Fig. 5.31]. The nerve carries information to the brain from the retina of the eye.

The third cranial nerve [Fig. 5.31]

The slender nerve that you will see piercing the dura mater between the anterior and posterior clinoid processes is the third cranial or **oculomotor nerve.** This nerve enters the orbit through the superior orbital fissure, and supplies most of the muscles of the eyeball.

The fourth cranial nerve [Fig. 5.31]

The only cranial nerve that emerges from the posterior surface of the brain stem is the fourth cranial or **trochlear nerve.** It is a very fine nerve, which you will find piercing the inner layer of dura mater on the under-surface of the tentorium cerebelli close to its free border, about 1.5 cm behind the anterior clinoid process. This nerve also reaches the orbit through the superior orbital fissure. It supplies one of the muscles of the eyeball (the superior oblique muscle).

The fifth cranial nerve [Fig. 5.31]

The fifth cranial or **trigeminal nerve** is the largest cranial nerve. It has a larger **sensory root** which innervates the skin

5.32

of the face and scalp, as well as the mucous coats of the nose and mouth, and a smaller **motor root** whose fibres supply muscles of mastication.

You will find the nerve as it enters a small out-pouching of the inner layer of the dura mater just below the medial end of the attached border of the tentorium cerebelli. The motor root of the nerve lies medial to the sensory root. The pouch, the **cavum trigeminale,** lies beneath the dura mater of the floor of the middle cranial fossa and contains a large ganglion of the trigeminal nerve, which will be dissected later.

The trigeminal nerve is so named because it divides into three parts, the **ophthalmic nerve,** the **maxillary nerve,** and the **mandibular nerve,** which leave the skull separately. You will not be able to see these nerves at this stage of your dissection.

The sixth cranial nerve [Fig. 5.31]

Look for a fine nerve that pierces the dura mater on the dorsum sellae near to the midline, and a little below the level of the trigeminal nerve. This is the sixth cranial or **abducent nerve** which, like the trochlear nerve, enters the orbit through the superior orbital fissure, to supply one muscle of the eyeball (the lateral rectus muscle).

The seventh and eighth cranial nerves [Fig. 5.31]

Below and postero-lateral to the trigeminal nerve you will see the seventh cranial, or **facial nerve,** and the eighth cranial, or **vestibulocochlear nerve,** passing laterally and entering the opening of a canal in the anterior wall of the posterior cranial fossa. Find this canal in the petrous part of the temporal bone of a skull [Fig. 5.30]. It is the **internal acoustic meatus.** The eighth nerve innervates the organs of hearing and balance, which are situated inside this bone. The seventh nerve takes a devious route through the petrous part of the temporal bone, and finally emerges from the skull through the **stylomastoid foramen,** which you should find on a skull medial to the anterior end of the mastoid process [Fig. 5.51]. You will dissect the facial nerve in its course through the temporal bone at a later stage, and when you dissect the face, you will see that the nerve supplies the sub-cutaneous muscles of facial expression.

As they enter the internal acoustic meatus, the facial nerve lies anterior to the vestibulocochlear nerve. Between the two you may see another nerve, which usually lies closer to the vestibulocochlear nerve. This is part of the facial nerve, and is called the **nervus intermedius.** A fine branch of the basilar artery also enters the internal acoustic meatus.

The ninth, tenth, and eleventh cranial nerves

Find a leash of nerves which pierce the dura mater below the internal acoustic meatus. These are the ninth cranial or **glossopharyngeal nerve,** the tenth cranial or **vagus nerve,** and the eleventh cranial or **accessory nerve,** which lie in that order from above down [Fig. 5.31]. They leave the skull through the **jugular foramen,** which lies below the point where they pierce the dura mater. Identify this foramen on the inner, and then on the outer surface of a skull [Fig. 5.30]. This complex of three nerves innervates the mucous coat and the striated and smooth muscles of the digestive and respiratory systems. The vagus nerve continues through the thorax into the abdominal cavity.

You will see a long slender nerve ascending from the vertebral canal, crossing the posterior aspect of the vertebral artery, and joining the ninth, tenth, and eleventh cranial nerves. It is formed from the **spinal roots of the accessory nerve,** which arise from the upper half of the cervical part of the spinal medulla. As can be seen, the spinal roots of the accessory join the **cranial roots of the accessory nerve** [Fig. 5.31]. The nerve fibres from the two sets of roots part company immediately outside the skull. Those from the spinal roots descend to supply the sternocleidomastoid and trapezius muscles. They have already been seen at the side of the neck [p. 5.11]. Those from the cranial roots of the accessory nerve join the vagus nerve.

The twelfth cranial nerve [Fig. 5.31]

The twelfth cranial or **hypoglossal nerve** will be found as a group of rootlets leaving the interior of the skull below and medial to the glossopharyngeal, vagus, and accessory nerves. It passes out of the skull through the **hypoglossal canal,** which should be examined on a skull [Fig. 5.30]. This canal lies immediately above the level of the foramen magnum. The nerve supplies the muscles of the tongue.

The further study of the dura mater and of the cranial nerves is now left until a later stage. Until then, leave a wet cloth inside the skull and place the two halves of the head together after each day's dissection, in order to prevent the dura mater from becoming dry and brittle.

The contents of the skull in general

Before returning to the dissection of the surface of the head and neck, note again that the anterior and middle cranial fossae of the skull are occupied by the cerebral hemispheres, and that the cerebellum lies in the posterior fossa, below the tentorium cerebelli. Remember that the attached border of the tentorium cerebelli is fixed to the posterior clinoid processes (in front of which the free border is fixed to the anterior clinoid processes) and the medial part of the petrous part of the temporal bone. Note, too, that the narrow anterior end of the falx cerebri is attached to the crista galli, and that its base is applied in the median plane to the whole width of the tentorium cerebelli. The falx cerebri separates the two cerebral hemispheres in the same way as the smaller falx cerebelli lies in the interval between the two cerebellar hemispheres. Look at the middle cranial fossa and try to visualize the temporal lobes of the cerebral hemispheres lying in front, with the occipital lobes behind, above the tentorium cerebelli. Recall, too, the sinuses of the dura mater which you have seen. The superior sagittal sinus usually runs into the right transverse sinus, and the straight sinus into the left transverse sinus. At a later stage you will dissect the sigmoid sinuses, which connect the transverse sinuses with the internal jugular veins, and the cavernous sinuses, which lie on either side of the hypophysial fossa. Finally, before turning from the interior of the skull, make sure that you can identify the cranial nerves and the foramina they traverse on their way out of the skull.

Section 5.6

The face and the temporal region

The dissection of the neck was interrupted at the stage where the deeper cervical structures were to be examined. They cannot, however, be seen before the mandible is displaced, and before this is done the superficial anatomy of the face must be examined.

The anterior third of the face is formed by the walls of the mouth. The muscle of the cheek is the **buccinator** [Fig. 5.32], and that of the lips the **orbicularis oris.** The fibres of these two muscles are joined at the angle of the mouth by those of a number of small fine muscles which lie in the fatty

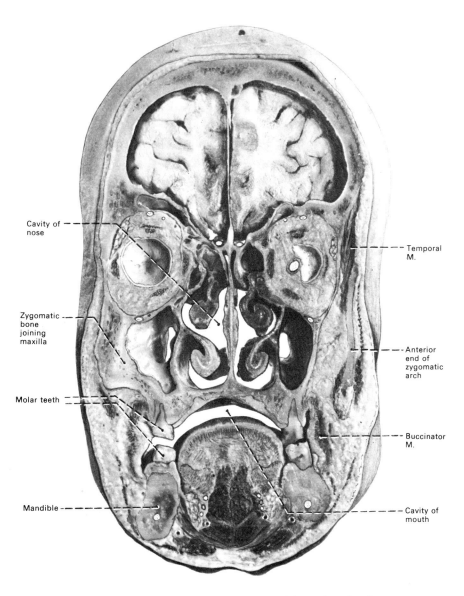

Cavity of nose

Zygomatic bone joining maxilla

Molar teeth

Mandible

Temporal M.

Anterior end of zygomatic arch

Buccinator M.

Cavity of mouth

Fig. 5.32 Frontal section of the head (anterior view).

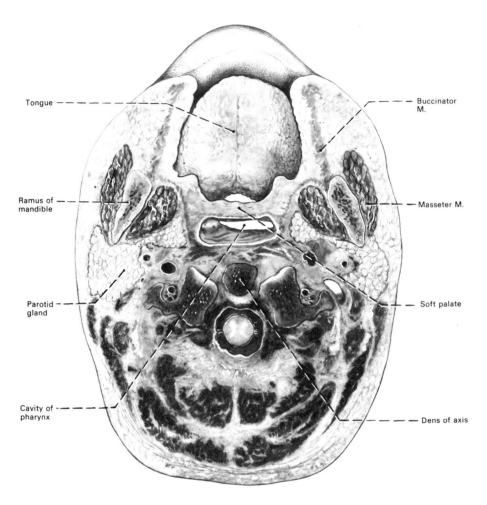

Tongue

Ramus of mandible

Parotid gland

Cavity of pharynx

Buccinator M.

Masseter M.

Soft palate

Dens of axis

Fig. 5.33 Horizontal section of the head. The head is sectioned at the level of the joint between the axis and the lateral mass of the atlas.

subcutaneous tissue of the cheek. These belong to a group of muscles known as the **muscles of facial expression,** since their pull determines the set of the skin of the face.

The buccinator muscle is attached to the lateral surfaces of the maxilla and mandible, some distance above and below those parts of their borders from which the molar teeth project.

The construction of the posterior two-thirds of the face is more complex than that of the anterior third. The posterior end of the cavity of the mouth narrows, and is continuous behind with the pharynx. The pharynx also has a muscular wall, with which the posterior border of the buccinator muscle is contiguous [Fig. 5.33]. A number of structures intervene between the wall of the pharynx and the skin of the side of the face. The principal one is the broad **ramus of the mandible,** whose upper end articulates with the squamous part of the temporal bone. The **muscles of mastication** pass from the skull to the ramus, and one of them, the masseter, covers most of its lateral surface. In addition, the **parotid gland** is wrapped round the posterior border

of the ramus, lying between it and the external acoustic meatus. Part of this gland overlies the masseter muscle, and is thus just beneath the skin.

The temporal region of the head is separated from the face by a bar of bone called the **zygomatic arch.** This runs forwards from the region of the auricle to the cheek or zygomatic bone, below and lateral to the eye. The temporal region lies at the side of the skull, and like the vertex above, consists of bone covered by skin, with a thin aponeurotic sheet intervening. From the temporal region one of the muscles of mastication, the temporal muscle, takes origin.

The cutaneous nerves of the region are branches of the trigeminal nerve. The facial nerve innervates the muscles of facial expression, and the motor root of the trigeminal nerve innervates the muscles of mastication. The vessels of the face are in two groups. The facial artery, which is a branch of the external carotid artery, and the facial vein serve the anterior part of the face. The artery supplying the posterior part of the face and the temporal region is the superficial temporal artery, one of the two terminal branches of the external carotid artery, the other terminal branch being the maxillary artery. This region is drained by the retromandibular vein.

Osteology and surface anatomy

The mandible [Fig. 5.34]

With a skull in front of you, so that you can correlate what you feel with what you see, palpate the lower border, or **base,** of the **body** of the mandible on yourself and follow it backwards. It ends at the **angle** of the mandible [Fig. 5.34]. From here trace the posterior border of the **ramus** or vertical part of the mandible. Its upper end lies immediately in front of the auricle. With a finger in the mouth, feel the anterior border of the ramus. On the skull, examine the two big processes that project from the upper border of the ramus. The anterior is the **coronoid process,** into which the temporal

muscle is inserted. The posterior is the **condylar process,** and the notch between them is called the **mandibular notch.** The condylar process carries the **head** and **neck** of the mandible. The head of the mandible articulates with the articular surface of the mandibular fossa on the under-surface of the temporal bone. This fossa is bounded anteriorly by a convexity called the articular tubercle. The joint is called the temporomandibular joint.

The teeth are set in the upper border of the body of the mandible. Identify the **mental foramen** on the outer surface of the body near its anterior end. It is the orifice of a canal in the bone, and through it passes a cutaneous branch of the trigeminal nerve.

The temporal bone [Fig. 5.35]

Examine the temporal bone. It consists of three parts. That which helps form the lateral wall of the middle cranial fossa is called the **squamous part** [Fig. 5.35]. The **zygomatic pro-**

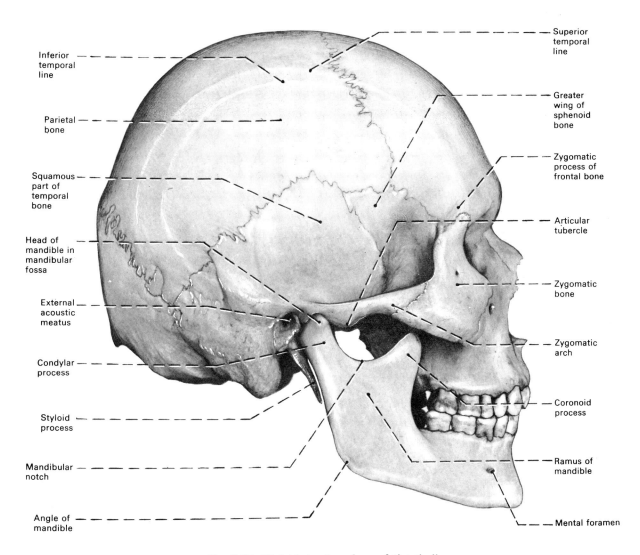

Fig. 5.34 Right lateral surface of the skull.

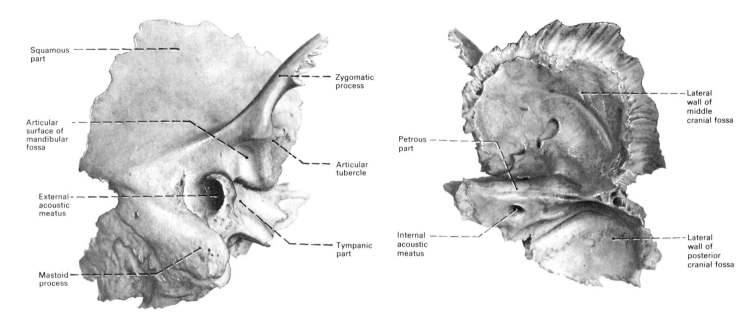

Squamous part

Zygomatic process

Articular surface of mandibular fossa

Articular tubercle

External acoustic meatus

Tympanic part

Mastoid process

a. *Lateral surface* Oblique view from below and in front.

Petrous part

Lateral wall of middle cranial fossa

Internal acoustic meatus

Lateral wall of posterior cranial fossa

b. *Medial surface* Oblique view from above and behind.

Fig. 5.35 The right temporal bone.

cess, **mandibular fossa,** and **articular tubercle** are parts of it. The large wedge of bone which projects medially and anteriorly from the squamous part, and which helps to form the base of the skull and the floor of the middle cranial fossa, is the **petrous part** of the temporal bone. Posteriorly, it forms part of the lateral wall of the posterior cranial fossa, and from it projects the **mastoid process,** behind the external acoustic meatus. The third part is the small **tympanic part** which forms the floor and anterior wall of the external acoustic meatus.

The zygomatic arch [Fig. 5.34]

The zygomatic arch begins at the lateral surface of the articular tubercle. Palpate the arch on yourself and follow it forwards to the **zygomatic bone.** On the skull you will see that this bone articulates behind with the zygomatic process of the temporal bone; above, with the frontal bone, so forming part of the lateral wall of the orbit; and below and medially, with the maxilla [Fig. 5.34].

The temporal fossa [Fig. 5.34]

Note that the upper border of the zygomatic arch continues anteriorly as the posterior border of the process of the zygomatic bone which articulates with the frontal bone. This becomes continuous with the posterior border of the corresponding short zygomatic process of the frontal bone, whence a ridge arches across the frontal and parietal bones and finishes above the mastoid process by becoming continuous with a posterior extension of the zygomatic process of the temporal bone. The elliptical area that has now been delineated is the temporal fossa. The ridge forming the upper

part of the boundary can be seen to consist of a **superior temporal line** and an **inferior temporal line** [Fig. 5.34].

You will recognize the frontal, parietal, temporal, and zygomatic bones in the floor of the temporal fossa. A fifth bone, the **greater wing of the sphenoid bone,** appears in its lower anterior corner. The temporal surface of this bone is interrupted below by a rough ridge called the **infratemporal crest.**

The teeth [Fig. 5.36]

Since the specimen you are dissecting is probably edentulous, you should examine the teeth of the skull, or at a convenient moment, examine your own teeth with the help of a mirror.

There are 32 permanent teeth. Eight pairs form a **superior dental arch,** which is set into the alveolar arch of the maxilla, and the other eight pairs an **inferior dental arch** which is set in the mandible [Fig. 5.36]. Each tooth has an exposed part, or **crown,** and one or more **roots** inserted into sockets, or **dental alveoli,** in the maxilla or mandible. The surfaces of the teeth which meet when the mouth is closed are called the occlusal or **masticatory surfaces.**

The four front teeth in each dental arch have chisel-shaped crowns and are called the **incisor teeth** (medial and lateral incisors). Lateral to the incisors are the **canine teeth** behind which are two **premolar teeth** (first and second premolars) and three **molar teeth** (first, second, and third molars). The masticatory surfaces of the molar teeth are broad, and are usually characterized by four irregular **dental cusps.** The premolars are smaller than the molars and have two cusps. The incisor, canine, and lower premolar teeth

5.38

have single roots, while the molars and upper premolars usually have more than one root.

The maxilla [Fig. 5.37]

Turn to the front of a skull and identify the large **infraorbital foramen** set in the anterior surface of the maxilla below the inferior margin of the orbit. The large depression below the foramen is known as the **canine fossa.** The elevation medial to the fossa corresponds to the root of the canine tooth. Further medially are slighter elevations related to the roots of the incisor teeth.

Trace the alveolar arch backwards and you will see that it extends beyond the third upper molar tooth before ending. This rounded projection of bone is called the **tuberosity of the maxilla** [Fig. 5.50].

The auricle [Fig. 5.38]

Turn now to the ear of your cadaver. The external ear consists of a flap-like structure, the auricle [Fig. 5.38] and the external acoustic meatus. The latter is the canal which runs towards the middle ear within the temporal bone.

The following features of the auricle should be identified: the **concha** of the auricle (or 'well of the ear'), which leads into the external acoustic meatus; the rim or **helix**, which begins in the concha and winds round to end at the soft lower end of the auricle, which is called the **lobule** of the auricle.

The **tragus** is the small process that overlaps the concha in front, like a small lid over the external acoustic meatus.

Reflection of the skin

The incision which was extended from the mastoid process to the lobule of the auricle must now be continued vertically upwards immediately in front of the auricle as far as the lower border of the zygomatic process of the temporal bone. From this point make a horizontal incision across the face to the side of the nose, along the lower border of the zygomatic arch. Continue the incision round the lower margin of the nose to just about the midpoint of the upper lip [Fig. 5.39].

Pick up the large flap of skin that has already been reflected from the neck, and continue reflecting it towards the midline of the face. Take care to reflect nothing more than skin. The skin flap should now be attached only at the borders of the lips. Leave it attached here so that the flap can be used to cover the dissection.

Superficial structures of the face

The muscles of facial expression [Fig. 5.40]

You may already be able to see some fibres of the **orbicularis oris,** which is the muscle of the lips. To reveal it more completely, stroke away the overlying fat and subcutaneous

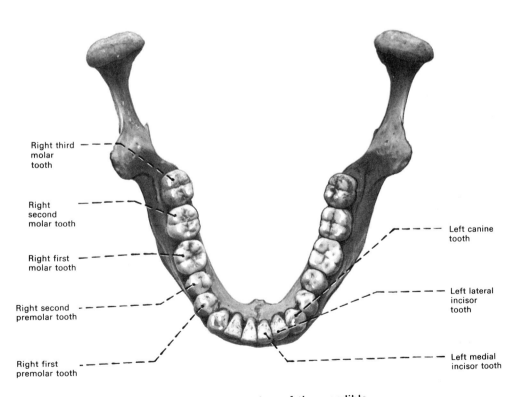

Right third molar tooth

Right second molar tooth

Right first molar tooth

Right second premolar tooth

Right first premolar tooth

Left canine tooth

Left lateral incisor tooth

Left medial incisor tooth

Fig. 5.36 Superior view of the mandible.

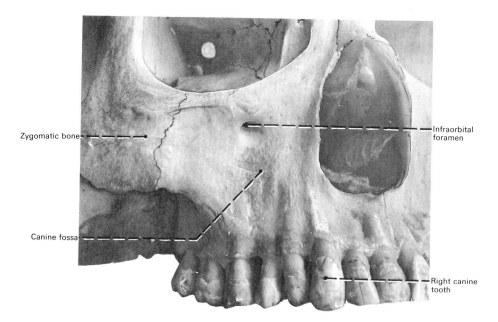

Zygomatic bone

Canine fossa

Infraorbital foramen

Right canine tooth

Fig. 5.37 The right maxilla.

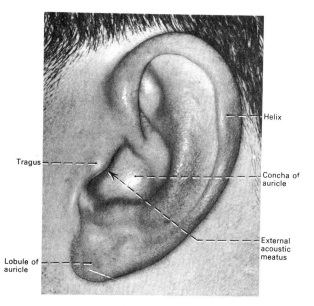

Tragus

Lobule of auricle

Helix

Concha of auricle

External acoustic meatus

Fig. 5.38 The auricle.

tissue in the direction of the muscle fibres, using the handle of a scalpel. Start at the angle of the mouth, where the muscle fibres run vertically, and follow them round into the upper and lower lips as far as you can.

It is tedious to dissect the muscles of facial expression, and their anatomy can be perfectly well appreciated from illustrations. The easiest muscle to demonstrate on the cadaver is the **depressor anguli oris,** which descends and fans out from the angle of the mouth to the base of the mandible [Fig. 5.40]. Other muscles run from the upper lip to the zygomatic bone and to the side of the nose, or laterally from

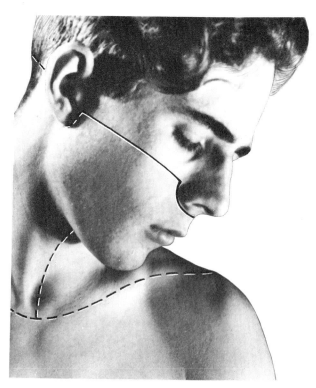

Fig. 5.39 Skin incision for the dissection of the face.

the angle of the mouth, to blend with the **platysma muscle,** whose posterior fibres ascend over the base of the mandible and curve forward into the lips.

Two muscles associated with the orbicularis oris lie too deep to be seen at this stage. They are the **buccinator muscle** of the cheek and the **levator anguli oris muscle,** which

5.40

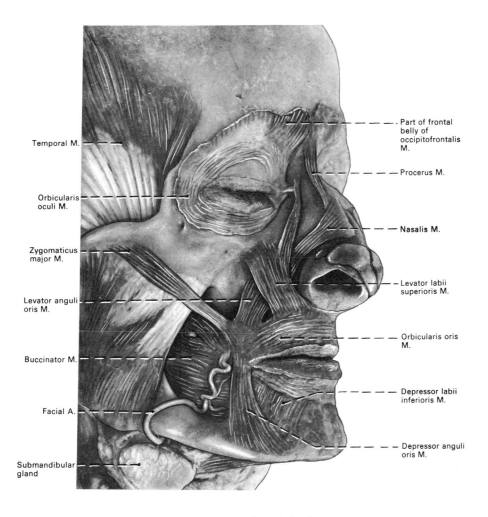

Temporal M.

Orbicularis
oculi M.

Zygomaticus
major M.

Levator anguli
oris M.

Buccinator M.

Facial A.

Submandibular
gland

Part of frontal
belly of
occipitofrontalis
M.

Procerus M.

Nasalis M.

Levator labii
superioris M.

Orbicularis oris
M.

Depressor labii
inferioris M.

Depressor anguli
oris M.

Fig. 5.40 The muscles of the face.

descends from the canine fossa of the maxilla to the angle of the mouth.

A number of small subcutaneous muscles are responsible for moving the auricle, and are grouped with the muscles of facial expression. They need not be dissected, but note that they are attached to the skeleton of the auricle which consists of a thin plate of elastic fibrocartilage continuous with the cartilage that surrounds the lateral half of the external acoustic meatus.

Precisely which muscles are responsible for each of the variety of 'faces' you can pull is not usually apparent. The orbicularis oris plays the major role in pursing the lips as in whistling. You should have little difficulty in observing in a mirror the actions of the elevators of your upper lip and of the angles of your mouth. You will also see that many facial expressions are accompanied by movements of the ears. You can also observe the action of the **orbicularis oculi muscle** which encircles the eye, although you will not expose this muscle on the cadaver until much later in your dissection [p. 5.100]. It is responsible for closing the eyelids, as in blinking. Its strong contraction shuts the eyes tight.

The facial artery and vein [Fig. 5.41]

Pick up the posterior border of the platysma muscle on the face where it crosses a bulky muscle, called the masseter muscle, which covers the ramus of the mandible. Using the handle of a scalpel, reflect the platysma muscle forwards as far as the anterior margin of the masseter. Take care not to destroy the fine branches of the facial nerve which you will find attached to the deep surface of the platysma. Now search for the facial artery and vein. They cross the lower border of the mandible just in front of the masseter muscle. With the aid of forceps and a blunt dissector, trace both vessels and their branches across the area exposed by the skin reflection. To do this you may have to reflect or divide the platysma but try to avoid damaging any of the other subcutaneous muscles of the face and, especially, the many fine nerves which you will encounter during this dissection.

As the facial artery and vein cross the lower border of the mandible they pierce the deep fascia of the neck to emerge on to the face deep to the platysma. They then run to the medial angle of the eye. Unless the cadaver has been

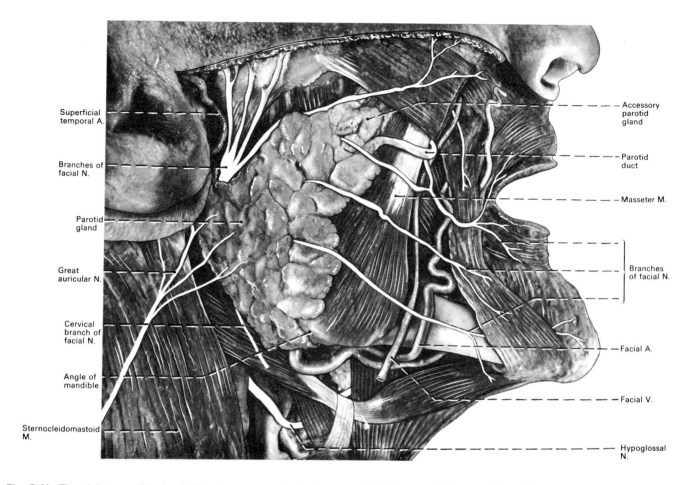

Superficial temporal A.

Branches of facial N.

Parotid gland

Great auricular N.

Cervical branch of facial N.

Angle of mandible

Sternocleidomastoid M.

Accessory parotid gland

Parotid duct

Masseter M.

Branches of facial N.

Facial A.

Facial V.

Hypoglossal N.

Fig. 5.41 The right parotid gland. The platysma muscle has been excised. The superficial part of the submandibular gland is absent. The same head and neck is shown in Figs 5.42, 5.44–5.47, 5.52–5.54.

particularly well injected, it will be easier to find the vein than the artery, behind which the vein runs a relatively straight course. The facial artery is tortuous and passes forwards towards the angle of the mouth, on its way to the medial angle of the eye. The artery sends branches to the upper and lower lips. There are corresponding tributaries that join the vein, which also has an important branch, the **deep facial vein** [Fig. 5.43], that runs backwards across the cheek and deep to the ramus of the mandible.

Surface anatomy

The surface markings of the facial vessels are easy to determine. Clench your jaw and determine the anterior limit of the insertion of the masseter into the mandible. At this point feel for a groove in the base of the bone and identify it on the skull. With the tip of a finger gently slide the skin to and fro over the groove and you should be able to feel a hard structure rolling backwards and forwards under your finger. This is the facial artery at the point where it winds round the base of the mandible to enter the face. If you do not press too hard, you will feel its pulsation in three places: as the artery passes over the mandible; near the angle of

the mouth when you hold the cheek between your finger and thumb; and at or near the medial angle of the eye.

A slight bluish tinge of the skin just medial to the medial angle of the eye is the only superficial evidence of the facial vein. This is where the vein starts.

The parotid gland [Fig. 5.41]

The parotid gland is a large, firm, lobulated structure which fits into the gap between the posterior border of the ramus of the mandible in front, the external acoustic meatus above, and the anterior borders of the mastoid process and sternocleidomastoid muscle behind [Fig. 5.41]. It overlaps the masseter muscle, which covers the ramus of the mandible. The **parotid duct** emerges from its anterior border and drains into the mouth, having pierced the buccinator muscle. If you clench your teeth and feel along the anterior border of the masseter muscle about a finger's breadth below the zygomatic arch, you should be able to feel the duct as a cord-like structure. It opens into the cavity of the mouth opposite the second upper molar tooth. Its opening can be readily seen.

On the cadaver, you will find the parotid duct on the level

5.42

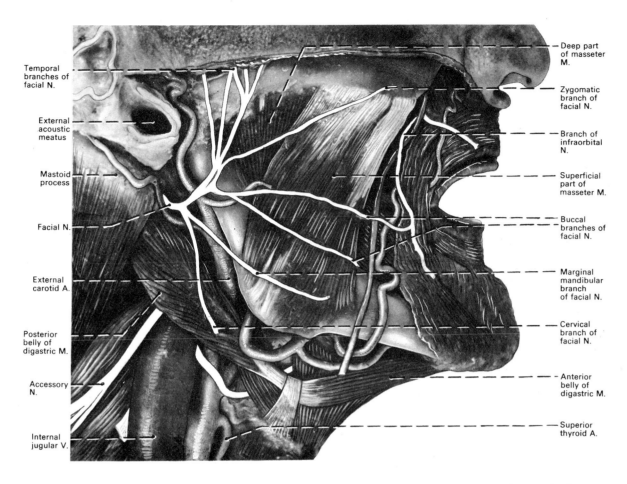

Temporal branches of facial N.

External acoustic meatus

Mastoid process

Facial N.

External carotid A.

Posterior belly of digastric M.

Accessory N.

Internal jugular V.

Deep part of masseter M.

Zygomatic branch of facial N.

Branch of infraorbital N.

Superficial part of masseter M.

Buccal branches of facial N.

Marginal mandibular branch of facial N.

Cervical branch of facial N.

Anterior belly of digastric M.

Superior thyroid A.

Fig. 5.42 The branches of the right facial nerve. The parotid gland and the auricle have been excised.

of a line drawn from the lobule of the auricle to a point midway between the red margin of the upper lip and the nose. Using blunt dissection, find the parotid duct at the point where it turns round the anterior border of the masseter; it is a fairly thick structure. Then search carefully just above and below it for branches of the facial nerve, which run parallel with it. Once these have been found, trace them and the duct backwards through a layer of fascia which covers the parotid gland. Almost immediately you will encounter lobules of the gland, and it will become impossible to trace either nerves or duct further. The lobules are finer, but otherwise similar in appearance to those of the pancreas.

Now continue reflecting the layer of fascia backwards over the gland. Use scissors to cut the numerous strands of tissue which leave the deep surface of the fascia to enter the gland. Cut the layer of fascia parallel with, and just below the zygomatic arch, and reflect it posteriorly to just beyond the posterior border of the ramus of the mandible. Also separate the sheet from the superficial surface of the masseter below the gland as far as the base of the mandible, to which it is attached.

You will now see that this sheet of fascia, which ensheathes the parotid gland, appears continuous with the platysma in the neck. The fascia is an upward extension of the superficial layer of the deep cervical fascia and can be separated from the platysma by which it is covered. Using blunt dissection, and starting anteriorly, detach the fascia from the mandible, keeping a look-out for the **cervical branch of the facial nerve** [Fig. 5.42] which enters the deep surface of the platysma, which it supplies, immediately below and behind the angle of the mandible. Follow the nerve a short distance into the fascial sheet and then divide it. The sheet of fascia can then be removed by cutting through it in front of the auricle.

Trace the **great auricular nerve,** which you found when you dissected the side of the neck [p. 5.11], towards the lobule of the auricle [Fig. 5.41]. You will find that branches of the nerve enter the lower part of the gland. Follow the two veins which form the external jugular vein upwards [p. 5.11]. One descends from behind the auricle, the other emerges from the parotid gland. Detach the former and then separate the latter from the surface of the sternocleidomastoid muscle. By means of blunt dissection, separate the upper end of the anterior border of the sternocleidomastoid from the parotid gland. Check for yourself that the gland is wedged between the posterior border of the ramus of the mandible in front and the sternocleidomastoid muscle and the mastoid process behind. To see this take a scalpel and, starting from below, cut off the auricle flush with the scalp.

Most of the superficial surface of the parotid gland can now be seen. Define its extent, removing, where necessary, any fascia by which it is still covered. Take special care not to damage branches of the facial nerve which emerge from the upper, lower, and anterior borders of the gland. You have seen how the gland is wedged in behind the mandible. Now note how the superficial surface of the gland overlaps the masseter muscle. Its anterior border extends forwards, particularly along the upper border of the parotid duct (the gland tissue here forms the **accessory parotid gland** [Fig. 5.41]). Above, the gland extends to the zygomatic arch, and below, it ends just behind the angle of the mandible, and on the sternocleidomastoid muscle.

Removal of the upper part of the sternocleidomastoid muscle

Now remove the remains of the upper part of the sternocleidomastoid muscle. Make sure, first, that the accessory nerve is entirely separated from the muscle. Then, by blunt dissection, separate the anterior border of the muscle from deeper structures. Turn the lower end of the muscle upwards and backwards as you do this. Scissors can be used to separate the posterior border of the muscle from the splenius capitis muscle, which it overlaps. You will see small arteries and veins entering and leaving the deep surface of the sternocleidomastoid. Cut these close to the muscle. As you approach the insertion of the sternocleidomastoid note the extension of its attachment backwards from the mastoid process along the superior nuchal line. Starting at the mastoid process, use a scalpel to sever the attachment.

The facial nerve [Fig. 5.42]

Return to the branch of the facial nerve which you should have found lying parallel to and above the parotid duct. Trace this nerve backwards into, and through, the parotid gland, using scissors to cut through the tissues covering the nerve. It is unnecessary to preserve any of the substance of the parotid gland. As the nerve is followed you will find that it is joined by others, or alternatively, that it divides and that the divisions are joined by other nerves. Whichever is the case, continue to follow the nerve or nerves backwards, picking up and not damaging any except the minute branches you encounter. By this means you will reach the main trunk of the facial nerve as it emerges from the stylomastoid foramen, medial to the mastoid process [Fig. 5.42].

Now follow all the branches of the facial nerve as they radiate through the parotid gland, cutting through and removing the substance of the gland superficial to the nerves. Do not cut or remove anything deep to the nerves.

You should have little difficulty in identifying the five main groups of branches to the muscles of facial expression. They emerge from the anterior and lower borders of the parotid gland, and are, from above down:

1. The **temporal branches,** which cross the zygomatic arch to supply the auricular muscles and the muscles of the forehead and upper eyelid.
2. The **zygomatic branches,** running above the parotid duct on to the zygomatic bone, to supply the muscles of the lower eyelid and the side of the nose.
3. The **buccal branches,** running below the parotid duct, to supply the buccinator muscle and the upper half of the orbicularis oris and its associated muscles.
4. The **marginal mandibular branch,** which runs along the mandible to the lower half of the orbicularis oris.
5. The **cervical branch,** which emerges from the lower end of the gland behind the angle of the mandible and which, earlier on, you detached from the deep surface of the platysma.

As you dissect you should notice that the zygomatic and buccal branches of the facial nerve are joined by branches of another nerve, which emerges on the face through the infraorbital foramen. This is the infraorbital nerve. It is a branch of the maxillary nerve, which is, itself, one of the three main branches of the trigeminal nerve. You will see the maxillary nerve at a much later stage of dissection [p. 5.116].

The buccinator muscle [Fig. 5.40]

Look for a nerve which runs forwards into the cheek from beneath the anterior border of the masseter. It lies deep to the masseter, somewhat closer to the mandible than to the maxilla, and breaks up into branches on the buccinator muscle. This is the **buccal nerve,** a branch of the mandibular nerve. It may not be easy to find, but when the nerve has been identified, clear away the loose encapsulated fat which lies on the buccinator muscle and which extends backwards between the buccinator and masseter muscles. This is part of the **buccal pad of fat** which intervenes between the masseter and temporal muscles on the one hand and the buccinator and deeper muscles of mastication on the other. The pad helps to stiffen the wall of the mouth, and being relatively much larger in infants than in adults, accounts for the rounded fullness of babies' cheeks.

Pick up the parotid duct and, at the point where it pierces the buccinator muscle, start removing the fairly tough **buccopharyngeal fascia** which overlies the muscle. Take care to preserve the buccal nerve and any veins you may encounter. Clean the buccinator muscle in order to follow the course of its fibres forwards into the lips. You will not be able to see the posterior attachments of the muscle at this stage of dissection.

The buccinator muscle is an important part of the cheek. Its fibres arise from the outer surfaces of the alveolar processes opposite the upper and lower molar teeth and from a ligament, the pterygomandibular raphe [p. 5.71], which passes from the mandible behind the last molar tooth to a bony projection behind the tuberosity of the maxilla. Anteriorly the fibres of the muscle blend with the orbicularis oris. Like the muscles of facial expression, the buccinator muscle is supplied by the facial nerve. The buccopharyngeal fascia which covers the muscle extends backwards to clothe the outer surface of the muscular wall of the pharynx.

The retromandibular vein [Fig. 5.43]

In the course of your dissection you will probably have seen a vein descending through the parotid gland, deep to the facial nerve and behind the posterior border of the ramus of the mandible. This is the retromandibular vein [Fig. 5.43]. By blunt dissection with forceps, trace the vein downwards, and you will find that it divides before leaving the gland.

The posterior branch joins a vein, the **posterior auricular vein,** running down behind the auricle, to form the **external jugular vein.** The anterior branch will be found joining the **facial vein** just below the mandible. Follow the facial vein from this point to where it ends in the **internal jugular vein.**

The arrangement of the facial and jugular veins varies considerably from one individual to another, and is usually different on the two sides of the same individual. For this reason the description given here may not accord with your specimen.

The masseter muscle [Fig. 5.42]

Isolate what remains of the superficial part of the parotid gland, and turn it forwards over the masseter muscle, so that it remains attached to the dissection only by the parotid duct.

Without damaging the branches of the facial nerve, clean the masseter muscle and identify its borders. It has a tendinous origin from the lower border of the zygomatic bone,

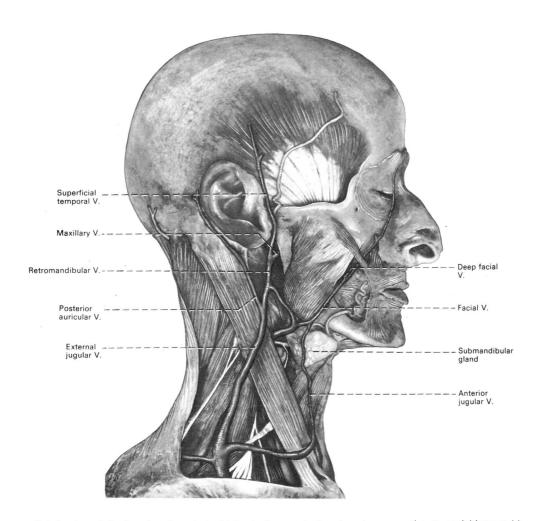

Fig. 5.43 **The superficial veins of the head and neck.** In this body the anterior jugular vein crosses the sternocleidomastoid muscle superficially.

and a fleshy one from the deep surface of the zygomatic arch. It is inserted into the lateral surface of the ramus of the mandible. The **superficial part** of the masseter passes downwards and backwards from origin to insertion; the **deep part,** some of which can be seen behind the superficial part, is vertical [Fig. 5.42]. The muscle entirely covers the ramus of the mandible except for the head and neck of the condylar process. The direction of the fibres of the masseter makes it obvious that its action would be to close the opened jaw. You will easily feel your own masseter if you clench your jaw.

The scalp

Make a vertical skin incision immediately behind the lateral border of the orbit, and extend it to the cut median surface of the half-head [Fig. 5.44]. Another incision should be made running upwards and backwards from a point above the external acoustic meatus but falling short of the cut median surface by 3 cm or so. (If you have chosen not to bisect the head as yet, make another incision extending forwards in the midline, from the external occipital protuberance to the point where the vertical incisions of each side meet each other.) Reflect the skin behind this incision upwards towards the midline, taking great care that you reflect no more than the skin. Leave the flap attached at its upper posterior corner, so that it can be replaced over the dissected area when the specimen is wrapped up.

The scalp consists of the soft structures which cover the skull between the temporal lines of the sides. It extends from the eyebrows in front to the superior nuchal line behind. The soft structures are arranged in five layers which, from the surface inwards, are:

1. Skin.
2. Dense subcutaneous tissue containing the nerves and vessels of the skin. Hair follicles abound in this layer.
3. The very thin **occipitofrontalis muscle,** which belongs to the muscles of facial expression. This flat muscle has a pair of **occipital bellies** behind, and a pair of **frontal bellies** in the forehead. The former are attached to the lateral

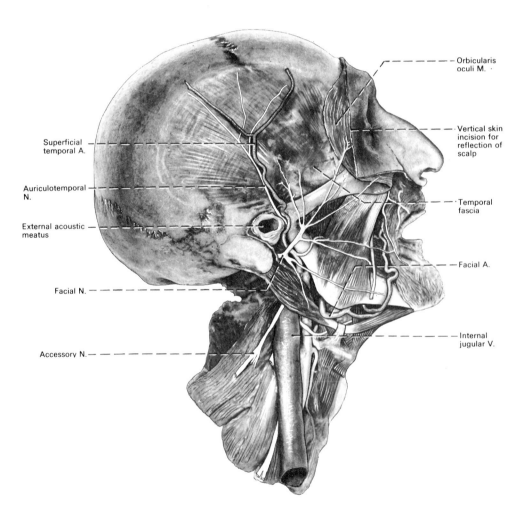

Fig. 5.44 Superficial structures of the head and neck.

part of the superior nuchal line on each side. The latter are attached to the skin over the eyebrows. The four bellies are connected by the thin fibrous **galea aponeurotica** or **epicranial aponeurosis.**

4. Loose areolar tissue, which allows movement between the overlying aponeurosis and the periosteum covering the bone.

5. The periosteum of the outer surface of the skull, which is also called the **pericranium.**

Vessels and nerves of the scalp

The vessels and nerves of the scalp approach it from various points. You have already found the **greater occipital nerve** entering the scalp posteriorly [p. 5.5], and you may have seen the **occipital artery,** a branch of the external carotid artery, accompanying it. A similar neurovascular bundle approaches the scalp in the temporal region from immediately in front of the external acoustic meatus. The vessels, the superficial temporal artery and vein, are more easily seen than the accompanying nerve, which is called the auriculotemporal nerve [Fig. 5.44].

The **superficial temporal artery** is a terminal branch of the external carotid artery and, in a living person, can be seen or felt where it crosses the zygomatic process of the temporal bone just in front of the auricle. This artery is often very tortuous, and an anterior branch which runs towards the forehead is often very conspicuous in middle and old age.

Dissect the superficial temporal vessels, and follow them down to where they cross the zygomatic process of the temporal bone. Do not use sharp instruments here because you may damage the **auriculotemporal nerve,** which lies behind the vessels. Follow the **superficial temporal vein** through the upper end of the deep part of the parotid gland. You may be able to demonstrate its continuity with the retromandibular vein. The stem of the superficial temporal artery and the auriculotemporal nerve lie deeper than the vein. At this stage do not try to trace them to their origins.

The superficial temporal artery supplies the tissues of the scalp over a wide area which extends to the midline superiorly; anteriorly as far forwards as the upper part of the forehead; and posteriorly to the vertex. It anastomoses freely with the other vessels of the scalp. The auriculotemporal nerve supplies the sense receptors and hair follicles of the skin over an area which does not extend as far anteriorly as that supplied by the superficial temporal artery.

Follow the **temporal branches of the facial nerve** superiorly over the zygomatic arch as far as the skin reflection allows [Fig. 5.42]. Most of the branches run anteriorly to supply the orbicularis oculi, the subcutaneous muscle surrounding the eye, and the frontal belly of the occipitofrontalis muscle. Some supply auricular muscles which arise from the surface of the galea aponeurotica and which are inserted into the auricle.

Now identify and, with the handle of a scalpel, separate the aponeurotic and periosteal layers of the scalp in the region from which the skin has been removed. It will be easy to do this if the specimen has not become too dry. Divide the galea aponeurotica in a frontal plane, carrying your incision to a point anterior to the external acoustic meatus. Pick up the aponeurosis on both sides of the incision and peel it back to the margins of the skin incisions. While doing so divide such branches of the facial nerve as you meet, and separate the attachment of the galea aponeurotica from the upper border of the zygomatic arch. At the side of the skull you will find that the reflection becomes difficult because the galea aponeurotica is firmly attached to the fascia covering the temporal muscle.

The temporal muscle and fascia

The temporal muscle arises from the bone of the temporal fossa and from the deep surface of a thick fascial layer which covers the muscle, and which is itself attached to certain of the boundaries of the fossa.

Starting at a point above the posterior end of the origin of the masseter, carry your scalpel superiorly and posteriorly at about 45° to the horizontal plane through the temporal fascia. Now make a curved incision through the fascia at its attachment to the superior temporal line, and reflect the fascia off the muscle [Fig. 5.45]. The attachment of the fascia to the upper border of the zygomatic arch will have to be cut with scissors to allow the reflection of the flap as far as the skin incisions permit.

You will now be able to see the fibres of the temporal muscle converging as they descend behind the zygomatic arch, to be inserted into the coronoid process of the mandible. Pass the handle of the scalpel down between the zygomatic arch and the muscle, push it forwards through the fascia and fat, and see it appear deep to the upper end of the anterior border of the masseter muscle.

Removal of the masseter muscle

To reveal the whole of the temporal muscle, the zygomatic arch and masseter muscle are removed together. Make sawcuts through the arch at each end of the origin of the masseter. The anterior cut will have to be made diagonally through the zygomatic bone. Use bone forceps to complete the section of the bone [Fig. 5.46].

During the process of removing the masseter, the nerve which supplies it can be dissected out, and the insertion of the muscle into the mandible examined. Lift the anterior border of the muscle, and separate its deep surface from the temporal muscle with the handle of a scalpel. Carefully turn the masseter and zygomatic arch back, tearing away any of the muscle fibres which run from the temporal muscle into the deep surface of the masseter. As you approach the posterior end of the masseter, search for the **masseteric nerve,**

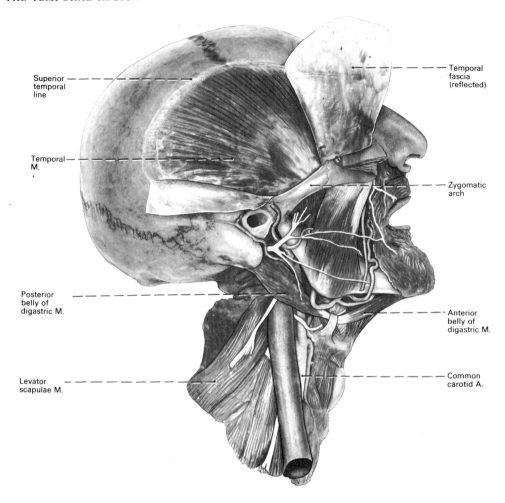

Superior temporal line

Temporal M.

Posterior belly of digastric M.

Levator scapulae M.

Temporal fascia (reflected)

Zygomatic arch

Anterior belly of digastric M.

Common carotid A.

Fig. 5.45 Reflection of the temporal fascia.

a branch of the mandibular nerve, which enters its deep surface [Fig. 5.47]. The nerve emerges from the mandibular notch behind the tendon of the temporal muscle and turns forwards as it enters the masseter. Trace the nerve a short distance into the masseter, and then dissect it out of the muscle, leaving a piece of muscle attached to the end of the nerve [see Fig. 5.52].

Complete the reflection of the masseter by scraping it off the mandible with the handle of a scalpel, and remove the muscle completely. In this way you will also remove the periosteum into which the muscle is inserted. As you do this, note the superior extension of the muscle's insertion into the ramus of the mandible. Any branches of the facial nerve which may interfere with the removal of the muscle should be divided.

The insertion of the temporal muscle [Fig. 5.47]

Now examine the insertion of the temporal muscle. The superficial fibres are inserted as tendon into the apex and anterior edge of the coronoid process of the mandible. Its deeper fibres are inserted as muscle into the deep surface of the coronoid process. Part of the insertion extends a considerable way down the anterior part of the ramus of the mandible and becomes tendinous.

The face and temporal region in general

Before proceeding to the next stage of dissection, which begins with the removal of a large part of the ramus of the mandible, rapidly revise the more important of the facial structures which you have already examined. The principal one was the parotid gland, which your dissection revealed as a prismatic structure wedged between the upper part of the sternocleidomastoid muscle and the posterior border of the ramus of the mandible. Above, it extended to the external acoustic meatus and the temporomandibular joint, and below to the angle of the mandible. The parotid duct emerged from the anterior border of the parotid gland,

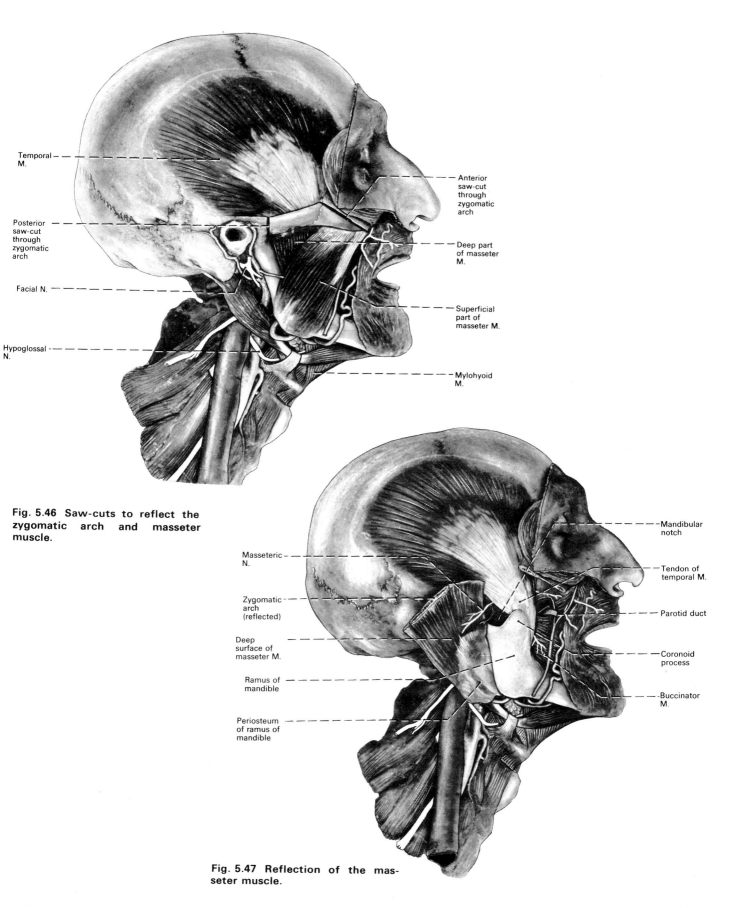

Temporal M.

Posterior saw-cut through zygomatic arch

Facial N.

Hypoglossal N.

Anterior saw-cut through zygomatic arch

Deep part of masseter M.

Superficial part of masseter M.

Mylohyoid M.

Fig. 5.46 Saw-cuts to reflect the zygomatic arch and masseter muscle.

Masseteric N.

Zygomatic arch (reflected)

Deep surface of masseter M.

Ramus of mandible

Periosteum of ramus of mandible

Mandibular notch

Tendon of temporal M.

Parotid duct

Coronoid process

Buccinator M.

Fig. 5.47 Reflection of the masseter muscle.

turned round the anterior border of the masseter muscle (where it could be palpated), and pierced the buccinator muscle opposite the second upper molar tooth.

You also saw that the deep part of the gland was traversed by the facial nerve, which divided into five divisions to supply the muscles of facial expression, including the muscles of the auricle, the occipitofrontalis muscle of the middle layer of the scalp, and the platysma. It also supplied the buccinator muscle. Associated with the nerve in the substance of the gland you found the retromandibular vein, which divided into an anterior branch that joined the facial vein, and a posterior branch which joined the posterior auricular vein to form the external jugular vein. Associated with the auriculotemporal nerve you also found the super-

ficial temporal artery, one of the two terminal branches of the external carotid artery. This vessel supplied the scalp, the posterior part of which you have already seen to be supplied by the occipital artery, another branch of the external carotid artery. You have also dissected the facial artery and vein for part of their course between the antero-inferior angle of the masseter muscle and the medial angle of the eye. Finally, recall again the arrangement of the fan-shaped temporal muscle, which arises from the bony floor of the temporal fossa and the overlying temporal fascia. It is inserted into the coronoid process and anterior border of the ramus of the mandible. Recall, too, the masseter muscle which arises from the zygomatic arch and is inserted into the lateral surface of the ramus of the mandible.

The infratemporal region

The next step in the dissection is to remove most of the ramus of the mandible, which makes it possible to see the other two principal muscles of mastication, the medial pterygoid muscle and the lateral pterygoid muscle. It also allows you to return to the dissection of the deeper structures in the upper part of the neck, and to see how they connect with some of those you have just been studying.

The infratemporal region does not have clearly-defined boundaries. It is the region between the ramus of the mandible and the side wall of the pharynx. Above, it is bounded by the under-surfaces of the greater wing of the sphenoid bone and the temporal bone. Below, as well as behind, it opens into the neck. In front, it is bounded by the infra-temporal surface of the maxilla and the backwardly-facing superficial surface of the posterior end of the buccinator muscle. The principal contents of the infratemporal region are the two pterygoid muscles, the mandibular nerve, and the maxillary artery, which is the larger of the two terminal branches of the external carotid artery.

Osteology

The mandible [Figs 5.48 and 5.49]

Turn to a skull and examine the medial surface of the **ramus** of the mandible. A prominent feature is the opening of the

mandibular canal which runs downwards into the bone. Through it run nerves and vessels to the pulp of the teeth of the mandible. The opening is called the **mandibular foramen** [Fig. 5.48]. A projection of bone from its anterior margin is called the **lingula** of the mandible. From the lower margin of the foramen a fine groove runs downwards and forwards on the surface of the bone. This is the **mylohyoid groove**, and in it runs the nerve which supplies the mylo-hyoid muscle and the anterior belly of the digastric, two muscles which you saw just before you interrupted your dis-section of the front of the neck [p. 5.21].

Look at the mandible from above, and note the **alveolar arch** into which the teeth are set [Fig. 5.49]. Just medial to the anterior border of the ramus, a medially-projecting butt-ress of bone develops in order to support the molar teeth. This forms a fairly broad area of bone, which widens as it sweeps down to the postero-lateral corner of the third molar tooth. It is into this area of bone that the deep fibres of the temporal muscle are inserted.

The pterygopalatine fossa

Now turn to the external surface of the base of the skull and, starting above the third molar tooth and the **tuberosity of the maxilla** behind, follow the surface of the maxilla upwards and backwards. You will find that this surface,

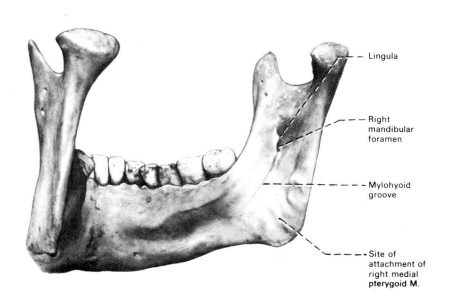

— Lingula

— Right mandibular foramen

— Mylohyoid groove

— Site of attachment of right medial pterygoid M.

Fig. 5.48 The mandible (viewed obliquely from behind and from the left).

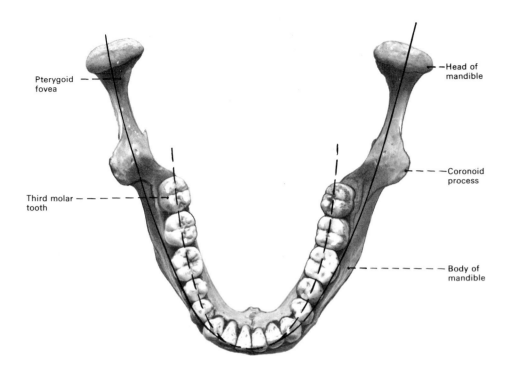

Pterygoid fovea

Third molar tooth

Head of mandible

Coronoid process

Body of mandible

Fig. 5.49 Superior view of the mandible. The alignment of the body and ramus of the mandible is shown by a continuous line. The broken line indicates the arrangement of the dental arch.

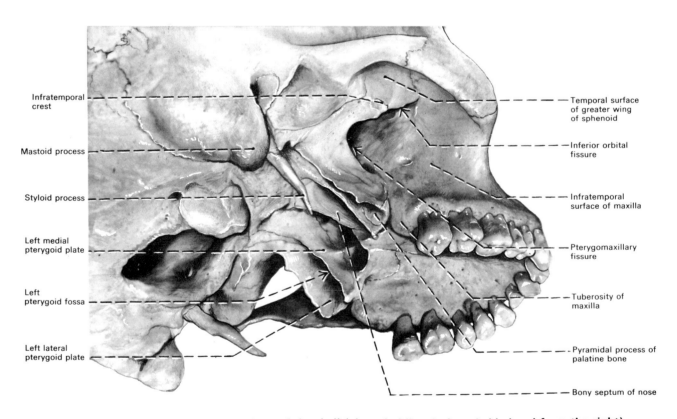

Infratemporal crest

Mastoid process

Styloid process

Left medial pterygoid plate

Left pterygoid fossa

Left lateral pterygoid plate

Temporal surface of greater wing of sphenoid

Inferior orbital fissure

Infratemporal surface of maxilla

Pterygomaxillary fissure

Tuberosity of maxilla

Pyramidal process of palatine bone

Bony septum of nose

Fig. 5.50 The external surface of the base of the skull (viewed obliquely from behind and from the right).

5.52

which faces laterally just above the molar teeth, becomes disposed posteriorly. This is the **infratemporal surface of the maxilla** [Fig. 5.50]. It runs into the posterior surface of the zygomatic process of the maxilla which articulates with the zygomatic bone, and it becomes continuous with the superior or **orbital surface of the maxilla** at the lower border of the **inferior orbital fissure**. The medial end of the infratemporal surface of the maxilla forms the anterior wall of a cleft called the **pterygopalatine fossa**. The posterior wall of the fossa is formed by the anterior border of a plate of bone which projects downwards from the under-surface of the skull behind. This is the **lateral pterygoid plate** which extends backwards from the downwardly-projecting **pterygoid process** of the sphenoid bone. Follow the lateral pterygoid plate upwards and you will find that it is continuous with the temporal surface of the greater wing of the sphenoid medial to the infratemporal crest. The entrance to the pterygopalatine fossa is called the **pterygomaxillary fissure.**

The pterygoid fossa [Fig. 5.50]

Look at the external surface of the base of the skull and identify the smaller **medial pterygoid plate,** lying to the medial side of the lateral plate. The gutter between the two is the pterygoid fossa. The bone joining the lower ends of the two pterygoid plates immediately behind the tuberosity of the maxilla belongs to neither the maxilla nor the sphenoid; it is the **pyramidal process of the palatine bone.** If you examine the skull carefully you may be able to see the sutural margins by which it is defined.

The foramen ovale and the foramen spinosum

Follow the posterior border of the lateral pterygoid plate upwards. This will lead you to a large elliptical foramen in the greater wing of the sphenoid. This is the foramen ovale [Fig. 5.51] through which the mandibular nerve passes from the middle cranial fossa. Immediately behind and lateral to

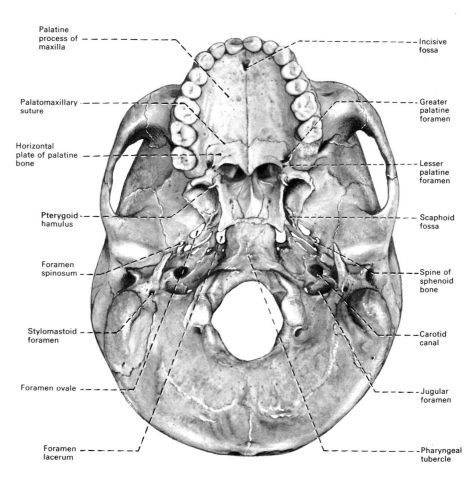

Fig. 5.51 The external surface of the base of the skull.

this foramen is a much smaller circular foramen, from the posterior margin of which a small spur of bone projects downwards. The spur of bone is the **spine of the sphenoid** and the foramen, consequently, is named the foramen spinosum. Through it run the middle meningeal artery, the middle meningeal veins, and a nerve to the meninges.

Reflection of the temporal muscle

Carefully remove the remains of the buccal pad of fat between the buccinator muscle and the temporal muscle. Feel the margin of the mandibular notch. Incise the periosteum of the superficial surface of the coronoid process of the mandible from the midpoint of the notch to the midpoint of the anterior border of the ramus of the mandible, and scrape or push it away for a short distance on either side of the incision. Without dividing any of the fibres of the temporal muscle deep to the coronoid process, try to carry out the same procedure on the deep surface of the bone. Cut through the bone along this line with bone forceps [Fig. 5.52]. Using force if necessary, turn the detached coronoid process upwards, taking with it the temporal muscle. This will entail separating the superficial fibres of the muscle from its many deeper fibres, which are inserted lower down on the ramus of the mandible. Continue the upward reflection of the superficial fibres of the muscle from the floor of the temporal fossa until the temporal muscle is folded back on the skull.

If you did not succeed in finding the **buccal nerve** earlier, search for it now by means of blunt dissection among the anterior fibres of the deeper part of the temporal muscle which are still attached to the mandible. It appears from under cover of the anterior border of the lower end of the temporal muscle and turns forwards on to the lower part of the superficial surface of the **buccinator muscle** [Fig. 5.53]. As the buccal nerve descends deep to the anterior border of the ramus of the mandible, it lies close to the temporal muscle and may actually traverse its substance. It is a sensory nerve and supplies the skin on the one side and the mucous coat of the mouth on the other side of the buccinator muscle. Remember that the muscle itself is supplied by the facial nerve.

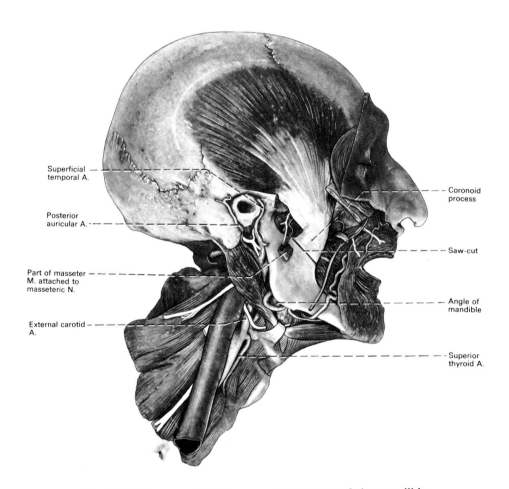

Superficial temporal A.

Posterior auricular A.

Part of masseter M. attached to masseteric N.

External carotid A.

Coronoid process

Saw-cut

Angle of mandible

Superior thyroid A.

Fig. 5.52 The removal of the coronoid process of the mandible.

5.54

Trace the buccal nerve upwards far enough to free it from the temporal muscle. Its ramifications on the buccinator muscle should be followed just enough to confirm that some of its fibres pierce the muscle to reach the mucous coat of the mouth on its deep surface. While doing this, preserve the largest of the veins you may encounter on the buccinator muscle, and trace it forwards. In all probability it will join the facial vein. It is the **deep facial vein,** which forms an anastomotic channel between the facial vein and a venous plexus which surrounds the pterygoid muscles. This **pterygoid plexus** is important because it communicates with the dural sinuses within the skull. The plexus will be seen when the pterygoid muscles are studied.

Divide any fibres of the temporal muscle that still remain attached to the mandible, and turn the deeper part of the muscle upwards, carefully pushing the muscle off the floor of the temporal fossa, but leaving its upper part attached to the bone. As you do this, look for two or three fine nerves which wind round the infratemporal crest of the sphenoid and sink into the deep surface of muscle. These are the **deep temporal nerves.** They are branches of the mandibular nerve

and supply the temporal muscle. The nerves are usually accompanied by fine arteries to the muscles.

Some pieces of the buccal pad of fat may still be found in the space now uncovered by the reflection of the coronoid process and tendon of the temporal muscle, and behind the zygomatic bone. Remove them.

Removal of the ramus of the mandible

Scrape the periosteum off the superficial surface of the ramus of the mandible. Take an amputation-saw and, from the angle of the mandible, make a shallow cut across this surface upwards to the midpoint of the anterior border of the ramus [Fig. 5.53]. The soft tissues covering the zygomatic bone will limit the depth of the cut.

Now scrape off the periosteum all the way round the lower part of the neck of the mandible, and saw through it horizontally, but not completely. You must now remove the bone between the two saw-cuts you have made, without damaging any of the structures which lie on the medial surface of the ramus, particularly the inferior alveolar nerve

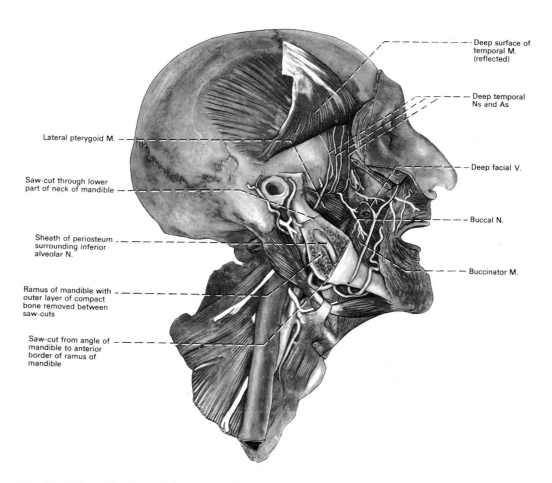

Fig. 5.53 The reflection of the temporal muscle and the removal of the ramus of the mandible.

which enters the mandibular foramen. Proceed as follows.

Starting at its posterior border, scrape away the periosteum from the deep surface of the lower end of the piece of bone between the two saw-cuts for a distance of about 5 mm from the posterior end of the lower saw-cut. With bone gouge forceps nibble along the lower saw-cut from its posterior end, until the spongy interior of the bone is reached. Then use them to remove the outer layer of compact bone between the two saw-cuts. As you do this look for the **inferior alveolar nerve** in the mandibular canal just below the mandibular foramen. When it has been seen, complete the section of the bone at the upper saw-cut with bone forceps. Having done this, carefully elevate the periosteum off the deep surface of the bone for a further 5 mm from the posterior end of the lower saw-cut, and nibble with bone forceps through the deep layer of compact bone along the saw-cut. Do not damage the inferior alveolar nerve.

The only other structure still in danger is the **mylohyoid nerve,** which leaves the inferior alveolar nerve just before the latter enters the mandibular foramen [Fig. 5.54]. When you examined the mandible [p. 5.51], you saw the groove

for the mylohyoid nerve on the deep surface of the ramus of the mandible. Bear the presence of this nerve in mind as you continue nibbling, and remove the remaining bone between the saw-cuts. Every time you insert the bone gouge forceps to bite off bone, be sure that the deep layer of the periosteum has already been elevated and, when removing loose pieces of bone, always peel them off the periosteum, which should thus remain in place.

When the bone has been removed, trim away any fibres of the temporal muscle which are inserted into the part of the mandible that still remains *in situ*, and then, by means of blunt dissection, carefully remove the deep periosteum from the underlying structures. It protected these structures when the bone was being removed, but it is now in the way.

The superficial contents of the infratemporal region

Follow the buccal nerve upwards until you find it sinking into a muscle—this is the **lateral pterygoid muscle** [Fig. 5.54]. Now trace the deep facial vein posteriorly and confirm that

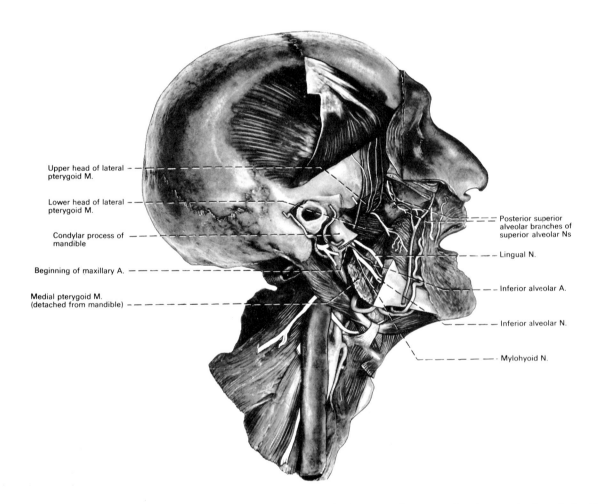

Fig. 5.54 The superficial contents of the infratemporal region. In this body the maxillary artery lies deep to the lateral pterygoid muscle.

Upper head of lateral pterygoid M.

Lower head of lateral pterygoid M.

Condylar process of mandible

Beginning of maxillary A.

Medial pterygoid M. (detached from mandible)

Posterior superior alveolar branches of superior alveolar Ns

Lingual N.

Inferior alveolar A.

Inferior alveolar N.

Mylohyoid N.

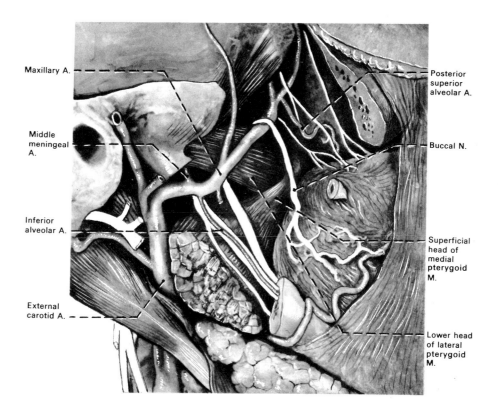

Fig. 5.55 The right maxillary artery.

it joins the pterygoid plexus, the network of veins overlying the muscles that are now exposed.

Identify the infratemporal surface of the maxilla, and preserve the fine vessels and nerves that cross it in a downward and lateral direction. These, the **posterior superior alveolar artery** and branches of the **superior alveolar nerves,** are dissected at a later stage.

The lateral pterygoid muscle [Figs 5.54 and 5.55]

By feeling with your finger, establish the position of the lateral pterygoid plate in relation to the infratemporal surface of the maxilla. The muscle covering the lateral pterygoid plate is the **lower head** of the lateral pterygoid muscle. The **upper head** of the muscle arises from the infratemporal crest and temporal surface of the greater wing of the sphenoid medial to the crest. Identify the upper head, and then clean and trace the two heads back towards the neck of the mandible, on to which they both converge. You will find that the buccal nerve emerges from between the two heads.

The maxillary artery [Fig. 5.55]

Crossing the lower head of the lateral pterygoid muscle obliquely or, less frequently, running deep to this head and emerging between the two heads of the muscle near their origin, you will come across a large artery that runs a horizontal though somewhat tortuous course. This is the maxillary artery [Fig. 5.55]. It is the larger of the two terminal branches of the external carotid artery (the smaller, as you should remember, being the superficial temporal artery). Trace the maxillary artery forwards to the point where it disappears into the pterygomaxillary fissure, and then posteriorly deep to the neck of the mandible. Do not pull the artery downwards in order to bring it into view. At the moment only one branch of the artery need be identified. This is the **inferior alveolar artery,** which accompanies the inferior alveolar nerve into the mandibular foramen, and which supplies the teeth and gums of the mandible.

The medial pterygoid muscle [Figs 5.54 and 5.55]

You may have noticed a few muscle fibres passing backwards and downwards from the origin of the lower head of the lateral pterygoid muscle. These comprise the very small **superficial head** of the medial pterygoid muscle, which takes origin from the pyramidal process of the palatine bone and the tuberosity of the maxilla. The **deep head** of the muscle arises from the medial surface of the lateral pterygoid plate, and will be found below the lateral pterygoid muscle as the two muscles diverge on their way to their insertions.

The inferior alveolar and lingual nerves

Do not clean the fascia off the medial pterygoid muscle at this stage lest you damage some important structures which descend from the lower border of the lateral pterygoid muscle, and which cross the lateral surface of the medial pterygoid muscle. The more important of them are the inferior alveolar nerve, which you have encountered already, and the lingual nerve, another sensory branch of the mandibular nerve [Fig. 5.54]. The lingual nerve descends anterior to the inferior alveolar nerve to supply the mucous coat of the floor of the mouth and the anterior two-thirds of the tongue.

Dissect at the lower border of the lateral pterygoid muscle and find and clean the lingual nerve. Then clean the inferior alveolar nerve, and search for the fine branch to the mylohyoid muscle, which leaves it posteriorly just above the mandibular foramen. Note, too, a thin ribbon-like ligament which lies deep to the inferior alveolar nerve. It is called the **sphenomandibular ligament,** and it runs upwards and slightly backwards from the lingula to the spine of the sphenoid [Fig. 5.56]. At this stage you will see its lower end only. It is pierced by the mylohyoid nerve.

Having cleaned and isolated the inferior alveolar and lingual nerves, clean the surface of the medial pterygoid muscle, removing any periosteum other than that into which the muscle is inserted. Define the two borders of the muscle, and note that its attachment to the medial surface of the mandible, which has already been removed, was partly tendinous.

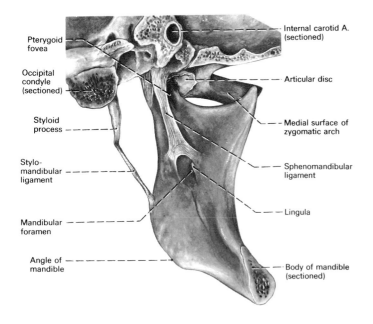

Pterygoid
fovea

Occipital
condyle
(sectioned)

Styloid
process

Stylo-
mandibular
ligament

Mandibular
foramen

Angle of
mandible

Internal carotid A.
(sectioned)

Articular disc

Medial surface of
zygomatic arch

Sphenomandibular
ligament

Lingula

Body of mandible
(sectioned)

Fig. 5.56 Medial view of the ligaments of the left temporomandibular joint. The medial parts of the occipital, temporal, and sphenoid bones have been removed.

The attachments of the pterygoid muscles

Though the origin of the medial pterygoid muscle and the insertion of the lateral pterygoid muscle cannot be easily studied on the cadaver until later, you should now look at a skull and define the attachments of these muscles.

The origins of the pterygoid muscles [Figs 5.50 and 5.51]

First, look at the infratemporal crest, the temporal surface of the greater wing of the sphenoid bone medial to the crest, and the lateral surface of the lateral pterygoid plate, from which, as you have seen, the two heads of the lateral pterygoid muscle arise. Then look at the medial surface of the lateral pterygoid plate, from which the deep head of the medial pterygoid muscle takes origin, and the tuberosity of the maxilla and pyramidal process of the palatine bone, from which its superficial and smaller head arises. Note that both pterygoid muscles arise from the lateral pterygoid plate, and that the smaller medial pterygoid plate is essentially a backward continuation of the side wall of the cavity of the nose.

The insertions of the pterygoid muscles

Examine the mandibular notch and the neck of the mandible. The small triangular-shaped depression on the anterior surface of the neck is the site of attachment of most of the lateral pterygoid muscle. It is called the **pterygoid fovea** [Fig. 5.49]. The medial pterygoid muscle is attached to the deep surface of the angle of the mandible behind the mylohyoid groove. This part of the bone is often ridged, because of the tendinous nature of the muscle's insertion [Fig. 5.48].

As they approach their insertions, the two pterygoid muscles pass both backwards and laterally. But while they arise from the skull fairly close together, their fibres diverge considerably on their way to their insertions. Their actions are, therefore, very different.

The temporomandibular joint

The articular surface of the mandibular fossa

Whenever the jaw opens, the head of the mandible automatically moves forward [Fig. 5.57]. Place your fingers just in front of the tragus of the auricle of your own ear, and open your own jaw. You will easily feel the head of your mandible moving forward. Return to the skull, and note again that the anterior wall of the mandibular fossa (on the squamous part of the temporal bone) is formed by the posterior face of the **articular tubercle,** which is a projection of the same bone. When the jaw is fully open, the head of the mandible lies on the summit of the tubercle, the two opposing surfaces of bone being cushioned from each other by an articular disc of fibrocartilage, which you will dissect later. Posteromedially the articular surface of the mandibu-

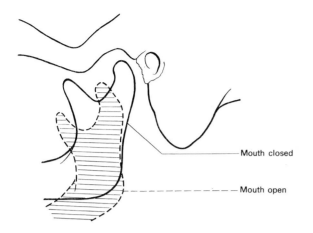

Fig. 5.57 Positions of the head of the mandible with the mouth open and closed. Superimposed tracings of radiographs.

— Mouth closed

— Mouth open

lar fossa is bounded by a narrow fissure, which separates it from the superior border of the tympanic part of the temporal bone. On the lateral side, this fissure is called the **tympanosquamous fissure** [Fig. 5.58]. More medially the fissure is occupied by what appears to be an independent spicule of bone. The latter is a downward extension of the petrous part of the temporal bone. Hence the medial part of the fissure is subdivided into two parallel fissures, an anterior **petrosquamous fissure** and a posterior **petrotympanic fissure.** The lateral part of the posterior border of the articular sur-

face is formed by an inferiorly-projecting part of the squamous part of the temporal bone, often called the **postglenoid tubercle** [Fig. 5.58].

Carefully note that the articular capsule of the temporomandibular joint is attached to this tubercle laterally, and into the tympanosquamous and petrotympanic fissures more medially; and that it is not attached to the inferior border of the tympanic part of the temporal bone. Laterally the capsule is attached to the margins of the mandibular fossa on the zygomatic process of the temporal bone, and anteriorly it passes on to the summit of the articular tubercle. Medially it is fixed to the medial margin of the mandibular fossa.

Note that the articular surface lies in the anterior part of the mandibular fossa, and that it does not include the tympanic part of the temporal bone in the posterior wall of the fossa.

The articular capsule

Remove the fascia which covers the side of the head and neck of the mandible, anterior to the superficial temporal artery. This will reveal a thickening of the articular capsule of the temporomandibular joint, called the **lateral ligament** [Fig. 5.59]. The ligament is attached above to the lateral side of the articular tubercle, and below to the side of the neck of the mandible. Its fibres run downwards and backwards.

Before opening the temporomandibular joint, once again identify the **masseteric nerve,** and trace it medially. You will

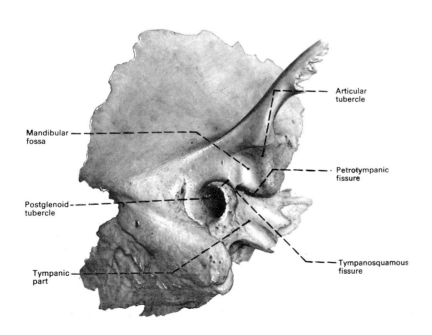

Mandibular fossa

Articular tubercle

Postglenoid tubercle

Petrotympanic fissure

Tympanic part

Tympanosquamous fissure

Fig. 5.58 Lateral surface of the right temporal bone (oblique view from below).

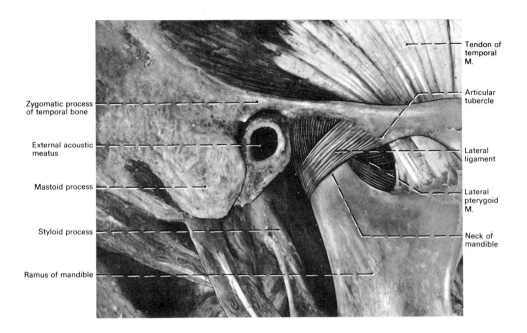

Zygomatic process
of temporal bone

External acoustic
meatus

Mastoid process

Styloid process

Ramus of mandible

Tendon of
temporal
M.

Articular
tubercle

Lateral
ligament

Lateral
pterygoid
M.

Neck of
mandible

Fig. 5.59 The lateral ligament of the right temporomandibular joint.

find that the nerve runs above the lateral pterygoid muscle, immediately anterior to the joint, to which it sends a branch.

The interior of the temporomandibular joint

Make an incision downwards and backwards from the side of the articular tubercle through the lateral part of the articular capsule. Cut as deeply as possible as your blade crosses the joint. Splay open your incision, and note that there are two joint cavities, one above the other, separated by an **articular disc** of fibrocartilage [Fig. 5.60]. The latter may be vertically-disposed at its posterior attachment. Move the head of the mandible in the joint, and notice that the articular disc also moves, and tends to straighten as the head of the mandible moves forwards. Insert one point of a pair of scissors into the upper joint cavity, and cut through the lateral part of the capsule, forwards and backwards. Do the same with the point of the scissors inserted into the lower cavity of the joint. You can now see that the surfaces of the interarticular disc correspond in shape to the articular surfaces of the temporal bone and mandible.

Pull the head of the mandible downwards and, with one point of the scissors in the upper joint cavity, cut through the rest of the articular capsule all the way round the articular surface of the temporal bone. In this way you will disarticulate the head of the mandible and articular disc from the skull.

Turn the head of the mandible laterally and forwards, using a blunt probe or the handle of a scalpel to free it from structures deep (i.e medial) to it. As the medial surface of the head comes into view you will see how the fibres of the

lateral pterygoid muscles converge and insert into the anterior surface of the neck of the mandible.

Removal of the lateral pterygoid muscle

The lateral pterygoid muscle is now to be detached from the greater wing of the sphenoid bone. Gently push the head of the mandible forwards beneath the maxillary artery, carefully separating it and the lateral pterygoid muscle from deeper structures. In doing so you will have to separate the muscle from the deep temporal nerves, which pass to the temporal muscle, and also the buccal nerve, which runs between the two heads of the lateral pterygoid muscle, and which, you will recall, is a sensory branch of the mandibular nerve. The nerve to the lateral pterygoid muscle, which is also a branch of the mandibular nerve, runs with the buccal nerve. When these nerves have been freed, detach first the lower, and then the upper head of the lateral pterygoid muscle from the lateral pterygoid plate and adjacent bone above. The head and neck of the mandible will now be completely free, and can be removed from the dissection.

The articular disc [Fig. 5.60]

The lower cavity of the temporomandibular joint and the articular disc have been removed with the mandible. Open the lower cavity at the back and sides. At its periphery the disc is attached to the inner surface of the articular capsule, and posteriorly to the tympanosquamous and petrotympanic fissures as well. Occasionally the articular disc is perforated, so that the upper and lower joint cavities communicate.

Now examine the attachment of the articular capsule.

5.60

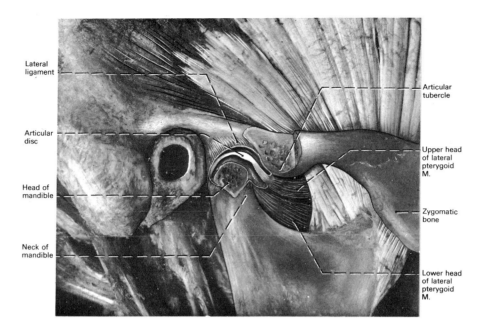

Lateral
ligament

Articular
disc

Head of
mandible

Neck of
mandible

Articular
tubercle

Upper head
of lateral
pterygoid
M.

Zygomatic
bone

Lower head
of lateral
pterygoid
M.

Fig. 5.60 The interior of the right temporomandibular joint. Most of the lateral ligament, and part of the head of the mandible and articular tubercle have been excised.

Note again that the tympanic part of the temporal bone takes no part in the formation of the joint.

Finally, carefully define the insertion of the lateral pterygoid muscle. The muscle is inserted into the pterygoid fovea of the neck of the mandible, but some of the upper fibres will be found to have a firm attachment to the anterior part of the articular capsule, and through this to the articular disc.

The movements of the mandible [Fig. 5.57]

When the mouth is closed and the jaw is at rest, the condylar process of the mandible lies just below the articular surface, and its posterior border is separated from the tympanic part of the temporal bone by the capsule of the joint and by a process of the parotid gland. When the jaw opens, the lateral pterygoid muscle contracts, and as a result, the condylar process is pulled forwards on the plate of fibrocartilage, which is stretched and straightened during the course of this process. When the muscles which keep the jaw closed are relaxed, gravity provides the force which opens the jaw. At the same time the mandible rotates on a transverse axis which passes through the upper part of the ramus of the mandible on both sides. The actual position of this transverse axis varies with every position of the mandible, but is never far removed from a line passing through the two mandibular foramina. This fact will be remembered if it is interpreted as implying that the inferior alveolar nerve and vessels will not become stretched as the jaw opens. It should be noted that the forward movement of the mandible occurs in the upper, and that rotation (the opening movement) occurs in the lower cavity of the temporomandibular joint.

The essential action of the lateral pterygoid muscle is, therefore, to pull the jaw forwards as it opens. That of the medial pterygoid muscle is obvious from its attachments. The muscle will be in a relaxed state when the jaw opens, and its contraction will help to close the jaw. It will also steady the mandible as the lateral pterygoid muscle acts.

Closing of the mouth is caused by the contraction of the temporal muscle, the masseter, and the medial pterygoid muscles, all of whose fibres are more or less vertically-disposed between the skull and the mandible. The movement is, however, also associated with the backward sliding of the head of the mandible into the mandibular fossa. This is brought about by the contraction of the almost horizontally-disposed posterior fibres of the fan-shaped temporal muscle. It is easy to see that these fibres pull in practically the same plane as those of the lateral pterygoid muscle, but in an opposite direction. Side to side or chewing movements of the jaw are brought about by the alternate action of all the muscles of mastication, but particularly of the pterygoid muscles.

If you place the tips of your index fingers immediately in front of your ears and just below the zygomatic process of the temporal bone, you can follow the movements of the heads of your mandible. Simply open and close your mouth, then protract and retract your jaw, and then make side to side movements, first with your mouth closed and then with it open.

To feel the contraction of your masseter and temporal muscles, place the tips of your fingers over the respective muscles and clench your teeth. The pterygoid muscles cannot be palpated.

Section 5.8

The upper part of the neck

Your dissection has now reached the stage when you can return to the study of the common carotid artery and its terminal branches. You have already exposed the structures that were enclosed in the carotid sheath. While doing so, you identified the ansa cervicalis [p. 5.19]. You also cleaned and divided the infrahyoid muscles.

Osteology

Certain additional features on the skull should be examined before you continue your dissection.

The temporal bone [Fig. 5.61]

Look at the temporal bone, and again examine the **mastoid process.** Medial to this is the deep **mastoid notch** from which the posterior belly of the digastric muscle arises, and medial

to the latter is the much narrower **groove for the occipital artery** [Fig. 5.61]. At the anterior end of the mastoid notch you will find the **stylomastoid foramen** [Fig. 5.51], with the long tapering **styloid process** anterior to it. The distal part of this process is often missing on macerated skulls.

The mandible [Fig. 5.61]

On the medial surface of the body of the mandible find a ridge running downwards and forwards from just below the third molar tooth; it fades out before the midline is reached. This is the **mylohyoid line,** from which the mylohyoid muscle arises [Fig. 5.61]. The small projections on the posterior surface of the junction of the two halves of the mandible form the **mental spine,** to which two pairs of muscles, the genioglossus above and the geniohyoid below, are attached. Below the anterior ends of the mylohyoid lines are a pair

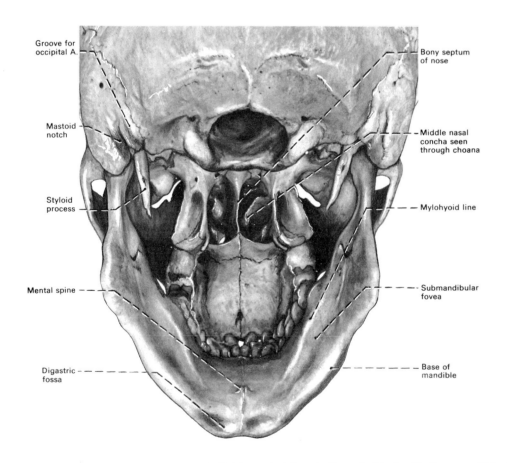

Fig. 5.61 The external surface of the base of the skull (viewed obliquely from behind with the mandible in position).

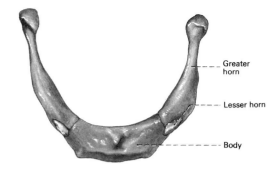

a. *From above*

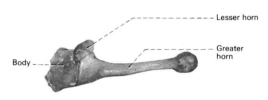

b. *From the left side*

Fig. 5.62 The hyoid bone.

of shallow impressions, the **digastric fossae,** for the attachment of the anterior bellies of the digastric muscles. Another shallow but larger depression lies below the posterior end of each mylohyoid line, and at the anterior end of the mylohyoid groove. This is the **submandibular fovea,** and within it, and subjacent to the bone, lies the submandibular gland.

The hyoid bone [Fig. 5.62]

If you cannot get an actual specimen, look at a picture of the hyoid bone. Identify its **body,** the longer posterior projecting arms or **greater horns,** and the shorter **lesser horns** superior to them [Fig. 5.62].

As you proceed with your dissection, you will learn about the structures that are attached to, or are in relation to these parts of the hyoid.

Structures in the upper part of the neck

On the half of the head which is attached to the remains of the trunk, free the inferior end of the **internal jugular vein,** and divide it about 1 cm above its termination. This will already have been done on the isolated half. On both halves of the head separate the superior part of the internal jugular vein from surrounding structures, and sever the **superior** and **middle thyroid veins,** which pass into the internal jugular vein from the thyroid gland. Also divide the **facial vein.** Thread the internal jugular vein through the ansa cervicalis, and separating it from deeper structures, reflect the whole

vein superiorly. Completely remove the vein up to the level of the angle of the mandible, and clear away the clotted blood from its upper and lower stumps.

Follow the **superior root of the ansa cervicalis** upwards through the fascia of the carotid sheath [Fig. 5.65]. You should be able to establish that it springs from the large **hypoglossal nerve,** which descends in the carotid sheath. You will find this nerve curving forwards across the internal and external carotid arteries, slightly above the level of the hyoid bone [Fig. 5.63].

Now pick up the **vagus nerve,** and trace it superiorly to the level of the hypoglossal nerve. Do the same with the **common carotid artery.** The artery divides into the **internal** and **external carotid arteries,** at the level of the superior border of the thyroid cartilage. Find the bifurcation of the common carotid artery, and note that the internal carotid artery is, at first, postero-lateral to the external carotid artery.

The superior thyroid vessels [Fig. 5.63]

Follow the external carotid artery upwards for a short distance, cleaning it as you do so, and find the first branch that it gives off from its anterior aspect. This is the **superior thyroid artery,** which loops down to the superior end of the thyroid gland [Fig. 5.63]. Follow and clean the artery as well as the associated **superior thyroid vein,** which you have already severed from the internal jugular vein. In order to do this, you will have to uncover the gland's concave postero-lateral surface, which lies in contact with, and overlaps the carotid sheath and its contents. The superior thyroid artery enters the gland on this surface. As you dissect, you will see that the artery gives off numerous small branches, some of which supply the larynx and the lower end of the pharynx.

Carefully remove the plexus of veins that connect the thyroid gland with the superior thyroid vein.

The digastric and stylohyoid muscles [Fig. 5.63]

Turn the cut end of the facial vein upwards towards the mandible, severing any small tributaries which enter its deep surface, but leaving the tributary from the retromandibular vein.

Deep to the facial and retromandibular veins you will see the **submandibular gland** [Fig. 5.63] encapsulated in fascia derived from the superficial layer of cervical fascia. Clean the fascia off the superficial surface and inferior border of the gland, and find the **intermediate tendon of the digastric muscle,** which the gland overlaps. The narrow muscle which you will see bestriding the tendon is the **stylohyoid muscle.** The tendon lies immediately above the hyoid bone, to which it is attached by a loop of fascia. When the two bellies of the digastric muscle contract, the bone is pulled upwards.

Define and clean the **anterior belly of the digastric muscle,** separating it from the underlying mylohyoid muscle. You may find a fine motor nerve entering the upper surface of

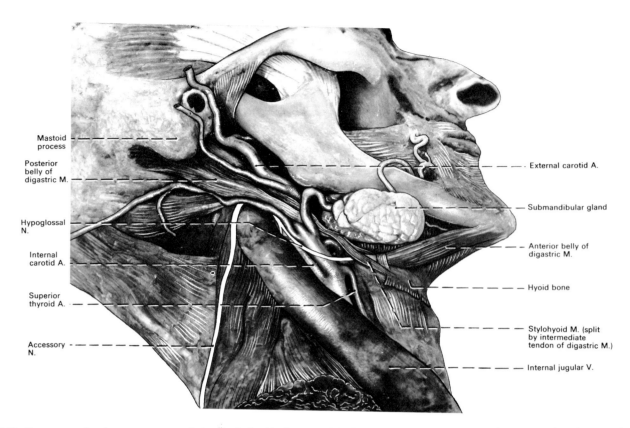

Mastoid process

Posterior belly of digastric M.

Hypoglossal N.

Internal carotid A.

Superior thyroid A.

Accessory N.

External carotid A.

Submandibular gland

Anterior belly of digastric M.

Hyoid bone

Stylohyoid M. (split by intermediate tendon of digastric M.)

Internal jugular V.

Fig. 5.63 Structures in the upper part of the neck. In this figure, and in Fig. 5.64, the facial artery is shown crossing the posterior belly of the digastric muscle and the stylohyoid muscle superficially. Usually the artery passes deep to these structures.

the anterior belly, whose origin from the digastric fossa on the mandible you should confirm. The nerve is a branch of the **mylohyoid nerve.**

Now follow the intermediate tendon of the digastric posteriorly. Do not disturb the stylohyoid muscle, but continue towards the **posterior belly of the digastric muscle.** This should be completely exposed and cleaned. Its superficial surface is, to some extent, overlapped by the parotid gland (which you have already removed). Blunt dissection only is to be used on the deep aspect of the muscle. You will find the upper end of the posterior belly of the digastric disappearing deep to the mastoid process, where it is attached to the mastoid notch. You may find the motor nerve to this belly running a short straight course from the facial nerve in the stylomastoid foramen.

The digastric muscle, particularly its posterior belly, is an important landmark in the superior part of the neck. The area which is bounded below by the two bellies of the muscle, and above by the base of the mandible and a line drawn from the angle of the mandible to the mastoid process, is call the **submandibular triangle.** The principal contents of the triangle are the submandibular gland and the facial artery. Note how closely the posterior belly lies to the transverse process of the atlas. Note especially that the two carotid arteries, the internal jugular vein and the vagus, ac-

cessory, and hypoglossal nerves, lie deep to the muscle, separated from it by a fairly thick layer of fascia.

Return to the intermediate tendon of the digastric muscle, and dissect the stylohyoid muscle, which you have already seen crossing the tendon obliquely. The upper end of the stylohyoid muscle is attached to the base of the styloid process. Feel for this process, and note that while the stylohyoid muscle, like the posterior belly of the digastric muscle, passes superficial to the large vessels of the neck, the styloid process itself projects downwards and forwards between the internal and external carotid arteries. This relationship will become clearer a little later in the dissection.

You will see that the inferior end of the stylohyoid muscle splits round the tendon of the digastric muscle, to be inserted into the hyoid bone [Fig. 5.63].

The occipital artery [Fig. 5.64]

Return to the external carotid artery, and follow it a little further superiorly. Above the point where it is crossed by the hypoglossal nerve, the artery gives off its first posterior branch, the occipital artery [Fig. 5.64]. This should now be traced as it runs superiorly and posteriorly across the internal carotid artery, the hypoglossal and accessory nerves, and the internal jugular vein. The occipital artery passes deep to the posterior belly of the digastric muscle and the

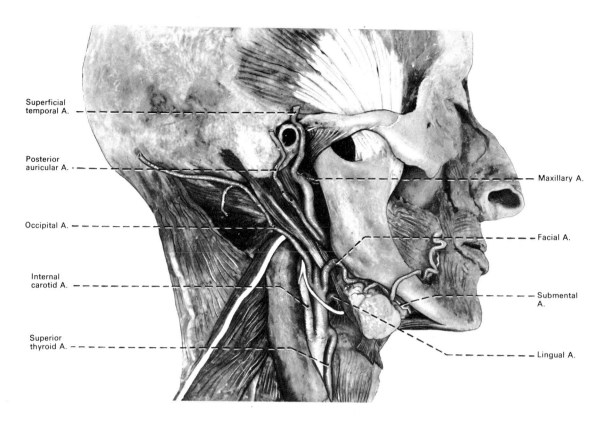

Superficial temporal A.

Posterior auricular A.

Occipital A.

Internal carotid A.

Superior thyroid A.

Maxillary A.

Facial A.

Submental A.

Lingual A.

Fig. 5.64 The right external carotid artery and its branches.

mastoid process. To follow the vessel further, reflect the splenius capitis and, working from below, cut through the tissue and muscle overlying the artery. You should be able to see the artery crossing the occipital bone just below the superior nuchal line, and then turning upwards to enter the scalp. Apart from the scalp, the artery supplies branches to the muscles between which it passes.

Carefully divide the posterior belly of the digastric muscle and the stylohyoid muscle as close to the base of the skull as you can, and reflect them anteriorly. This will ease your dissection of the structures deep to them, but the muscles should be replaced from time to time in order to study their relationships.

In subsequent dissection do not hesitate to remove the small and variable veins that ramify in this region. They roughly correspond to the arteries, and communicate with one or both of the jugular veins.

The hypoglossal nerve [Fig. 5.65]

Identify the hypoglossal nerve where it crosses the external carotid artery, and follow it anteriorly. Lift the submandibular gland, and define the lower end of the posterior border of the mylohyoid muscle. Working above the intermediate tendon of the digastric muscle, confirm that the hypoglossal nerve disappears from view deep to this border of the mylohyoid muscle [Fig. 5.65].

The facial artery [Figs 5.41 and 5.64]

Now look for the lingual and facial arteries [Fig. 5.64]. They are anterior branches of the external carotid artery, and arise at about the level where the artery is crossed by the hypoglossal nerve, just above the greater horn of the hyoid bone. Not uncommonly these two vessels arise from the external carotid artery by a single trunk.

For the present the facial artery only is to be followed. It lies above the lingual artery, and at first runs deeply and upwards, under cover of the posterior belly of the digastric muscle. The facial artery then loops forwards in a groove in the posterior end of the submandibular gland, and passes downwards, forwards, and laterally between the gland and the inner surface of the body of the mandible where a branch, the **submental artery** runs forward. It then turns round the base of the mandible, just anterior to the insertion of the masseter muscle. You have already dissected its further course [p. 5.41].

The mylohyoid nerve [Fig. 5.65]

Now free the submandibular gland from the inner surface of the mandible, and look for the fine mylohyoid nerve which, further forwards, accompanies the submental artery. Trace the nerve anteriorly, and you will see it forming a spray of branches, all but one of which enter the superficial surface of the **mylohyoid muscle.** The remaining branch

5.65

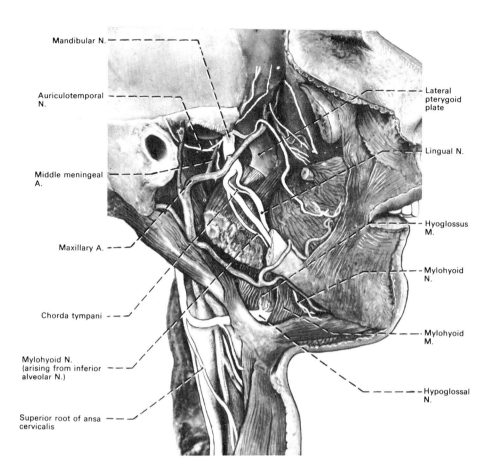

Mandibular N.

Auriculotemporal
N.

Middle meningeal
A.

Maxillary A.

Chorda tympani

Mylohyoid N.
(arising from inferior
alveolar N.)

Superior root of ansa
cervicalis

Lateral
pterygoid
plate

Lingual N.

Hyoglossus
M.

Mylohyoid
N.

Mylohyoid
M.

Hypoglossal
N.

Fig. 5.65 The right infratemporal region after the removal of the lateral pterygoid muscle.

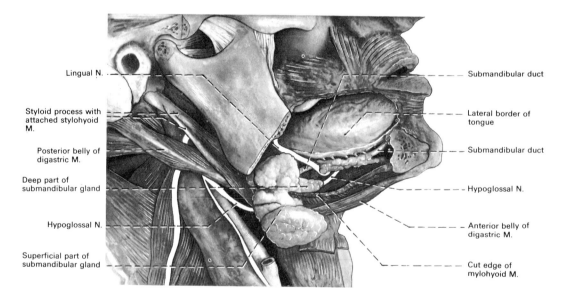

Lingual N.

Styloid process with
attached stylohyoid
M.

Posterior belly of
digastric M.

Deep part of
submandibular gland

Hypoglossal N.

Superficial part of
submandibular gland

Submandibular duct

Lateral border of
tongue

Submandibular duct

Hypoglossal N.

Anterior belly of
digastric M.

Cut edge of
mylohyoid M.

Fig. 5.66 The right submandibular gland. The body of the mandible and part of the cheek have been removed to expose the tongue. The external carotid artery has also been removed.

continues its course to supply the **anterior belly of the digastric muscle.**

Now trace the mylohyoid nerve superiorly and posteriorly to the point where it leaves the **inferior alveolar nerve** [Fig. 5.65]. To do this, lift the periosteum off the deep surface of the angle of the mandible as far forwards as is necessary, and thus, at the same time, complete the detachment of the medial pterygoid muscle. To ease the dissection of the mylohyoid nerve, remove what remains of the angle of the mandible with bone forceps.

The submandibular gland [Fig. 5.66]

Turn the submandibular gland forwards and upwards to separate its deep surface from the underlying muscles. You will find that part of the gland hooks under the deep surface of the mylohyoid muscle, and that it is from here that the duct of the gland, the **submandibular duct,** emerges. Since the mylohyoid muscles form the floor of the mouth, the duct is inside the cavity of the mouth from the start [Fig. 5.66].

The superficial part of the submandibular gland comprises the bulk of the gland. Identify its three surfaces. They are: an infero-lateral or superficial surface; a lateral surface, which lies deep to the mandible and the inferior attachment of the medial pterygoid muscle; and a medial surface, which overlaps the two bellies of the digastric muscle and lies, anteriorly, on the mylohyoid muscle. Posterior to the mylohyoid muscle, the medial surface lies on the hyoglossus muscle.

The hyoglossus muscle [Fig. 5.67]

The hyoglossus muscle arises from the greater horn of the hyoid bone, and its fibres run vertically upwards into the side of the tongue [Fig. 5.67]. In shape the hyoglossus is a thin quadrangular sheet. Close to its inferior border it is crossed by the hypoglossal nerve, which is passing forwards between it and the mylohyoid muscle. Start cleaning the muscle in an upward direction from the level of the nerve, using great care. At the superior border of the muscle you will find that its vertically-running fibres intermingle with a series of horizontal muscle fibres. The latter constitute the **styloglossus muscle,** which is descending from the styloid process. Do not clean this muscle yet.

Since the hyoglossus muscle runs into the side of the tongue, and the mylohyoid is attached to the inner surface of the mandible, it follows that if you inserted the handle of a scalpel between the two muscles, you would bring it into contact with the mucous coat of the mouth at the side of the tongue. Confirm that this is so.

Now follow the **lingual artery,** and you will find that it very soon disappears by passing deep to the lower end of the posterior border of the hyoglossus muscle. At this point the artery lies deep (medial) to the hypoglossal nerve.

The posterior auricular artery [Fig. 5.64]

One more branch of the external carotid artery must be found before the artery is traced to its termination. This is

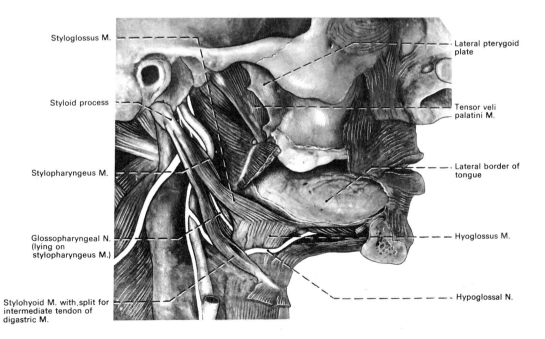

Fig. 5.67 The right infratemporal region after removal of the mandible and both pterygoid muscles. Most of the cheek and buccinator muscle have been removed to expose the tongue. The submandibular gland and the digastric muscle have also been removed.

the posterior auricular artery, which is smaller than any of the branches you have already examined. It ascends posteriorly, above the posterior belly of the digastric muscle, towards the stylomastoid foramen, into which it sends a branch. The posterior auricular artery then runs behind the auricle to supply it and part of the scalp. The artery was probably cut when the auricle was removed.

The termination of the external carotid artery

You should now follow and clean the external carotid artery as far as its termination.

Having crossed the styloid process on its lateral side, you will find that the external carotid artery enters the parotid gland, where it runs deep to the retromandibular vein. It ends behind the neck of the mandible, by dividing into the maxillary artery and superficial temporal artery [Fig. 5.64]. The superficial temporal artery usually looks as though it is the continuation of the external carotid artery, and may be confused with it.

Any branches of the facial nerve which still remain attached to facial structures will now have to be divided at their peripheral ends, and the nerve turned back. Some of the remaining cartilage of the external acoustic meatus may have to be cut away to allow the superficial temporal artery to be followed.

Remove the remains of the parotid gland so that you may establish the continuity of the external carotid artery with those parts of the superficial temporal and maxillary arteries which have already been displayed.

The superficial temporal artery

As you have seen, the superficial temporal artery ascends over the posterior root of the zygomatic process of the temporal bone to pass into the scalp. In addition to the scalp, the artery helps to supply the auricle, the parotid gland, the mandibular joint, and the temporal and masseter muscles.

The maxillary artery

The maxillary artery passes anteriorly across the infratemporal fossa. At first it lies close to the medial border of the neck of the mandible. Here it gives off two small but important branches: the inferior alveolar artery which you have followed into the mandibular canal, and an artery which you will find ascending and entering the skull medial to the articular eminence of the temporal bone. This is the **middle meningeal artery.** It runs upwards and passes into the middle cranial fossa through the foramen spinosum [Fig. 5.51] to supply the meninges. The middle meningeal artery lies deep to the lateral pterygoid muscle and could not be dissected before this muscle had been removed.

You have already traced the maxillary artery in its further course across the inferior head of the lateral pterygoid muscle, to the point where it leaves the infratemporal fossa

by passing through the pterygomaxillary fissure. Its terminal branches will be dissected at a later stage.

Also note and then remove the maxillary veins. These drain blood from the pterygoid venous plexus into the retromandibular vein.

The mandibular nerve [Fig. 5.65]

The mandibular nerve emerges from the foramen ovale. It is the largest of the divisions of the trigeminal nerve. In addition to sensory fibres it incorporates the whole of the motor root of the trigeminal nerve, the latter being distributed to the four main muscles of mastication, to the mylohyoid muscle and to the anterior belly of the digastric muscle. The mandibular nerve supplies the mucous coat of the mouth, the lower teeth, and skin of the face and scalp, through the lingual, the inferior alveolar (which lies posterior to the lingual), the buccal, and the auriculotemporal nerves. Trace the **inferior alveolar, lingual, buccal, deep temporal,** and **masseteric nerves** towards the foramen ovale, and find the mandibular nerve, from which they all spring. As you do this, dissect away the pterygoid plexus and the emissary veins which connect it, through foramina in the base of the skull, with the sinuses of the dura mater.

The auriculotemporal nerve [Fig. 5.65]

Find and trace a moderately large nerve which runs in a posterior direction from the mandibular nerve, close to the point where the latter emerges from the foramen ovale. This is the auriculotemporal nerve. It is directed laterally behind the temporomandibular joint, and passes, with the superficial temporal vessels, into the scalp, where it has already been identified [p. 5.47]. The nerve supplies the temporomandibular joint, the parotid gland, the skin of the auricle and the external acoustic meatus, the ear-drum or tympanic membrane, and the scalp.

Close to the point where it joins the mandibular nerve, the auriculotemporal nerve splits to enclose the middle meningeal artery. This vessel runs upwards through the foramen spinosum, behind and lateral to the foramen ovale. Clean the artery carefully, and you will find the fibres of the auriculotemporal nerve which loop around its deep side. The artery thus appears to pierce the nerve.

The chorda tympani [Fig. 5.65]

Now find a small but very important branch of the facial nerve, the chorda tympani, which joins the posterior border of the lingual nerve, just below the foramen ovale [Fig. 5.65]. The chorda tympani lies above and deep to the auriculotemporal nerve and the middle meningeal artery, and leaves the skull through the petrotympanic fissure, posterior to the attachment of the capsule of the temporomandibular joint.

Removal of the medial pterygoid muscle

To remove the medial pterygoid muscle, first use the handle of a scalpel to free the muscle from surrounding structures. Then thread it under the inferior alveolar and lingual nerves. The lateral pterygoid plate was revealed when the lateral pterygoid muscle was removed. You will now be able to see how the medial pterygoid muscle arises from the medial surface of this plate.

Use bone gouge forceps to remove the lateral pterygoid plate, and carefully detach the muscle. As you turn the muscle forwards you may see the nerve to the medial pterygoid, a branch of the motor root of the trigeminal nerve, entering its deep surface. If so, divide it. Clean away what remains of the origin of the muscle from the base of the lateral pterygoid plate.

The removal of the medial pterygoid muscle reveals a thin triangular muscle whose fibres pass downwards and forwards to converge on a glistening tendon. This is the **tensor veli palatini muscle** [Fig. 5.67], which will be studied at a later stage of dissection.

To obtain a better exposure of deeper structures, divide the posterior auricular artery and any vessels which run posteriorly from the superficial temporal artery and prevent you freeing the external carotid artery.

The styloid process and related structures

Feel the styloid process, and look for a fibrous band which is attached to its tip. This, the **stylohyoid ligament,** should be traced inferiorly and anteriorly, to the point where it disappears behind the hyoglossus muscle. The inferior end of the ligament is attached to the lesser horn of the hyoid bone. The ligament follows the course of an embryological structure, the cartilage of the second visceral arch, from which the styloid process and the lesser horn are derived.

The **styloglossus muscle** descends from the lower end of the styloid process and the stylohyoid ligament. Its fibres have already been seen mingling with those of the hyoglossus muscle on the side of the tongue [p. 5.67 and Fig. 5.67]. As you remove a sheet of fascia which is attached along the muscle's inferior border, and which overlies the external carotid artery, be careful lest you detach the styloglossus muscle from the styloid process.

The third muscle which arises from the styloid process descends medial to the tip of the process. This is the **stylopharyngeus.** Follow it a short distance inferiorly and look for a nerve, the **glossopharyngeal nerve,** which winds round its posterior border and descends obliquely across its lateral surface. The stylopharyngeus disappears from view deep to a sheet of muscle, the middle constrictor muscle of the pharynx, whose superior border winds round the stylopharyngeus in much the same way as does the glossopharyngeal nerve [Fig. 5.68].

Trace the glossopharyngeal nerve forwards and downwards. You will find it disappearing deep to the posterior border of the hyoglossus muscle above the level of the lingual artery and the stylohyoid ligament, both of which pass under the muscle. If the facial artery makes it difficult for you to follow the nerve, free the facial artery by cutting through its branch, the **ascending palatine artery,** which springs from the facial artery close to its origin. As usual, do not hesitate to remove any small veins you encounter. Now trace the glossopharyngeal nerve posteriorly and superiorly as it winds round the stylopharyngeus muscle. Separate the nerve from the muscle, and you may be able to see the fine branch which the nerve sends to the muscle. Note that the hypoglossal nerve is at a lower level, just above the greater horn of the hyoid bone.

The proximal parts of the last four cranial nerves [Fig. 5.68]

The internal carotid artery and the last four cranial nerves are now to be dissected deep to the styloid process and its associated muscles. If the dissection is too difficult with the styloid process in place, divide the process near its base with bone forceps, and turn it forwards and downwards with the stylopharyngeus and styloglossus muscles still attached to it.

Start with the **accessory nerve,** and trace it upwards. You will find it gaining the interval between the internal carotid artery and the internal jugular vein by passing upwards and crossing the vein either superficially or deeply at the level of the transverse process of the atlas. Note again how closely the nerve lies to this process. Then trace the internal jugular vein, the **hypoglossal nerve,** and the **vagus nerve.** At this level the nerves are between the artery and the vein, the vagus lying medial to the hypoglossal nerve. At the level of the transverse process of the atlas, you will find a branch of the vagus which passes forwards deep to the internal carotid artery. This is the **superior laryngeal nerve** [Fig. 5.68]. Now look for a fine branch of the vagus which turns forwards superficial to the internal carotid artery. This is the largest of the **pharyngeal branches of the vagus.** It crosses the artery below the **glossopharyngeal nerve.**

Now turn to a skull, and identify, on the external surface of its base, the opening of the carotid canal for the internal carotid artery in the petrous part of the temporal bone, with the larger jugular foramen posterior to it [Fig. 5.69], and the small hypoglossal canal medial to the latter. This will help you to appreciate that near the base of the skull, the internal carotid artery lies in front of the internal jugular vein, with the last four cranial nerves between them. As the nerves descend, the accessory nerve turns posteriorly, and the glossopharyngeal and hypoglossal nerves anteriorly, the former between, and the latter lateral to the internal and external carotid arteries. The vagus nerve continues along the course of the vessels throughout the neck.

It is useful at this point to note the structures which pass

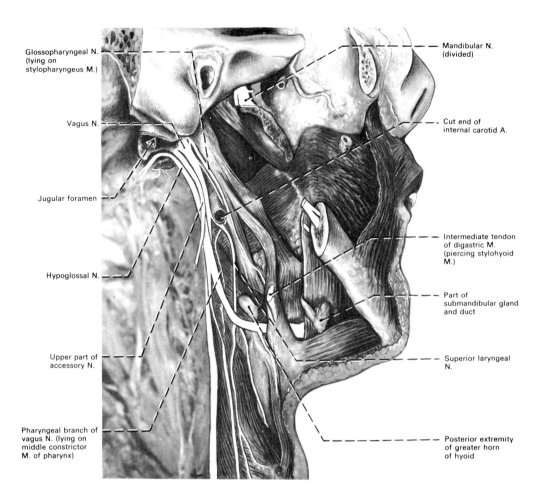

Glossopharyngeal N.
(lying on
stylopharyngeus M.)

Vagus N.

Jugular foramen

Hypoglossal N.

Upper part of
accessory N.

Pharyngeal branch of
vagus N. (lying on
middle constrictor
M. of pharynx)

Mandibular N.
(divided)

Cut end of
internal carotid A.

Intermediate tendon
of digastric M.
(piercing stylohyoid
M.)

Part of
submandibular gland
and duct

Superior laryngeal
N.

Posterior extremity
of greater horn
of hyoid

Fig. 5.68 The right glossopharyngeal, vagus, accessory, and hypoglossal nerves (postero-lateral view). A posterior view of a similar dissection is shown in Fig. 5.78. The vertebral column and the part of the skull behind the hypoglossal canal have been removed. In this body the hypoglossal nerve passes below the greater horn of the hyoid bone; it normally passes above.

or intervene between the external and internal carotid arteries. The most prominent is the styloid process, and since the external carotid artery ends in the parotid gland, a part of the gland also intervenes. Three other structures which do so are the stylopharyngeus muscle, the glossopharyngeal nerve, and the pharyngeal branches of the vagus. Confirm these points on your dissection.

The stylohyoid muscle, which is innervated by the facial nerve, passes lateral to the vessels. The styloglossus is a muscle of the tongue and is supplied by the hypoglossal nerve. It arises from the styloid process anterior to the vessels.

The external carotid artery

Confirm once more that the common carotid artery divides into external and internal carotid arteries at about the level of the upper border of the thyroid cartilage; that the superior thyroid, lingual, and facial arteries, branches of the external carotid artery, pass anteriorly, the occipital and

posterior auricular arteries posteriorly; and that the two terminal branches of the external carotid artery (the superficial temporal and the maxillary arteries) start behind the neck of the mandible [Fig. 5.64]. The smallest branch of the external carotid artery, the **ascending pharyngeal artery,** need not be dissected. It arises close to the beginning of the external carotid artery, and ascends the neck at the side of the pharynx, deep to the internal carotid artery. Note the tortuous course of the facial artery as it passes round the submandibular gland, to emerge at the antero-inferior angle of the masseter muscle. Observe especially that the hypoglossal nerve crosses lateral to both the external and internal carotid arteries, just above the level of the greater horn of the hyoid bone (which is also the level at which the lingual artery arises), and that it passes lateral to the hyoglossus muscle and medial to the mylohyoid muscle, that is to say, between these two muscles. Finally, again examine the styloid process, the stylohyoid muscle, and the anterior and posterior bellies of the digastric muscle, and check their relations to all the vessels and nerves in their vicinity.

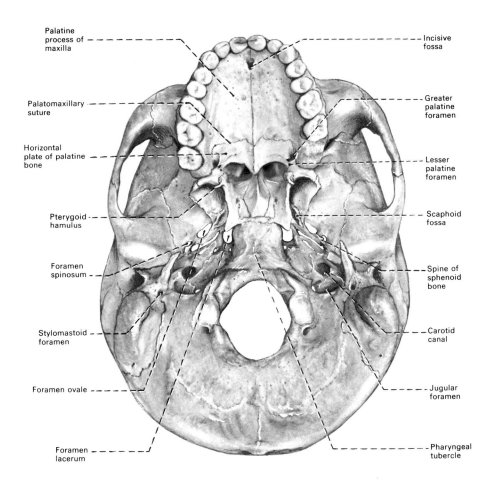

Palatine process of maxilla

Palatomaxillary suture

Horizontal plate of palatine bone

Pterygoid hamulus

Foramen spinosum

Stylomastoid foramen

Foramen ovale

Foramen lacerum

Incisive fossa

Greater palatine foramen

Lesser palatine foramen

Scaphoid fossa

Spine of sphenoid bone

Carotid canal

Jugular foramen

Pharyngeal tubercle

Fig. 5.69 The external surface of the base of the skull.

Section 5.9

The mouth and the upper pharynx

Osteology

The bony palate

Examine the bony palate on a skull. All but the posterior quarter consists of the horizontal **palatine process of the maxilla** [Fig. 5.69]. A fine ridge or groove marks the union of the two processes in the midline. The bulky tooth-bearing **alveolar process of the maxilla** projects downwards on each side. Behind the medial incisor teeth you will find the **incisive fossa.** In this fossa you will see the openings of a pair of **incisive canals,** one each side of the midline. Each incisive canal opens above into the corresponding half of the nasal cavity.

The posterior quarter of the palate is formed on each side by the **horizontal plate of the palatine bone,** the transverse suture between these plates and those of the maxillae being visible in most skulls. Identify the **greater palatine foramen** immediately behind the **palatomaxillary suture** at the postero-lateral corner of the palate. Behind it are the **lesser palatine foramina.**

The sphenoid and temporal bones [Fig. 5.69]

Identify the **pterygoid hamulus,** a curved projection of bone from the postero-inferior corner of the medial pterygoid plate [Fig. 5.69]. A fibrous band called the **pterygomandibular raphe** connects the tip of the pterygoid hamulus with the mandible just behind the third molar tooth. This raphe anchors the posterior border of the buccinator in front, and the anterior border of the superior constrictor muscle of the pharynx, which forms the upper part of the pharynx, behind.

Examine the skull just above and behind the medial pterygoid plate. The small ovoid **scaphoid fossa** which you will see, gives origin to the tensor veli palatini, one of the muscles of the soft palate. The irregular gap posterior and medial to the scaphoid fossa, between the body of the sphenoid bone, the petrous part of the temporal bone, and the basilar part of the occipital bone, is the **foramen lacerum.** Posterior to this is the opening of the **carotid canal,** through which the internal carotid artery enters the skull.

The **cartilaginous part of the auditory tube** lies in the gutter formed by the posterior border of the greater wing of the sphenoid and the petrous part of the temporal bone, the **bony part of the auditory tube** entering the temporal bone between the foramen spinosum and the external opening of the carotid canal. The auditory tube thus lies medial to both the foramen ovale and the foramen spinosum.

About a centimetre anterior to the foramen magnum, in the midline, is the **pharyngeal tubercle.** The upper end of the median raphe of the pharynx is attached to it. This raphe joins the muscles of the two sides of the pharynx in the midline posteriorly.

Surface anatomy

You can study most of the superficial anatomy of the mouth with the aid of a mirror.

The lips

With your lips closed, note that in the midline of the upper lip there is a shallow gutter which extends from the nose to the red zone of the lip. This indentation is called the **philtrum.** The slight protrusion of the red zone of the lip at the lower end of the philtrum is called the **tuberculum** of the upper lip.

Evert your upper lip with your fingers and you will see in the midline a fold of mucous membrane, the **frenulum of the upper lip,** connecting the lip to the maxilla. Evert the lower lip and you will see a similar but smaller frenulum attaching it to the mandible.

The cavity of the mouth [Fig. 5.70]

The part of the cavity of the mouth between the lips and cheeks on the one hand, and the teeth and gums on the other, is the **vestibule of the mouth.** The vestibule is limited above and below where the mucous coat on the inner surfaces of the lips and cheeks folds back on itself as it passes on to the alveolar processes. When the teeth are in the biting position (called occlusion), the vestibule and the **cavity of the mouth proper** communicate with each other behind the molar teeth. You will remember that the parotid duct opens into the vestibule opposite the second upper molar tooth.

Now examine the mucous membrane coating the alveolar processes of the maxilla and mandible. It is divided into two zones. The paler zone immediately close to the teeth is the **gum** or gingiva, while the smooth redder zone further away is called the **alveolar mucous membrane.** Pull your lip about

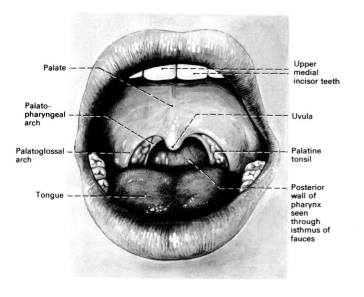

Fig. 5.70 The cavity of the mouth.

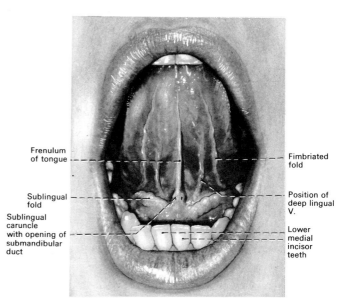

Fig. 5.71 The under-surface of the tongue.

with your fingers to establish that the alveolar mucosa is mobile. In contrast, the gingival mucosa covering the gum is firmly attached to underlying periosteum. It is also thicker than the alveolar mucosa. The boundary between the two zones follows an irregular course parallel to that of the free margin of the gum.

The palate [Figs 5.70 and 5.76]

Look at the roof of your mouth. Anteriorly it is formed by the **hard palate** which, at the front and sides, curves downwards to the gum margin in which the teeth are set. Posterior to the hard palate is the **soft palate** which arches backwards and downwards with the **uvula** projecting in the midline from its free postero-inferior border.

The pale low ridge in the midline of the hard palate is the **palatine raphe.** Anteriorly it ends behind the central incisor teeth in an oval elevation, the **incisive papilla.** Feel your own incisive papilla with the tip of your tongue, and look at the papilla in someone else's mouth. Extending laterally from the incisive papilla and the palatine raphe are irregular folds of the mucous membrane called the **palatine rugae.**

With the tip of a finger, follow the posterior border of your hard palate laterally until you feel a small bony projection at the postero-lateral angle of the hard palate. This is the **pterygoid hamulus.** It lies behind and medial to the maxillary tuberosity. Open your mouth widely and you may see a fold of mucous membrane extending obliquely downwards and outwards from the region of the pterygoid hamulus towards the mandible behind the third lower molar tooth. This, the **pterygomandibular fold,** marks the posterior boundary of the cheek, and corresponds to the pterygomandibular raphe.

The tongue [Fig. 5.71]

In the floor of the mouth is the tongue, separated from the gums on each side by a gutter. The anterior end of the tongue is free, and on its inferior surface can be seen a median fold of the mucous coat called the **frenulum** of the tongue [Fig. 5.71]. The bulge in the mucous coat of the floor of the mouth on each side of the base of this fold forms the **sublingual fold.** At the medial end of the fold is a papilla, the **sublingual caruncle,** where the submandibular duct opens.

The presence of large tortuous veins close to the mucous membrane accounts for the bluish coloration of the undersurface of the tongue on each side of the frenulum.

Now examine the texture of the upper surface or dorsum of the tongue. It is densely studded with minute papillae, **filiform papillae,** which are responsible for the tongue's slightly rough or furry appearance. Scattered chiefly at the tip and along the margins of the tongue are the **fungiform papillae,** which appear as bright red spots. Posteriorly, the dorsal surface of the tongue disappears from view as it curves downwards into the pharynx.

The fauces [Fig. 5.70]

The cavity of the mouth becomes continuous with the pharynx at the **isthmus of the fauces,** which is bounded on each side by a ridge of the mucous coat called the **palatoglossal arch,** which passes from the soft palate to the side of the tongue [Fig. 5.70]. Behind it is another ridge called the **palatopharyngeal arch.** The **palatine tonsil** lies between the two arches. The posterior wall of the pharynx can easily be seen by depressing the tongue with a spatula, or by contracting the muscles of the faucial isthmus, as when slowly making the sound 'Ah' with the mouth wide open.

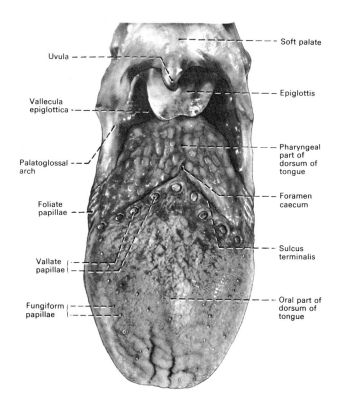

Soft palate

Uvula

Epiglottis

Vallecula
epiglottica

Pharyngeal
part of
dorsum of
tongue

Palatoglossal
arch

Foramen
caecum

Foliate
papillae

Sulcus
terminalis

Vallate
papillae

Fungiform
papillae

Oral part of
dorsum of
tongue

Fig. 5.72 The dorsum of the tongue.

The tongue and the floor of the mouth

The tongue [Figs 5.72, 5.74, and 5.77]

Look at the medial surface of your specimen and examine the tongue. It is a mass of muscle covered with mucosa, and its movements are controlled not only by muscles attached to the hyoid bone and each styloid process posteriorly, and to the mental spine of the mandible anteriorly, but also by its intrinsic muscles. The two halves of the tongue are imperfectly separated by the median fibrous septum of the tongue.

The dorsum of the tongue [Fig. 5.72]

The mucous coat of the dorsum of the tongue is provided with special taste receptors, as well as with ordinary touch and pressure receptors. These mostly occur in the papillae, of which you have already identified the fungiform type on your own tongue. In the dissection identify the **vallate papillae,** which are arranged in a V-shaped row, the point of the V being in the midline towards the posterior end of the tongue. Each papilla is about 1 to 2 mm in diameter, and is surrounded by a fine circular groove [Fig. 5.72]. In a median section you will be able to make out only one limb of the V, running laterally and forwards. It marks the boundary between the **oral part,** or anterior two-thirds, and the **pharyngeal part,** or posterior one-third, of the dorsum of the tongue. These two parts of the tongue have different embryological origins, and the line of the vallate papillae

roughly corresponds to the **sulcus terminalis,** by which the two are demarcated during one stage of embryonic development. The point of the V in the midline also has an embryological significance. It is the **foramen caecum** of the tongue, and marks the site from which the thyroid gland developed in a diverticulum (the **thyroglossal duct**) from the cavity of the mouth.

You may be able to identify the **foliate papillae** which lie at the sides of the tongue, at the junction of its oral and pharyngeal parts. The smaller **filiform papillae** cannot be seen by the naked eye.

The muscles of the tongue

The muscles of the tongue are conveniently divided into two groups: the **intrinsic muscles,** whose fibres run entirely within the tongue, and with whose detailed arrangement you need not be concerned, and the **extrinsic muscles,** which have an external attachment. All the intrinsic muscles and all the extrinsic muscles, except the palatoglossus, which is supplied by the pharyngeal plexus, are supplied by the hypoglossal nerve.

Look at the cut surface of the tongue and identify the fan-shaped **genioglossus muscle** [Fig. 5.77]. It has a pointed attachment to the mental spine [Fig. 5.61]. The uppermost fibres curve anteriorly towards the tip of the tongue, while the lowest fibres pass horizontally backwards towards its base to become attached to the body of the hyoid bone, whose cut surface you should identify. On each side of the midline is a genioglossus muscle. Posteriorly these are separated from each other by a median fibrous septum; but this cannot be identified on the bisected specimen.

Identify and separate from the inferior surface of the genioglossus the small **geniohyoid muscle,** which passes from the mental spine to the body of the hyoid bone. Identify the cut edge of the **mylohyoid muscle** below the geniohyoid muscle.

The floor of the mouth

Using scissors, cut through the mucous coat of the floor of the mouth close to the gum, starting in the midline in front of the tongue and carrying the incision as far back as the position of the lower third molar tooth. Gently push the tongue over towards the midline, and use the handle of a scalpel to separate the structures on the side of the tongue from the medial surface of the mandible and the mylohyoid muscle. Slide a seeker forwards lateral to the genioglossus, and divide the muscle close to its origin from the mandible. This will allow the tongue and attached structures to be swung medially, leaving only the geniohyoid and mylohyoid muscles in position [Fig. 5.73]. As you do this, cut any blood vessels which pierce the mylohyoid. Continue the dissection backwards, clearing the deep surface of the mylohyoid until you reach its posterior border.

You can now see that together the two mylohyoid muscles

5.74

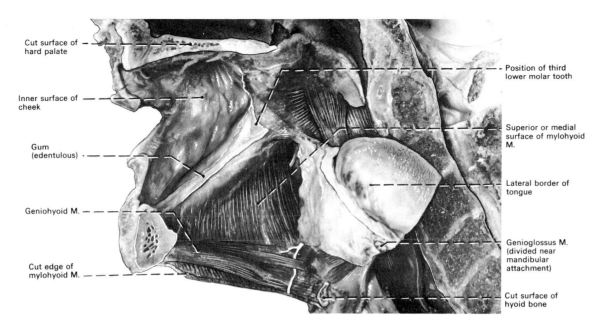

Cut surface of hard palate

Inner surface of cheek

Gum (edentulous)

Geniohyoid M.

Cut edge of mylohyoid M.

Position of third lower molar tooth

Superior or medial surface of mylohyoid M.

Lateral border of tongue

Genioglossus M. (divided near mandibular attachment)

Cut surface of hyoid bone

Fig. 5.73 Dissection of the right half of the floor of the mouth. The tongue has been turned aside. The soft palate has already been dissected.

form a trough-like floor to the mouth [Fig. 5.73]. When they contract they raise the hyoid bone and the floor of the mouth; or when the position of the hyoid is fixed by the contraction of the infrahyoid muscles [p. 5.20], they help in the opening of the mouth.

The hypoglossal nerve [Fig. 5.75]

Follow the hypoglossal nerve from the neck to the floor of the mouth, and dissect out its branches until you find them sinking into the musculature of the tongue [Fig. 5.75].

The lingual nerve [Figs 5.74 and 5.75]

Find the lingual nerve just below and medial to the position of the lower third molar tooth, and trace it forwards by blunt dissection. You will find that it turns medially and superiorly, and that it branches to supply the mucous coat of the anterior two-thirds of the dorsum of the tongue. Remember that as the lingual nerve passes to the tongue, it first lies between the ramus of the mandible and the medial pterygoid muscle, and anterior to the mandibular foramen. Having passed close to the lower third molar tooth, it comes to lie between the mylohyoid and hyoglossus muscles. Near the third molar tooth the lingual nerve is only covered by the mucous coat of the gum.

The submandibular duct [Fig. 5.75]

Search for the submandibular duct in the connective tissue at the side of the tongue, just above the point where the lingual nerve swings upwards towards the dorsum of the tongue. When you have found the duct, trace it backwards to the deep part of the submandibular gland, from which

it emerges, and forwards to the papilla where it opens into the mouth at the medial end of the sublingual fold.

The hypoglossal nerve, the lingual nerve, and the submandibular duct pass forwards into the mouth, above and medial to the mylohyoid muscle, between it and the hyoglossus muscle which is attached to the side of the tongue. Posteriorly the lingual nerve lies above the duct, but where the nerve loops down at the side of the tongue it crosses the duct superficially and, passing beneath the duct, ascends towards the dorsum of the tongue on the medial side of the duct. The hypoglossal nerve lies in the same muscular interval but at a lower level, immediately above the hyoid bone.

The sublingual gland [Fig. 5.74]

Now dissect the sublingual gland. It lies at the side of the genioglossus muscle and is the smallest of the three salivary glands. The sublingual fold in the floor of the mouth is formed by its superior edge, which immediately underlies the mucous coat. The gland has some eight to twenty ducts, most of which enter the cavity of the mouth independently along the summit of the sublingual fold. A few may either join the submandibular duct, or join together to form a **greater sublingual duct** which opens separately into the mouth on the sublingual caruncle.

Nerve supply of the submandibular and sublingual glands

All the salivary glands have a parasympathetic secretomotor nerve supply. The submandibular and sublingual glands receive their supply from the **chorda tympani** by way of the lingual nerve. If you trace the submandibular duct

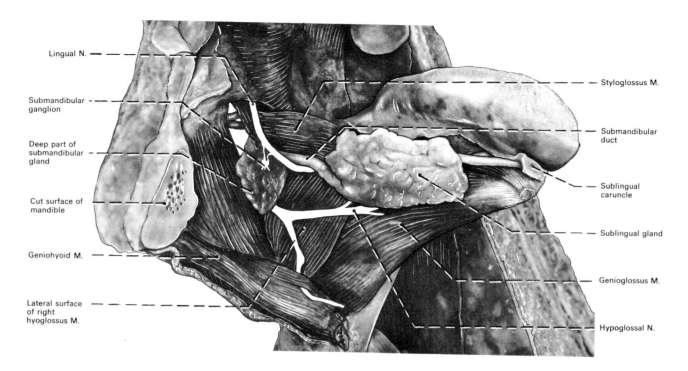

Lingual N.

Submandibular ganglion

Deep part of submandibular gland

Cut surface of mandible

Geniohyoid M.

Lateral surface of right hyoglossus M.

Styloglossus M.

Submandibular duct

Sublingual caruncle

Sublingual gland

Genioglossus M.

Hypoglossal N.

Fig. 5.74 The right sublingual gland. The tongue has been turned back in such a way that the figure shows its right lateral border. The sublingual gland is abnormally large. The soft palate has already been dissected.

posteriorly to the deep part of the submandibular gland, you will encounter fine nerve fibres which run towards the gland from a mass of tissue suspended from the lingual nerve. This tissue need not be dissected. Within it is the **submandibular ganglion** [Fig. 5.74], which receives pre-ganglionic fibres from the lingual nerve, and sends post-ganglionic fibres to the submandibular and sublingual glands.

The lingual artery [Fig. 5.75]

The artery to the tongue, the lingual artery, was seen passing from the external carotid artery to the posterior border of the hyoglossus muscle [p. 5.67]. Its further course should now be followed. First find the anterior border of the hyoglossus, and separate it gently from the genioglossus, which lies on its medial side. The artery lies between the two

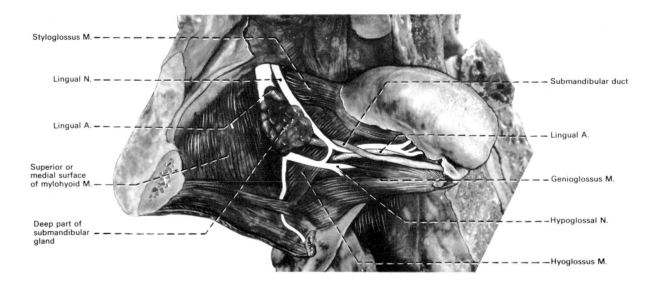

Styloglossus M.

Lingual N.

Lingual A.

Superior or medial surface of mylohyoid M.

Deep part of submandibular gland

Submandibular duct

Lingual A.

Genioglossus M.

Hypoglossal N.

Hyoglossus M.

Fig. 5.75 Structures at the right side of the tongue. The sublingual gland has been removed and the tongue has been turned back in such a way that the figure shows its right lateral border. The soft palate has already been dissected.

muscles and sends branches to both. It ends by turning superiorly along the anterior border of the hyoglossus to enter the inferior surface of the free part of the tongue [Fig. 5.75].

Blood from the tongue drains mainly through veins which accompany either the lingual artery or the hypoglossal nerve as far as the posterior border of the hyoglossus muscle, where they unite to join either the facial vein or the internal jugular vein.

The nerve supply of the tongue

Refresh your memory about the styloglossus, hyoglossus, and genioglossus muscles, which are supplied by the hypoglossal nerve. These are the main extrinsic muscles of the tongue, and their names indicate the different structures to which the tongue is attached. The small palatoglossus muscle, which is supplied by pharyngeal branches of the vagus nerve, is a further extrinsic muscle of the tongue.

Note that the extrinsic and intrinsic muscles of the tongue have a nerve supply entirely different from that of the mucous coat of the tongue. The mucous coat of the anterior two-thirds of the dorsum of the tongue receives its general sensory innervation through the lingual nerve, a branch of the mandibular nerve. That of the posterior one-third is supplied by the glossopharyngeal nerve. The taste receptors of the anterior two-thirds of the dorsum of the tongue are innervated by the facial nerve, the fibres from the receptors leaving the tongue by way of the lingual nerve and reaching the facial nerve through the chorda tympani. Both the taste and ordinary receptors in the posterior one-third of the dorsum of the tongue are innervated by the glossopharyngeal nerve, which also supplies the vallate papillae, although these lie in the anterior two-thirds of the dorsum of the tongue.

The glands of the mouth

On the superficial surface of the buccinator muscle, and around the parotid duct, are a number of small mucous glands which you do not dissect. These are called the **molar glands.** They are mentioned here only in order to call your attention to the fact that, in addition to the large salivary glands, innumerable small glands are closely associated with the mucous coat of the mouth, tongue, and pharynx. The mucous glands which lie deep to the buccinator muscle are called **buccal glands,** and others lying in the submucous tissue of the lips are called **labial glands.** The glands of your own lips and cheeks can be felt with the tip of the tongue as slight irregularities beneath the mucous coat.

The parts of the pharynx

Look at the medial surface of your specimen. The palatoglossal arch can be easily demonstrated by pulling the tongue gently towards the midline. Behind it is the **cavity**

of the pharynx, which ends at the back of the cricoid cartilage by running into the oesophagus. The part of the pharynx behind the cavity of the mouth is called the **oral part** of the pharynx, and the parts above and below are the **nasal part** and the **laryngeal part** respectively [Fig. 5.76].

The upper boundary of the oral part of the pharynx is formed by the free border of the soft palate, and the lower boundary by the superior border of the **epiglottis,** the stiff leaf-like structure which projects upwards behind the tongue.

The nasal part of the pharynx

On the half of the head on which the septum of the nose lies, you will be able to see the boundaries of the posterior apertures of the nasal cavity, or **choanae.** Through the choanae the nasal cavity communicates with the nasal part of the pharynx. Inferior to the nasal cavity, the soft palate, which faces upwards as well as backwards, forms an anterior wall to the lower part of the nasal part of the pharynx. The roof and posterior wall of the nasal part of the pharynx are formed by the inferior surfaces of the sphenoid and occipital bones anterior to the pharyngeal tubercle.

Identify the **pharyngeal opening of the auditory tube,** on the side wall of the nasal part of the pharynx [Fig. 5.77]. Its posterior margin is a prominent projection called the **tubal elevation.** Posterior to the tubal elevation is the **pharyngeal recess,** bounded anteriorly by the **salpingopharyngeal fold.**

The nasal part of the pharynx communicates with the oral part of the pharynx through the **pharyngeal isthmus.** Beneath the mucous coat of the posterior wall of the pharynx, above this isthmus, one often finds a mass of lymphoid tissue, called the **pharyngeal tonsil,** or adenoids.

The oral part of the pharynx

The posterior one-third of the dorsum of the tongue, behind the V, forms part of the anterior wall of the oral part of the pharynx. Note the fossa for the **palatine tonsil,** between the **palatoglossal** and the **palatopharyngeal** arches. The tonsil consists of lymphoid tissue and may not be prominent in your specimen. Determine the lateral relations of the tonsil by placing the tip of a finger between the two arches and turning the specimen over. The immediate relation is the superior constrictor muscle, on which lies the styloglossus muscle and the facial artery, which supplies the palatine tonsil. The glossopharyngeal nerve passes just below the tonsillar fossa. More laterally is the internal carotid artery.

The muscle fibres within the palatopharyngeal and palatoglossal arches form the **palatopharyngeus** and **palatoglossus muscles.** These can be seen by incising and reflecting the mucous coat along the arches.

The little pocket which lies on each side between the epiglottis and the tongue is the **vallecula epiglottica** [Fig. 5.72]. The midline fold which separates the two valleculae is the

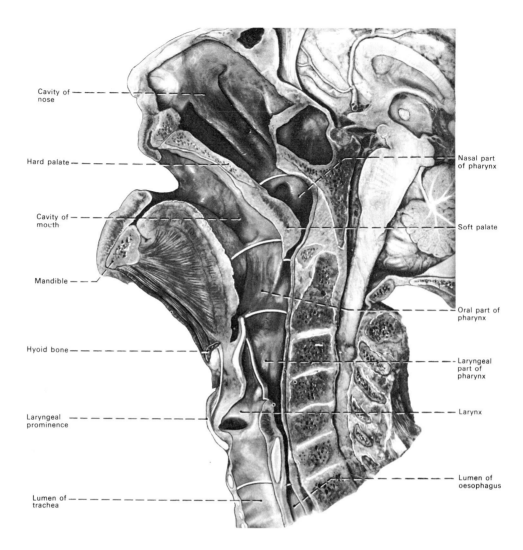

Cavity of nose

Hard palate

Cavity of mouth

Mandible

Hyoid bone

Laryngeal prominence

Lumen of trachea

Nasal part of pharynx

Soft palate

Oral part of pharynx

Laryngeal part of pharynx

Larynx

Lumen of oesophagus

Fig. 5.76 Median section of the head and neck. The boundaries of the parts of the pharynx are outlined in white.

median glosso-epiglottic fold. Laterally the valleculae are bounded by the **lateral glosso-epiglottic folds,** which extend from the sides of the epiglottis to the side walls of the pharynx at their junction with the tongue [Fig. 5.77].

The external surface of the pharynx

Using the handle of a scalpel, and working from the midline, separate the posterior wall of the pharynx from the muscles covering the vertebral column behind. You will find the separation is easy to begin with, but that the fascia becomes tough as you push laterally. The artificial space you have created is called the **retropharyngeal space.** Break through its lateral boundary so that the handle of your scalpel emerges in the deep part of the side of the neck. Complete the separation of the pharynx from the muscles covering the vertebral column, as far down as the level of the thyroid cartilage.

The external surface of the pharynx is covered by fairly

tough fascia called the **buccopharyngeal fascia.** Before you start to peel off this fascia, in which the nerves and vessels supplying the pharynx ramify, return to the lateral surface of the specimen and pick up the main **pharyngeal branch of the vagus** [p. 5.69]. Follow this nerve forwards between the external and internal carotid arteries, and see how it branches in the buccopharyngeal fascia and forms a plexus, the **pharyngeal plexus,** to supply the muscles of the wall of the pharynx and the mucous coat of the pharynx [Fig. 5.78]. If the pharyngeal branches have not yet been successfully identified, this can now be done by finding their terminal branches in the buccopharyngeal fascia and tracing them upwards.

Now strip the fascia off the back and sides of the nasal and oral parts of the pharynx so as to reveal the underlying muscle fibres. Remove any veins that obscure the dissection, but try not to detach the pharyngeal branches of the vagus nerve.

Clean the buccopharyngeal fascia off the posterior part

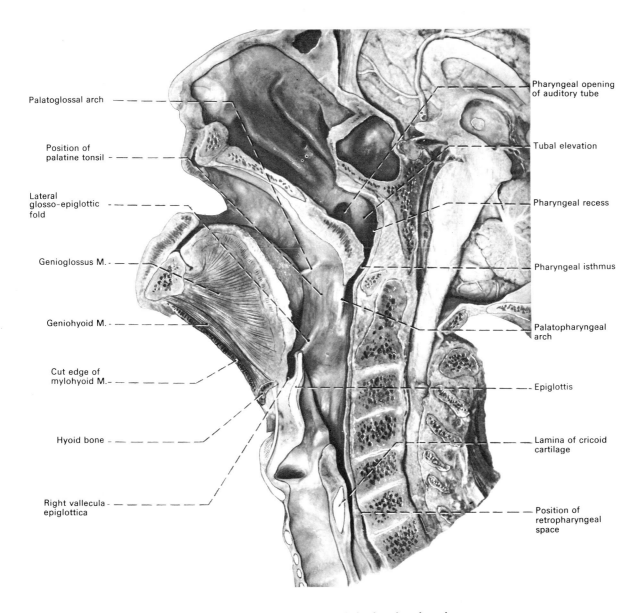

Palatoglossal arch

Position of palatine tonsil

Lateral glosso-epiglottic fold

Genioglossus M.

Geniohyoid M.

Cut edge of mylohyoid M.

Hyoid bone

Right vallecula epiglottica

Pharyngeal opening of auditory tube

Tubal elevation

Pharyngeal recess

Pharyngeal isthmus

Palatopharyngeal arch

Epiglottis

Lamina of cricoid cartilage

Position of retropharyngeal space

Fig. 5.77 Median section of the head and neck.

of the buccinator muscle and try to identify the **pterygo-mandibular raphe.** It forms a thin fibrous junction between the buccinator muscle and the muscle fibres of the upper part of the pharyngeal wall, and its lower end will probably have been detached from the mandible. Try to avoid damaging the pharyngeal wall during this dissection.

The constrictor muscles of the pharynx [Fig. 5.78]

The posterior and lateral walls of the pharynx are formed almost entirely by three sheet-like overlapping muscles, called the **superior, middle,** and **inferior constrictor muscles of the pharynx.** The upper border of the inferior constrictor muscle overlaps the lower border of the middle constrictor, and the latter overlaps the superior constrictor in the same way.

Anteriorly, each constrictor muscle is attached to bony or cartilaginous structures, while posteriorly, each unites with the muscle of the other side in a median seam, the **raphe of the pharynx,** which is attached above to the pharyngeal tubercle. Confirm that the pharyngeal wall is attached to the skull at this point in your specimen.

The superior constrictor muscle [Fig. 5.78]

The muscle fibres of the pharyngeal wall that are attached to the pterygomandibular raphe are part of the superior constrictor muscle. This muscle is also attached to the pterygoid hamulus and the adjacent parts of the medial pterygoid plate, and to the mandible behind the lower third molar tooth, while a few of its lowermost fibres are attached to the tongue and to the floor of the mouth.

5.79

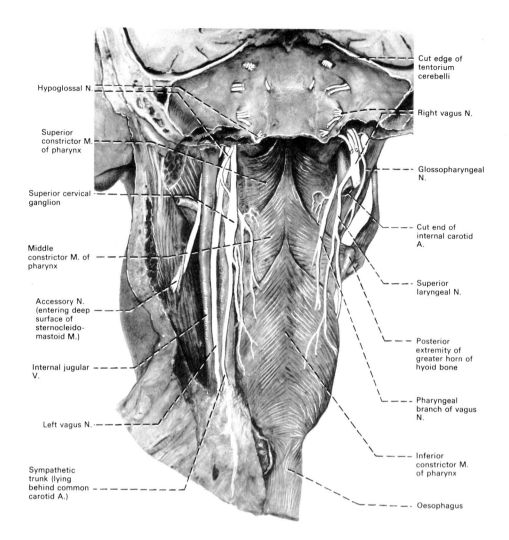

Hypoglossal N.

Superior constrictor M. of pharynx

Superior cervical ganglion

Middle constrictor M. of pharynx

Accessory N. (entering deep surface of sternocleido-mastoid M.)

Internal jugular V.

Left vagus N.

Sympathetic trunk (lying behind common carotid A.)

Cut edge of tentorium cerebelli

Right vagus N.

Glossopharyngeal N.

Cut end of internal carotid A.

Superior laryngeal N.

Posterior extremity of greater horn of hyoid bone

Pharyngeal branch of vagus N.

Inferior constrictor M. of pharynx

Oesophagus

Fig. 5.78 The posterior aspect of the pharynx. Note that this specimen has not been bisected. The vertebral column and its attached muscles, most of the occipital bone, as well as the structures on the right side of the neck, have been removed.

Working posteriorly from the pterygoid hamulus, carefully define the upward extent of the superior constrictor muscle. You will find that it does not reach the base of the skull but that it has a superior margin which curves upwards and backwards from the pterygoid hamulus to the pharyngeal tubercle, passing below the fan-shaped tensor veli palatini muscle that was exposed when the medial pterygoid muscle was removed [p. 5.69].

Between the superior constrictor muscle and the base of the skull the pharyngeal wall lacks a muscular coat, which is replaced here by a connective tissue membrane, the **pharyngobasilar fascia,** which is lined by a mucous coat. Below, the pharyngobasilar fascia is continuous with a fibrous coat which intervenes between the mucous and the muscular coats of the pharyngeal wall.

Now clean the lower border of the superior constrictor. You will find that it is crossed by the styloglossus and stylopharyngeus muscles, and that only its anterior end can be made out [Fig. 5.80]. Posterior to the stylopharyngeus

muscle, the lower border of the superior constrictor muscle of the pharynx is covered by the middle constrictor muscle of the pharynx, whose upper border has already been seen winding round the stylopharyngeus.

The glossopharyngeal nerve [Figs 5.67 and 5.68]

Again identify the glossopharyngeal nerve and trace it forwards to the point where it passes under the hyoglossus muscle [Fig. 5.67]. Both the glossopharyngeal nerve and the stylopharyngeus muscle, which lies medial to it, pass through the interval between the lower and upper borders of the superior and middle constrictor muscles respectively. In this way the glossopharyngeal nerve reaches the submucous tissues of the pharynx and posterior one-third of the dorsum of the tongue, which it innervates.

On the medial surface of the specimen note that the point where the nerve passes between the two constrictors lies between the two palatal arches, about halfway between the soft plate and the floor of the vallecula epiglottica.

5.80

The glossopharyngeal nerve is the sensory nerve to most of the mucous coat of the nasal and oral parts of the pharynx. The trigeminal nerve is responsible for the sensory innervation of the mucous coat of the nose, the oral cavity, and the roof of the nasal part of the pharynx.

The palate

Turn to the medial surface of your specimen and examine the palate. Except for its nerve and blood supply, there is little of the anatomy of the hard palate that cannot be learned from the macerated skull.

The soft palate

The levator veli palatini muscle [Figs 5.79 and 5.80]

Pull the soft palate downwards, and identify on its dorsal surface a faint broad ridge, the **levator elevation,** running from the palate to the pharyngeal opening of the auditory tube. Take a pair of scissors and, starting from the midline, cut through the mucous coat on the dorsal surface of this ridge until you reach the pharyngeal opening. Hold the points of the scissors upwards so as to avoid damaging the underlying muscle, which is called the levator veli palatini [Fig. 5.79]. Strip the mucous coat from the surface of the muscle, which you will see passes downwards and forwards to become inserted into the dorsal surface of the soft palate. The muscle arises from the under-surface of the petrous part of the temporal bone anterior and medial to the carotid canal, and from the cartilage which forms the medial wall of the auditory tube.

The action of the levator veli palatini muscle is to raise the posterior part of the soft palate and pull it slightly backwards. The levator veli palatini is supplied by the pharyngeal branches of the vagus nerve, in common with all the other pharyngeal and palatal muscles except the tensor veli palatini muscle, which is supplied by the mandibular nerve, and the stylopharyngeus which is supplied by the glossopharyngeal nerve.

The tensor veli palatini muscle [Figs 5.79 and 5.80]

Make a second incision, about 1 cm long, just through the mucous coat of the side wall of the nasal part of the pharynx, starting at the upper end of the first incision, and cutting forwards and slightly upwards into the nasal cavity. Reflect the mucous coat in front of the first incision off the dorsal surface of the soft palate, and off the side wall of the pharynx, until you reach the hard palate and the medial pterygoid plate. Careful blunt dissection antero-lateral to the levator veli palatini muscle will reveal the deep surface of the tensor veli palatini muscle. Gently separate the two muscles and pass the handle of a scalpel backwards and downwards between them. Turn the specimen over and you will see the handle appearing from below the lower border of the tensor veli palatini. You first saw the lateral surface of the tensor veli palatini when you removed the medial pterygoid muscle [Fig. 5.67]. Note once more how the fibres of this small muscle pass downwards and forwards to converge on a tendon which winds round the **pterygoid hamulus.**

The tensor veli palatini muscle has a linear origin which extends from the scaphoid fossa to the medial surface of

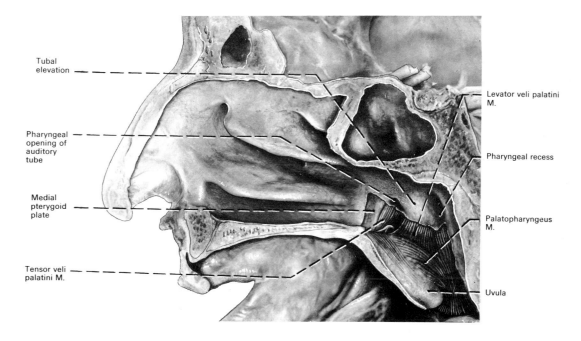

Tubal elevation

Pharyngeal opening of auditory tube

Medial pterygoid plate

Tensor veli palatini M.

Levator veli palatini M.

Pharyngeal recess

Palatopharyngeus M.

Uvula

Fig. 5.79 Dissection of the soft palate (right side of median section).

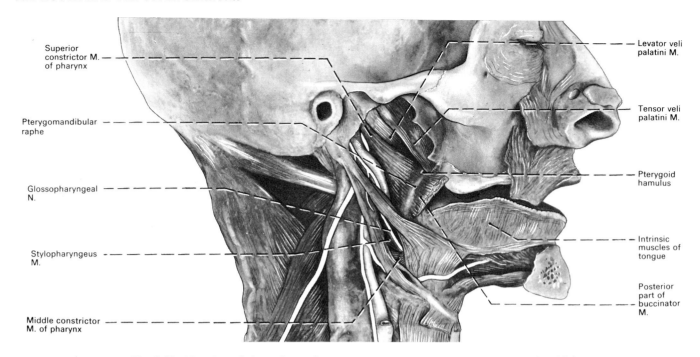

Superior constrictor M. of pharynx

Pterygomandibular raphe

Glossopharyngeal N.

Stylopharyngeus M.

Middle constrictor M. of pharynx

Levator veli palatini M.

Tensor veli palatini M.

Pterygoid hamulus

Intrinsic muscles of tongue

Posterior part of buccinator M.

Fig. 5.80 Muscles of the palate, pharynx, and tongue (viewed from the right side).

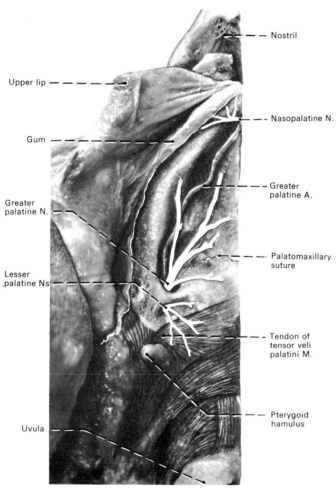

Upper lip

Gum

Greater palatine N.

Lesser palatine Ns.

Uvula

Nostril

Nasopalatine N.

Greater palatine A.

Palatomaxillary suture

Tendon of tensor veli palatini M.

Pterygoid hamulus

Fig. 5.81 The nerves of the right half of the palate (viewed from below). The body was edentulous.

the spine of the sphenoid. Identify these bony points on a skull. Between them, the muscle arises from the antero-lateral wall of the auditory tube. After curving round the pterygoid hamulus, the tendon of the tensor veli palatini muscle fans out to form a thin horizontal membrane in the soft palate, which is known as the **palatine aponeurosis.** You may see the palatine aponeurosis on your dissection if you carefully remove the overlying layers of the soft palate, starting near the pterygoid hamulus. Anteriorly, the aponeurosis is attached to the posterior border of the bony palate; posteriorly, it blends with connective tissue of the soft palate.

The tensor veli palatini muscle is innervated by a branch of the mandibular nerve. When the two tensor veli palatini muscles act together they tighten the soft palate. In con-junction with the levator veli palatini muscles they transform the soft palate into a taut horizontal plate which seals off the nasal part from the oral part of the pharynx. Those fibres of the tensor veli palatini which are attached to the auditory tube have an additional action in so far as they open the tube by pulling on its wall.

The auditory tube

Insert a seeker into the auditory tube, turn the specimen over, and note that the tube lies above the upper borders of the tensor and levator veli palatini muscles. Identify the upper free edge of the superior constrictor muscle of the pharynx. The tube and the levator veli palatini muscle pass through the side wall of the pharynx above the upper edge of the superior constrictor muscle, while the tensor veli pala-tini muscle passes just behind the origin of the upper end of the buccinator muscle as it turns round the pterygoid hamulus [Fig. 5.80].

From the pharynx the auditory tube passes upwards, backwards and laterally to the **middle ear** in the temporal bone. The base of a triangular plate of cartilage in its postero-medial wall lies directly under the mucous coat of the pharyngeal wall, where it forms the tubal elevation. The antero-lateral wall of the tube is membranous. Posteriorly, the tube narrows and continues as a bony canal in the petrous part of the temporal bone. Look again at the base of the skull and once again identify the gutter in which the cartilaginous part of the auditory tube lies.

The nerve supply of the palate [Fig. 5.81]

Incise the mucous coat of the roof of the mouth along the inner (lingual) gum margin, or on the ridge of the gum if your cadaver has no teeth, starting posteriorly and ending anteriorly in the midline. Reflect the mucous coat medial to the incision, and search in the submucous tissue opposite the molar teeth for a nerve that runs parallel with the gum. When it has been found, trace this nerve, the **greater palatine nerve,** posteriorly, and you will find it emerging from the greater palatine foramen at the postero-lateral angle of the hard palate [Fig. 5.81]. Do not preserve the artery which accompanies the nerve, but dissect the nerve through the soft tissues which cover the bone. These tissues are thick, because of the numerous glands which underlie the mucous coat. The greater palatine nerve supplies the medial (lingual) surface of the gum and the hard palate, except for a small part opposite the upper incisor and canine teeth, which is supplied by the **nasopalatine nerve.** The latter nerve descends on the side of the nasal septum to the incisive canal, which it traverses. The incisive canal, which pierces the hard palate and opens on its inferior surface at the incisive fossa, may have been opened when the head was divided. The **lesser palatine nerves,** which emerge behind from the lesser palatine foramina and supply the soft palate, need not be dissected.

The laryngeal part of the pharynx, the larynx, and the thyroid gland

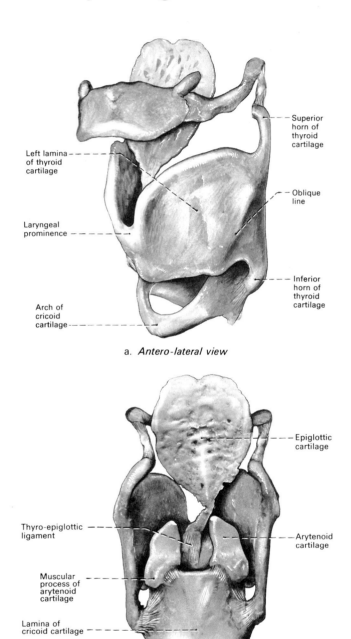

a. *Antero-lateral view*

b. *Posterior view*

The lowest or laryngeal part of the pharynx lies below the level of the hyoid bone and is continuous at its inferior end with the oesophagus, which begins at the level of the sixth cervical vertebra, opposite the lower border of the cricoid cartilage. In the upper half of its anterior wall, the laryngeal part of the pharynx communicates with the larynx through the inlet of the larynx. The larynx lies anterior to the laryngeal part of the pharynx, and at its lower end is continuous with the trachea.

The laryngeal cartilages

The skeletal anatomy of these structures is important to the understanding of the anatomy of their soft tissues. Apart from the hyoid bone, the framework of the larynx is primarily cartilaginous. Patches of cartilage may undergo ossification in later life, but the cartilaginous framework is practically never preserved during the preparation of dry skeletons. If specially prepared specimens cannot be obtained, the anatomy of the cartilages concerned should be studied from diagrams, and by palpation of the dissected specimen.

The thyroid cartilage [Fig. 5.82]

The thyroid cartilage consists of two lateral **laminae** whose

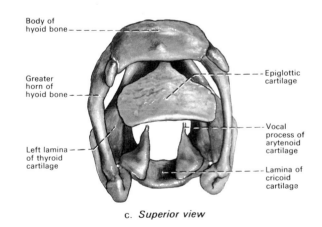

c. *Superior view*

Fig. 5.82 The hyoid bone and the cartilages of the larynx.

anterior borders fuse in the midline to form the **laryngeal prominence,** or Adam's apple [Fig. 5.82]. The angle at which the two laminae meet is more acute in men than women. This accounts for the greater prominence of the cartilage in the male. The two laminae are roughly quadrilateral, and their posterior borders are prolonged upwards and downwards as two processes called the **superior** and **inferior horns.** You will have no difficulty in palpating the superior horn on your dissection. On the lateral surface of each lamina there is a faint ridge called the **oblique line.** This runs from a point just anterior to the root of the superior horn, downwards and a little forwards to the inferior border of the lamina. The sternothyroid muscle, the thyrohyoid muscle, and the inferior constrictor muscle of the pharynx are attached to the cartilage along, or close to, this line.

The cricoid cartilage [Fig. 5.82]

The cricoid cartilage lies between the inferior horns of the thyroid cartilage, and forms a ring of cartilage shaped like a signet-ring, with a quadrate posterior **lamina** and a narrow anterior **arch.** On your specimen identify the cut surfaces of the arch and the lamina. The lower border of the cartilage is horizontal, but the upper border runs upwards and posteriorly because of the great depth of the lamina. There is a small facet on the posterior part of each lateral surface of the cartilage for its articulation with the inferior horn of the thyroid cartilage.

The arytenoid cartilages [Fig. 5.82]

On each side of the midline, on the upper border of the lamina of the cricoid cartilage, is a pyramidal arytenoid cartilage. The concave base of each arytenoid cartilage articulates with the cricoid cartilage by a synovial joint, and is roughly triangular in shape. One corner of the base is directed anteriorly, and is called the **vocal process.** To it is attached the posterior end of the vocal ligament. Another corner projects laterally, and is called the **muscular process,** since some of the muscles of the larynx are attached to it. The third corner is ill-defined. You should be able to make out the position, and approximate size and shape of the arytenoid cartilage on your specimen by palpating it between your thumb and finger. This will help you appreciate that any movement it makes on the cricoid cartilage would be reflected in a change in the disposition of the vocal ligament, which is attached anteriorly to the posterior aspect of the laryngeal prominence of the thyroid cartilage.

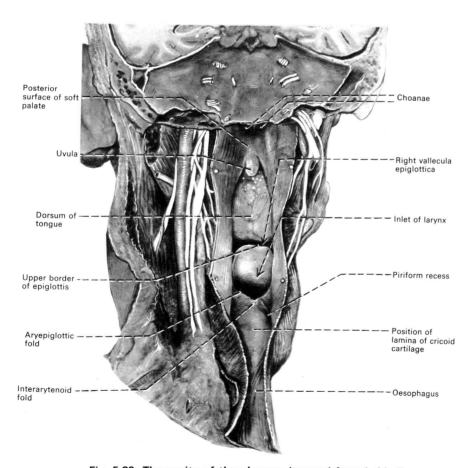

Fig. 5.83 The cavity of the pharynx (opened from behind).

Posterior surface of soft palate

Uvula

Dorsum of tongue

Upper border of epiglottis

Aryepiglottic fold

Interarytenoid fold

Choanae

Right vallecula epiglottica

Inlet of larynx

Piriform recess

Position of lamina of cricoid cartilage

Oesophagus

The epiglottic cartilage [Fig. 5.82]

The epiglottic cartilage is a thin petal-like plate of elastic fibrocartilage with a stem attached to the thyroid cartilage below, and a broad free border above.

The laryngeal part of the pharynx and the oesophagus

The inlet of the larynx [Figs 5.83, 5.86, and 5.88]

Examine the boundaries of the inlet of the larynx. Above is the upper border of the epiglottis [Fig. 5.83]. At each side is a prominent fold of mucosa, called the **aryepiglottic fold,** which is attached to the lateral border of the epiglottis above and anteriorly, and which sweeps downwards and posteriorly to the apex of the arytenoid cartilage. Posteriorly the inlet is completed by a small **interarytenoid fold** of mucosa, which was divided when the head was bisected.

Note that on each side of the inlet of the larynx the cavity of the pharynx extends a short distance anteriorly to form the **piriform recess.** The mucous coat of the lateral wall of

the lower part of the recess clothes the posterior part of the thyroid cartilage. Above the thyroid cartilage the lateral wall of the recess is formed by the thyrohyoid membrane, which stretches from the upper border of the thyroid cartilage to the body and greater horn of the hyoid bone.

Below the inlet of the larynx note that the anterior wall of the pharynx is formed by the posterior surfaces of the arytenoid and cricoid cartilages, and the muscles and mucous coat by which they are covered.

The superior laryngeal nerve [Figs 5.78 and 5.84]

The middle and inferior constrictor muscles of the pharynx are the chief supporting structures of the mucous coat of the lateral and posterior walls of the laryngeal part of the pharynx. Before these two muscles are cleaned further, find the superior laryngeal nerve, a branch of the vagus which you saw earlier [p. 5.69], and trace it on its course deep (medial) to the internal carotid artery. The nerve divides into a thicker **internal branch,** which you will find disappearing deep to the posterior border of the thyrohyoid muscle, and a finer **external branch,** which runs downwards [Fig. 5.84]. If you turn the sternothyroid muscle back and dis-

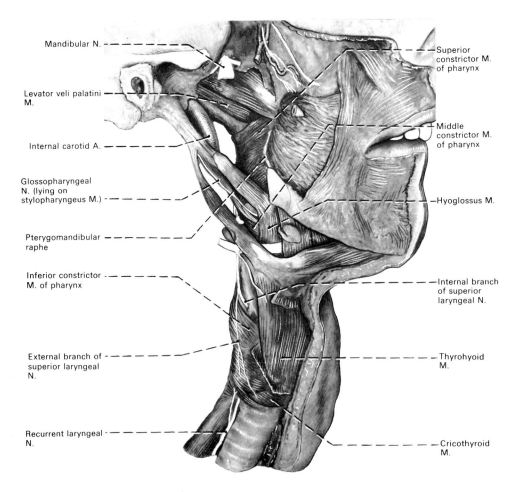

Fig. 5.84 Right lateral view of the pharynx.

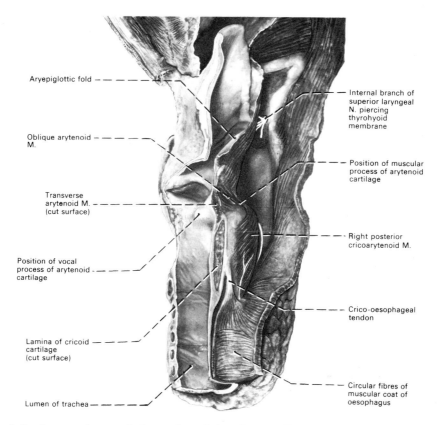

Aryepiglottic fold

Oblique arytenoid M.

Transverse arytenoid M. (cut surface)

Position of vocal process of arytenoid cartilage

Lamina of cricoid cartilage (cut surface)

Lumen of trachea

Internal branch of superior laryngeal N. piercing thyrohyoid membrane

Position of muscular process of arytenoid cartilage

Right posterior cricoarytenoid M.

Crico-oesophageal tendon

Circular fibres of muscular coat of oesophagus

Fig. 5.85 The relations of the laryngeal part of the cavity of the pharynx. The figure shows the medial aspect of the right half of a bisected larynx and pharynx from which the mucous coat of the pharynx and oesophagus has been removed.

lodge the thyroid gland, you can trace this nerve to its termination in the small **cricothyroid muscle,** which overlies the arch of the cricoid cartilage. The external branch of the superior laryngeal nerve also supplies part of the inferior constrictor muscle of the pharynx.

The inferior constrictor muscle of the pharynx [Figs 5.78 and 5.84]

Now examine the origin of the inferior constrictor muscle of the pharynx from the oblique line of the thyroid cartilage, and also the attachments of the sternothyroid and thyrohyoid muscles to the line. The inferior constrictor of the pharynx is also attached to the side of the cricoid cartilage. Between the thyroid and cricoid cartilages it has a short anterior border, which arches over the cricothyroid muscle. The latter arises from the front and lateral part of the arch of the cricoid cartilage, and its fibres diverge as they run posteriorly, deep to the inferior constrictor. They are inserted into the lower border of the lamina of the thyroid cartilage and the anterior border of its inferior horn.

The middle constrictor muscle of the pharynx [Figs 5.78 and 5.84]

Without damaging the superior laryngeal nerve and its branches, clean enough of the buccopharyngeal fascia off the superficial surface of the two lower constrictor muscles

of the pharynx to see their fibres. Once again define the upper border of the fan-shaped middle constrictor, where it crosses the stylopharyngeus muscle. Trace it backwards to the midline, and establish that it overlaps the fibres of the superior constrictor. Then trace it forwards and note that it passes deep to the posterior border of the hyoglossus, together with the glossopharyngeal nerve and the lingual artery. The middle constrictor arises from the hyoid bone in the angle between the lesser and greater horns.

The origin of the oesophagus

Turn to the medial surface of the dissection, and carefully remove the mucous coat from the posterior surface of the lamina of the cricoid cartilage and the adjoining anterior wall of the oesophagus. Use scissors for this purpose, cutting through the mucous coat along the aryepiglottic fold to allow it to be reflected laterally. When you have reflected the mucous coat for about 5 mm, separate the oesophagus from the back of the trachea. The outer muscular fibres of the oesophagus are longitudinally-disposed, and are attached by a tendinous band, the **crico-oesophageal tendon,** to the median ridge on the back of the lamina of the cricoid cartilage [Fig. 5.85]. This tendinous band will have been divided when the head was sectioned, but there should be little difficulty in identifying what remains of it. The longitudinal muscle fibres of the oesophagus descend from it, and

5.87

fan out so that, about 3 cm below the lower border of the cricoid cartilage, they completely invest the oesophagus. Deep to them you may be able to see a layer of circularly-disposed fibres, which are continuous above with the lower fibres of the inferior constrictor muscle of the pharynx. Because the oesophagus tends to deviate to the left of the midline, this dissection will probably be easier to carry out on the left half of the neck.

The muscles of the pharynx in general

Now quickly revise the anatomy of the whole pharynx. The mucous coat of its posterior and lateral walls is supported by the three overlapping **constrictor muscles** of the pharynx. Anteriorly these muscles take origin, from above down-wards: from the medial pterygoid plate and pterygo-mandibular raphe (superior constrictor), the stylohyoid ligament and hyoid bone (middle constrictor), and the thyroid and cricoid cartilages (inferior constrictor) [Fig. 5.84]. All are inserted into the posterior median **raphe of the pharynx,** which is attached above to the **pharyngeal tubercle** on the under-surface of the basilar part of the occipital bone [Fig. 5.69]. Laterally there are three places in this muscular wall through which important structures 'enter' the pharynx. The uppermost is between the superior constrictor and the base of the skull, and through it pass the auditory tube and the levator veli palatini muscle. Between the superior and middle constrictors the stylopharyngeus muscle and the glossopharyngeal nerve gain the deep surface of the muscular lamina. The internal branch of the superior laryngeal nerve passes between the middle and inferior constrictors [Fig. 5.84].

In addition to the three constrictor muscles, there are three minor pharyngeal muscles, of which only the **stylo-pharyngeus,** which arises from the styloid process, has already been dissected. The other two, on whose dissection you need not spend any time, are the **salpingopharyngeus,** which arises from the cartilage of the auditory tube, and the **palatopharyngeus,** which arises from the palate. These two make folds in the mucous coat. All three minor pharyngeal muscles either blend with the constrictors of the pharynx, or are inserted into the posterior border of the thyroid cartilage.

The innervation of the pharynx

The muscles of the pharynx are innervated by branches of the **glossopharyngeal** and **vagus nerves,** and the **cranial roots of the accessory nerve.** The motor fibres in the pharyngeal branches of these nerves arise in the **nucleus ambiguus,** which is a well-defined collection of nerve cells in the medulla oblongata. The branch of the glossopharyngeal nerve supplies only the stylopharyngeus muscle. The fibres of the cranial roots of the accessory nerve join the vagus, and are distributed to the pharyngeal muscles by way of the **pharyn-geal plexus.** This plexus lies in the buccopharyngeal fascia on the middle constrictor muscle, and is formed by the pharyngeal branches of the vagus, the external branch of the superior laryngeal nerve, and branches from the glosso-pharyngeal nerve and the sympathetic trunk. Do not spend time on the dissection of this plexus.

The trigeminal and glossopharyngeal nerves are respon-sible for the sensory innervation of the nasal part of the pharynx, while the sensory innervation of the oral part of the pharynx is almost entirely provided by the glosso-pharyngeal nerve. The mucous coat of the laryngeal part of the pharynx is supplied by the internal branch of the superior laryngeal nerve, which pierces the thyrohyoid

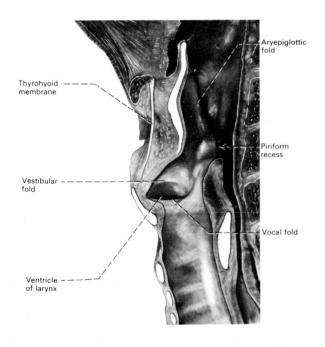

Fig. 5.86 Median section of larynx (right half).

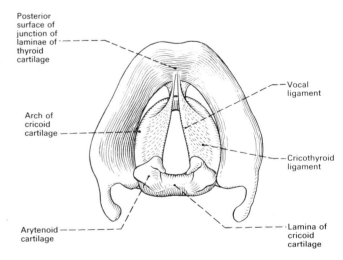

Fig. 5.87 The cricothyroid ligament (schematic view of larynx from above).

membrane under cover of the thyrohyoid muscle, to reach the submucosal tissues in the piriform recess [Fig. 5.85].

The larynx

The mucous coat of the larynx

Now examine the mucous coat of the larynx. It presents two ridges with an elliptical depression, the **ventricle of the larynx,** between them [Fig. 5.86]. The upper ridge is called the **vestibular fold,** and the lower the **vocal fold.** The vocal folds are usually called the **vocal cords.** Each consists of a fold of mucosa which is firmly adherent to the **vocal ligament** which, as already noted, is attached in front to the inner surface of the thyroid cartilage close to its fellow, and behind to the vocal process of the arytenoid cartilage. The two vocal ligaments are the thickened upper free borders of the **cricothyroid ligament,** which is a thin sheet of fibro-elastic tissue that closes the interval between the thyroid and cricoid cartilages [Fig. 5.87]. The membrane extends upwards from the upper border of the arch of the cricoid cartilage, to the under-surface of the arytenoid cartilage and its vocal process, and to the internal surface of the angle of the thyroid cartilage. The anterior part of the crico-thyroid ligament, together with the vocal ligament, is called the **conus elasticus.** It is thickened in the midline anteriorly.

The vestibular fold encloses a feeble ligament which is the inferior free border of a fibrous sheet that stretches from the lateral margin of the epiglottis in front, to the lateral border of the arytenoid cartilage behind. This sheet thus lies within the aryepiglottic fold.

The narrow fissure between the vocal folds, and extending back between the arytenoid cartilages, is called the **rima glottidis** [Fig. 5.88]. Changes in its shape and in the tension of the vocal folds play a part in the production of different sounds, and are brought about by the action of the muscles of the larynx.

The muscles of the larynx [Figs 5.85 and 5.89]

To expose the muscles of the larynx, reflect the mucous coat off the back of the cricoid and arytenoid cartilages as far as the posterior border of the thyroid cartilage. Clean the **posterior cricoarytenoid muscle,** which arises on each side of the midline from the posterior surface of the cricoid cartilage [Fig. 5.85]. You will see that the fibres of the muscle converge towards the laterally-projecting muscular process of the arytenoid cartilage above. You can easily feel this process.

The unpaired **transverse arytenoid muscle** passes between the posterior surfaces of the arytenoid cartilages. You should have no difficulty in identifying its cut surface in the plane in which the larynx was sectioned. Carefully remove the thin fascia off its posterior surface. While you do this, you may see on its posterior surface a few obliquely-running muscle fibres which cross each other near the midline. These form the **oblique arytenoid muscles,** which run from the muscular process of one arytenoid cartilage to the apex of the opposite cartilage. Some fibres of the oblique arytenoid muscles continue beyond the arytenoid cartilages into the aryepiglottic folds.

Lateral to the cricothyroid ligament and the ventricle of the larynx lies a sheet of muscle, the **thyroarytenoid muscle,** which stretches from the deep surface of the thyroid cartilage in front, to the arytenoid cartilage behind. To expose this muscle, detach the vocal and vestibular folds at their anterior ends and reflect them medially, together with the mucous coat of the larynx, the plane of separation being as close as possible to the deep surface of the thyroid cartilage [Fig. 5.89]. This will detach the thyroarytenoid muscle

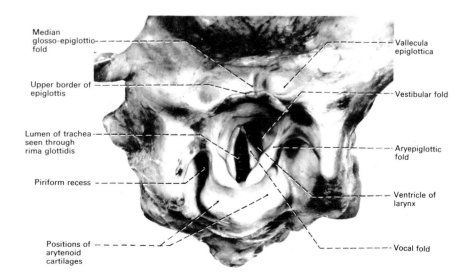

Fig. 5.88 The larynx (from above).

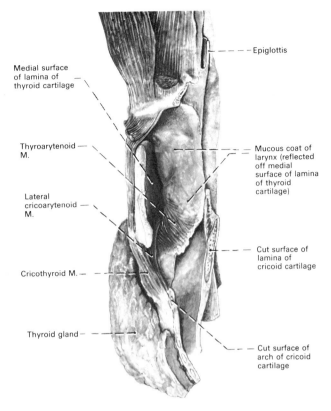

Epiglottis

Medial surface of lamina of thyroid cartilage

Thyroarytenoid M.

Lateral cricoarytenoid M.

Cricothyroid M.

Thyroid gland

Mucous coat of larynx (reflected off medial surface of lamina of thyroid cartilage)

Cut surface of lamina of cricoid cartilage

Cut surface of arch of cricoid cartilage

Fig. 5.89   The thyroarytenoid muscle (antero-medial view of right half of bisected larynx).

from the thyroid cartilage. Reflect the muscle medially, and note that some of its fibres sweep upwards into the ary-epiglottic fold. The lower deeper fibres of the muscle are applied to the vocal ligaments, and are called the **vocalis muscle.**

Inferior to the thyroarytenoid muscle look for the small **lateral cricoarytenoid muscle.** It arises from the upper border of the arch of the cricoid cartilage laterally, and runs upwards and backwards to the muscular process of the arytenoid cartilage. Lateral (superficial) to it is the **cricothyroid**

muscle. Note how this muscle is inserted into the lower border of the lamina of the thyroid cartilage and into the anterior surface of its inferior horn.

The actions of the muscles of the larynx [Fig. 5.90]

The muscles of the larynx modify:

1. The shape of the rima glottidis.
2. The tension of the vocal folds.
3. The shape of the inlet of the larynx.

The posterior and lateral cricoarytenoid muscles and the transverse and oblique arytenoid muscles belong to the group of muscles which change the shape of the rima glottidis. Of these, only the posterior cricoarytenoid muscles abduct the vocal folds, and so widen the rima. They do this by rotating the arytenoid cartilages [Fig. 5.90a]. All other muscles of the larynx which affect the shape of the rima glottidis tend to close it. The most important of those which do so are the lateral cricoarytenoid and transverse arytenoid muscles. The former adduct the vocal folds by rotating the arytenoid cartilages [Fig. 5.90b]; the latter closes the posterior third of the rima glottidis by drawing the arytenoid cartilages together [Fig. 5.90c].

The tension of the vocal folds is increased by the contraction of the cricothyroid muscles, which pull and rotate the thyroid cartilage downwards and forwards in relation to the cricoid cartilage [Fig. 5.90d]. This movement increases the distance between the angle of the thyroid cartilage and the arytenoid cartilages, which are situated on the lamina of the cricoid cartilage. In general, the thyroarytenoid muscles relax the vocal folds [Fig. 5.90e], but segments of the folds may be tightened by the deep fibres of the muscles.

The muscle fibres in the aryepiglottic folds, aided by the transverse and oblique arytenoid muscles, close the inlet of the larynx during swallowing, and so prevent particles of food getting into the trachea and bronchi. They do this by drawing the arytenoid cartilages together and pulling them upwards and forwards into contact with the epiglottis.

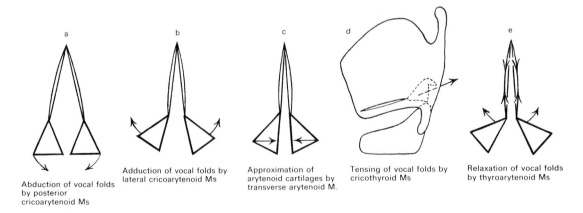

a

b

c

d

e

Abduction of vocal folds by posterior cricoarytenoid Ms

Adduction of vocal folds by lateral cricoarytenoid Ms

Approximation of arytenoid cartilages by transverse arytenoid M.

Tensing of vocal folds by cricothyroid Ms

Relaxation of vocal folds by thyroarytenoid Ms

Fig. 5.90 Actions of the muscles of the larynx. The arrows show the direction of movement of the arytenoid cartilages.

The innervation of the larynx

Now study the nerves of the larynx. The cricothyroid muscle is innervated by the **external branch of the superior laryngeal nerve** [Fig. 5.84]. All the remaining muscles of each side of the larynx are supplied by the **recurrent laryngeal nerve,** which is a branch of the vagus nerve. The left recurrent laryngeal nerve was seen in the thorax winding round the ligamentum arteriosum and the arch of the aorta, before it ascended in the groove between the oesophagus and the trachea [pp. 3.22, 3.44]. The right recurrent laryngeal nerve turns upwards at a much higher level, by hooking round the right subclavian artery [p. 3.19]. The dissectors of the right half of the body should find the nerve at this point [Fig. 3.44].

On both sides separate the thyroid gland from the oesophagus and trachea. Entering the lower part of the posterior surface of the gland you will find the inferior thyroid artery. Close to the artery you will see the recurrent laryngeal nerve in the groove between the oesophagus and trachea [Fig. 5.91]. Trace the nerve upwards, and you will see that it disappears deep to the lower border of the inferior constrictor muscle of the pharynx, posterior to the cricoid cartilage. On the left side, where the head is still attached to the trunk, follow the whole course of the nerve from the vagus to the larynx.

The most important sensory nerve to the larynx is the **internal branch of the superior laryngeal nerve** which, as you have seen [p. 5.88], pierces the thyrohyoid membrane in the side wall of the piriform recess [Fig. 5.85]. This nerve innervates the mucous coat of the larynx down to the vocal fold. Below this, the mucous coat is supplied by afferent fibres running in the recurrent laryngeal nerve.

The act of swallowing

The first part of the act of swallowing is voluntary. The tongue pushes the bolus of food backwards into the oral part of the pharynx. The stimulation of the sense receptors of the mucous coat of the oral part of the pharynx sets in motion a complex pattern of involuntary movement which completes the act. The pharyngeal isthmus closes, the larynx and the laryngeal part of the pharynx are drawn upwards behind the hyoid bone, the inlet to the larynx is closed, and breathing is temporarily arrested. The bolus then descends into the lowest part of the pharynx, whence it is propelled into the oesophagus.

Confirm by feeling your neck that when you swallow, the hyoid bone and the thyroid and cricoid cartilages all move upwards.

Identify and then try to work out the functions of each of the muscles and nerves involved in the act of swallowing. This will entail reviewing the muscles of the tongue, palate, pharynx, and larynx, and the suprahyoid and infrahyoid muscles.

Note that the parts of the mucous coat of the pharynx and larynx which normally come into contact with food, are all clothed with a stratified squamous epithelium. The mucous coat of the purely respiratory parts is clothed with a ciliated columnar epithelium. An exception is the mucous coat of the vocal folds, which has a stratified squamous epithelium.

The thyroid gland

The anatomy of the thyroid gland should now be reviewed. Little dissection will be necessary to establish the following points.

The gland consists of two **lobes** connected by the **isthmus of the thyroid gland,** which crosses the second and third tracheal cartilages [Fig. 5.92]. Often there is an additional **pyramidal lobe,** which projects upwards as a thin strand from the upper border of one side of the isthmus. This is connected to the hyoid bone by the **levator glandulae thyroideae muscle,** a fibrous or fibromuscular band, which you may have noticed earlier in your dissection [p. 5.21]. Each lobe has a postero-medial surface, which is applied below to the sides of the trachea and oesophagus, and above to the larynx and lower part of the pharynx; a superficial antero-lateral surface, which is covered by the infrahyoid and sternocleido-

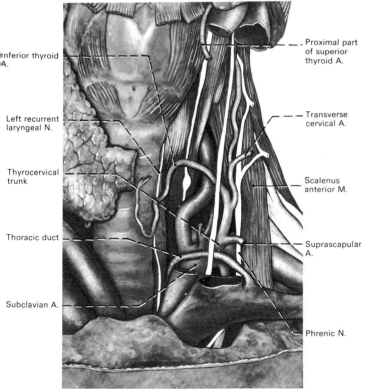

Inferior thyroid A.

Left recurrent laryngeal N.

Thyrocervical trunk

Thoracic duct

Subclavian A.

Proximal part of superior thyroid A.

Transverse cervical A.

Scalenus anterior M.

Suprascapular A.

Phrenic N.

Fig. 5.91 The left side of the root of the neck. Most of the common carotid artery and the internal jugular vein have been removed.

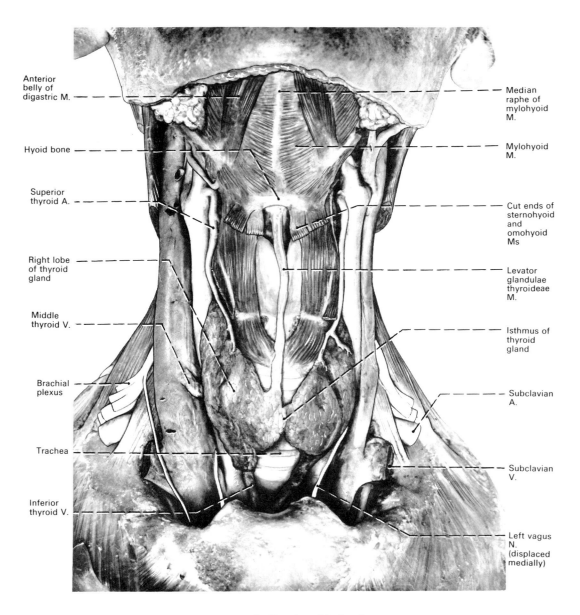

Anterior belly of digastric M.

Hyoid bone

Superior thyroid A.

Right lobe of thyroid gland

Middle thyroid V.

Brachial plexus

Trachea

Inferior thyroid V.

Median raphe of mylohyoid M.

Mylohyoid M.

Cut ends of sternohyoid and omohyoid Ms

Levator glandulae thyroideae M.

Isthmus of thyroid gland

Subclavian A.

Subclavian V.

Left vagus N. (displaced medially)

Fig. 5.92 The thyroid gland.

mastoid muscles; and a postero-lateral surface, which overlaps the carotid sheath.

The thin **pretracheal layer of cervical fascia** [see p. 5.22] ensheathes the larynx and lower pharynx, trachea, and oesophagus. It also encapsulates the thyroid gland which is thereby bound to these structures and moves with them in swallowing.

The blood supply of the thyroid gland [Figs 5.91 and 5.92]

The gland is very vascular, and derives its blood supply from the **superior** and **inferior thyroid arteries.** You have already seen the superior thyroid artery [p. 5.63].

The left inferior thyroid artery should now be dissected throughout its course. Begin at the scalenus anterior muscle at the root of the neck, and identify the phrenic nerve. Find

and clean the subclavian artery medial to the muscle, taking particular care not to damage a grey tubular structure, the thoracic duct [see p. 5.94], which lies anterior to the vessel. Look for a short branch of the artery which ascends along the medial border of the muscle and almost immediately divides. This is the **thyrocervical trunk** [Fig. 5.91]. Its branches are the suprascapular artery, the transverse cervical artery, and the inferior thyroid artery. The first two lie anterior to the scalenus anterior muscle in front of the phrenic nerve, and then cross the posterior triangle of the neck, where they have already been seen [p. 5.14].

Now follow the inferior thyroid artery, which will have been divided on the right side of the head when it was separated from the trunk. The artery reaches the posterior border of the thyroid gland by turning medially behind the carotid sheath. It supplies the gland as well as neighbouring structures, including the larynx, trachea, and oesophagus. The branches of the thyroid arteries anastomose freely on their own side but, apart from a small artery which runs along the upper border of the isthmus, they anastomose only slightly with the vessels of the other side.

Blood is drained from the thyroid gland by the superior, middle, and inferior thyroid veins, which you will already have seen and removed [p. 5.63]. The **superior thyroid vein** may join the facial vein, or run straight to the internal jugular vein, as does the **middle thyroid vein,** which is very short [Fig. 5.92]. The **inferior thyroid veins** descend on the front of the trachea to join the brachiocephalic veins in the superior mediastinum [p. 3.19].

The parathyroid glands

The **superior** and **inferior parathyroid glands** are small ovoid masses of tissue, often not more than 5 mm in length, which are usually impossible to identify in a dissection. They lie close to, or embedded in, the posterior part of each lobe of the thyroid gland near the border between the postero-lateral and postero-medial surfaces. In all, there are usually four parathyroid glands, but they vary in their number and exact positions. Although they are functionally important, you should not spend time looking for them.

Section 5.11

Deep structures of the neck

Only a few structures remain to be dissected in the neck. Each dissector should study both sides of the head and neck, as some structures will be demonstrated more easily on one side than the other.

The thoracic duct

On the left side look for the termination of the thoracic duct [Fig. 5.93], which, at an earlier stage, was traced from the abdomen and through the thorax [p. 3.45]. It should have been identified in the last part of your dissection, when the root of the left subclavian artery was cleaned [p. 5.92]. The duct is a slender thin-walled vessel and may be mistaken for a vein. Note that it ascends into the neck along the left border of the oesophagus, and that about a finger's breadth below the cricoid cartilage it arches laterally behind the

carotid sheath. It then descends in front of the subclavian artery and opens into the left brachiocephalic vein at the junction of the internal jugular vein with the subclavian vein.

Tributaries of the brachiocephalic vein

Now identify the **vertebral vein,** which is a tributary of the brachiocephalic vein. The vertebral vein is formed from the veins accompanying the vertebral artery. You will find that it emerges from the foramen transversarium of the sixth cervical vertebra, and that it descends in front of the subclavian artery to open into the posterior aspect of the brachiocephalic vein a little below its commencement. Other tributaries of the brachiocephalic vein include the **inferior thyroid** and **internal thoracic veins,** but by this stage of the dissection they will have been removed.

Branches of the subclavian artery

Turn your attention to the branches of the subclavian artery. For descriptive purposes the subclavian artery is divided into a first part, which lies medial to the scalenus anterior muscle, a second part, which lies behind, and a third part, which lies lateral to the muscle. Almost all the branches of the artery arise from the first part, which you must now clean. Of these you have already seen the **internal thoracic artery** in the thorax [p. 3.9], and the **thyrocervical trunk** [p. 5.92]. Find the slender **costocervical trunk** on the left side, arising from the first part of the subclavian artery [Fig. 5.93] (on the right side this artery comes from the second part of the subclavian artery). Clean and follow this vessel upwards and backwards, and establish that it reaches the neck of the first rib. Here it divides into the **highest intercostal artery** and the **deep cervical artery,** which you need not dissect. The first of these branches supplies the upper two intercostal spaces [p. 3.21]; the second goes on to supply the muscles of the back of the neck.

The vertebral artery

Medial to the costocervical trunk you will find the origin of the vertebral artery, which is the first branch of the subclavian artery [Fig. 5.93]. Identify and clean it on both sides of the body. The artery springs from the back of the subclavian artery and ascends towards the foramen transversarium of the sixth cervical vertebra, lying deeply behind

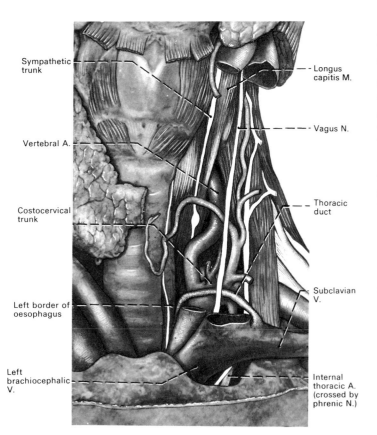

Sympathetic trunk

Vertebral A.

Costocervical trunk

Left border of oesophagus

Left brachiocephalic V.

Longus capitis M.

Vagus N.

Thoracic duct

Subclavian V.

Internal thoracic A. (crossed by phrenic N.)

Fig. 5.93 The left side of the root of the neck. Most of the common carotid artery and the internal jugular vein have been removed.

the common carotid artery. It enters this foramen and then ascends through the **foramina transversaria** of all the superjacent cervical vertebrae, lying in front of the cervical nerves which issue from the intervertebral foramina. This part of the course of the vertebral artery need not be dissected, as it can be understood sufficiently well after a glance at the cervical vertebrae. After the artery emerges from the foramen transversarium of the atlas, it passes medially round the posterior surface of the lateral mass to enter the vertebral canal. This part of its course has already been dissected [p. 5.7]. The artery then passes in front of the **posterior atlanto-occipital membrane,** which is a fibrous membrane attached above to the posterior margin of the foramen magnum, and below to the posterior arch of the atlas.

Divide the posterior atlanto-occipital membrane, then the spinal dura mater, which is adherent to its deep surface, and also the two small muscles, rectus capitis posterior major and rectus capitis posterior minor, so as to see this part of the artery's course. The artery pierces the dura mater

and the arachnoid, and ascends through the **foramen magnum** into the skull. You have already seen that it ends by joining its fellow on the posterior surface of the basilar part of the occipital bone to form the **basilar artery** [p. 5.28]. The vertebral artery gives off branches to muscles, to the spinal medulla and to the hindbrain.

The cervical part of the sympathetic trunk

Now examine the sympathetic trunk in the neck. It runs parallel with, and medial to, the vagus nerve behind the common and internal carotid arteries [Figs 5.93 and 5.94]. You will have to search for it in the fascia deep to the carotid, as it lies outside the carotid sheath. The sympathetic trunk is usually thinner than the vagus, but is easily distinguished from it by its irregular thickness, and by the long spindle-shaped swelling at its upper end. This is the **superior cervical ganglion.** There may be two or more other smaller ganglia along the course of the trunk, of which the **stellate**

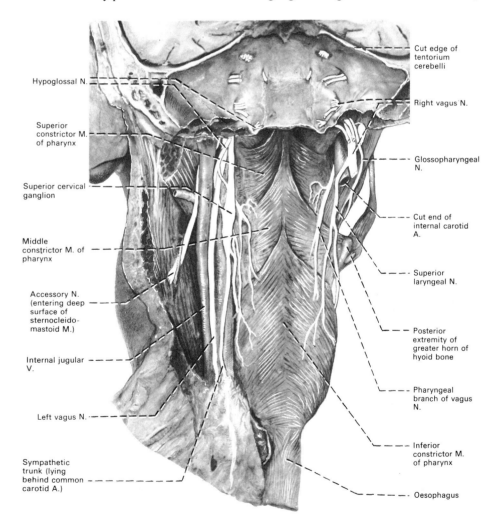

Hypoglossal N.

Superior constrictor M. of pharynx

Superior cervical ganglion

Middle constrictor M. of pharynx

Accessory N. (entering deep surface of sternocleidomastoid M.)

Internal jugular V.

Left vagus N.

Sympathetic trunk (lying behind common carotid A.)

Cut edge of tentorium cerebelli

Right vagus N.

Glossopharyngeal N.

Cut end of internal carotid A.

Superior laryngeal N.

Posterior extremity of greater horn of hyoid bone

Pharyngeal branch of vagus N.

Inferior constrictor M. of pharynx

Oesophagus

Fig. 5.94 The posterior aspect of the pharynx. The vertebral column and its attached muscles, most of the occipital bone, as well as the structures on the right side of the neck, have been removed.

5.95

ganglion at the root of the neck can usually be identified. This ganglion is irregularly shaped, and lies close behind the vertebral artery, between the transverse process of the seventh cervical vertebra and the neck of the first rib. The stellate ganglion is formed by the fusion of the **inferior cervical ganglion** and the **first thoracic ganglion,** which are, however, sometimes separate. Demonstrate the continuity of the cervical and thoracic parts of the sympathetic trunk.

As with the other ganglia of the sympathetic trunk, the cervical ganglia send postganglionic fibres in the form of grey rami communicantes to the ventral rami of the cervical nerves, but exactly where they come off varies from body to body. So, too, do the origin and number of the fine **cervical cardiac nerves** which descend into the thorax [see p. 3.43]. Other branches of the cervical part of the sympathetic trunk form plexuses around arteries in the neck, and so pass to structures like the thyroid gland and trachea. In addition, the superior cervical ganglion communicates with the glossopharyngeal, vagus, and hypoglossal nerves, and with the pharyngeal plexus. It also provides a rich plexus of sympathetic nerves which accompanies the internal carotid artery into the skull, and which is called the **internal carotid plexus.**

The longus colli and longus capitis muscles

Taking care not to damage the nerves, lift the fascia covering the cervical plexus and the scalenus anterior muscle, and peel it in a medial direction off the structures lying deep to it. This is the **prevertebral layer of cervical fascia** [Fig. 5.23]. Medial to the transverse processes of the cervical vertebrae you will uncover the longus colli and longus capitis muscles, which lie in front of, and arise from, the cervical vertebrae [Figs 5.93 and 5.133]. Do not spend time on their dissection. The longus capitis is inserted into the inferior surface of the basilar part of the occipital bone, and the longus colli into the anterior surfaces of the bodies of the vertebrae. Both muscles flex the head and neck, the longus capitis acting on the atlanto-occipital joint, and the longus colli on the joints of the vertebral column.

Section 5.12

The orbit

The eyeball, which is connected with the brain by the optic nerve, is situated in the orbit, within which it is rotated by the muscles of the eyeball, or extrinsic muscles, a term which distinguishes them from the intrinsic muscles within the eyeball. The specialized epidermis, or conjunctiva, overlying the eyeball is thin, translucent, and, over the front of the eye, transparent. It is protected against injury by the eyelids and by the lacrimal fluid which, when secreted in excess, forms tears. The lacrimal gland, which secretes this lacrimal fluid, is situated mainly in the upper lateral corner of the front of the orbit.

In the following dissection you will be examining the eyelids, the conjunctiva, the lacrimal apparatus, the eyeball and the optic nerve, the muscles of the eyeball and their nerve supply, and the branches of the ophthalmic nerve and artery, all of which traverse the orbit.

Osteology

Examine the orbit on a skull. It may be likened to a four-sided pyramid lying on one side, with the base, which is bounded by the supraorbital and infraorbital margins, facing anteriorly. The **supraorbital margin** is formed by the frontal bone, and is marked by a **supraorbital foramen** or **notch** [Fig. 5.95], which you can feel above your own eye. The zygomatic bone forms most of the lateral margin and the lateral half of the **infraorbital margin.** The medial half of the infraorbital margin is formed by the maxilla. An upward-projecting frontal process of the maxilla meets the downward-projecting nasal part of the frontal bone about the midpoint of the medial margin of the orbit.

The walls of the orbit

The superior wall [Fig. 5.95]

Now look at the four walls of the orbit. The superior wall, or roof, is formed by the same **orbital part of the frontal bone** which forms the floor of the anterior cranial fossa. Posteriorly, the frontal bone articulates with the **lesser wing of the sphenoid bone,** which you have already identified inside the skull. The medial end of the lesser wing of the sphenoid is pierced by the **optic canal,** which you will see at the back of the orbit.

The lateral wall [Fig. 5.95]

Most of the lateral wall of the orbit is formed by the **greater wing of the sphenoid,** which, externally, helps to form the temporal fossa. The rest of the lateral wall is formed by the **zygomatic bone.** The two wings of the sphenoid are separated by a fissure, the **superior orbital fissure,** which is obliquely placed at the back of the orbit. Below and laterally, the greater wing of the sphenoid forms the upper boundary of the **inferior orbital fissure,** which intervenes between the greater wing of the sphenoid and the part of the maxilla which forms the inferior wall, or floor, of the orbit. Look at the infratemporal surface of the maxilla [Fig. 5.50] to see how closely the inferior orbital fissure is related to the pterygomaxillary fissure. The small foramen you will see on the orbital surface of the zygomatic bone is the **zygomatico-orbital foramen** [Fig. 5.95].

The inferior wall [Fig. 5.95]

Note the **infraorbital groove** on the inferior wall, or floor, of the orbit. Anteriorly it continues into the infraorbital canal which opens on to the anterior surface of the maxilla at the **infraorbital foramen.**

The medial wall [Fig. 5.95]

Most of the medial wall of the orbit is made up of a rectangular plate of bone, the **orbital plate of the ethmoid bone,** which articulates above with the frontal bone and below with the maxilla. Behind, the orbital plate of the ethmoid meets the side of the body of the sphenoid. In front of it lie first, a small bone, the **lacrimal bone,** and then the frontal process of the maxilla. If you look down on the anterior medial corner of the inferior wall of the orbit from above, you will see the **nasolacrimal canal** bounded by the maxilla and the lacrimal bone. Two small foramina which lie in the sutures between the orbital plate of the ethmoid and the frontal bone are the **anterior** and **posterior ethmoidal foramina** [Fig. 5.95].

Surface anatomy

Use a mirror to study the surface anatomy of the contents of the orbit on yourself.

The eye [Fig. 5.96]

The white of the eye is called the **sclera,** and is part of the tough external **fibrous coat of the eyeball.** The visible part of the sclera is covered by a thin transparent membrane called the **conjunctiva** [Fig. 5.96a]. Anteriorly, the fibrous coat of the eyeball is transparent and fuses with the

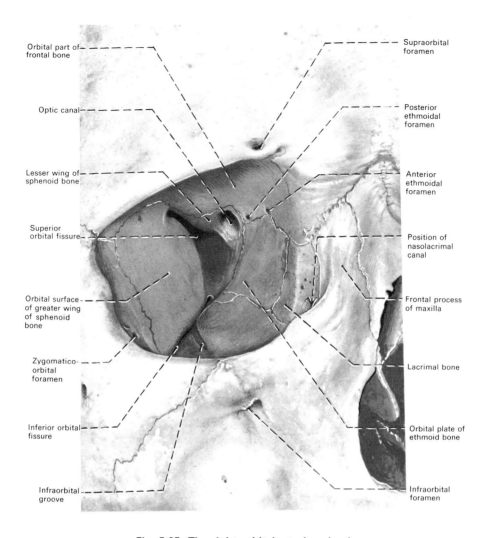

Orbital part of frontal bone

Optic canal

Lesser wing of sphenoid bone

Superior orbital fissure

Orbital surface of greater wing of sphenoid bone

Zygomatico- orbital foramen

Inferior orbital fissure

Infraorbital groove

Supraorbital foramen

Posterior ethmoidal foramen

Anterior ethmoidal foramen

Position of nasolacrimal canal

Frontal process of maxilla

Lacrimal bone

Orbital plate of ethmoid bone

Infraorbital foramen

Fig. 5.95 The right orbit (anterior view).

conjunctiva to form a circular window, the **cornea,** through which you can see the coloured **iris,** with its many radial striations.

In the centre of the iris is the black **pupil.** The iris is like the diaphragm of a camera, and controls the amount of light that enters the eye through the pupil. As more light strikes the eye, the pupil constricts. This movement of the iris is brought about by smooth circular muscle fibres which constitute the **sphincter of the pupil.** The action of this muscle is opposed by the **dilator of the pupil,** whose smooth muscle fibres are arranged radially in the iris. By directing a beam of light through the pupil with an ophthalmoscope it is possible to see a part of the internal coat of the eyeball called the **retina,** which lies at the back of the eyeball.

Beyond the **margin of the cornea** the conjunctiva has only a loose connection with the eyeball. Above and below, it lines the inner surface of the eyelids, at whose margins it becomes continuous with the skin of the face. When the eyelids are closed, the conjunctiva forms the **conjunctival sac.**

The eyelids [Fig. 5.96]

The **upper eyelid** is much larger than the lower. The elliptical fissure between the margins of the two eyelids is called the **palpebral fissure,** and its inner and outer ends, the **medial** and **lateral angles of the eye.** Each eyelid contains a thin but stiff plate of fibrous tissue called the **tarsus,** which is anchored to the walls of the orbit by the **medial** and **lateral palpebral ligaments.** The medial palpebral ligament can be felt as a rounded horizontal cord if a finger is placed between the nose and the medial angle of the eye. Immediately beneath the skin, and superficial to the tarsi, lies the **orbicularis oculi** muscle. Its fibres are arranged circularly like a sphincter; when they contract the eye becomes tightly shut.

Pull the **lower eyelid** down (evert it), and you will see that its inner surface (which is lined by conjunctiva), is coarsely striated at right-angles to the free border of the lid. The pale streaks are **tarsal glands,** whose ducts open on to the **posterior palpebral margin** of the free border of the lid [Fig. 5.96b]. Tarsal glands are arranged in the same way in

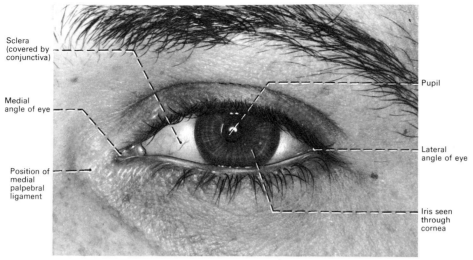

a. *With the eye open*

Sclera (covered by conjunctiva)

Medial angle of eye

Position of medial palpebral ligament

Pupil

Lateral angle of eye

Iris seen through cornea

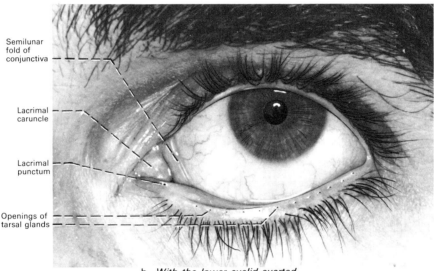

b. *With the lower eyelid everted*

Fig. 5.96 The left eye.

Semilunar fold of conjunctiva

Lacrimal caruncle

Lacrimal punctum

Openings of tarsal glands

the upper lid. The **eyelashes** project from the **anterior palpebral margins.** They are important receptors for initiating the 'blink reflex'.

The lacrimal apparatus

The lacrimal fluid washes over the surface of the eyeball, downwards and medially from the supero-lateral corner of the conjunctival sac, into which it is secreted by the **lacrimal gland.** The fluid is normally evaporated, or is drained from the surface of the conjunctiva by capillary attraction through two **lacrimal canaliculi.** One of these opens on to the summit of a small **lacrimal papilla** at the medial end of each posterior palpebral margin. Identify the papilla on each eyelid and its fine opening, the **lacrimal punctum.** Each lacrimal canaliculus passes medially to the **lacrimal sac,** which lies behind the medial palpebral ligament. Note that the pink fleshy mass, the **lacrimal caruncle,** which can be

seen in the medial angle of the eye, is not the lacrimal sac. It is a small node of skin containing sebaceous glands. From the lacrimal sac a duct, called the **nasolacrimal duct,** drains the lacrimal fluid into the nose. When the lacrimal glands secrete too profusely, this normal process of drainage becomes insufficient, and tears result.

Reflection of the skin

Continue the skin incision you made across the face [see p. 5.39] to the midline of the nose. Make another horizontal incision from the lateral angle of the eye to the margin of the skin remaining on the face and forehead [Fig. 5.97]. Reflect all this skin except that covering the lower half of the nose, making further incisions along the free borders of the eyelids to complete its removal. You should now be able to see the thin quadrilateral **frontal belly of the occipito-**

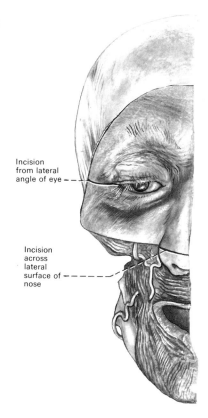

Incision from lateral angle of eye

Incision across lateral surface of nose

Fig. 5.97 Skin incisions for the dissection of the orbit.

frontalis muscle on the forehead. Inferiorly the muscle blends with the **orbicularis oculi.** The fibres of this elliptical muscle arise from the medial palpebral ligament and the bone adjacent to it. At the side of the nose you may encounter other subcutaneous muscles descending from near the medial angle of the eye. You need not dissect them. They are all innervated by the facial nerve.

Now strip the scalp downwards and forwards, removing periosteum as well. As you approach the supraorbital margin look for the **supraorbital nerve,** which is a branch of the ophthalmic nerve [Fig. 5.98]. It emerges from the supraorbital foramen or notch. Trace it upwards for 2 or 3 cm. Its branches pierce the occipitofrontalis muscle, and are then distributed to the skin of the scalp near the midline as far back as the vertex.

Removal of the superior wall of the orbit

Strip from the skull all that remains of the scalp and periosteum above the plane of the lesser wing of the sphenoid, removing, as you do so, what is left of the temporal muscle and the temporal fascia. Within the skull, incise the dura mater of the brain along the lateral margin of the cribriform plate of the ethmoid bone, and carry the incision anteriorly

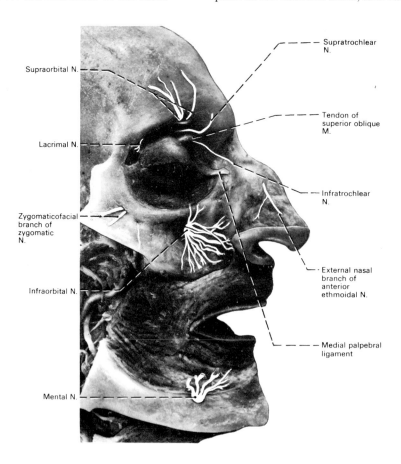

Supraorbital N.

Lacrimal N.

Zygomaticofacial branch of zygomatic N.

Infraorbital N.

Mental N.

Supratrochlear N.

Tendon of superior oblique M.

Infratrochlear N.

External nasal branch of anterior ethmoidal N.

Medial palpebral ligament

Fig. 5.98 Cutaneous nerves of the face and forehead. The scalp and the orbicularis oculi muscle have been removed.

5.100

and medially to the cut median surface. Use the handle of a scalpel to peel the dura mater off the calvaria and off the floor of the anterior cranial fossa, but do not disturb the dura mater over the cribriform plate. With a frame-saw remove the calvaria by placing the half-head with its superficial surface uppermost. Without damaging the dura mater saw through the head in a horizontal plane, just above the level of the superior wall of the orbit anteriorly [Fig. 5.99], and above the transverse sinus of the dura mater, in the attached border of the tentorium cerebelli posteriorly. Use an amputation-saw to remove the superior wall of the orbit and the supraorbital margin by making two sagittal saw-cuts through the frontal bone above each end of the orbital margin. Apply bone forceps or a chisel to the supraorbital margin between the two saw-cuts and fracture the intervening bone. As you remove the bone, take care not to damage the supraorbital nerve in the supraorbital foramen, which will have to be opened with bone forceps. The periosteum of the superior wall of the orbit strips off the bone very easily and is left behind.

Using bone gouge forceps, remove the rest of the superior wall, back to and including the lesser wing of the sphenoid bone. Each time you use the forceps, see that the bone you are about to nibble away is completely bare of periosteum and dura mater. Only in this way can you be sure of not damaging any of the underlying soft structures. When you get to the lesser wing of the sphenoid, remove all but the margins of the optic canal and the medial half of the anterior clinoid process, and so open the superior orbital fissure. With bone forceps remove the upper half of the lateral orbital margin.

It is likely that you will have opened up the ethmoidal sinuses along the medial wall of the orbit. If so, their lining mucous coat will be exposed. They communicate with the cavity of the nose.

The contents of the orbit

The frontal nerve [Fig. 5.100]

You should be able to trace the course of the **supraorbital nerve** through the periosteum of the superior wall of the orbit, back towards the superior orbital fissure. Using scissors, cut forwards through the periosteum and expose the nerve in the orbit. The smaller **supratrochlear nerve** lies medial to it. Trace both back to the frontal nerve from which they branch [Fig. 5.100]. Then trace the frontal nerve to the superior orbital fissure, taking care not to damage the fine trochlear nerve which lies on its medial aspect. The supratrochlear nerve supplies an area of skin around the medial angle of the eye.

Reflect the periosteum on each side of the incision you made to expose the frontal nerve, and remove the two flaps of periosteum so formed by cutting their attachments along the medial and lateral margins of the orbital roof.

The lacrimal gland [Fig. 5.100]

Find the lacrimal gland, which is a lobular structure situated behind the lateral end of the supraorbital margin. The deep surface of the gland is separated from the eyeball by the lateral rectus muscle. Lift the gland off the structures underlying it, and then place a blunt probe into the lateral part of the **superior fornix of the conjunctiva** (the angle of reflection of the conjunctiva from the sclera to the eyelid). You will then be able to appreciate how close the gland lies to

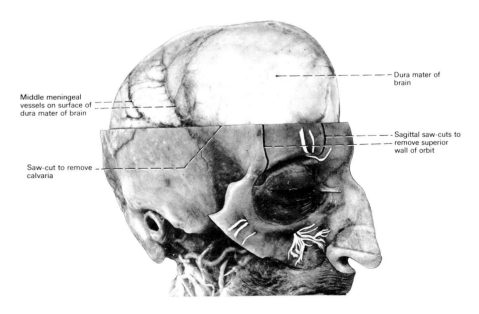

Fig. 5.99 Saw-cuts to remove the superior wall of the orbit.

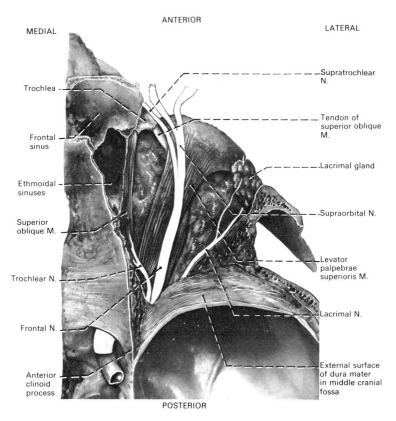

MEDIAL · ANTERIOR · LATERAL

Trochlea

Frontal sinus

Ethmoidal sinuses

Superior oblique M.

Trochlear N.

Frontal N.

Anterior clinoid process

Supratrochlear N.

Tendon of superior oblique M.

Lacrimal gland

Supraorbital N.

Levator palpebrae superioris M.

Lacrimal N.

External surface of dura mater in middle cranial fossa

POSTERIOR

Fig. 5.100 The frontal nerve and the levator palpebrae superioris muscle. Superior view of the right orbit after the removal of the superior wall of the orbit and the lesser wing of the sphenoid bone.

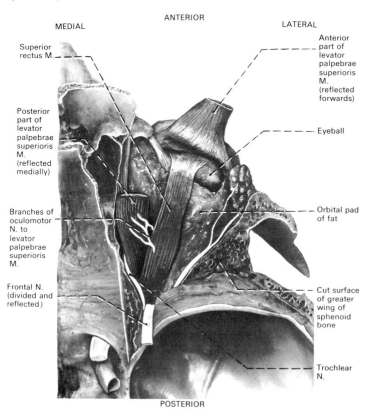

MEDIAL · ANTERIOR · LATERAL

Superior rectus M.

Posterior part of levator palpebrae superioris M. (reflected medially)

Branches of oculomotor N. to levator palpebrae superioris M.

Frontal N. (divided and reflected)

Anterior part of levator palpebrae superioris M. (reflected forwards)

Eyeball

Orbital pad of fat

Cut surface of greater wing of sphenoid bone

Trochlear N.

POSTERIOR

Fig. 5.101 The superior rectus muscle. Superior view of the right orbit after the reflection of the levator palpebrae superioris muscle.

5.102

the fornix. The ducts of the gland open into this part of the fornix.

The lacrimal nerve [Fig. 5.100]

Search for the fine lacrimal nerve behind the postero-lateral border of the lacrimal gland. This nerve is a branch of the ophthalmic nerve. You should trace it from the superior orbital fissure along the lateral wall of the orbit to the point where it passes below the gland. The nerve supplies the gland and the skin of the lateral part of the upper eyelid.

The levator palpebrae superioris muscle [Fig. 5.100]

Now define the borders of the long, narrow muscle underlying the frontal nerve. This is the levator palpebrae superioris, the elevator of the upper eyelid. It arises from the superior wall of the orbit immediately in front of the optic canal, a fact you will no longer be able to confirm. To demonstrate the insertion of the muscle, separate it from another muscle on which it rests, and divide it about the middle. Turn the anterior end forwards [Fig. 5.101], and you will see how the levator palpebrae superioris is inserted as a broad aponeurosis into the upper eyelid. The levator palpebrae superioris muscle is peculiar in consisting of smooth as well as striated muscle fibres.

The parts of the lacrimal gland

The lateral edge of the aponeurosis of the levator palpebrae superioris indents the lacrimal gland, subdividing the gland into an upper and larger **orbital part,** and a lower and smaller **palpebral part.** It is the palpebral part of the gland which lies in close relationship with the upper conjunctival fornix.

The superior rectus muscle [Fig. 5.101]

Beneath the levator palpebrae superioris lies the superior rectus muscle, which arises from the upper margin of the optic canal and is inserted into the eyeball [Fig. 5.101]. Define the borders of this narrow muscle, separate it from the structures below it, and divide it across its middle. Turn the anterior end of the muscle up, and trace it forwards. This will bring you to the eyeball, but the actual tendinous insertion of the muscle to the sclera cannot be seen, because the eyeball is loosely invested by thin fascial membranes called the **sheaths of the eyeball.** By blunt dissection remove only sufficient of these sheaths to see the insertion of the muscle. Note the axis of the muscle with respect to the sagittal plane. You will realize the importance of this point when you come to consider the movements of the eyeball.

The trochlear nerve [Fig. 5.100]

The trochlear nerve should now be found crossing the levator palpebrae superioris muscle close to its origin. It enters the orbit through the superior orbital fissure, medial to the frontal and lacrimal nerves. Trace the nerve as it turns medially above the muscle to enter the upper border of the superior oblique muscle, which will be found lying along the medial wall of the orbit.

The superior oblique muscle [Figs 5.100 and 5.103]

Clean the superior oblique muscle, and note that it arises from the superior wall of the orbit close to the upper and medial margin of the optic canal. You will have difficulty in tracing the muscle forwards to its insertion, because its tendon passes through a small fibrocartilaginous sheath and then turns backwards and laterally over the eyeball, under cover of the superior rectus muscle, to be inserted into the sclera behind the equator of the eyeball. Lift the anterior cut end of the superior rectus muscle in order to find the insertion of the tendon of the superior oblique muscle into the sclera. Establish the continuity of the muscle and tendon by pulling gently backwards and forwards on them. You will see that the fibrocartilaginous sheath, or **trochlea,** through which the tendon passes, acts like a pulley. The trochlea itself is attached to a small fossa, the **fovea trochlearis** (sometimes an elevation, the **spina trochlearis**) on the frontal bone at the upper end of the medial margin of the orbit.

The lateral rectus muscle [Fig. 5.102]

Carefully peel the dura mater off the anterior wall and floor of the middle cranial fossa as far back as the anterior clinoid process. Now nibble away the part of the greater wing of the sphenoid that lies below the superior orbital fissure, and find the lateral rectus muscle [Fig. 5.102]. This muscle arises by an upper and a lower head from two tendinous bands which pass from the upper and lower margins of the optic canal to a small tubercle at the medial end of the infero-lateral margin of the superior orbital fissure. In this way the origin of the lateral rectus spans part of the superior orbital fissure near its medial end. The lateral rectus muscle is inserted into the lateral aspect of the eyeball in approximately the same plane as the superior rectus muscle. Do not try as yet to examine the muscle's attachments closely.

The origins of the rectus muscles

From the medial and inferior margins of the optic canal, the medial rectus muscle and the inferior rectus muscle respectively take origin. These two muscles, which you will see later, are inserted into the eyeball in a way similar to the superior and lateral rectus muscles. The four rectus muscles are arranged like a cone [Fig. 5.103]. A **common tendinous ring** at the apex of the cone provides an origin for the four muscles. The ring encircles the optic canal and part of the superior orbital fissure. Within the cone lie the eyeball, certain blood vessels and nerves, and the **orbital pad of fat,** which fills the remaining space. The vessels and nerves leave or enter the cone, either through the optic canal, or through the part of the superior orbital fissure which lies between the two heads of the lateral rectus muscle, and so

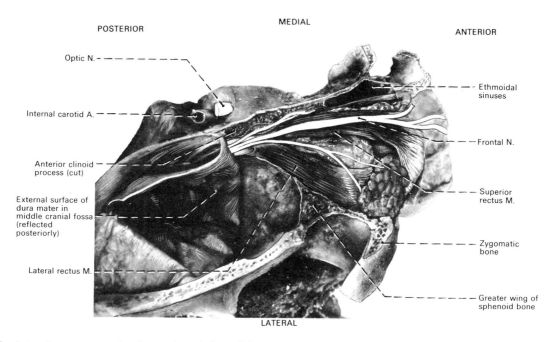

POSTERIOR   MEDIAL   ANTERIOR

Optic N.

Internal carotid A.

Anterior clinoid
process (cut)

External surface of
dura mater in
middle cranial fossa
(reflected
posteriorly)

Lateral rectus M.

Ethmoidal
sinuses

Frontal N.

Superior
rectus M.

Zygomatic
bone

Greater wing of
sphenoid bone

LATERAL

Fig. 5.102 The lateral rectus muscle. Supero-lateral view of the right orbit from which the superior wall and most of the lateral wall have been removed.

within the common tendinous ring. So far you have dissected only three nerves, the lacrimal, frontal, and trochlear nerves. These pass through the superior orbital fissure lateral to, and outside the origin of the lateral rectus, and they should be traced backwards as far as the reflection of the dura mater allows.

The optic nerve [Figs 5.103 and 5.104]

Carefully remove the orbital pad of fat to reveal the optic nerve running forwards and laterally from the optic canal to the eyeball, and also the fine nasociliary nerve, which crosses the optic nerve from its lateral to its medial side as it passes forwards [Fig. 5.104]. As you do this, remove any veins that may be in the way, but preserve the arteries you encounter.

The nasociliary nerve [Fig. 5.104]

The nasociliary nerve is one of the three branches of the ophthalmic nerve, the others being the lacrimal and frontal nerves. The nasociliary nerve enters the orbit through the superior orbital fissure within the common tendinous ring which gives origin to the rectus muscles. Trace the nerve forwards, and pick up its branches above or medial to the optic nerve. The nasociliary nerve ends near the medial wall of the orbit below the superior oblique muscle. Here it divides into the **infratrochlear nerve,** which passes forwards under the trochlea to supply the skin of the eyelids and the upper half of the nose, and the **anterior ethmoidal nerve** [Fig. 5.105], which leaves the medial wall of the orbit through the anterior ethmoidal foramen to reach the mucous coat of the anterior and middle cells of the ethmoidal sinuses and

the nasal cavity. You may also find the **posterior ethmoidal nerve,** another branch of the nasociliary nerve, which traverses the posterior ethmoidal foramen, to innervate the posterior cells of the ethmoidal sinuses, and the sphenoidal sinus.

More important than these terminal branches of the nasociliary nerve are the two **long ciliary nerves** which leave the trunk of the nasociliary nerve as it crosses the optic nerve. These fine nerves run forwards to the eyeball, and are mainly sensory to the cornea [Fig. 5.105].

The abducent nerve [Fig. 5.104]

Trace the nasociliary nerve backwards through the superior orbital fissure, using scissors to cut through the upper head of the lateral rectus muscle. Lying below the nasociliary nerve at the superior orbital fissure you will find the abducent nerve. Trace it into the medial surface of the lateral rectus muscle, which it supplies.

The oculomotor nerve [Fig. 5.104]

Medial to the nasociliary nerve, at the superior orbital fissure, lie the two chief branches of the oculomotor nerve, one above the other. The **superior branch** [Fig. 5.104] enters the inferior surface of the superior rectus muscle, which it supplies, some of the fibres of the nerve passing through the muscle to innervate the overlying levator palpebrae superioris. Now find the **inferior branch** of the oculomotor nerve and trace it forwards to where it divides. One branch passes forwards, and the other passes medially, below the optic nerve. You will see that the forward-directed branch almost immediately gives off a short stoutish twig which

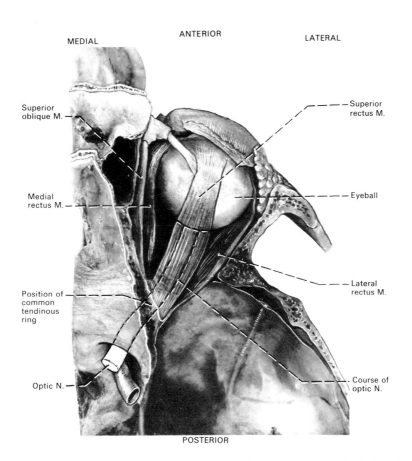

ANTERIOR

MEDIAL   LATERAL

Superior
oblique M.

Superior
rectus M.

Medial
rectus M.

Eyeball

Lateral
rectus M.

Position of
common
tendinous
ring

Optic N.

Course of
optic N.

POSTERIOR

Fig. 5.103 The muscles of the right eyeball (viewed from above). The inferior rectus muscle lies below the optic nerve and is hidden by the superior rectus muscle.

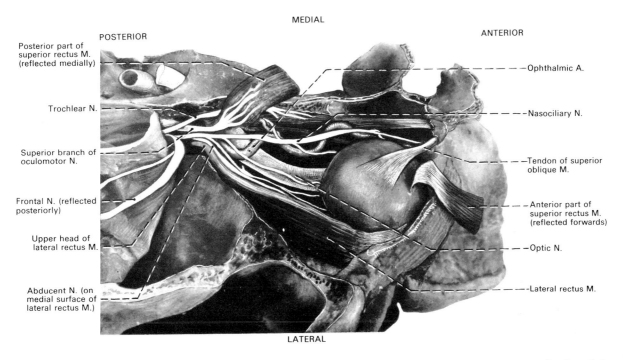

MEDIAL

POSTERIOR   ANTERIOR

Posterior part of
superior rectus M.
(reflected medially)

Ophthalmic A.

Trochlear N.

Nasociliary N.

Superior branch of
oculomotor N.

Tendon of superior
oblique M.

Frontal N. (reflected
posteriorly)

Anterior part of
superior rectus M.
(reflected forwards)

Upper head of
lateral rectus M.

Optic N.

Abducent N. (on
medial surface of
lateral rectus M.)

Lateral rectus M.

LATERAL

Fig. 5.104 The nasociliary, abducent, and oculomotor nerves. Supero-lateral view of the right orbit after the reflection of the superior rectus muscle. The upper head of the lateral rectus muscle has been turned laterally to expose the structures passing through the common tendinous ring.

turns upwards and ends in a slight swelling. This swelling is the **ciliary ganglion.**

The ciliary ganglion [Fig. 5.105]

You can confirm that you have found the ciliary ganglion by dissecting out a branch it receives from the nasociliary nerve, and also by identifying some of the numerous fine **short ciliary nerves** which it sends to the eyeball. The ciliary ganglion is important. Parasympathetic motor fibres from the oculomotor nerve relay in it, and the postganglionic fibres which arise in the ganglion run through the short ciliary nerves into the eyeball to supply the sphincter of the pupil and the ciliary muscle, which focuses the lens of the eye. The branch from the nasociliary nerve transmits sensory fibres, which pass back from the eyeball through the ganglion. This branch also contains postganglionic sympathetic fibres from the internal carotid plexus.

The ophthalmic artery [Fig. 5.104]

During the dissection of the nasociliary nerve you will have encountered the ophthalmic artery (a branch of the internal carotid artery), which winds round the optic nerve from its lateral side [Fig. 5.104]. Trace the artery backwards and note that it enters the orbit through the optic canal below the nerve. Its most important branch, the **central artery of the retina,** enters the optic nerve, and is, therefore, obscured from view. It is the only artery supplying the inner layers of the retina. Other branches of the ophthalmic artery supply the outer coats of the eyeball, the muscles of the eyeball, the eyelids, and the lacrimal gland.

The ophthalmic veins

The various veins you have removed usually pass into two veins, the **superior ophthalmic** and **inferior ophthalmic veins,** which leave the orbit through the superior orbital fissure. Their tributaries communicate with the veins of the face at the medial angle of the eye. Sometimes the inferior ophthalmic vein passes to the pterygoid plexus [p. 5.55] through the inferior orbital fissure.

The medial and inferior rectus muscles

To see the medial and inferior rectus muscles [Figs 5.103 and 5.106], which have already been described, cut the optic nerve as far posteriorly from the eyeball as possible, and turn it forwards. Remove all remaining fat, sacrificing the ophthalmic vessels if necessary. Now trace the branches of the oculomotor nerve to these muscles, and to the superior rectus and levator palpebrae superioris muscles.

The inferior oblique muscle [Fig. 5.106]

Only one orbital structure remains to be seen, the inferior oblique muscle. Pull down (evert) the lower eyelid, and incise the inferior fornix of the conjunctiva. Blunt dissection will soon reveal the muscle arising from the antero-medial part of the inferior wall of the orbit [Fig. 5.106]. Strip the fascial sheath off the postero-lateral aspect of the eyeball in order to see the insertion of the muscle. The muscle is supplied by the oculomotor nerve. Note that the direction of the fibres of the inferior oblique muscle is similar to that of the tendon of the superior oblique muscle as the latter approaches its insertion.

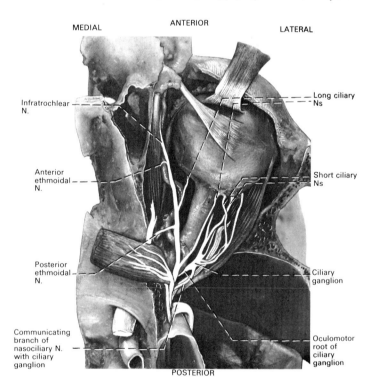

MEDIAL   ANTERIOR   LATERAL

Infratrochlear N.

Anterior ethmoidal N.

Posterior ethmoidal N.

Communicating branch of nasociliary N. with ciliary ganglion

POSTERIOR

Long ciliary Ns

Short ciliary Ns

Ciliary ganglion

Oculomotor root of ciliary ganglion

Fig. 5.105 The ciliary ganglion. Superior view of the right orbit. The superior rectus muscle has been divided and reflected, and the upper head of the lateral rectus muscle has been turned laterally.

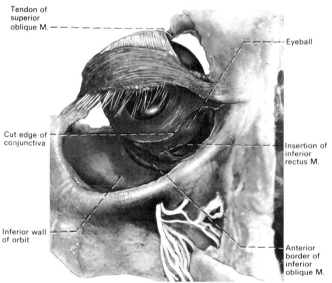

Tendon of superior oblique M.

Cut edge of conjunctiva

Inferior wall of orbit

Eyeball

Insertion of inferior rectus M.

Anterior border of inferior oblique M.

Fig. 5.106 The inferior oblique muscle. Anterior view of the right orbit. The lower eyelid and the inferior fornix of the conjunctiva have been removed.

The muscles of the eyeball

The actions of the muscles of the eyeball

The actions of the medial and lateral rectus muscles are obvious; they turn the eye medially or laterally [Fig. 5.107]. The superior and inferior rectus muscles, however, approach the eyeball at an angle to the sagittal plane. As a result the superior rectus turns the eye upwards and somewhat medially, and also slightly rotates it around its antero-posterior axis. A point on the upper surface of the eyeball would, therefore, move medially as the muscle contracts. The inferior rectus turns the eye downwards, somewhat medially, and rotates it slightly in the direction opposite to that of the superior rectus. The inferior oblique muscle turns the eye upwards and laterally, while the superior oblique muscle turns it downwards and laterally. Both of these muscles also rotate the eye slightly around its antero-posterior axis, but in opposite directions. Upward movement of the eye in the sagittal plane is produced by the combined actions of the superior rectus and inferior oblique muscles. In a similar fashion, the superior oblique muscle corrects the medial deviation and rotation produced by the inferior rectus when the eye is turned downwards.

The innervation of the muscles of the eyeball

It is important that you should remember the nerves supplying these muscles. The **trochlear nerve** supplies the superior oblique muscle; the **abducent nerve** the lateral rectus muscle; the **oculomotor nerve,** all the remaining muscles of the eyeball and also, by way of the **ciliary ganglion,** two intrinsic muscles, the sphincter of the pupil and the ciliary muscle. The dilator of the pupil is supplied by postganglionic sympathetic fibres which arise from the **superior cervical ganglion** and join the internal carotid plexus. They leave the plexus in the cavernous sinus, accompany the nasociliary nerve, and pass either through the long ciliary branches of that nerve, or through the ciliary ganglion and short ciliary nerves, to the eyeball.

The levator palpebrae superioris elevates the upper eyelid. The smooth muscle fibres in the muscle are innervated by postganglionic sympathetic nerve fibres from the superior cervical ganglion. They reach the muscle by way of the internal carotid plexus and the oculomotor nerve. If these fibres become paralysed the upper eyelid droops. The striated muscle fibres of the levator palpebrae superioris are supplied by the oculomotor nerve.

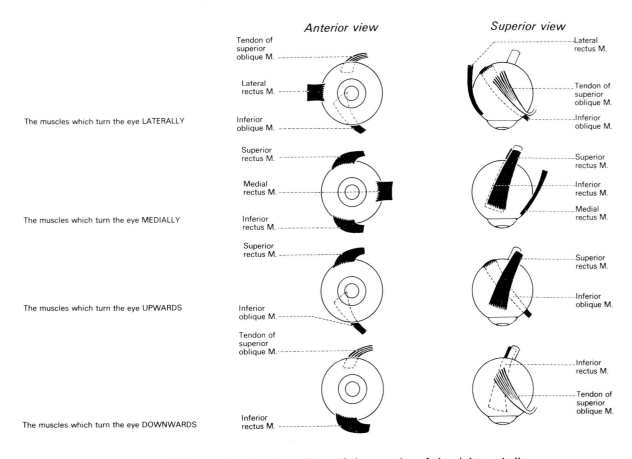

Fig. 5.107 Schema showing the actions of the muscles of the right eyeball.

Section 5.13

The sinuses of the dura mater

The blood that passes to the brain through the internal carotid and vertebral arteries is drained through numerous cerebral veins which connect directly with the nearest venous sinus of the dura mater. These sinuses are capacious channels that lie between the two layers of the dura mater of the skull. The principal sinuses are represented diagrammatically in Fig. 5.108. You examined the superior and inferior sagittal sinuses and the straight sinus in the margins of the falx cerebri after the head was bisected [p. 5.30]. At the same time you saw the commencement of at least one of the transverse sinuses. You should now examine the remaining venous sinuses of the dura mater.

The transverse and sigmoid sinuses

Working entirely beneath the tentorium cerebelli, slit open the **transverse sinus** along its length, first using scissors and then a scalpel. On the skull you will see how the bony groove which corresponds to the sinus first runs laterally round the wall of the skull and then makes an S-shaped curve as it descends to the jugular foramen. This S-shaped part of the sinus is known as the **sigmoid sinus** [Fig. 5.109]. Bearing its course in mind, continue to slit the sinus open until you reach the jugular foramen. Take care not to damage the glossopharyngeal, vagus, and accessory nerves as they leave the skull at this point. In the jugular foramen the sigmoid sinus becomes continuous with the internal jugular vein.

The cavernous and petrosal sinuses

The cavernous sinus is a venous sinus which lies between the layers of dura mater at the side of the body of the sphenoid. In its lateral wall lie the oculomotor, trochlear, ophthalmic, and maxillary nerves. The abducent nerve and the internal carotid artery, surrounded by the internal carotid plexus, lie within the sinus. All these structures are separated from the blood in the sinus by endothelium. Lateral to the posterior end of the sinus is the ganglion of the trigeminal nerve, called the trigeminal ganglion.

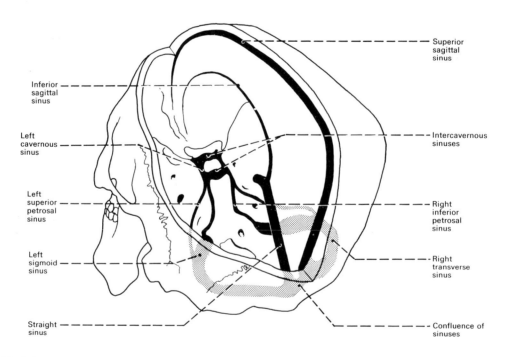

Fig. 5.108 Schema of the sinuses of the dura mater (oblique superior view from the left of interior of skull).

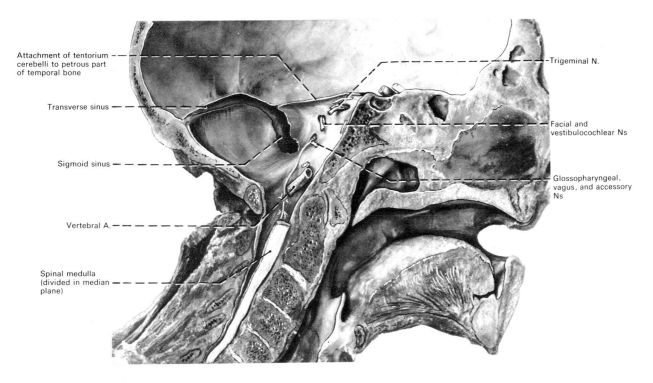

Attachment of tentorium cerebelli to petrous part of temporal bone

Transverse sinus

Sigmoid sinus

Vertebral A.

Spinal medulla (divided in median plane)

Trigeminal N.

Facial and vestibulocochlear Ns

Glossopharyngeal, vagus, and accessory Ns

Fig. 5.109 The left posterior cranial fossa. The tentorium cerebelli has been excised.

Dissection of the cavernous sinus [Fig. 5.110]

Using scissors, cut through the free border of the tentorium cerebelli immediately lateral to the point at which it is pierced by the trochlear nerve, and carry the incision towards the opening of the **cavum trigeminale** [p. 5.33], into which the trigeminal nerve can be seen disappearing. If you can no longer see the point where the trochlear nerve pierces the tentorium cerebelli, begin the cut behind the cavum trigeminale. When the cavum trigeminale has been reached, continue the cut forwards, across the floor of the middle cranial fossa, by inserting the lower point of the scissors into the cavum trigeminale above the trigeminal nerve, and continue cutting until you reach the dura mater that has already been separated from the middle and anterior cranial fossae. Insert scissors above the point where the oculomotor nerve pierces the dura mater, and cut forwards for 5 mm. Then carefully strip the dura mater medial to the first scissor-cut in a backward direction, following the trochlear nerve from the superior orbital fissure as you do so. Be careful not to damage the nerve, which should be traced to the point where it pierces the dura mater [Fig. 5.110].

The superior petrosal sinus [Fig. 5.110]

The cavernous sinus and the cavum trigeminale will now be open. Gently free the trochlear nerve from dura mater and from the other nerves with which it lies in the side wall of the cavernous sinus, and turn it forwards. Examine the cut edges of the dura mater which forms the roof of the

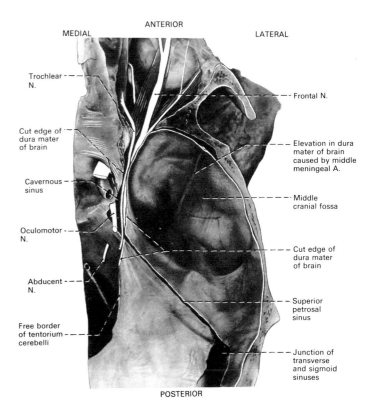

MEDIAL

ANTERIOR

LATERAL

Trochlear N.

Cut edge of dura mater of brain

Cavernous sinus

Oculomotor N.

Abducent N.

Free border of tentorium cerebelli

Frontal N.

Elevation in dura mater of brain caused by middle meningeal A.

Middle cranial fossa

Cut edge of dura mater of brain

Superior petrosal sinus

Junction of transverse and sigmoid sinuses

POSTERIOR

Fig. 5.110 The right cavernous and superior petrosal sinuses. Superior view of a bisected head.

cavum trigeminale. You will find that you have transected a small sinus of dura mater, the superior petrosal sinus, which runs along the attached border of the tentorium cerebelli and grooves the petrous part of the temporal bone, where the latter forms the posterior border of the middle cranial fossa. Trace this sinus postero-laterally by inserting into it the lower point of a pair of scissors and cutting open its roof. Confirm that the superior petrosal sinus communicates laterally with the beginning of the sigmoid sinus. Medially you will find that it connects with the cavernous sinus.

Dissection of the cavum trigeminale [Fig. 5.111]

Remove the dura mater that forms the roof of the cavum trigeminale by making an additional cut through the free border of the tentorium cerebelli parallel with and about 5 mm lateral to your first incision, continuing the cut anteriorly along the lateral margin of the cavum trigeminale. Finish this cut by turning your scissors medially along the anterior margin of the cavum trigeminale, until it joins the first incision. Take care, when cutting, not to damage the flat **trigeminal ganglion** which will now be

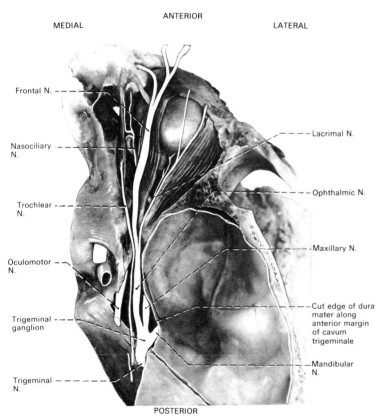

Fig. 5.111 The right trigeminal ganglion and the ophthalmic nerve. Superior view of a bisected head.

exposed [Fig. 5.111]. The three nerves into which the trigeminal nerve divides leave the antero-lateral border of the ganglion.

The contents of the cavernous sinus [Fig. 5.112]

Follow the **ophthalmic nerve** into the cavernous sinus, and confirm that it divides into the lacrimal, frontal, and nasociliary nerves. Trace the **oculomotor nerve** through the cavernous sinus (you have already traced the **trochlear nerve** [p. 5.109]). Then find the **abducent nerve.** To do so, clear out any blood clot in the sinus medial to the ophthalmic nerve, and look for the **internal carotid artery** as it pursues a sinuous course through the sinus. The abducent nerve is closely applied to the lateral side of the artery, but follows a straighter course [Fig. 5.112]. Trace the nerve forwards from the point where it pierces the dura mater, using scissors to cut the dura mater that forms the posterior wall of the sinus.

Connections of the cavernous sinus

It is important to know the connections of the cavernous sinus. The **ophthalmic veins** enter it at its anterior end; veins from the brain enter its superior surface; from its posterior end the **superior petrosal sinus** and the **inferior petrosal sinus** connect it with the beginnings of the sigmoid sinus and internal jugular vein respectively. In addition, **emissary veins,** which run through the foramen lacerum, connect the sinus with the pterygoid plexus. Some of these veins may pass either through the foramen ovale, or through inconstant foramina in the greater wing of the sphenoid. Through these emissary veins, and through the ophthalmic veins, the cavernous sinus is connected with the facial vein. Note that the sella turcica and the hypophysis lie between the two cavernous sinuses, which are connected to each other by **anterior** and **posterior intercavernous sinuses.** These cross the upper part of the sella turcica, one in front of and the other behind the infundibulum.

The inferior petrosal sinus [Fig. 5.113]

The inferior petrosal sinus will be seen to run downwards, backwards, and slightly laterally from the cavernous sinus towards the jugular foramen [Fig. 5.113]. It passes through the anterior end of the jugular foramen, to enter the beginning of the internal jugular vein in the **jugular fossa.** Identify this fossa on the external surface of the base of a skull. It lies in the temporal bone immediately lateral to the jugular foramen, with which it is continuous. Feel the inferior petrosal sinus below the dura mater with the blunt end of a probe. When you have outlined its course, open the sinus by slitting the dura mater with a scalpel. Take care not to divide the glossopharyngeal, vagus, and accessory nerves which accompany the sinus through the jugular foramen.

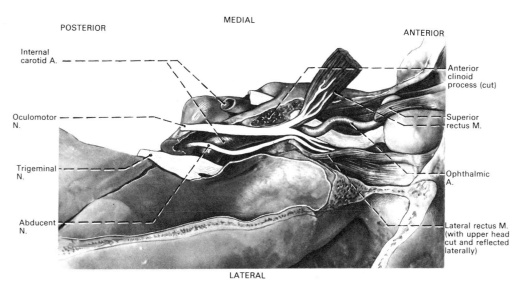

MEDIAL

POSTERIOR   ANTERIOR

Internal   Anterior
carotid A.   clinoid
                                                             process (cut)

Oculomotor   Superior
N.   rectus M.

Trigeminal   Ophthalmic
N.   A.

Abducent   Lateral rectus M.
N.   (with upper head
                                                             cut and reflected
                                                             laterally)

LATERAL

Fig. 5.112 The right cavernous sinus. Oblique lateral view of the dissection after removal of the trochlear and ophthalmic nerves.

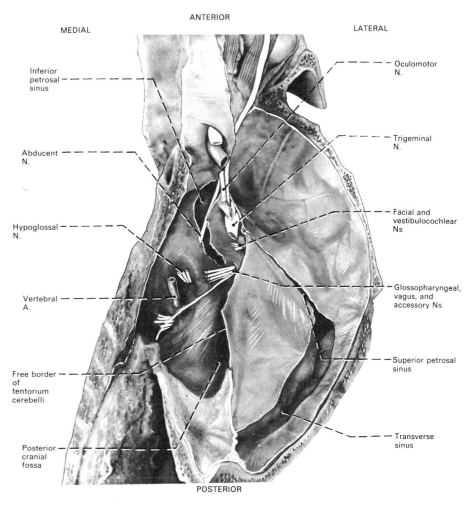

ANTERIOR

MEDIAL   LATERAL

Inferior   Oculomotor
petrosal   N.
sinus

                                                             Trigeminal
                                                             N.

Abducent
N.

                                                             Facial and
                                                             vestibulocochlear
                                                             Ns

Hypoglossal
N.

                                                             Glossopharyngeal,
                                                             vagus, and
Vertebral   accessory Ns
A.

                                                             Superior petrosal
                                                             sinus

Free border
of
tentorium
cerebelli

Posterior   Transverse
cranial   sinus
fossa

POSTERIOR

Fig. 5.113 The right inferior petrosal sinus. Oblique superior view of a bisected head.

5.111

Section 5.14

The nose

The cavity of the nose is divided into right and left halves by the septum of the nose, which only rarely lies exactly in the median plane. Each half of the cavity opens anteriorly through the nostril, and communicates posteriorly with the nasal part of the pharynx. The nasal cavity is lined with the mucous coat of the nose, which is closely adherent to the subjacent periosteum. This mucous coat pouches out to line the paranasal sinuses in the bones that form the walls of the nasal cavity. You have already seen some of these sinuses in the frontal, ethmoid, and sphenoid bones [Fig. 5.25].

Osteology and surface anatomy

The anatomy of the external nose is best examined on yourself or your partner, with a skull available for reference.

The lower part of the nose is movable, and consists of skin and cartilage. The upper part is rigid, and has a bony skeleton.

Look at the skull, and identify the two small **nasal bones** between the **frontal processes of the maxillae,** and articulating above with the frontal bone [Fig. 5.114]. Look through the anterior bony aperture of the nasal cavity, called the **piriform aperture,** and note that, except at the base, there is no

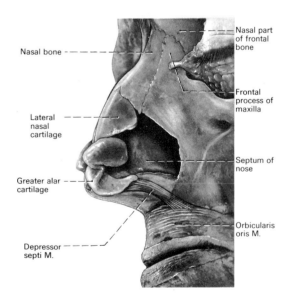

Fig. 5.114 Skeleton of the external nose.

bone in the front part of the **nasal septum.** If you now examine your specimen, you will see that a plate of cartilage makes up the missing part of the septum. On your own nose you can feel that the skin is more adherent to the cartilage forming the lower half of the external nose than to the bone above.

The part of the nasal cavity above the **nostril** is the **vestibule of the nose.** Its wall is slightly expanded and forms the wing or **ala of the nose.** Unlike the rest of the nasal cavity, the vestibule is lined with skin, from which stout hairs, the **vibrissae,** grow across the nostril. Subcutaneous muscles are inserted into the ala and septum of the nose. The size and shape of the nostril and vestibule vary as these muscles contract.

Dissection of the nasal cavity

Because of the close relation of the soft tissues to the bones, there is no advantage in studying the skeletal anatomy of the nose before beginning your dissection. A skull should, however, be available for reference.

The choanae [Fig. 5.61]

On one half of the head the nasal septum is probably intact, and on this side you will be able to examine the boundaries of the choanae, or posterior apertures of the nasal cavity. Refer to a skull and note that the choanae are bounded above by the body of the sphenoid bone; laterally by the medial pterygoid plate; and below by the posterior part of the hard palate formed by the horizontal plate of the palatine bone. They are separated from each other by the vomer, a bone of the nasal septum.

The nasal septum [Fig. 5.115]

The nasal septum has a **bony part,** which is formed by two plates of bone (the vomer and the perpendicular plate of the ethmoid bone), a **cartilaginous part,** and a small **membranous part** [Fig. 5.115]. The bone at the posterior end of the septum is the **vomer,** which articulates superiorly with the body of the sphenoid bone; inferiorly with the hard palate, which also forms the floor of the nasal cavity; and anteriorly with the cartilaginous part of the septum below, and the **perpendicular plate of the ethmoid bone** above. The latter lies within the upper half of the nasal septum. Identify the vomer and the perpendicular plate of the ethmoid in the skull.

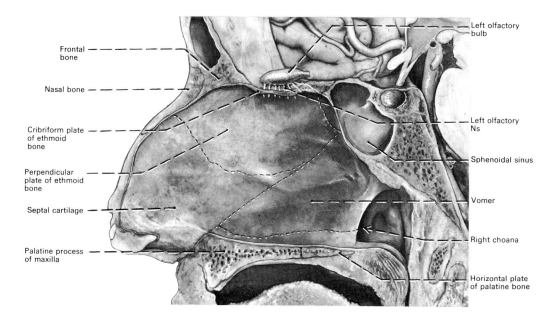

Frontal bone

Nasal bone

Cribriform plate of ethmoid bone

Perpendicular plate of ethmoid bone

Septal cartilage

Palatine process of maxilla

Left olfactory bulb

Left olfactory Ns

Sphenoidal sinus

Vomer

Right choana

Horizontal plate of palatine bone

Fig. 5.115 The septum of the nose.

The roof of the nasal cavity [Fig. 5.115]

Using scissors, remove the septum of the nose, and examine the roof of the nasal cavity. It is divided into an anterior sloping part, formed by the **nasal bones;** a middle horizontal part, formed by the **cribriform plate of the ethmoid bone;** and a posterior sloping part, mostly formed by the **body of the sphenoid bone.** Carefully reflect the dura mater that was left covering the cribriform plate. As you do so, you may see **olfactory nerves** traversing the foramina in the plate and piercing the dura mater. They innervate a a small olfactory region of the mucous coat at the upper end of the lateral and septal walls of the cavity.

The floor of the nasal cavity [Fig. 5.115]

The floor of the nasal cavity is formed on each side by the upper surfaces of the **palatine process of the maxilla** in front, and the **horizontal plate of the palatine bone** behind. It is much wider than the roof.

The lateral wall of the nasal cavity [Figs 5.116 and 5.117]

On the lateral wall of the nasal cavity are three overhanging projections, each of which consists of a curled plate of bone covered with a thick mucous coat. These are the **superior, middle,** and **inferior nasal conchae,** and they partially divide the nasal cavity into three horizontal channels, the **superior, middle,** and **inferior nasal meatuses** [Fig. 5.116]. Each meatus is bounded above by the attachment of its corresponding concha. The part of the nasal cavity above the superior concha is called the **spheno-ethmoidal recess;** the part between the vestibule in front and the meatuses behind is the **atrium of the middle meatus.**

Most of the lateral wall of the nasal cavity is formed by the maxilla, the ethmoid, and the inferior nasal concha. The inferior nasal concha is a separate bone; the middle and superior conchae are parts of the ethmoid bone. The posterior part of the lateral wall is formed by the **perpendicular plate of the palatine bone** and the **medial pterygoid plate.**

Use scissors to cut through the attachment of the inferior nasal concha to the wall of the cavity. Below the attachment of the anterior end of the concha, find the opening of the **nasolacrimal duct** into the inferior nasal meatus [Fig. 5.117]. The duct drains the lacrimal fluid from the lacrimal sac. It occupies the nasolacrimal canal [see p. 5.97]. On the dry skull, confirm that the nasolacrimal canal opens into the inferior meatus.

Now remove the middle nasal concha. On the lateral wall of the middle meatus you will see a curved groove, the **hiatus semilunaris,** running forwards and upwards to continue into a passage called the **ethmoidal infundibulum.** The bulge above the hiatus semilunaris is termed the **ethmoidal bulla.**

The paranasal sinuses [Fig. 5.117]

The ethmoidal infundibulum communicates with the **frontal sinus.** Use a soft flexible wire or seeker to confirm this fact. The numerous small **ethmoidal sinuses** are interposed in the ethmoid bone between the lateral wall of the nasal cavity and the medial wall of the orbit. You saw them when removing the superior wall of the orbit [p. 5.101]. They are divided into **anterior, middle,** and **posterior cells.** The anterior cells open into either the anterior end of the hiatus semilunaris, or the ethmoidal infundibulum; the middle, on to the surface of the ethmoidal bulla; and the posterior, into the superior nasal meatus. Examine these openings with a seeker. Find the slit-like opening of the maxillary sinus in the lower and posterior end of the hiatus semilunaris. The **sphenoidal sinus** opens into the spheno-ethmoidal recess.

All these paranasal sinuses lighten the bones surrounding the nose by replacing what would otherwise be cancellous bone.

The maxillary sinus [Fig. 5.118]

Starting at the posterior end of the attachment of the middle concha, make a vertical cut in the mucous coat as far as the floor of the nasal cavity. Scrape the mucous coat forwards, off the lateral wall of the inferior and middle meatuses. Open the maxillary sinus by breaking down and removing its thin medial wall (the lateral wall of the nasal cavity) except for 5 mm in front of the incision. Remove the mucosal lining of the sinus.

The maxillary sinus is the largest of the paranasal sinuses. It occupies the body of the maxilla and may even extend laterally into the zygomatic bone. Its floor is formed by the alveolar process of the maxilla into which the upper teeth are set. The roots of the first and second upper molar teeth

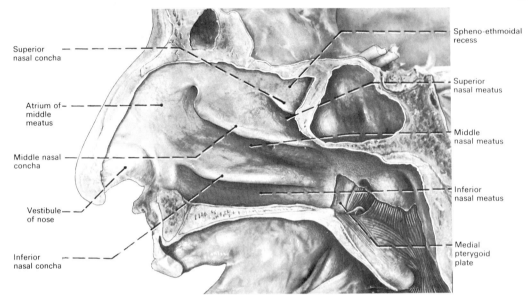

Fig. 5.116 The right lateral wall of the nasal cavity.

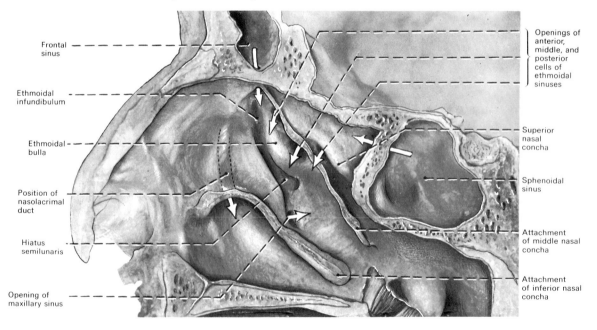

Fig. 5.117 The right lateral wall of the nasal cavity after removal of the middle and inferior nasal conchae. The arrows indicate openings into the nasal cavity.

5.114

produce elevations on the floor of the sinus, and occasionally the thin layer of bone between their dental alveoli and the mucous coat of the sinus may be deficient. Note that the floor of the sinus lies below the level of the floor of the nasal cavity, and that the opening of the sinus into the cavity is high up on its medial wall.

The mucous coat of the nose

The mucous coat which lines the paranasal sinuses is supplied with mucous glands, and is covered with ciliated columnar epithelium. In each sinus the movement of the cilia sweeps the mucus secreted by the glands towards the aperture through which the sinus communicates with the nasal cavity.

Note, too, that the mucous coat of the nose is continuous with the mucous coat of the paranasal sinuses, the mucous coat of the pharynx (and thus with the mucous coat of the auditory tube and middle ear), the skin of the vestibule and, by way of the nasolacrimal duct, with the conjunctiva. It is divisible into two areas: a small upper **olfactory region,** over and above the superior concha, and a large **respiratory region** below this. The latter part of the mucous coat contains venous sinuses and numerous mucous glands, and is thick and spongy in the living body. Its function is to warm and moisten inhaled air, and to trap dust particles on its moistened surface, the area of which is increased by the presence of the conchae. Its epithelium is formed of ciliated columnar cells. The cilia beat in such a way as to produce

a flow of mucus towards the choanae.

The innervation of the nasal mucosa

In addition to the **olfactory nerves,** which innervate the olfactory region, the mucous coat of the nose is supplied with ordinary sensory nerves. Except for the **anterior ethmoidal nerve** (a branch of the nasociliary nerve) which supplies the roof and anterior part of the lateral and septal walls, these sensory nerves are branches of the maxillary nerve, and most of them reach the mucous coat by passing through the **sphenopalatine foramen.**

Identify this foramen on the skull. It lies in the lateral wall of the nasal cavity immediately behind the posterior end of the middle nasal concha [Fig. 5.118], and can be seen by looking either through the choana, or through the pterygomaxillary fissure.

Find the foramen on your specimen, reflecting mucous coat if necessary. Do not spend time dissecting the nerves of the nasal cavity, but note that the **posterior superior nasal branches of the pterygopalatine ganglion,** which will be dissected later, and the **nasopalatine nerve** traverse the sphenopalatine foramen to supply most of the mucous coat of the nasal cavity. The nasopalatine nerve crosses the roof of the nasal cavity, and descends on the nasal septum towards the incisive canal in front. The terminal branches of the nasopalatine nerve traverse the canal to supply the anterior part of the hard palate and the internal surface of the gum. Branches of the **greater palatine nerve** also supply nasal mucosa [Fig. 5.121].

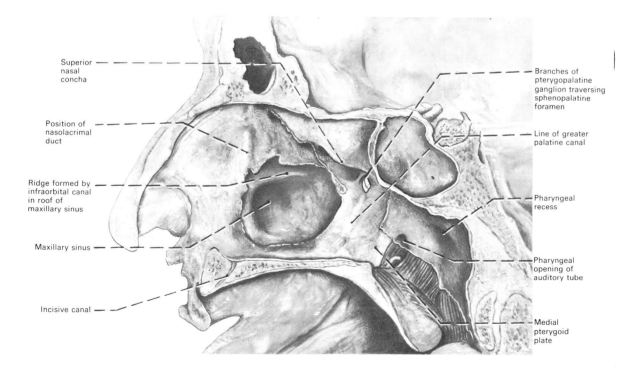

Fig. 5.118 The right maxillary sinus. The medial wall of the maxillary sinus and the mucous coat of the nasal cavity have been removed.

Section 5.15

The trigeminal nerve

The trigeminal nerve has three main branches. Of these, the ophthalmic and mandibular nerves have already been dissected, and the maxillary nerve should now be studied.

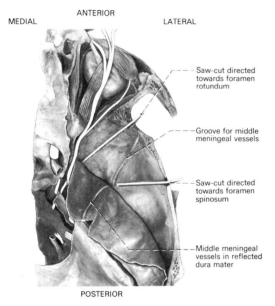

Fig. 5.119 **The right middle cranial fossa (showing saw-cuts to expose the maxillary nerve).** The dura mater has been reflected posteriorly and a card has been placed in each saw-cut.

Dissection of the maxillary nerve

When dissecting the cavernous sinus, you incised the dura mater of the middle cranial fossa in a sagittal plane, and stripped the dura mater medial to your incision [Fig. 5.111]. Now strip the dura mater lateral to the incision, as far back as the foramen spinosum. The **middle meningeal artery** and **veins,** which pass through this foramen, will be seen embedded in the dura mater [Fig. 5.119]. They groove the inner surface of the skull. The middle meningeal veins lie lateral to the artery (i.e. on its outer side) and are often completely embedded in bone for parts of their courses.

With the lateral side of the half-head uppermost, make a saw-cut in the frontal plane through the articular tubercle of the temporal bone, towards, but not quite reaching, the foramen spinosum. Make another saw-cut about 3 cm in front of the first, but passing slightly backwards as well as medially. The second cut should almost reach the foramen rotundum, which is situated just below the medial end of the superior orbital fissure [Fig. 5.30]. Remove the bone between the two saw-cuts with bone forceps, taking care not to fracture the body of the sphenoid bone. Remove the lateral margins of the foramen spinosum, foramen ovale, and foramen rotundum without damaging the structures passing through them. Remove what remains of the lateral

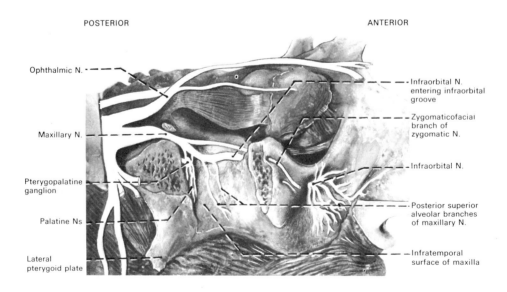

Fig. 5.120 **The right maxillary nerve.** Lateral view of the dissection after the greater wing of the sphenoid bone has been excised.

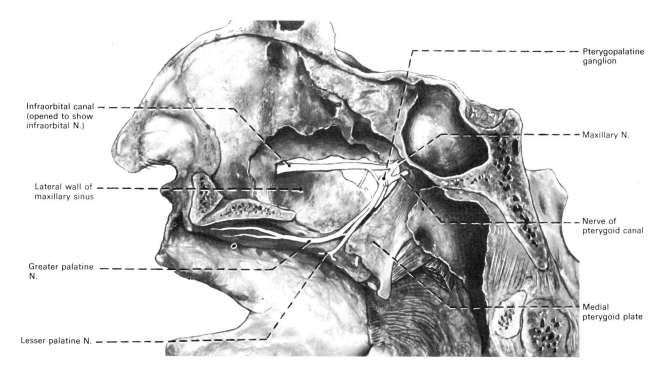

Pterygopalatine
ganglion

Infraorbital canal
(opened to show
infraorbital N.)

Maxillary N.

Lateral wall of
maxillary sinus

Nerve of
pterygoid canal

Greater palatine
N.

Medial
pterygoid plate

Lesser palatine N.

Fig. 5.121 **The right pterygopalatine ganglion.** Medial view of the dissection after the medial wall of the maxillary sinus and most of the palate have been excised. The palatine and infraorbital canals have been opened.

wall of the orbit and of the greater wing of the sphenoid lateral to these foramina. If the bone should fracture, first gently free all attached soft structures before removing the isolated bits of bone.

Now trace the maxillary nerve through the **foramen rotundum** into the **pterygopalatine fossa,** where you will see the nerve bending laterally to reach the **infraorbital groove** of the maxilla. Here it becomes the **infraorbital nerve** [Fig. 5.120]. By tearing the periosteum you should be able to find the two **posterior superior alveolar branches** of the maxillary nerve, which descend on to the infratemporal surface of the maxilla. They enter small canals in the bone and supply the molar teeth and the associated outer or labial surface of the gum.

Turn to the medial surface of the dissection. Again identify the **greater palatine nerve** emerging from the greater palatine foramen at the postero-lateral corner of the hard palate. Trace the nerve backwards by removing the medial wall of the canal in which it is running, the **greater palatine canal,** as far up as the sphenopalatine foramen [Fig. 5.121]. Bone forceps will be required to remove some of the hard palate at the lower end, but use dissecting forceps to nibble away the side wall of the nasal cavity. When you have removed the posterior part of the medial wall of the maxillary sinus, remove the anterior wall of the greater palatine canal. Now identify the ridge in the anterior part of the roof of the maxillary sinus caused by the **infraorbital canal** [Fig. 5.118]. Working from inside the sinus, use dissecting forceps

to remove the floor of the canal. Start at the front and work backwards. Finally, remove the upper half of the infratemporal surface of the maxilla, still working from inside the sinus.

You should now have little difficulty in seeing the whole course of the maxillary nerve from the trigeminal ganglion behind, to the infraorbital canal in front.

The pterygopalatine ganglion [Fig. 5.121]

Follow the greater palatine nerve upwards to the pterygopalatine fossa, and make out its connection with the maxillary nerve, removing any blood vessels which you may encounter. Most of these will be branches of the maxillary artery. Firm dissection will reveal that the greater palatine nerve is connected to a small mass of tissue, the pterygopalatine ganglion, which, in turn, is connected to the maxillary nerve by a pair of short nerves, the **pterygopalatine nerves** [Fig. 5.121]. These comprise the sensory fibres from the nasal and palatal mucosa. They traverse the ganglion after passing through its **posterior superior nasal branches,** the **greater** and **lesser palatine nerves,** and the **nasopalatine nerve.**

Now look posterior to the ganglion for a nerve which emerges from a canal, the **pterygoid canal,** in the root of the pterygoid process, and which runs forward to join the ganglion. This, the **nerve of the pterygoid canal,** carries parasympathetic fibres from the facial nerve [see p. 5.133] which relay in the ganglion. The nerve also contains some postganglionic sympathetic fibres from the internal carotid plexus. These autonomic fibres, of which only the parasympathetic synapse in the pterygopalatine ganglion, are distributed to the mucous glands of the nasal cavity and palate and, by a devious route, to the lacrimal gland.

The zygomatic nerve [Figs 5.120 and 5.122]

In addition to its posterior superior alveolar branches and the pterygopalatine nerves, the maxillary nerve also gives off a zygomatic nerve, which passes through the inferior orbital fissure along the lateral wall of the orbit and into the zygomatic bone, where it divides, sending one branch to the skin over the zygomatic bone [Fig. 5.122], and the other to the skin over the anterior part of the temporal fossa. Do not spend time dissecting these nerves.

The infraorbital nerve [Figs 5.120 and 5.122]

The infraorbital nerve, which is the continuation of the maxillary nerve, emerges from the infraorbital canal at the infraorbital foramen on the anterior surface of the maxilla. Turn to the face and dissect the nerve at this point. It will be found deep to the subcutaneous muscles which arise from the bone above the foramen. Trace its branches far enough to define the area to which they are distributed. They supply the skin of the lower eyelid and the side of the nose, and the skin and mucous coat of the upper lip [Fig. 5.122].

Within the infraorbital canal the infraorbital nerve gives off **middle** and **anterior superior alveolar branches,** which descend in the wall of the maxillary sinus and supply the premolar, canine, and incisor teeth. The anterior branch also supplies some nasal mucosa. These nerves need not be dissected. You should note that almost every branch of the maxillary nerve is accompanied by a branch of the maxillary artery which, itself, ends in the pterygopalatine fossa.

The mandibular nerve

Dissection of the mental nerve

The only important branch of the mandibular nerve which remains to be dissected is the mental nerve [Fig. 5.122]. It arises from the **inferior alveolar nerve** in the mandibular canal and emerges from the mental foramen on the superficial surface of the body of the mandible, below the second premolar tooth. You will find the nerve if you search deep to the posterior border of the depressor anguli oris muscle. It supplies the skin over the body of the mandible, the skin and mucous coat of the lower lip, and the external or labial

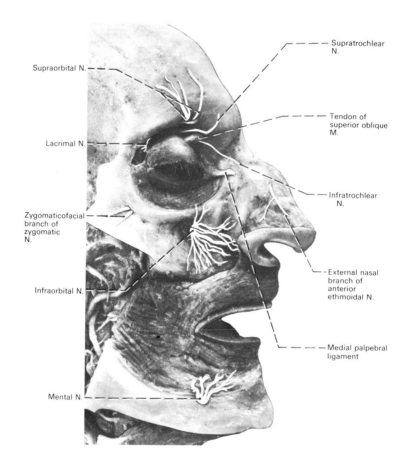

Fig. 5.122 Cutaneous nerves of the face and forehead. The scalp and the orbicularis oculi muscle have been removed.

Supraorbital N.

Lacrimal N.

Zygomaticofacial branch of zygomatic N.

Infraorbital N.

Mental N.

Supratrochlear N.

Tendon of superior oblique M.

Infratrochlear N.

External nasal branch of anterior ethmoidal N.

Medial palpebral ligament

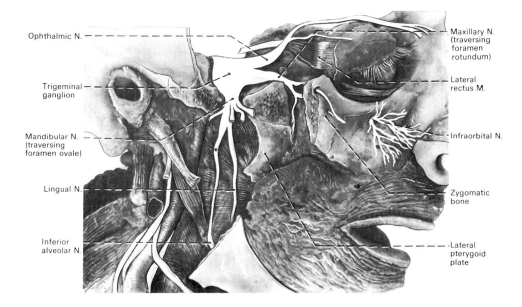

Fig. 5.123 The three parts of the right trigeminal nerve. Antero-lateral view of the dissection shown in Fig. 5.120.

surface of the gum related to the lower incisor and canine teeth.

The distribution of the trigeminal nerve

The distribution to muscles

You should now review the branches of the three parts of the trigeminal nerve and their distribution [Fig. 5.123]. Only the mandibular nerve carries any fibres from the motor root of the trigeminal nerve. You have seen all the muscles it supplies [see p. 5.68], except for one small muscle of the middle ear, the tensor tympani muscle.

The distribution to skin

The ophthalmic, maxillary, and mandibular nerves supply areas of skin on the face and scalp. The ophthalmic nerve does so through its branches, the lacrimal, supraorbital, supratrochlear, and infratrochlear nerves, and through the external nasal branch of the anterior ethmoidal nerve. The latter nerve is the terminal branch of the anterior ethmoidal nerve, and it supplies the skin of the lower half of the nose [Fig. 5.122]. The maxillary nerve divides into the infra-orbital nerve and the two branches of the zygomatic nerve, which innervate the intermediate part of the face, while the mandibular nerve supplies the region of the ear, and the lower part of the face, through the auriculotemporal, buccal, and mental nerves.

The distribution to mucosa

The three main nerves also supply the mucous coat of the nasal cavity and paranasal sinuses, and the mucous coat of the mouth. The ophthalmic nerve supplies that of the upper part of the nasal cavity and upper sinuses; the maxillary nerve, that of the lower and larger part of the nasal cavity, as well as the maxillary sinus and palate; and the mandibular nerve, the mucosa of the cheek and floor of the mouth.

The distribution to the teeth

The upper incisor, canine, and premolar teeth are supplied by the anterior and middle branches of the superior alveolar nerves; the upper molar teeth, by the posterior superior alveolar branches. All the lower teeth are supplied by the inferior alveolar nerve [Fig. 5.123].

The distribution to the gums

The internal or lingual surface of the gum related to the upper molars and premolars is supplied by the greater palatine nerve. The rest of this surface is supplied by the naso-palatine nerve. The labial surface of the gum is innervated posteriorly, lateral to the upper molar teeth, by the posterior superior alveolar nerves and anteriorly by the infraorbital nerve. The lingual nerve supplies all of the internal or lingual surface of the gum of the lower jaw. The labial surface of the gum of the lower jaw is supplied, behind, by the buccal nerve, and in front by the mental nerve.

The vertebral column and spinal medulla

The vertebral column supports the head, neck, and trunk. To it is attached the thoracic cage and, at its lower or sacral end, it articulates with the hip-bones to form the pelvis.

The subdivision of the vertebral column into vertebrae permits the column a certain degree of flexibility, which varies in the different parts of the column in accordance with the nature of the joints between the vertebrae.

In the articulated vertebral column, the combined vertebral foramina form the vertebral canal, through which the spinal medulla descends to the level of the lower border of the first lumbar vertebra. From the spinal medulla arise thirty-one pairs of spinal nerves grouped as follows: eight cervical nerves, twelve thoracic nerves, five lumbar nerves, five sacral nerves, and the coccygeal nerve. The spinal medulla and the roots of the spinal nerves are enclosed by the three layers of the meninges.

The parts of a vertebra and the principal features which distinguish the vertebrae belonging to the different sections of the vertebral column are dealt with on pages 3.2 to 3.4. The atlas and axis are described on pages 5.3 and 5.4. See if you are still able to tell a cervical vertebra from a thoracic vertebra, and a thoracic vertebra from a lumbar vertebra.

The deep muscles of the back

You have already dissected most of the muscles of the back of the neck, and you also encountered, at different stages of dissection, the group of muscles which form the erector spinae. This mass of muscle lies in the groove at the side of the spinous processes of the vertebrae, and is covered, particularly in the lumbar and sacral regions, by the posterior layer of the thoracolumbar fascia.

The erector spinae [Fig. 5.124]

Examine the erector spinae, without spending time on any details. Note that it has a thick broad superficial tendon by which it is attached to the spinous processes of the lumbar vertebrae, the median sacral crest, the lower end of the dorsal surface of the sacrum, the lateral sacral crest, which lies lateral to the dorsal sacral foramina, and the adjacent part of the iliac crest [Fig. 5.124]. From this U-shaped origin the muscle fibres ascend and split into three longitudinal columns which, medio-laterally, are called the spinalis, longissimus, and iliocostalis muscles. The **spinalis muscles** are

inserted into the spinous processes up to the level of the fifth cervical vertebra; the **longissimus muscles** into the transverse processes of the thoracic and cervical vertebrae. (One longissimus muscle is inserted into the skull, forming the **longissimus capitis muscle** [Fig. 5.124].) The **iliocostalis muscles** are inserted into the angles of the ribs and into the transverse processes of the cervical vertebrae. Each column of muscle is reinforced by fresh muscle fibres which arise where the lower fibres of the muscle column are inserted.

The transversospinalis muscle

Deep to the erector spinae lies the transversospinalis muscle, which is subdivided into three more muscle groups, dis-

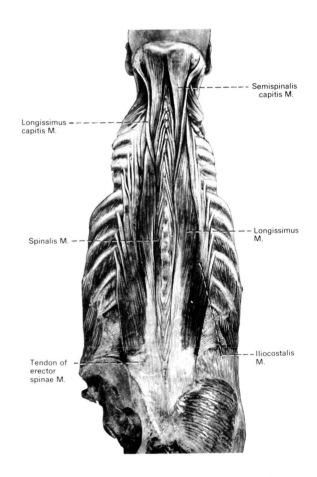

Longissimus capitis M.

Semispinalis capitis M.

Spinalis M.

Longissimus M.

Iliocostalis M.

Tendon of erector spinae M.

Fig. 5.124 The deep muscles of the back.

posed in layers and named: the **semispinalis, multifidus,** and **rotatores muscles.** The semispinalis group is the most superficial; the rotatores the deepest. Their fibres all lie more obliquely than those of the erector spinae, running upwards and medially from the transverse processes of the vertebrae to the spinous processes (or skull), the deeper being the more oblique and shorter. Except for the **semispinalis capitis** and **cervicis,** which you examined when you dissected the back of the neck [see p. 5.7], they do not warrant close study.

You have also already dissected the deep muscles of the suboccipital region [p. 5.6] and the splenius capitis [p. 5.5]. Remember that all the deep muscles of the back are supplied by the dorsal rami of the spinal nerves.

The spinal medulla, meninges, and nerves

To open the vertebral canal, remove the deep muscles of the back so as to expose the dorsal surface of the sacrum, and the spinous processes and laminae of the vertebral arches of the lumbar and thoracic vertebrae, preserving, where possible, the dorsal rami of one or two spinal nerves. Using a saw, cut through the laminae of the vertebral arches close to the medial side of the articular processes, slanting the saw slightly towards the midline [Fig. 5.125]. This operation will be made easier by flexing the back, but in the lumbar region it is probable that bone forceps, or a chisel and mallet, will have to be used. As far as possible, remove the spinous processes and laminae in one piece. Do not discard them. Make sure that the vertebral canal is opened as far as its inferior limit.

The epidural space

The spinal dura mater is now exposed [Fig. 5.126]. You will see that, unlike the dura mater of the brain, it is only loosely attached to the walls of the vertebral canal. Within the intervening epidural space lie networks of veins and minute arteries which, from above downwards, enter the canal from the vertebral artery, the costocervical trunk, and the posterior intercostal, lumbar, and lateral sacral arteries. The arteries supply the spinal medulla, the meninges and the vertebrae. The veins form what are called the **internal vertebral venous plexuses.** These ramify on the anterior as well as the posterior surface of the dura mater, and extend through the length of the vertebral canal. The plexuses drain blood from the vertebrae and spinal medulla, and have connections with the sinuses of the dura mater in the skull, a plexus of veins on the posterior surface of the laminae of the vertebral arches, and with the vertebral, posterior intercostal, lumbar, and lateral sacral veins.

The spinal dura mater [Fig. 5.126]

The spinal dura mater forms a membranous tube, which you can easily see is both firmly adherent to the margins of the foramen magnum above, and anchored along its length by

the spinal nerves as they emerge from it. The width of the tube corresponds to the width of the vertebral canal. Thus, it is wider in the cervical and lumbar parts of the canal than in the thoracic part.

Clean the outer surface of the dura mater and define its lower limit. In the sacral canal the dura mater rapidly tapers

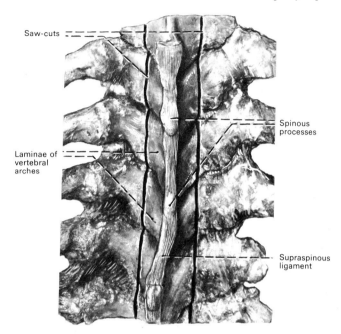

Fig. 5.125 Saw-cuts to open the vertebral canal.

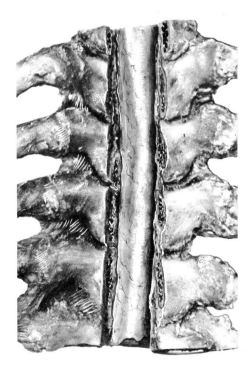

Fig. 5.126 Posterior view of the spinal dura mater. The spinous processes and the laminae of the vertebral arches have been excised.

to end at the level of the second or third sacral vertebra. You may be able to find a fibrous thread, the **filum of the spinal dura mater,** extending from the end of the tube of dura mater to the back of the coccyx [Fig. 5.127].

The spinal arachnoid

Using scissors, slit the dura mater open along its length. If you take great care you may not damage the underlying arachnoid. Peel the dura mater back to reveal the tube of arachnoid. The arachnoid is closely applied to the deep surface of the dura mater, the two being separated by a capil-

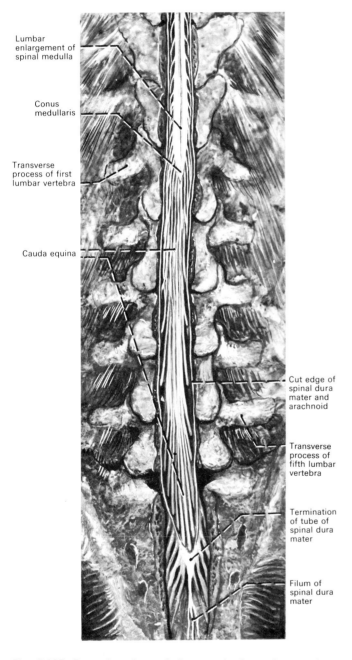

Fig. 5.127 Posterior view of the vertebral canal opened to show the cauda equina.

lary interval, the **subdural space.** The tube of arachnoid ends at the same level as the dural tube. It forms a loose investment for the spinal medulla, from which it is separated by the relatively wide **subarachnoid space.**

The spinal pia mater

Slit the arachnoid open along the midline, and expose the spinal medulla with its covering of vascular pia mater. The spinal pia mater is thicker than the pia mater of the brain, and firmly adheres to the spinal medulla. Down each side of the spinal medulla runs a series of fine tooth-like projections of pia mater called the **denticulate ligaments** [Fig. 5.128]. Carefully displace the spinal medulla to one side and identify one or two of these ligaments. Their lateral tips are attached to the deep surface of the arachnoid and dura mater midway between the exits of the adjacent spinal nerves. They help to anchor the spinal medulla in the dural tube, and are useful landmarks for the surgeon who wishes to make a selective division of the fibre tracts of the spinal medulla.

The spinal medulla [Figs 5.127 and 5.128]

The spinal medulla is continuous above with the medulla oblongata of the brain. Below, it ends by rapidly tapering at the level of the lower border of the first lumbar vertebra, though its pial covering is continued as a fibrous thread, the **filum terminale.** In infants, the spinal medulla extends

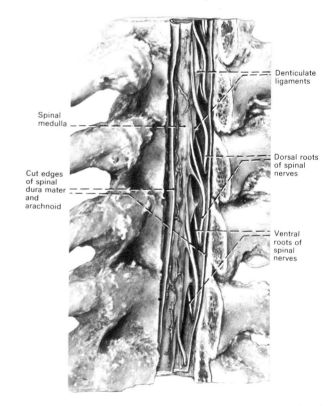

Fig. 5.128 The spinal medulla *in situ* (left posterior view).

5.122

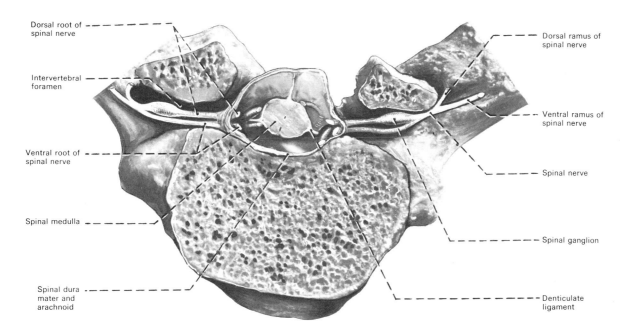

Dorsal root of spinal nerve

Intervertebral foramen

Ventral root of spinal nerve

Spinal medulla

Spinal dura mater and arachnoid

Dorsal ramus of spinal nerve

Ventral ramus of spinal nerve

Spinal nerve

Spinal ganglion

Denticulate ligament

Fig. 5.129 Transverse section of the thoracic part of the vertebral column and spinal medulla. The laminae of the vertebral arches and the rami communicantes have been removed.

down to the third lumbar vertebra. At the second or third sacral vertebra the arachnoid and dural tubes terminate, but the filum terminale continues, ensheathed by dura mater, to form the filum of the spinal dura mater. The tapered end of the spinal medulla is called the **conus medullaris** [Fig. 5.127].

In the mid-thoracic region the spinal medulla is roughly cylindrical in shape, but in both the cervical and lumbar regions it is expanded so that its breadth exceeds its antero-posterior diameter. These expansions are called the **cervical enlargement** and the **lumbar enlargement,** and correspond to the sites of attachment of the spinal nerves supplying the upper and lower limbs respectively.

The spinal nerves [Figs 0.3 and 5.129]

Each of the thirty-one pairs of spinal nerves is attached to the spinal medulla by a **ventral root,** which is motor (efferent) in function, and a **dorsal root** which is sensory (afferent) [Fig. 5.128]. Both roots split up into **rootlets** as they approach the spinal medulla. If you examine the spinal medulla as it lies *in situ*, you will see the dorsal roots of the spinal nerves entering the postero-lateral surface of the medulla on each side as a continuous series of rootlets arranged in a straight line. On each dorsal root is a ganglion, the **spinal ganglion,** in which are situated the cell bodies of the afferent nerve fibres. The cell bodies of the efferent fibres in the ventral roots are situated in the **anterior horn of grey matter** of the spinal medulla.

Follow the roots of one or two thoracic nerves out of their corresponding intervertebral foramina. To do this, re-move the bone of the articular processes with bone forceps.

As the roots pass laterally and downwards from the spinal medulla towards their points of exit from the vertebral canal, they pass through the arachnoid and dura mater, from both of which they receive coverings. The spinal nerves proper are formed by the junctions of the ventral and dorsal roots immediately beyond the spinal ganglia, most of which lie in the intervertebral foramina [Fig. 5.129]. The spinal nerves themselves are very short, and divide almost immediately into **ventral** and **dorsal rami.** On the nerves you are tracing, identify the ganglia on the dorsal roots; the separate exits from the dura mater of the ventral and dorsal roots; the formation of the spinal nerves, and their division into rami.

This general pattern is modified in certain parts of the spinal medulla. The **first** and **second cervical nerves** do not traverse intervertebral foramina. The first cervical nerve passes between the posterior arch of the atlas and the occipital bone, and the second emerges below the atlas, passing behind the superior articular process of the axis. The **sacral** and **coccygeal nerves** both form and divide within the sacral canal, and their rami traverse the pelvic sacral foramina, the dorsal sacral foramina, and the lower opening of the sacral canal, called the hiatus sacralis.

The cauda equina [Fig. 5.127]

The length and obliquity of the roots of the spinal nerves increase progressively from above downwards. Since the spinal medulla ends in the upper lumbar region, the lower lumbar, sacral, and coccygeal roots have to travel a relatively long way to their exits from the vertebral canal, within which they collectively form what is called the cauda equina.

Before turning from this part of your dissection, examine the spinal medulla and the cauda equina after you have removed them from the vertebral canal. To do this, divide the spinal medulla and the meninges horizontally at the top of the vertebral column, and cut the nerve roots outside the dura mater, close to the wall of the canal. Note the cervical and lumbar enlargements particularly.

The joints and ligaments of the vertebral column

Now examine the joints of the vertebral column. They consist of a series of cartilaginous joints between the bodies of the vertebrae, and a series of synovial joints between the articular processes of the vertebral arches.

The joints of the vertebral bodies

Between the adjacent surfaces of the bodies of the vertebrae are interposed **intervertebral discs** of fibrocartilage. You can see some of these in section in the neck. They form pads between the vertebrae and, all told, contribute about one-quarter of the length of the vertebral column.

The principal ligaments of the joints between the bodies of the vertebrae are the **anterior** and the **posterior longitudinal ligaments** [Fig. 5.130a and b]. The anterior longitudinal ligament is the ligament that covers the anterior surfaces of the vertebral bodies. It extends down the length of the

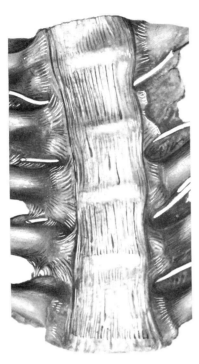

a. *The anterior longitudinal ligament* Anterior view of the bodies of thoracic vertebrae

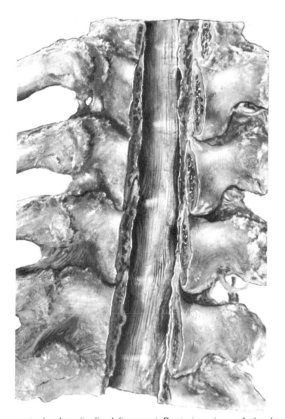

b. *The posterior longitudinal ligament* Posterior view of the bodies of thoracic vertebrae

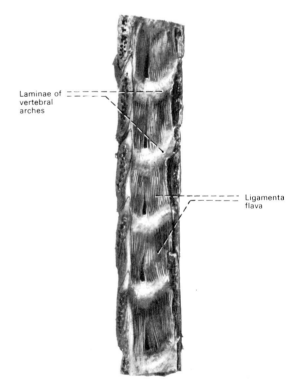

Laminae of vertebral arches

Ligamenta flava

c. *Anterior surface of a segment of spinous processes and laminae*

Fig. 5.130 Ligaments of the vertebral column.

5.124

vertebral column, from the occipital bone to the sacrum. It adheres to the intervertebral discs and to the upper and lower borders of the vertebrae. In a similar fashion the posterior longitudinal ligament extends throughout the vertebral canal and is attached to the posterior aspects of all the vertebral bodies except the atlas.

The joints of the vertebral arches

The articular processes of the vertebral arches form plane synovial joints with each other and are enclosed within articular capsules. In order to examine the ligaments between the arches, turn to the spinous processes and laminae which you removed in one piece when you opened the vertebral canal, and clean and define the ligaments connecting any two or three arches. The broad ligament connecting adjacent laminae is the **ligamentum flavum** [Fig. 5.130c]. This is made up of yellow elastic fibres, and assists the erector spinae muscles in controlling the movements of the vertebral column.

Tease out the **interspinous ligaments** between some of the spinous processes, and the **supraspinous ligament** which overlies the spinous processes. Between the tip of the spinous process of the seventh cervical vertebra (vertebra prominens) and the external occipital protuberance, the supraspinous ligament is represented by the **ligamentum nuchae,** which, as you already know [p. 1.7], is not a true ligament but a fibrous membrane which lies in the sagittal plane at the back of the neck. The **intertransverse ligaments** between adjacent transverse processes are the only ligaments of the vertebral arches which you have not seen. Do not spend time dissecting them.

Note that in the thorax are also found the joints of the heads of the ribs together with the costotransverse joints [see pp. 3.49–3.50].

The atlanto-occipital and atlantoaxial joints

The **atlanto-occipital joint,** the **median atlantoaxial joint,** and the **lateral atlantoaxial joint** and their ligaments require

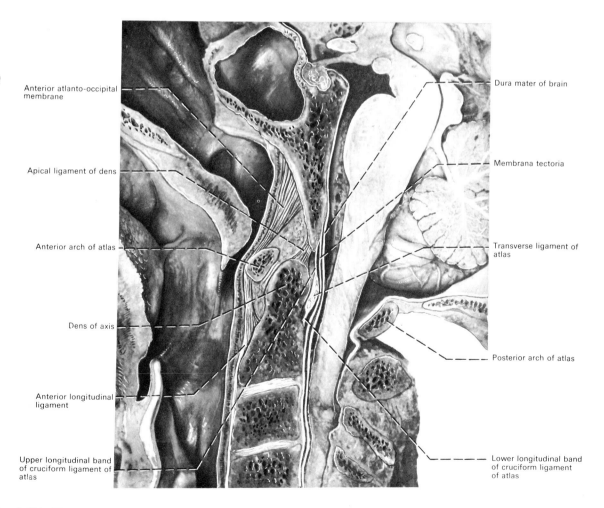

Anterior atlanto-occipital membrane

Apical ligament of dens

Anterior arch of atlas

Dens of axis

Anterior longitudinal ligament

Upper longitudinal band of cruciform ligament of atlas

Dura mater of brain

Membrana tectoria

Transverse ligament of atlas

Posterior arch of atlas

Lower longitudinal band of cruciform ligament of atlas

Fig. 5.131 The ligaments connecting the skull to the vertebral column. Part of a median section of the head and neck.

special study. Working on the medial surface of your dis-section, tease out the tissues between the anterior arch of the atlas and the occipital bone, and identify the ligamen-tous membrane that stretches between these bones. This is the **anterior atlanto-occipital membrane,** with the narrow upper end of the anterior longitudinal ligament in front of it [Fig. 5.131]. The **posterior atlanto-occipital membrane,** which is the broad ligamentous sheet attached to the pos-terior margin of the foramen magnum above, and the pos-terior arch of the atlas below, was divided when you traced the course of the vertebral artery.

Identify the dens of the axis projecting upwards behind the anterior arch of the atlas. Immediately behind its upper half you will find the cut surface of the thick **transverse liga-ment of the atlas,** which holds the dens in contact with the anterior arch of the atlas. Look carefully for the synovial cavity between the ligament and the dens, and for another cavity between the dens and the anterior arch of the atlas. These are the synovial cavities of the median atlantoaxial

joint. You may not be able to make out two small ligamen-tous bands which run longitudinally from the upper and lower borders of the transverse ligament to the occipital bone and to the body of the axis respectively. These two **longitudinal bands** and the transverse ligament are, collec-tively, called the **cruciform ligament of the atlas** [Fig. 5.132]. Do not spend time on their dissection.

Follow the cut edge of the posterior longitudinal ligament upwards, and you will find that, at its upper end, it passes from the back of the body of the axis through the foramen magnum to be attached to the occipital bone in front of the foramen. Between the axis and the occipital bone this liga-mentous sheet is called the **membrana tectoria.** There are three other ligaments which connect the axis to the occipital bone: a midline **apical ligament of the dens** [Fig. 5.131] attached to the tip of the dens, which you will find blending with the anterior atlanto-occipital membrane in front and the upper longitudinal band of the cruciform ligament behind; and a pair of stout **alar ligaments,** one on each side

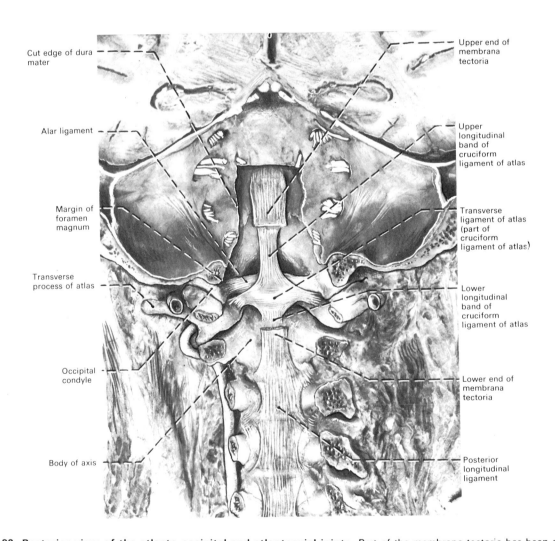

Fig. 5.132 Posterior view of the atlanto-occipital and atlantoaxial joints. Part of the membrana tectoria has been excised.

of the dens, which attach it to the medial borders of the occipital condyles [Fig. 5.132].

To examine the alar ligament, disarticulate the atlanto-occipital joint on the separated half of the head and neck. Begin by pulling away and separating from the vertebral column all the soft structures in front of it (the pharynx and oesophagus and the structures in front of them, together with the nerves of the neck, the sympathetic trunk, the carotid arteries, and the internal jugular vein). You will have to divide branches of cervical nerves, some suboccipital muscles, the meninges, and what may remain of the spinal medulla. As you cut the ligaments connecting the skull to the vertebral column, in order to complete the disarticulation, you will be able to identify the alar ligament.

The rectus capitis lateralis and anterior muscles

The disarticulation also allows you to identify the cut ends of two small muscles which are attached between the atlas and the skull. These muscles are the **rectus capitis lateralis,** which is inserted lateral to the occipital condyle, and the **rectus capitis anterior,** which is inserted in front of the condyle [Fig. 5.133]. Both arise from the transverse process of the atlas.

The articular surfaces of the atlanto-occipital, atlanto-axial, and of the other intervertebral joints are best studied on the skeleton. It is important to know how they are disposed, in order to appreciate the limitations which they impose on the movements of the vertebral column.

The structure of the intervertebral discs

To examine the structure of an intervertebral disc, disarticulate one of the intervertebral joints in the thorax or the lumbar region. The horizontal section through the intervertebral disc will reveal that it is made up of an outer ring of concentrically-disposed laminae of fibrous tissue and fibrocartilage (the **annulus fibrosus**), and a central mass of softer fibrogelatinous tissue (the **nucleus pulposus**).

Removal of the temporal bone

Apart from the dissection of the brain and eyeball for which you should be supplied with further specimens, there only remains the auditory and vestibular apparatus to dissect. To make its dissection easy, the temporal bone and the adjacent parts of the sphenoid and occipital bones have to be decalcified.

Remove the temporal bone from your specimen by mak-

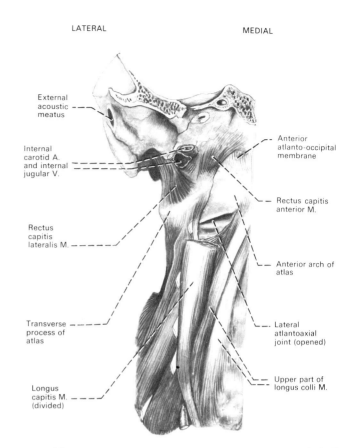

LATERAL · MEDIAL

External acoustic meatus · Anterior atlanto-occipital membrane · Internal carotid A. and internal jugular V. · Rectus capitis anterior M. · Rectus capitis lateralis M. · Anterior arch of atlas · Transverse process of atlas · Lateral atlantoaxial joint (opened) · Longus capitis M. (divided) · Upper part of longus colli M.

Fig. 5.133 Prevertebral muscles. Anterior view of the right half of a bisected vertebral column with part of the skull, and attached muscles.

ing two saw-cuts in the coronal plane, one in front of and the other behind the temporal bone. The anterior saw-cut should be a continuation of the cut that was directed towards the foramen spinosum [p. 5.116]. The posterior saw-cut should bisect the lateral margin of the foramen magnum. Divide the soft tissues that connect the temporal bone with the rest of your specimen, but do not detach them from the temporal bone.

The temporal bone is decalcified by immersing it in a 10 per cent solution of concentrated nitric acid for 7 to 14 days, the solution being changed twice weekly. To test for completion of decalcification, stick a needle into the bone. It should sink in when pressure is applied. When decalcification is complete, wash the specimen in running water for 24 hours and store it in a 50 per cent solution of alcohol in water.

Since decalcification takes about two weeks you may be supplied with a decalcified temporal bone taken from a cadaver dissected a year ago.

Section 5.17

The eyeball

You will be unable to obtain a clear idea of the internal structure of the eyeball from the eyes of the cadaver you are dissecting. You should therefore be given the fresh eyeball of an ox to examine.

The eye is a highly specialized sense organ designed to transmit visual stimuli to the brain. An optical system of transparent refracting media brings images of external objects to focus on a complex light-sensitive membrane, called the retina, at the back of the eyeball. From here nerve fibres pass to the brain through the optic nerve, conveying information about the images that have been received. Other parts of the eye are responsible for the focusing of the optical system, and for controlling the amount of light falling on the retina.

Dissection of the eyeball

Remove the muscles, fat, fascia, and **conjunctiva** from the ox's eyeball with which you have been provided. This is best done with a pair of scissors, starting behind where the **optic nerve** pierces the outer coat of the eyeball (the **sclera**), and working forwards and round the globe [Fig. 5.134]. The conjunctiva will have been cut close to the margin of the anterior transparent part of the outer coat of the eyeball (the **cornea).** As you clean the outer surface of the eyeball you may be able to see where the **ciliary arteries** and the **ciliary nerves** pierce the sclera close to the optic nerve [Fig.

5.105]. A little farther forwards you may also see the points of emergence of veins, the **venae vorticosae.**

The centre of the cornea in front is called the **anterior pole** of the eyeball; the corresponding point at the back of the eyeball is the **posterior pole;** the line joining the poles coincides with the **optic axis** of the eyeball [Fig. 5.134]. Note that the optic nerve pierces the sclera to the nasal (i.e. medial) side of the posterior pole. The widest circle round the eyeball with its plane at right-angles to the optic axis is called the **equator,** and planes passing through both poles are called **meridians** [Fig. 5.134].

Squeeze the eyeball gently, holding it with a finger and thumb at the poles. With a sharp scalpel make a short incision along the equator, cutting just deeply enough to penetrate the coats of the eyeball. Now place the eyeball with the cornea downwards, and insert one point of a fine pair of scissors into the incision you have made. Cut right round the equator, keeping the scissors close to the sclera, and steadying the eyeball by holding it by the optic nerve. Include in your cut the dark pigmented layer which you will find deep to the sclera, but be careful not to cut much more deeply than this. Gently remove the posterior half of the eyeball, turn it, and place it with the posterior pole downwards.

The coats of the eyeball [Fig. 5.135]

You can now see that the eyeball consists of a capsule con-

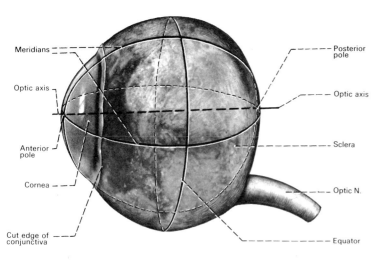

Fig. 5.134 Lateral view of the ox's eyeball.

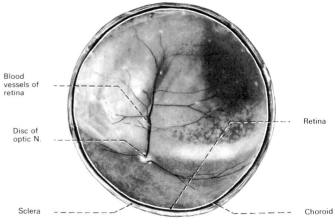

Fig. 5.135 Posterior half of the ox's eyeball (viewed from the front).

taining transparent material. Examine the posterior part of the capsule which you have just removed, and identify the three coats by which it is formed [Fig. 5.135]. The outermost coat is the **fibrous coat of the eyeball** of which the posterior five-sixths comprises the tough whitish **sclera.** The **internal coat of the eyeball** is the translucent grey **retina.** (It is transparent during life.) Between them lies the deeply pigmented **vascular coat of the eyeball.** In the posterior part of the eyeball the vascular coat is called the **choroid.**

The retina [Fig. 5.135]

You will see fine blood vessels ramifying over the retina [Fig. 5.135]. These are branches of the **central artery of the retina** and their accompanying veins. They radiate from a pale slightly-raised spot on the retina called the **disc of the optic nerve.** Though you cannot see them, it is to this point that the very numerous nerve fibres which arise in the retina converge. The fibres then pass through a number of minute holes in the sclera into the optic nerve, which you can see is attached to the eyeball at this point. The sclera is continuous with the tough fibrous **external sheath of the optic nerve,** which you will see clearly if you section the nerve with a sharp scalpel. The external sheath of the optic nerve is, in turn, continuous with the inner layer of the dura mater of the brain.

The retina can be studied in the living subject by means of an ophthalmoscope. (This is an exercise you should carry out in another part of your course.) Seen in this way, the human retina appears red, the coloration being due to the blood in the vessels of the inner layers of the choroid. The optic disc appears as a pale slightly-cupped elevation, the depression in the centre of the disc being called the **excavatio papillae.** Though the nerve fibres cannot be seen converging upon the disc, the branches of the retinal vessels are clearly visible as they ramify over the retina.

The central artery of the retina and its accompanying veins are the only blood vessels that supply the inner layers of the retina. Posterior to the eyeball, they lie, for part of their course, within the fibrous external sheath of the optic nerve [Fig. 5.141], which forms a relatively indistensible sheath for the vessels. As a result, the venous drainage of the retina is liable to become obstructed by an increase in the pressure of the contents of the sheath. This frequently occurs when there is a rise in the pressure of the cranial contents (e.g. when there is a tumour of the brain). It results in a swelling of the optic disc, called papilloedema.

At the point where the optic axis intersects the retina, there is a specialized area responsible for 'central' vision. In the human eye this appears as an oval yellowish area, the **macula,** in the centre of which is a minute depression, the **fovea centralis.** The ox's retina has no fovea centralis, and you will not be able to recognize the macula, because it is both diffuse and lacks a yellow colour. Note that the optic disc is insensitive to light and that it lies, in the human

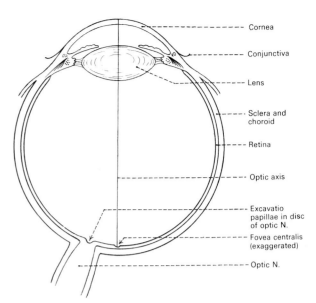

Fig. 5.136 Schematic horizontal section of the right human eyeball (viewed from above).

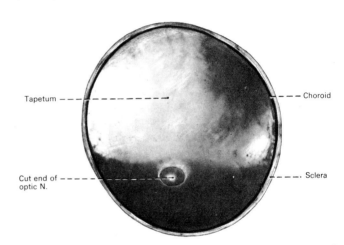

Fig. 5.137 Posterior half of the ox's eyeball after the removal of the retina (viewed from the front).

eye, on the nasal (medial) side of the optic axis [Fig. 5.136]. There is consequently a **'blind spot'** in the temporal half of the visual field.

Lift the retina with a pair of forceps, and you will find that it is attached to the choroid only at the optic disc. Sever this attachment and remove the retina. You can now examine the choroid, which is composed chiefly of blood vessels which supply the outer layers of the retina. The most obvious feature of the choroid of the ox is a roughly semicircular and irridescent area called the tapetum [Fig. 5.137]. Although this is a common feature in vertebrate eyes, it is not present in man.

The lens and the vitreous body [Fig. 5.139]

Now put to one side the posterior part of the eyeball and look at the anterior part, which you left lying with the

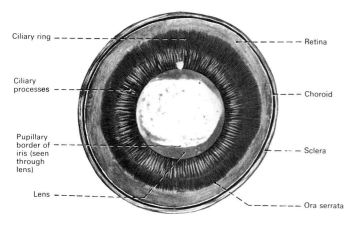

Ciliary ring

Ciliary processes

Pupillary border of iris (seen through lens)

Lens

Retina

Choroid

Sclera

Ora serrata

Fig. 5.138 Anterior half of the ox's eyeball (viewed from behind).

cornea downwards. It is filled with a mass of clear watery jelly, called the **vitreous body,** through which you will see the sharply-defined circular margin of the lens of the eye [Fig. 5.138]. Surrounding the lens is a frill of meridionally-placed deeply-pigmented ridges, the **ciliary processes.** Encircling the frill of ciliary processes, called the **corona ciliaris,** is a finely-grooved pigmented band called the **ciliary ring,** whose peripheral border runs into the anterior part of the retina. The indented margin between the ciliary ring and the retina is called the **ora serrata.**

With a quick movement turn the anterior part of the eyeball over, and gently lift the cornea and sclera, carefully separating them from the vitreous body and lens with the handle of a scalpel. The vitreous body and lens will be left behind, with the lens uppermost. Lay the cornea, sclera and their attached structures aside for later study.

The vitreous body consists of a mesh of very fine transparent fibres, the **vitreous stroma,** filled with fluid, the **vitreous humour,** which is enclosed within a thin capsular membrane, the **vitreous membrane.** The vitreous body of your specimen will be distorted, but the vitreous membrane prevents it from collapsing completely.

You will see that the anterior surface of the lens projects further anteriorly than the vitreous body [Fig. 5.139]. The

posterior surface lies in a depression in the vitreous body, called the **hyaloid fossa.** The lens is held in position by the **ciliary zonule,** which may be regarded as a thickened part of the vitreous membrane encircling the lens. The position of the zonule is clearly marked by a layer of pigment, which is adherent to it and which was detached from the ciliary processes when the cornea and sclera were removed. The ciliary zonule splits into two layers: a thin posterior layer which lines the hyaloid fossa, and a thicker anterior layer which is attached to the lens.

On one side depress the margin of the lens. Then, on the opposite and elevated side, cut with fine scissors at the inner border of the ring of pigment, between the lens and the vitreous body. Cut more than halfway round the perimeter of the lens. In this way you will sever the connection between the ciliary zonule and the lens, and you will also have divided the highly elastic **capsule of the lens,** which can now be peeled off the anterior surface of the **lens substance.**

Remove the substance of the lens. Divide it in half with a sharp scalpel; you may then see that it has a faint laminar structure. Pick up one half with your fingers and note that the lens substance has a soft sticky **cortex** and a firmer centre, or **nucleus.** Squeeze it and you will find that the lens substance is plastic, but not elastic. The shape of the lens is normally determined by its elastic capsule and not by the structure of its substance.

The transparent membrane lining the hyaloid fossa of the vitreous body can be clearly seen. Pick it up with a pair of forceps and lift up the vitreous body, so demonstrating that the vitreous humour is contained by the vitreous membrane.

The iris and the chambers of the eyeball [Figs 5.140 and 5.141]
Now gently wash the inner surface of the anterior part of the eyeball in running water, and remove the many pigment cells that will have been scattered by your dissection. The anterior part of the retina should also be detached and removed at the same time.

Identify the **iris** and note that in the ox's eye the pupil is oval, and not circular as in the human eye. Using scissors divide the anterior half of the eyeball along a meridian. You

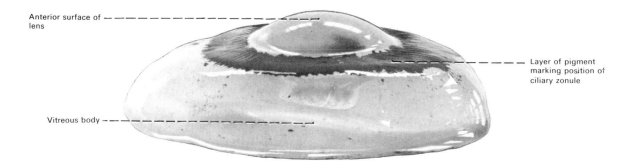

Anterior surface of lens

Layer of pigment marking position of ciliary zonule

Vitreous body

Fig. 5.139 The lens and the vitreous body. The vitreous body is lying on a plane surface and its shape is therefore distorted.

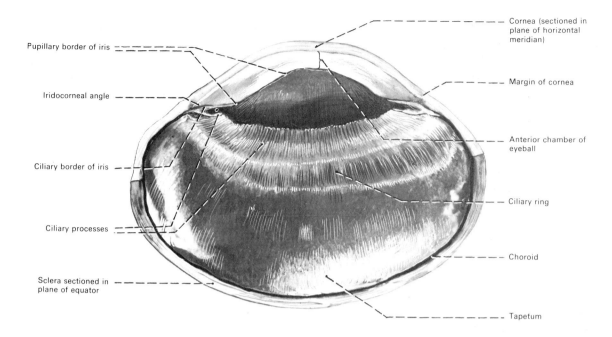

Pupillary border of iris

Iridocorneal angle

Ciliary border of iris

Ciliary processes

Sclera sectioned in plane of equator

Cornea (sectioned in plane of horizontal meridian)

Margin of cornea

Anterior chamber of eyeball

Ciliary ring

Choroid

Tapetum

Fig. 5.140 Oblique view of an anterior quadrant of the ox's eyeball. The lens, vitreous body, and retina have been removed and loose pigment cells have been washed away.

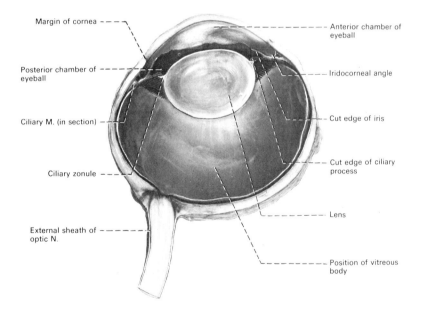

Margin of cornea

Posterior chamber of eyeball

Ciliary M. (in section)

Ciliary zonule

External sheath of optic N.

Anterior chamber of eyeball

Iridocorneal angle

Cut edge of iris

Cut edge of ciliary process

Lens

Position of vitreous body

Fig. 5.141 Meridional section of the ox's eyeball through the optic nerve. The vitreous body has been removed.

can now see that the sclera is continuous with the cornea at the **margin of the cornea** [Fig. 5.140]. The cornea has a smaller radius of curvature than the sclera, and so it appears as a low dome projecting forwards in front of the sclera. The junction of the two is marked by a slight furrow called the **sulcus sclerae.** The most superficial layer of cells, or **anterior corneal epithelium,** is continuous with the conjunctiva just beyond the margin of the cornea [see p. 5.97].

Examine the cut surface of the iris. If the lens were in position, you would find that the free **pupillary border of the iris**

rests on the anterior surface of the lens. The iris partially subdivides the space between the lens and cornea into the **anterior** and **posterior chambers of the eyeball** [Fig. 5.141] which intercommunicate through the pupil. The lens and the ciliary zonule form the posterior boundary of the posterior chamber of the eyeball.

The muscles of the iris

Smooth muscle fibres in the iris regulate the amount of light falling on the retina by opening (dilating) or closing constricting) the pupil. The muscle fibres are arranged in two groups: one forming the **dilator of the pupil,** the other forming the **sphincter of the pupil.** The dilator muscle of the pupil is supplied by sympathetic fibres; the sphincter by parasympathetic fibres, both sets of nerve fibres running in the ciliary nerves [p. 5.106]. The outer or **ciliary border of the iris** is attached to the ring of ciliary processes. In section you will see that the blunt free margins of the ciliary processes just overlap the ciliary border of the iris. The iris, the ciliary processes, the ciliary ring, and the choroid are all parts of the vascular coat of the eyeball.

The aqueous humour

The ciliary processes form a circumferential boundary to the posterior chamber of the eyeball, into which they secrete a watery fluid, the aqueous humour, which slowly circulates through the pupil into the anterior chamber, where it is absorbed into veins in the angle between the anterior surface of the ciliary border of the iris and the cornea. Identify this, the **iridocorneal angle** [Fig. 5.141]. It forms the circumferential boundary of the anterior chamber and lies close to the margin of the cornea.

Occasionally the aqueous humour is absorbed more slowly than it is secreted, and there is a consequent rise in intra-ocular pressure which causes great pain. The condition is known as glaucoma.

The ciliary body [Fig. 5.142]

Light entering the eye passes through four refracting media: the cornea, the aqueous humour, the lens, and the vitreous body. It becomes focused on to the retina by changes in the shape of the lens brought about by the contraction or relaxation of a ring of smooth muscle fibres, the ciliary muscle. The **ciliary muscle,** the **ciliary ring,** and the **ciliary processes** comprise the ciliary body. If you examine the cut surface of the meridional section with a hand lens, you should see the ciliary muscle as a triangular pale zone behind the iridocorneal angle and between the ciliary processes and the sclera [Fig. 5.141]. Carefully peel the choroid off the deep surface of the sclera, using the handle of your scalpel. Continue forwards to the margin of the cornea, when the choroid, ciliary

body, and iris will come away in one piece. Examine the outer surface of the ciliary body, and you will see the pale circular band of the ciliary muscle.

The ciliary muscle comprises inner **circular fibres** and outer **meridional fibres** [Fig. 5.142]. The former lie close to the peripheral border of the iris; the latter are attached anteriorly to the deep surface of the sclera, immediately behind the margin of the cornea at the iridocorneal angle. The meridional fibres pass backwards from their origin to be inserted into the ciliary processes and ring, which are, in turn, attached to the ciliary zonule. When the ciliary muscle relaxes, the pressure of the ocular contents keeps the ciliary zonule stretched, and the lens is thus held under tension. Contraction of both parts of the ciliary muscle constricts the ciliary ring and processes, drawing them towards the periphery of the lens. This movement slackens both the ciliary zonule and the capsule of the lens, whose elasticity then causes the plastic lens to assume a more spherical shape. This, in turn, shortens the focal length of the optical system of the eye and brings images of near objects into focus on the retina. When the ciliary muscle relaxes, the intra-ocular pressure again makes the ciliary zonule tense, and the lens flattens. This process of focusing the eye is called accommodation.

Parasympathetic fibres from the oculomotor nerve supply the ciliary muscle through the ciliary ganglion and the short ciliary nerves. It is useful to remember that these fibres supply both the ciliary muscle and the sphincter of the pupil, and that the two muscles often contract simultaneously, so that accommodation for near objects is usually accompanied by constriction of the pupil.

The ciliary nerves [Fig. 5.105]

The **long** and **short ciliary nerves** pierce the sclera close to the optic nerve and run forwards between the sclera and choroid in grooves on the inner surface of the sclera. Peel the choroid off the sclera of the posterior part of the eyeball and wash the inner surface of the sclera of both the posterior and anterior parts of the eyeball in running water. If you now examine the sclera, you should find either the nerves themselves or, at least, the grooves in which they run. Trace the nerves forwards and you may be able to see that they branch to form a plexus in the region of the ciliary body, from which nerve fibres run to the ciliary muscle, the iris and the cornea. Both groups of ciliary nerves contain sensory fibres from the nasociliary nerve to supply the sclera and cornea, and sympathetic fibres from the internal carotid plexus to supply the blood vessels of the eye. The sympathetic fibres to the dilator of the pupil run in the long ciliary nerves. The parasympathetic fibres to the sphincter of the pupil and the ciliary muscle run from the ciliary ganglion through the short ciliary nerves. Refer back to pages 5.106 and 5.107 for a description of the course of these nerves outside the eyeball.

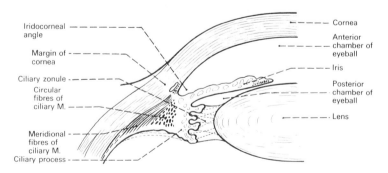

Fig. 5.142 Schematic meridional section of the ciliary body and adjacent structures of the human eyeball.

The auditory and vestibular apparatus

The ear is divided into three parts: the **external ear,** which consists of the auricle and the external acoustic meatus; the **middle ear** or tympanic cavity, which is a narrow air-filled chamber lying between the external and internal ear; and the **internal ear** [Fig. 5.143], which comprises a complex system of canals in the petrous part of the temporal bone, called the bony labyrinth. The labyrinth is lined by periosteum, and filled with fluid called perilymph. Within the bony labyrinth, and mostly surrounded by perilymph, lie membranous tubes and sacs, the membranous labyrinth, which are filled with endolymph, and in which are located the receptors for the sensations of hearing and balance.

Sound waves enter the ear through the external acoustic meatus and impinge on a thin tense membrane, the **tympanic membrane,** which closes the inner end of the meatus and separates it from the tympanic cavity. The vibration of the membrane is transmitted across the tympanic cavity by a bridge of three small jointed bones, the **auditory ossicles,** to a point on the medial wall of the cavity where the cavity is separated from the perilymph of the labyrinth by only a thin membrane. The vibration set up in the fluid of the labyrinth stimulates receptors in the cochlea which are supplied by fibres of the cochlear part of the vestibulocochlear nerve, along which the resulting nervous impulses pass from the inner ear through the internal acoustic meatus to the brain.

The 'balance' receptors in the internal ear are stimulated when the endolymph in the membranous labyrinth moves either as the position of the head is changed, or as a result of gravitational pull. They are the terminal elements of the vestibular part of the vestibulocochlear nerve.

The **tympanic cavity** develops as an off-shoot of the cavity of the nasal part of the pharynx and maintains its connection with the latter through the auditory tube. This connection serves to equalize the pressures on the two sides of the tympanic membrane. From a backward extension of the tympanic cavity, called the mastoid antrum, arise numerous small air-spaces, the mastoid cells. The mastoid cells, mastoid antrum, tympanic cavity, and auditory tube are all lined with a mucous coat which is continuous at the pharyngeal opening of the auditory tube with the mucous coat of the nasal part of the pharynx. This mucous coat is supplied by the tympanic nerve, a branch of the glosso-pharyngeal nerve, the same cranial nerve which supplies

most of the mucous coat of the oral and nasal parts of the pharynx [p. 5.88]. Apart from the auditory and vestibular (balance) apparatus, the only other important anatomical feature of the temporal bone which you will now study is the course followed by the facial nerve from the internal acoustic meatus to the stylomastoid foramen.

Dissection of the decalcified temporal bone

You can carry out the following dissection of the temporal bone on a specimen which has been decalcified by treatment with acid [p. 5.127]. You will need a magnifying glass to see some of the structures your dissection displays.

The petrosal nerves [Fig. 5.144]

Refer to a skull in order to orientate your specimen correctly. In the skull, identify on the upper surface of the petrous part of the temporal bone a small foramen from which a fine groove runs antero-medially to the foramen lacerum. The small foramen and groove lodge the **greater petrosal nerve** [Fig. 5.144], which leaves the facial nerve in the temporal bone and runs forwards across the foramen lacerum to join sympathetic fibres from the internal carotid plexus, and so form the **nerve of the pterygoid canal** [see p. 5.117].

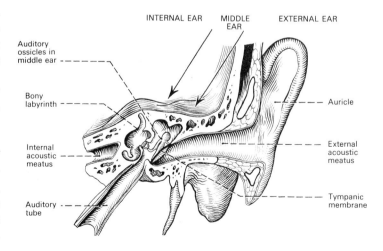

Fig. 5.143 Schematic section through the left ear. The arrows indicate the boundaries between the internal, middle, and external ear.

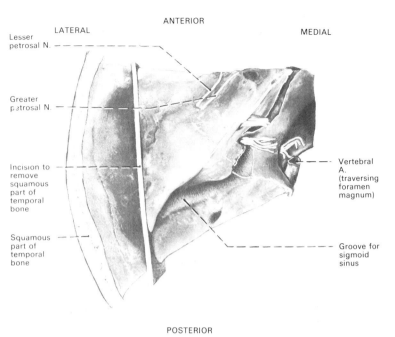

ANTERIOR

LATERAL — MEDIAL

Lesser petrosal N.

Greater petrosal N.

Incision to remove squamous part of temporal bone

Squamous part of temporal bone

Vertebral A. (traversing foramen magnum)

Groove for sigmoid sinus

POSTERIOR

Fig. 5.144 Superior view of a decalcified left temporal bone. A card has been placed in the incision used to remove the squamous part.

Examine the same region of your decalcified specimen. With the help of a pair of fine dissecting forceps you should be able to identify the greater petrosal nerve. It is difficult to separate the nerve cleanly from the overlying dura mater.

You should also be able to isolate another nerve lateral to, and almost parallel with, the greater petrosal nerve. This, the **lesser petrosal nerve,** emerges from another small opening in the temporal bone. It runs towards the foramen ovale

through which it passes to the **otic ganglion** (it sometimes emerges from the skull through a separate unnamed canal). This very small ganglion, for which you should not search, is situated just below the foramen ovale and deep to the mandibular nerve. It is a relay station for parasympathetic fibres from the **tympanic nerve,** which reach the ganglion through the lesser petrosal nerve. The postganglionic fibres from the ganglion are distributed to the parotid gland through the auriculotemporal nerve [see p. 5.68].

The external ear and tympanic membrane

With a sharp scalpel make a vertical incision parallel to the median plane, in order to remove the squamous part of the temporal bone of your decalcified specimen [Fig. 5.144]. Start anteriorly, close to the medial surface of the squamous part, and extend the cut backwards to cross the beginning of the sigmoid sinus. Use a pair of scissors to remove the anterior wall of the **external acoustic meatus,** taking care not to damage the tympanic membrane which closes off the medial end of the meatus [Fig. 5.145]. As you do this you will remove most of the **tympanic part of the temporal bone.** Clear out any wax and examine the **tympanic membrane,** which is now exposed to view. Note that the outer surface of the tympanic membrane is concave and that the membrane lies obliquely to the sagittal plane, so that it faces not only sideways but also downwards and forwards. To the deepest point of the concavity of the membrane (the **umbo** of the tympanic membrane) is attached the lower end of a slender spicule of bone, the **handle of the malleus,** which runs upwards and slightly forwards almost to the circumference of the membrane [Fig. 5.146].

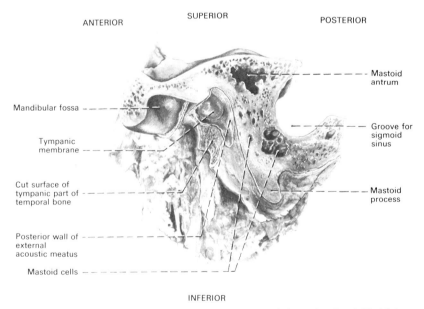

ANTERIOR — SUPERIOR — POSTERIOR

Mandibular fossa

Tympanic membrane

Cut surface of tympanic part of temporal bone

Posterior wall of external acoustic meatus

Mastoid cells

Mastoid antrum

Groove for sigmoid sinus

Mastoid process

INFERIOR

Fig. 5.145 The external acoustic meatus and the tympanic membrane. Lateral view of a decalcified left temporal bone after the removal of its squamous part and the excision of the anterior wall of the external acoustic meatus.

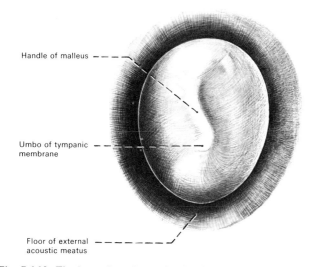

Handle of malleus --- --

Umbo of tympanic --- --
membrane

Floor of external --- --- --- --/
acoustic meatus

Fig. 5.146 The lateral surface of the left tympanic membrane.

The middle ear

Behind the external acoustic meatus, the temporal bone and its mastoid process are honeycombed with the small **mastoid cells,** which vary in size and extent from one temporal bone to another. These cells communicate with the large cavity, called the **mastoid antrum,** which you can see just posterior to the external acoustic meatus [Fig. 5.145]. Antero-medially the antrum communicates with the **tympanic cavity.** Examine the squamous part of the temporal bone

which you removed, and try to identify on it the lateral wall of the mastoid antrum. Note how closely this wall is related to the superficial surface of the bone. The antrum lies deep to a depression immediately above and behind the external acoustic meatus. This depression is sometimes called the **suprameatal triangle.** It is a useful guide to the surgeon.

The tympanic cavity [Fig. 5.147]

To open up the tympanic cavity use a pair of fine dissecting forceps to remove the bony roof of the mastoid antrum. Carefully follow the cavity forwards and medially, removing the roof as you proceed. As you do this, the small **auditory ossicles** will come into view. At this stage the most easily recognized bone is the small spherical **head of the malleus** [Fig. 5.147]. It lies in the **epitympanic recess** (or upper part) of the tympanic cavity.

Complete the removal of the thin bony roof of the tympanic cavity, using the anterior margin of the tympanic membrane as a guide to the anterior limit of the cavity. The roof of the tympanic cavity forms part of the floor of the middle cranial fossa, and is called the **tegmen tympani.**

Antero-medially the tympanic cavity is continuous with the **bony part of the auditory tube.** Do not try to open up the auditory tube. A very small slender muscle, the **tensor tympani,** is attached to the walls of a canal immediately above and in line with this part of the tube. Posteriorly, the tendon

LATERAL   ANTERIOR   MEDIAL

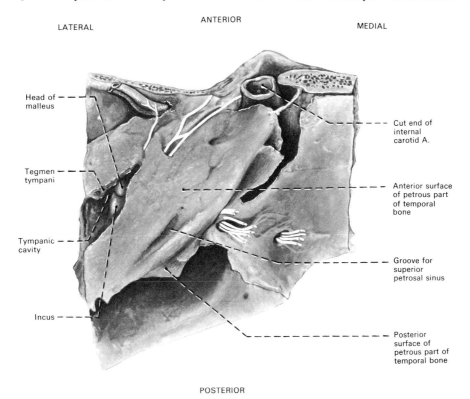

Head of --- --
malleus

Tegmen --- --
tympani

Tympanic --- --
cavity

Incus --- ---

Cut end of
internal
carotid A.

Anterior surface
of petrous part
of temporal
bone

Groove for
superior
petrosal sinus

Posterior
surface of
petrous part
of temporal
bone

POSTERIOR

Fig. 5.147 The tympanic cavity. Superior view of a decalcified left temporal bone after the removal of the squamous part, and part of the tegmen tympani.

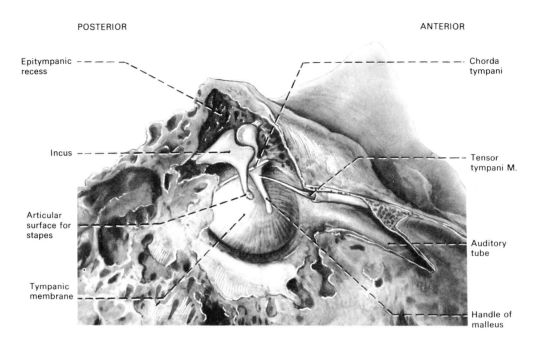

POSTERIOR   ANTERIOR

Epitympanic recess — Chorda tympani

Incus — Tensor tympani M.

Articular surface for stapes

Tympanic membrane — Auditory tube

Handle of malleus

Fig. 5.148 The lateral wall of the left tympanic cavity (looking laterally).

of this muscle turns laterally and is inserted into the malleus below its head [Fig. 5.148]. Try to identify the tendon, and then pass a stiff bristle, or a piece of fine wire, into the tympanic cavity forwards and medially below the tendon of the tensor tympani. The wire should traverse the auditory tube. If enough of the mucous coat of the pharynx has been left on the specimen to allow you to identify the **pharyngeal opening of the auditory tube,** you will be able to confirm that the two ends of the tube are continuous.

Look into the tympanic cavity through the opening you have made in its roof, and examine more closely the head of the malleus. Note that it articulates with another ossicle, the **incus** [Fig. 5.147]. Look for a downwardly-projecting process of the incus which articulates in turn with a very fine stirrup-shaped bone, the **stapes,** whose foot-piece, the **base of the stapes,** is applied to the medial wall of the tympanic cavity.

To study the tympanic cavity more closely, use a sharp scalpel to divide the specimen vertically down the middle of the cavity. By so doing you separate the medial and lateral walls. As you do this try to cut across the chain of ossicles at the articulation between the incus and the stapes.

The lateral wall of the tympanic cavity [Fig. 5.148]
First examine the lateral wall of the tympanic cavity [Fig. 5.148]. You will see that the tympanic membrane, to which the handle of the malleus is attached, forms almost the whole of the lateral wall. You may be able to see the insertion of the tensor tympani muscle into the upper end of the handle. The muscle is supplied by the mandibular nerve. Above the insertion of the tensor tympani you should see

a fine thread-like structure crossing the medial side of the malleus in an antero-posterior direction. This is the **chorda tympani** which, in your dissection of the infratemporal region, you saw joining the lingual nerve [p. 5.68]. Do not attempt to follow the course of the chorda tympani through the temporal bone, but note that the nerve arises from the facial nerve a short distance above the stylomastoid foramen, and that it runs upwards and forwards through a narrow canal to enter the tympanic cavity, across which it passes just medial to the upper part of the tympanic membrane and the malleus. The chorda tympani enters another narrow canal near the anterior margin of the membrane, and passes along the lateral wall of the auditory tube, to emerge from the petrotympanic fissure at the medial end of the tympanosquamous fissure [see p. 5.59].

The medial wall of the tympanic cavity [Fig. 5.149]
Now identify the stapes in the medial wall of the tympanic cavity [Fig. 5.149]. Its base fits into a window, the **fenestra vestibuli,** in the medial wall of the tympanic cavity. If you use a magnifying glass you should have no difficulty in seeing the minute thread-like tendon of the **stapedius muscle,** which is attached to the stapes near its articulation with the incus. Posteriorly, the tendon emerges from the tip of a very small projection of bone called the **pyramidal eminence,** within which the stapedius muscle is lodged. The stapedius and tensor tympani muscles usually act together to damp the more intense vibrations of the ossicles caused by loud sounds.

The relatively large bulge of the medial wall of the tympanic cavity below the stapes is called the **promontory.** You may be able to make out one or two fine strands of the **tympanic plexus** of the glossopharyngeal nerve on the surface of the promontory. The lesser petrosal nerve is a branch of this plexus.

In one of the depressions below and behind the promontory is another small bony window, the **fenestra cochleae,** which is closed by a membrane. You will not find it easy to identify this window correctly. The slight antero-posterior ridge above the stapes is produced by the canal for the facial nerve, and is called the **prominence of the facial canal.** The bone here is so thin that the nerve can be seen within the canal. The elevation above and behind the facial canal lies in the medial wall of the **aditus to the antrum** (the entrance to the mastoid antrum), and forms the **prominence of the lateral semicircular canal.**

Relations of the tympanic cavity

It is necessary to know the relations of the tympanic cavity and its extensions in order to understand the possible complications which may arise as a result of the spread of infection from an inflammation of the middle ear, which is a common condition in children. Note that only the thin tegmen tympani separates the tympanic cavity and mastoid antrum from the meninges of the middle cranial fossa and the temporal lobe of the brain. If you pick up the internal

jugular vein in the jugular fossa, below and behind the tympanic cavity, you will see that only a thin lamina of bone separates the tympanic cavity and mastoid antrum from this important vein. The antrum is also related, posteriorly, to the sigmoid sinus. Below and in front of the tympanic cavity it is likely that the lateral wall of the carotid canal has been shaved off. Identify the internal carotid artery inside its canal and note that this, too, is closely related to the floor of the tympanic cavity. You have already noted the relation of the mastoid antrum to the suprameatal triangle on the superficial surface of the temporal bone.

The intrapetrous part of the facial nerve

Examine the facial and vestibulocochlear nerves where they enter the **internal acoustic meatus**; the facial nerve is the one that is uppermost. Now remove the roof of the internal acoustic meatus with scissors [Fig. 5.150]. Insert one blade of the scissors into the meatus, keeping it above the nerves and applied to the anterior wall of the meatus, and cut in the direction of the foramen from which the greater petrosal nerve emerges. Make a similar cut with the scissors applied to the posterior wall of the meatus, again directing your cut to the same foramen. Remove the piece of bone you have isolated, and then use dissecting forceps to trace the course

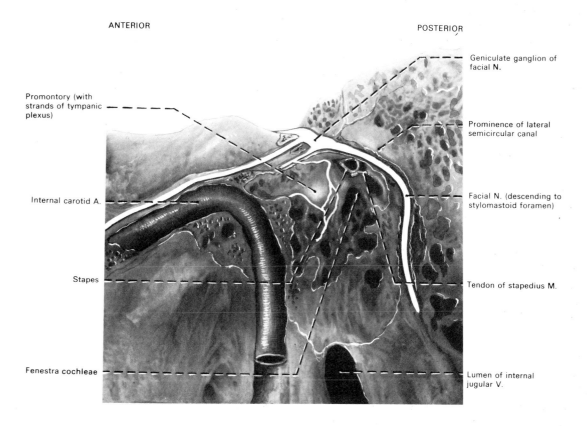

ANTERIOR   POSTERIOR

Promontory (with strands of tympanic plexus)

Internal carotid A.

Stapes

Fenestra cochleae

Geniculate ganglion of facial N.

Prominence of lateral semicircular canal

Facial N. (descending to stylomastoid foramen)

Tendon of stapedius M.

Lumen of internal jugular V.

Fig. 5.149 The medial wall of the left tympanic cavity (looking medially). The internal carotid artery and the facial nerve have been exposed.

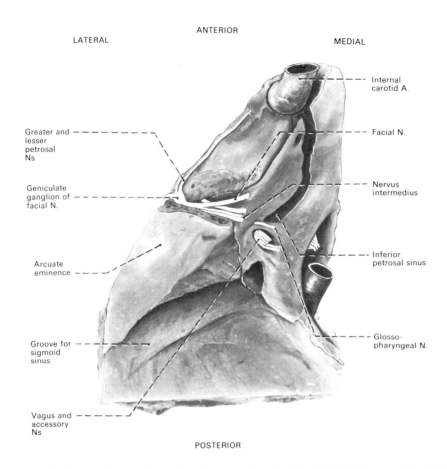

ANTERIOR

LATERAL   MEDIAL

Internal
carotid A.

Greater and
lesser
petrosal
Ns

Facial N.

Geniculate
ganglion of
facial N.

Nervus
intermedius

Arcuate
eminence

Inferior
petrosal sinus

Groove for
sigmoid
sinus

Glosso-
pharyngeal N.

Vagus and
accessory
Ns

POSTERIOR

Fig. 5.150 The facial nerve in the internal acoustic meatus. Superior view of a decalcified left temporal bone from which the parts lateral to the tympanic cavity have been excised. The internal acoustic meatus has been laid open.

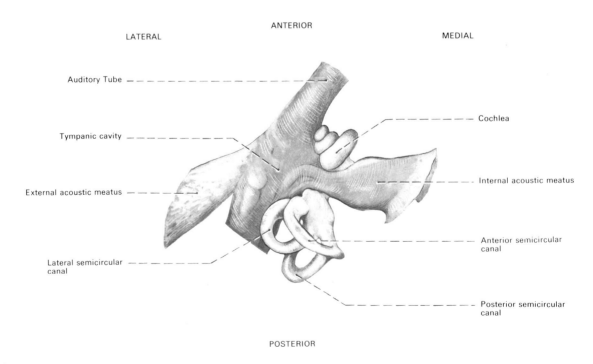

ANTERIOR

LATERAL   MEDIAL

Auditory Tube

Cochlea

Tympanic cavity

External acoustic meatus

Internal acoustic meatus

Anterior semicircular
canal

Lateral semicircular
canal

Posterior semicircular
canal

POSTERIOR

Fig. 5.151 Superior view of a cast of the cavities of the left temporal bone.

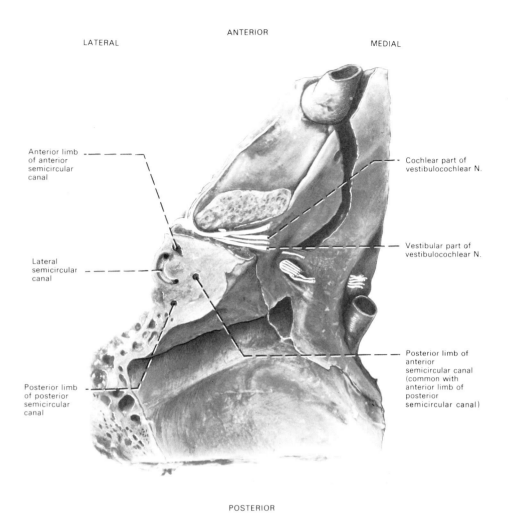

LATERAL   ANTERIOR   MEDIAL

Anterior limb of anterior semicircular canal

Lateral semicircular canal

Posterior limb of posterior semicircular canal

Cochlear part of vestibulocochlear N.

Vestibular part of vestibulocochlear N.

Posterior limb of anterior semicircular canal (common with anterior limb of posterior semicircular canal)

POSTERIOR

Fig. 5.152 The semicircular canals. Superior view of the dissection shown in Fig. 5.150 after section in the plane of the lateral semicircular canal.

of the facial nerve to a point immediately posterior to the foramen. Here the nerve turns sharply backwards to run postero-laterally in the **facial canal** just deep to the medial wall of the tympanic cavity above the stapes. Use dissecting forceps to expose this part of the nerve. As it passes backwards, it turns gently to descend vertically to the **stylo-mastoid foramen.**

The point where the nerve abruptly turns from an antero-lateral to a postero-lateral course is called the **geniculum** of the facial nerve, and is marked by a small swelling, the **geniculate ganglion,** in which are located the cell bodies of the sensory (taste) fibres that join the facial nerve in the chorda tympani [see p. 5.76]. Between the geniculate ganglion and the brain stem the sensory (taste) and para-sympathetic fibres of the facial nerve form the **nervus inter-medius** [see p. 6.6], which runs alongside but separately from the fibres supplying the muscles of facial expression. Identify the nervus intermedius on your dissection. You should also see that the greater petrosal nerve leaves the facial nerve at the geniculate ganglion.

The internal ear

You should be able to establish some of the following facts on your dissection.

The bony labyrinth [Fig. 5.151]

The system of canals in the petrous part of the temporal bone, which comprises the bony labyrinth, is divided into three parts: the **vestibule,** the **cochlea,** and the **bony semi-circular canals,** all of which are lined by periosteum. The vestibule is a small chamber which lies between the medial wall of the middle ear and the bottom of the internal acoustic meatus. In its lateral wall is the fenestra vestibuli, which is closed by the periosteal lining, and into which the base of the stapes fits. The vestibule communicates, in front, with the coiled bony canal, the cochlea; behind, with the semicircular canals. The cochlea is a tapering spiral tube which makes about two and one-half turns around a cen-tral bony pillar, the **modiolus.** The first turn of the cochlea is responsible for the elevation on the medial wall of the tympanic cavity called the promontory.

The semicircular canals [Fig. 5.151]

There are three semicircular canals, and in order to understand their function you should know in what planes they lie [Fig. 5.151]. The **anterior semicircular canal** and the **posterior semicircular canal** are both vertical, the former at right-angles to, and the other parallel with the long axis of the petrous part of the temporal bone. The anterior semicircular canal lies beneath an elevation, called the arcuate eminence, on the upper surface of the petrous part of the temporal bone, about 1 cm behind the internal acoustic meatus. The **lateral semicircular canal** lies in the angle between the other two canals and beneath the prominence on the medial wall of the aditus to the antrum, immediately above the facial nerve.

Make an almost horizontal incision with a sharp scalpel through the centre of this prominence, keeping your blade parallel with the subjacent facial nerve. Complete the incision but do not discard the small piece of bone that you have separated. This incision will lay open most of the lateral semicircular canal [Fig. 5.152]. Immediately anterior to it you should see where the anterior semicircular canal has been cut across at two points. Identify the same two points on the small piece of bone you have just removed, and then divide it so as to lay open the anterior canal. Make another incision in the same piece of bone at right-angles to the last incision and passing through the posterior limb of the anterior canal. This incision should open up the posterior semicircular canal.

Each bony semicircular canal possesses a slight dilatation or **bony ampulla** at one end. You may be able to make out the ampulla at the lateral end of the lateral canal.

The membranous labyrinth

You will not be able to study the more detailed anatomy of the membranous labyrinth on your specimen. For this, special preparations suitable for microscopic examination are required. If they are not available, you will have to content yourself, for the present, with a textbook description. You should note now that the membranous labyrinth, containing the **endolymph,** lies within the bony labyrinth, from which it is separated by **perilymph.** Its chief parts, which are all continuous with each other, correspond to the parts of the bony labyrinth, and are: two sacs called the **utricle** and the **saccule,** which lie in the vestibule; the **cochlear duct;** and the **semicircular ducts.**

The auditory receptors are located in the cochlear duct. The nerve fibres from these receptors traverse minute canals in the modiolus before they emerge from its base at the bottom of the internal acoustic meatus. The nerve fibres collectively form the cochlear part of the vestibulocochlear nerve; their cell bodies are situated in the modiolus and form the **spiral ganglion of the cochlea.** Examine the vestibulocochlear nerve in the internal acoustic meatus and note that it is divided longitudinally into two parts. The anterior one is the cochlear part. Pick this up with a pair of forceps and pull it gently but firmly out of the internal acoustic meatus. It should come away with the coiled cochlear duct attached to it.

The receptors which respond to gravitational pull and to movements of the head lie in the utricle, the saccule, and in the swellings (the **membranous ampullae**) of the semicircular ducts. The nerve fibres from these receptors form the vestibular part of the vestibulocochlear nerve. Their cell bodies are collected together in the **vestibular ganglion** which lies within the internal acoustic meatus.

Chart of contents of the brain

COMPONENTS	SUBDIVISIONS					
	Forebrain		Midbrain	Hindbrain		
	Cerebrum	Diencephalon		Pons	Medulla oblongata	Cerebellum
Grey matter	cerebral cortex basal nuclei	thalamic nuclei hypothalamic nuclei	nuclei of the cranial nerves central grey matter red nucleus substantia nigra	pontine nuclei	nucleus gracilis nucleus cuneatus inferior olivary nucleus	cerebellar cortex cerebellar nuclei
White matter	association fibres commissural fibres corpus callosum anterior commissure projection fibres internal capsule fornix		superior cerebellar peduncle basis pedunculi	middle cerebellar peduncle longitudinal fibres	inferior cerebellar peduncle pyramid	cerebellar peduncles
Ventricles	lateral	third	cerebral aqueduct	fourth		
		interventricular foramen				
Cranial Nerves	I olfactory	II optic	III oculomotor IV trochlear	V trigeminal VI abducent	IX glossopharyngeal X vagus XI accessory XII hypoglossal	
				VII facial VIII vestibulocochlear		
Arteries	branches from cerebral arterial circle			branches from vertebral and basilar arteries		

Part 6

The brain

Some of the main features of the brain were examined when the skull was dissected [p. 5.27], and at some other time in your course the central nervous system will be studied in detail. In the following dissection you examine such macroscopic characters of the brain as can be easily seen in the dissecting room.

The method of choice in the study of the brain requires that each group of students should dissect two brains. These would have been fixed in formalin and stored in a 50 per cent solution of alcohol in water. Each brain, to which the cerebral arteries and veins, and the twelve pairs of cranial nerves will still be attached, will have been severed from the spinal medulla, and will be enveloped by arachnoid.

If, because of the scarcity of specimens, it is difficult to provide every four or six students with more than one brain, teachers should decide whether to increase the size of the group so as to abide by what is much the preferred method of study, or to follow the modified, and less revealing course of dissection appropriate for the examination of a single brain [p. 6.30 onwards]. Whichever course is followed the instructions are fortunately the same over a considerable part of the dissection. In order to avoid unnecessary repetition of the text, the sequence of procedures set out for the one-brain study therefore refers, wherever possible, to the more detailed instructions outlined for two brains. In either case it would help if students were able to refer, as they dissect, to mounted specimens of different parts of the brain that have been specially prepared and stained to display particular features.

Section 6.1
The 'two-brain' dissection

The major subdivisions of the brain

You already know that a longitudinal fissure, the **longitudinal fissure of the cerebrum,** which contains the falx cerebri [p. 5.27], divides the cerebrum into right and left **hemispheres.** You have also noted that the cerebral hemispheres lie in the part of the cranial cavity above the tentorium cerebelli, and that they form the major part of the **forebrain,** which is connected by the **midbrain** to the **hindbrain** below the tentorium cerebelli. You will also remember that the tentorium cerebelli lies in the **transverse fissure of the cerebrum** between the cerebral hemispheres and the **cerebellum.** Recall, too, that the anterior extremity of the frontal lobe [p. 5.27] is the **frontal pole,** and that of the temporal lobe, the **temporal pole** [Fig. 6.1]. The posterior extremity of the cerebral hemisphere is the **occipital pole.**

Note that all parts of the central nervous system are made up of what are called **grey matter** and **white matter.** The grey matter consists of aggregations of cell-bodies of neurons. The white matter, which preponderates in the central nervous system, consists of nerve fibres. The surface of the cerebral hemispheres and of the cerebellum comprises a thin layer of grey matter. Other concentrations of nerve-cell bodies form large ganglia deep in the brain.

The ventral surface of the brain

Lay the brain on its superior surface and study its ventral aspect. In the midline behind is the terminal part of the brain stem, formed by the almost cylindrical **medulla oblongata** [Fig. 6.2]. Inferiorly, the medulla oblongata is continued into the spinal medulla, which usually begins a little below the foramen magnum. Superiorly the medulla oblongata is bounded by the lower horizontal border of the **pons.** This is the swollen part of the brain stem which is marked by transversely-running striations. On each side the pons is connected to the cerebellum by a thick bundle called the **middle cerebellar peduncle.** The medulla oblongata, pons, and cerebellum collectively form the hindbrain. The term

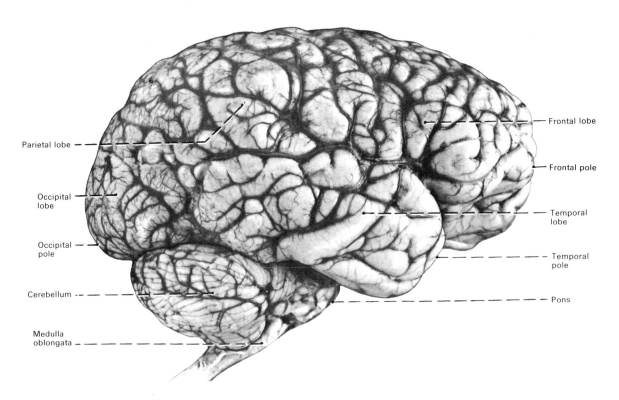

Fig. 6.1 The right side of the brain. The midbrain is hidden from view.

'brain stem' is used to refer collectively to the medulla oblongata, pons, and midbrain.

On the base of the brain, at the rostral (upper) border of the pons, are two small protuberances, the **mamillary bodies,** on either side of the midline. In front of these is the pituitary stalk or **infundibulum,** which you saw in your dissected cadaver [p. 5.27]. (The **hypophysis** itself will have been left in the skull from which the brain was removed.) Immediately anterior to the infundibulum is a thick transverse bar of nervous tissue, called the **optic chiasma,** which connects the posterior ends of the **optic nerves.** The mamillary bodies and the infundibulum belong to a part of the forebrain called the **diencephalon,** which is joined to the pons by the midbrain, which is so short that it is not easy to see at this stage.

Using forceps, carefully remove the arachnoid that stretches between the optic chiasma and the mamillary bodies, and identify the **optic tracts,** which extend posterolaterally from the optic chiasma on each side of the infundibulum and mamillary bodies.

The arteries and veins of the brain [Fig. 6.3]

Examine the **basilar artery,** which you will see in the midline on the anterior surface of the pons [Fig. 6.3]. You have already noted [p. 5.28] that this artery is formed by the junction of the two **vertebral arteries,** and you will now see that it terminates at the rostral (upper) border of the pons by

dividing into two parallel pairs of arteries. The upper pair are the right and left **posterior cerebral arteries,** and the lower the **superior cerebellar arteries.** To see these arteries more clearly, remove the arachnoid that covers them, taking care not to pull away any nerve roots as you do so. The posterior cerebral arteries turn backwards above the tentorium cerebelli, to supply the posterior parts of the cerebral hemispheres. The superior cerebellar arteries pass posterolaterally below the tentorium cerebelli, to supply the upper parts of the cerebellum.

Try to find a branch from each vertebral artery which passes laterally to ramify on the inferior surface of the cerebellum. These are the **posterior inferior cerebellar arteries.** The basilar artery also gives off two **anterior inferior cerebellar arteries** at the lower border of the pons, as well as a number of smaller arteries which pass laterally to the pons itself.

On each side of the infundibulum and optic chiasma identify the cut end of the **internal carotid artery.** Carefully nibbling away the arachnoid, find the large branch each internal carotid artery sends forwards and medially to the medial surface of each hemisphere. This is the **anterior cerebral artery.** Look for the short **anterior communicating artery,** which crosses the midline above the optic chiasma, and forms a communicating channel between the two anterior cerebral arteries [Fig. 6.3].

The continuation of the internal carotid artery beyond

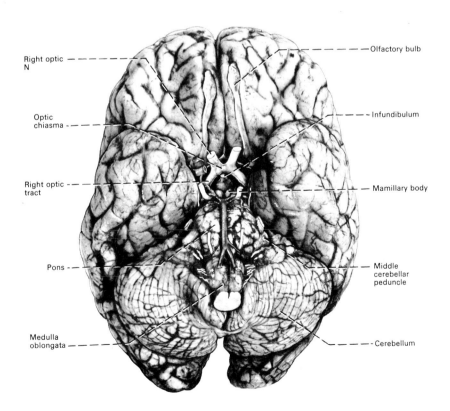

Right optic
N

Optic
chiasma

Right optic
tract

Pons

Medulla
oblongata

Olfactory bulb

Infundibulum

Mamillary body

Middle
cerebellar
peduncle

Cerebellum

Fig. 6.2 The ventral surface of the brain.

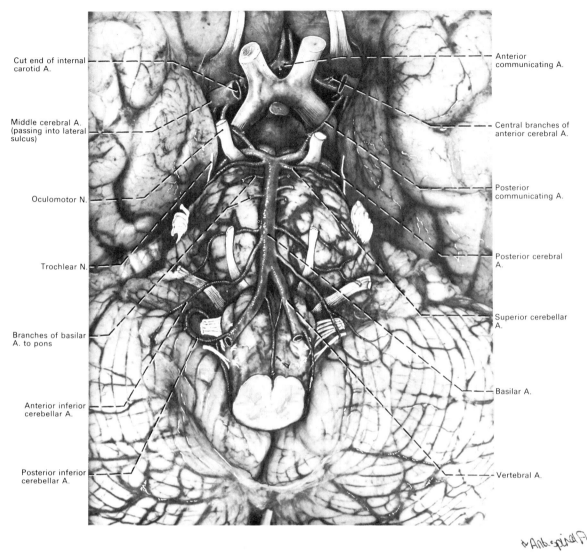

Cut end of internal carotid A.

Middle cerebral A. (passing into lateral sulcus)

Oculomotor N.

Trochlear N.

Branches of basilar A. to pons

Anterior inferior cerebellar A.

Posterior inferior cerebellar A.

Anterior communicating A.

Central branches of anterior cerebral A.

Posterior communicating A.

Posterior cerebral A.

Superior cerebellar A.

Basilar A.

Vertebral A.

Fig. 6.3 The arteries on the ventral surface of the brain.

the origin of the anterior cerebral artery is called the **middle cerebral artery.** The middle cerebral artery disappears from view as it passes laterally into the depths of a deep fissure, called the **lateral sulcus,** in the supero-lateral or convex surface of the cerebrum.

Now look carefully on each side for a fine branch each internal carotid artery sends posteriorly to join the posterior cerebral artery. These branches are the **posterior communicating arteries.** The anastomoses formed by the anterior and posterior communicating arteries complete an arterial ring, known as the **cerebral arterial circle,** whose other components are the proximal parts of the posterior cerebral arteries, the internal carotid arteries, and the proximal parts of the two anterior cerebral arteries.

Gently displace the optic nerves, and carefully examine the proximal parts of the anterior and middle cerebral arteries. Note the leash of fine branches which these arteries

send directly into the subjacent cerebral substance at the sides of the optic chiasma. These are their ganglionic or **central branches** [Fig. 6.3]. The area they pierce on each side is called the **anterior perforated substance** [Fig. 6.4].

The vessels which you can see ramifying beneath the arachnoid on the supero-lateral surfaces of the cerebral hemispheres are either **cerebral veins** or the terminal branches of cerebral arteries. The veins around the frontal pole and over the upper parts of each hemisphere pass into the superior sagittal sinus; those from the occipital pole pass to the superior petrosal and transverse sinuses; while those from the inferior part of the supero-lateral surface, between the frontal and occipital poles, pass downwards, forwards, and then medially to form the **superficial middle cerebral vein,** which drains into the cavernous sinus. Large anastomotic channels connect the veins on the supero-lateral surface of each hemisphere.

6.4

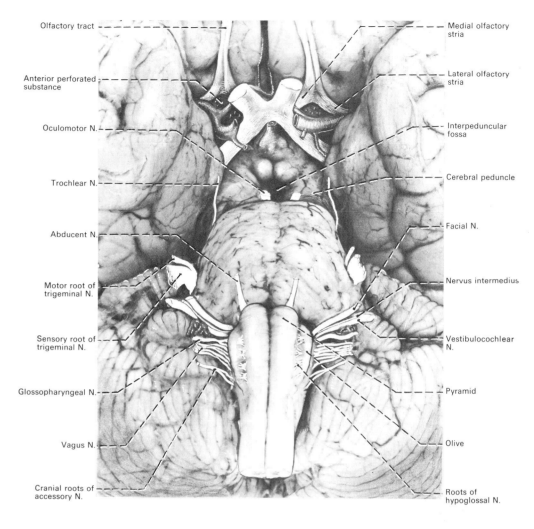

Olfactory tract

Anterior perforated substance

Oculomotor N.

Trochlear N.

Abducent N.

Motor root of trigeminal N.

Sensory root of trigeminal N.

Glossopharyngeal N.

Vagus N.

Cranial roots of accessory N.

Medial olfactory stria

Lateral olfactory stria

Interpeduncular fossa

Cerebral peduncle

Facial N.

Nervus intermedius

Vestibulocochlear N.

Pyramid

Olive

Roots of hypoglossal N.

Fig. 6.4 The cranial nerves. The basilar artery and its branches have been removed.

The cranial nerves

Examine the origins of the cranial nerves, nibbling away and displacing the arachnoid where necessary. You noted the points of exit of the nerves from the interior of the skull when you removed the brain from your dissected cadaver [pp. 5.31–5.33].

The olfactory (1st cranial) nerves [Fig. 5.115]

Close to the midline, on the inferior surface of the cerebral hemisphere, behind the frontal pole, find the flat and narrow **olfactory tracts.** Anteriorly, each tract terminates in a small mass of tissue, the **olfactory bulb** [Fig. 6.2] which, with the brain in position in the skull, lies on the cribriform plate of the ethmoid. The bulbs are connected with the olfactory region of the mucous coat of the nose by the olfactory nerves, which pass through the perforations of the cribriform plate. Follow each olfactory tract posteriorly from the olfactory bulb towards the anterior perforated substance,

where it terminates by dividing into two diverging ridges, the **medial** and **lateral olfactory striae** [Fig. 6.4], which quickly fade into the surrounding cerebral substance.

The optic (2nd cranial) nerve [Fig. 6.2]

You have already identified the optic nerves. The fibres which make up the medial parts of each optic nerve cross the midline (decussate) in the **chiasma,** and so enter the **optic tract** of the opposite side. The decussating fibres come from the medial or nasal half of each retina, i.e. that part of the retina in each eye that lies medial to a vertical line passing through the macula [see p. 5.129].

The oculomotor and trochlear nerves [Figs 6.3 and 6.4]

The nerve which emerges from the midbrain on each side, between the posterior cerebral and superior cerebellar arteries, is the oculomotor nerve (3rd cranial nerve) [Fig. 6.3]. In a much more lateral position between these two

6.5

arteries look for the very fine trochlear nerve (4th cranial nerve), winding round the side of the midbrain. When you have identified the trochlear nerves, carefully displace the terminal branches of the basilar artery, and tear the arachnoid, if necessary, in order to trace the oculomotor nerves to their attachments to the brain. You will see that they spring from the sides of a deep groove in the midline of the midbrain, called the **interpeduncular fossa** [Fig. 6.4]. This extends from the upper border of the pons caudally to the mamillary bodies rostrally (anteriorly). On each side the groove is bounded by a large longitudinally-striated column, called the **cerebral peduncle,** which joins the pons and the forebrain.

The trigeminal nerve [Fig. 6.4]

The large nerve which you will find emerging from the side of the pons is the trigeminal nerve (5th cranial nerve). Identify its **sensory root,** and its smaller and more medial **motor root.**

The abducent, facial, and vestibulocochlear nerves [Fig. 6.4]

The thin nerve, which runs longitudinally upwards from its attachment near the midline at the lower border of the pons, is the abducent nerve (6th cranial nerve). At the same level, but more laterally, emerge the facial nerve (7th cranial nerve) and the vestibulocochlear nerve (8th cranial nerve). The facial nerve lies medial to the vestibulocochlear nerve, and between the two you should be able to see the small **nervus intermedius,** in which run the sensory and visceral motor fibres of the facial nerve. Note that at their origins these two cranial nerves are closely related to the adjacent cerebellum. Their site of attachment is often referred to as the **cerebellopontine angle.**

The glossopharyngeal, vagus, and accessory nerves [Fig. 6.4]

The contiguous rootlets which are attached in a vertical series to the side of the medulla oblongata, in line with the facial nerve, form the glossopharyngeal nerve (9th cranial nerve), the vagus nerve (10th cranial nerve), and the cranial roots of the accessory nerve (11th cranial nerve), in that order from above downwards. They lie behind a swelling of the antero-lateral surface of the medulla oblongata, called the **olive.** The uppermost one or two rootlets form the glossopharyngeal nerve, and the most caudal the **cranial roots of the accessory nerve.** You are not likely to see the **spinal roots of the accessory nerve,** which you should, however, have found in the cadaver you dissected [p. 5.33]. They arise from the upper five cervical segments of the spinal medulla.

The hypoglossal nerve [Fig. 6.4]

Note the two longitudinal ridges, called **pyramids,** on either side of the midline on the anterior surface of the medulla oblongata, and between them the **anterior median fissure.**

The upper end of each pyramid is separated from the olive by a shallow groove. The series of nerve rootlets that emerge from this groove become the hypoglossal nerve (12th cranial nerve).

The corpus callosum and dorsal surface of the midbrain

Remove the basilar artery, dividing its branches close to their origins, and taking care not to damage the cranial nerves that you have just identified.

Turn the brain over so that it lies on its base, or ventral surface, and carefully separate the cerebral hemispheres in order to look into the longitudinal fissure. You will see that the floor of the fissure is formed by the upper surface of a thick band of nervous tissue which connects the two hemispheres. This band is striated transversely, and is called the **corpus callosum.** It is the largest of a number of commissures that connect the two hemispheres.

Now look at the brain from behind. If you separate the occipital poles you will see the large rounded posterior border or **splenium of the corpus callosum** [Fig. 6.5]. Holding the occipital poles apart, lift the brain gently from the table so as to allow the cerebellum to fall away from the cerebral hemispheres. Now clear away the arachnoid between the splenium of the corpus callosum and cerebellum by perforating it and then enlarging the hole with a blunt probe; but do not pull off any arachnoid.

Identify the **great cerebral vein,** which emerges in the midline from beneath the splenium of the corpus callosum. You will remember that this vein drains into the straight sinus, which starts immediately behind the posterior border of the corpus callosum [p. 5.30]. As you clear away the arachnoid in the more caudal part of the interval between the splenium and the cerebellum, take care that you do not remove the very fine **trochlear nerve** [Fig. 6.5], which, as you can now see, arises from the lower border of the posterior surface of the midbrain. This surface presents two pairs of small swellings, called the **corpora quadrigemina.** The upper pair are the **superior colliculi,** and the lower, the **inferior colliculi.** Between the splenium of the corpus callosum and the superior colliculi, and below the great cerebral vein, is a small oval body, called the **pineal body,** which is attached by a stalk to the diencephalon [Fig 6.5 and 6.6].

(If you are dissecting one brain, you will now study the brain stem, the instructions for which start on page 6.30.)

The medial surface of the bisected brain

Place one of the two brains, with which you have been provided, on its ventral (basal) surface. Insert a long-bladed knife (the blade should be 30 cm or more in length) into the longitudinal fissure between the two hemispheres and completely divide the brain in the median plane, cutting through the corpus callosum and the brain stem. In the subsequent instructions the parts of this brain will be referred to as 'BRAIN A'. The unbisected brain will be referred to as 'BRAIN B'.

Grey and white matter

Examine the cut surface of the pons of BRAIN A and note the numerous pale longitudinal streaks by which it is marked. These streaks are bundles of nerve fibres, which form the **white matter** of the brain stem [Fig. 6.6]. The darker **grey matter** between them comprises aggregations of the cell bodies (perikarya) of neurons.

Now look at the cut surface of the cerebellum. Note the small central core of white matter which branches towards the highly-folded surface from which, however, it is always

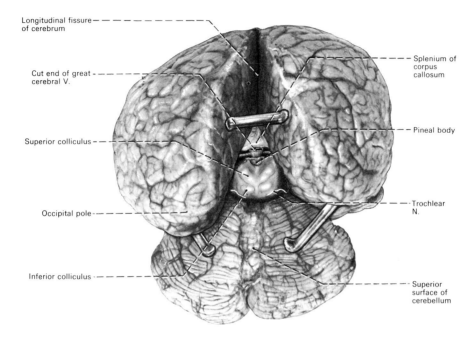

Fig. 6.5 **The dorsal surface of the midbrain.** Posterior view of the brain with the hemispheres and cerebellum separated by glass rods.

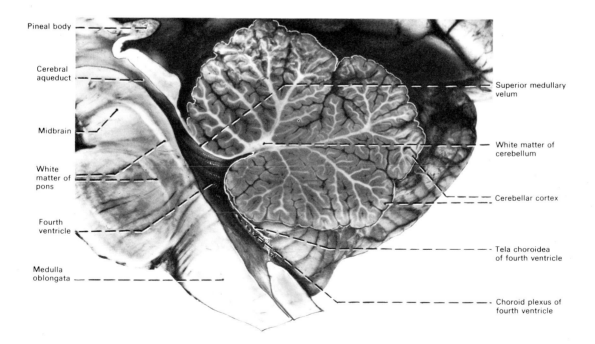

Fig. 6.6 **Median section of the brain stem.** Right half of BRAIN A.

separated by a thin rind or **cortex** of grey matter, the cerebellar cortex. A corresponding arrangement of grey and white matter characterizes the cerebral hemispheres, the surface of which is not as finely folded as is that of the cerebellum. The full extent of the folded surfaces greatly exceeds that of the cranial cavity.

The ventricular system

The fourth ventricle [Fig. 6.6]

The brain and spinal medulla develop in the embryo from a tubular structure called the **neural tube,** whose lumen contains **cerebrospinal fluid.** In the brain the lumen never becomes occluded, except in rare pathological conditions. If you look at the cut surface of the brain you bisected (BRAIN A), you can see an expanded part of this lumen, called the fourth ventricle [Fig. 6.6], between the cerebellum posteriorly and the pons and medulla oblongata anteriorly. The posterior wall or **roof of the fourth ventricle** has an apex which is formed by the white core of the cerebellum. Rostral to this, the roof is formed by a thin sheet of white matter, the **superior medullary velum.** Now gently separate the cerebellum and medulla oblongata, and you will see that the inferior part of the roof of the fourth ventricle is formed by a delicate membrane which has probably been torn. This membrane consists only of the lining epithelium of the ventricle, called **ependyma,** and the pia mater on its external surface. This particular area of pia mater is rich in blood vessels and is called the **tela chorioidea of the fourth ventricle.** In the membrane is a relatively large median aperture, through which cerebrospinal fluid can escape into the subarachnoid space. (The **inferior medullary velum** is a narrow and thin sheet of white matter which is interposed between the ependyma and pia mater at the upper lateral margin of the tela chorioidea.)

Cerebrospinal fluid is secreted in the fourth ventricle, and in all the other dilatations or ventricles of the brain, by vascular structures called choroid plexuses, which comprise tufts of vessels which invaginate the thin membranes formed where ependyma and pia mater come into apposition. The **choroid plexus of the fourth ventricle** is the long dark granular structure which you will find attached to the thin part of the roof of the ventricle.

The cerebral aqueduct [Fig. 6.6]

At its caudal end, the fourth ventricle connects with a very narrow central canal that traverses the length of the spinal medulla. If you follow the cavity of the ventricle rostrally (upwards) into the midbrain, you will find that it again narrows into a small canal, the cerebral aqueduct. At the upper boundary of the midbrain, the cerebral aqueduct opens into the third ventricle.

The third ventricle [Figs 6.7 and 6.8]

The third ventricle is a slit-like space which forms the cavity of the diencephalon. Note that in front of the mamillary bodies the ventricle extends down into the **infundibulum,** anterior to which you will find the cut surface of the **optic chiasma,** forming the inferior part of the ventricle's anterior wall. Above the level of the chiasma is the thin **lamina terminalis** [Fig. 6.7], which forms the main part of the anterior

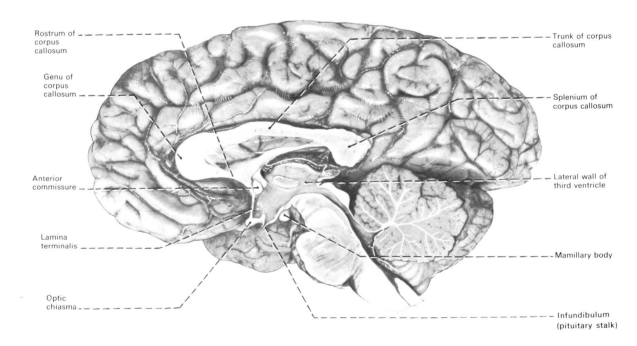

Fig. 6.7 Median section of the brain. Right half of BRAIN A.

wall. It is connected above to the anterior end or **genu of the corpus callosum** by the **rostrum of the corpus callosum.** Embedded in the posterior surface of the lamina terminalis you will find a rounded bundle of fibres, the **anterior commissure,** which you divided when you cut the brain in two, and which connects the two hemispheres [Fig. 6.7].

Note that the space between the inferior surface of the anterior half of the corpus callosum and its rostrum is occupied by a sagittally-disposed membrane, called the **septum pellucidum** [Fig. 6.8], which, in spite of its thinness, consists of two sheets of tissue enclosing a minute closed cavity, the **cavity of the septum pellucidum.** On either side of the curved postero-inferior border of the septum pellucidum runs a bundle of fibres which passes forwards from the under-surface of the posterior part of the corpus callosum and curves downwards, to sink into the lateral wall of the third ventricle, immediately above and behind the anterior commissure. This bundle is called the **fornix.** The fibres of the fornix extend backwards through the substance of the lateral wall of the ventricle to the **mamillary bodies** [Fig. 6.7].

Most of the lateral wall of the third ventricle is formed by a mass of grey matter called the **thalamus,** which you will shortly examine in detail. The two thalami are sometimes attached to each other across the ventricular cavity, and it is possible that you will be able to make out the cut surface of the connection, which is called the **interthalamic adhesion** [Fig. 6.8]. A shallow horizontal groove on the surface of the lateral wall of the ventricle, at about the level of the anterior commissure, separates the thalamus above from another part of the brain called the **hypothalamus,** below.

The hypothalamus includes the mamillary bodies and the infundibulum.

Pass a probe obliquely upwards, forwards, and laterally through the small foramen which you will find behind the anterior end of the fornix. This foramen is called the **interventricular foramen,** and the tip of your probe is entering the main or **lateral ventricle** of the cerebral hemisphere. If you divided the brain in such a way that the septum pellucidum is missing on one side, you should be able to see into the ventricle of that side.

A diverticulum of the subarachnoid space extends forwards from the lower border of the splenium of the corpus callosum to the interventricular foramen. This diverticulum is lined by pia mater which coats the under-surface of the corpus callosum and fornix above, and the upper surfaces of the thalami below, and is called the **tela chorioidea of the third ventricle.** Between the thalami the pia mater comes into contact with the ependyma of the third ventricle and so forms a thin roof to the ventricle. This roof is invaginated by the **choroid plexus of the third ventricle.**

At the posterior end of the roof of the third ventricle is the attachment of the **pineal body** [Fig. 6.6]. Note that a recess of the ventricular cavity extends into the **pineal stalk.** Carefully examine the cut edge of the ventricular roof just below the entrance to this recess. Here you should be able to make out the cut surface of another small commissure, the **posterior commissure** [Fig. 6.8], which also connects the two hemispheres.

(The 'one-brain' dissector should return to page 6.35 and continue his study of the ventricles of the forebrain.)

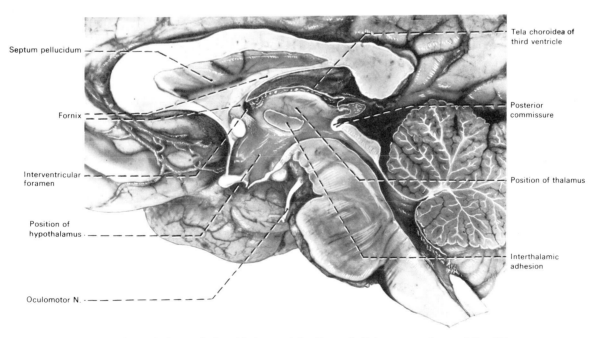

Septum pellucidum

Fornix

Interventricular foramen

Position of hypothalamus

Oculomotor N.

Tela choroidea of third ventricle

Posterior commissure

Position of thalamus

Interthalamic adhesion

Fig. 6.8 The relations of the third ventricle. BRAIN A. Enlargement of part of Fig. 6.7.

The brain stem

You must now separate the brain stem from the cerebral hemispheres. To do this, divide each half of the bisected brain (BRAIN A) transversely just below the middle of the superior colliculus, and at right-angles to the long axis of the brain stem, taking care not to damage the hemispheres, which you will study later. To do the same to the whole brain (BRAIN B) lay the brain down on its superior surface so that you are looking at its base. Your cut will be made between the mamillary bodies and the oculomotor nerves. Place the heel of the blade of your scalpel against the ventral surface of one of the two cerebral peduncles with the point of the blade directed laterally. Begin your cut by moving the point of the blade backwards, then across the midline through the dorsal part of the midbrain. Then cut forwards through the other peduncle and complete the separation of cerebrum from the cerebellum and the brain stem.

Now examine the unbisected brain stem (BRAIN B), on which you have already identified the anterior median fissure, the pyramids, and the olives of the medulla oblongata.

The pyramids are made up of longitudinal bundles of nerve fibres. Chief among these are the **corticospinal tracts** of motor nerve fibres, which arise from cells in the cerebral cortex and end by forming connections with neurons at all levels of the grey matter of the spinal medulla. Towards the lower end of the medulla oblongata the greater part of each corticospinal tract crosses over the midline to the opposite side.

Splay open the rostral end of the anterior median fissure by inserting the closed points of a pair of blunt forceps. Follow the fissure downwards, opening it up as you go. If the brain stem was cut off low enough when the brain was removed from the cadaver, you will see that the lower end of the anterior median fissure is interrupted by the decussation of the two corticospinal tracts, called the **pyramidal decussation.**

Now examine the posterior aspect of the medulla oblongata. Its lower part resembles the spinal medulla, but the **posterior median sulcus,** by which it is marked, soon splays open into the caudal part of the fourth ventricle.

Gently separate the cerebellum and medulla oblongata so as to expose the thin roof, or tela chorioidea, of the caudal end of the fourth ventricle. It might no longer be intact. Remove this lower part of the roof, together with the choroid plexus that invaginates it, noting as you do so that it extends laterally on each side until it meets a thick bundle of nervous tissue, which diverges from the posterior median sulcus of the medulla oblongata to enter the cerebellum higher up. These bundles are the two **inferior cerebellar peduncles.**

The rhomboid fossa [Fig. 6.10]

Your next step is to remove the cerebellum from the brain stem of the unbisected specimen (BRAIN B). On each side incise the middle cerebellar peduncle just posterior to the roots of the trigeminal, facial, and vestibulocochlear nerves, cutting in a postero-medial direction and trying not to damage the surface of the cerebellum [Fig. 6.9]. Hold the brain stem so that the cerebellum tends to fall away from it, and cut the structures that still connect them across the interval between the anterior border of the superior cerebellar surface and the midbrain. The detached cerebellum will be studied later.

The floor of the fourth ventricle is now exposed [Fig.

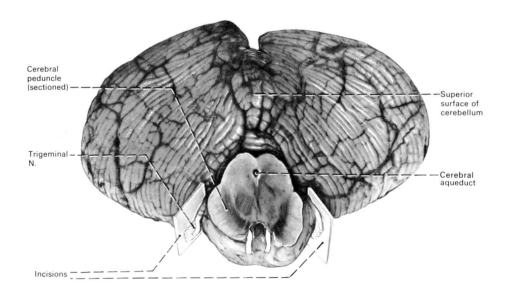

Fig. 6.9 Incisions to remove the cerebellum from the brain stem. BRAIN B, viewed from above. A card has been placed in each incision.

6.10]. Because of its shape it is called the rhomboid fossa. At the level of the junction between the medulla oblongata and the pons are two lateral angles, called the **lateral recesses of the fourth ventricle.** There is a superior angle where the ventricle continues into the cerebral aqueduct, and an inferior angle where it joins the central canal of the lower part of the medulla oblongata.

Carefully nibble away the tightly-adherent pia mater off the posterior surface of the lower part of the medulla oblongata and try to make out on the infero-lateral boundaries of the ventricle two slight elevations on each side, formed by aggregations of nerve cells (nuclei). The medial elevation is the **tubercle of the nucleus gracilis,** and the lateral elevation, the **tubercle of the nucleus cuneatus.** These two nuclei are relay stations for the tracts of nerve fibres, the one the **fasciculus gracilis,** the other the **fasciculus cuneatus,** which ascend in the white matter of the posterior part of the spinal medulla. You can easily make out these tracts just caudal to the tubercles.

The inferior cerebellar peduncle [Fig. 6.10]

Examine the inferior cerebellar peduncle which, as you will now see clearly, lies between the upper part of the infero-lateral boundary of the fourth ventricle and the groove from which the rootlets of the glossopharyngeal, vagus, and accessory nerves emerge behind the olive. The peduncle passes up from the medulla oblongata into the cerebellum, where it lies on the medial side of the much larger **middle cerebellar peduncle.** At this point it has been divided obliquely by the incision used to separate the brain stem and cerebellum.

The superior cerebellar peduncle [Fig. 6.10]

The supero-lateral boundary of the ventricle is mostly formed by the superior cerebellar peduncle. This is a flat bundle of fibres which passes fowards and upwards from the cerebellum to the midbrain. Like the inferior cerebellar peduncle, this peduncle will also have been divided obliquely.

Stretching between the well-defined medial borders of the superior cerebellar peduncles, and forming the roof of the ventricle in this region, is the thin **superior medullary velum,** which you have already identified on the bisected brain stem. Lying on the upper surface of the superior medullary velum you may find a thin layer of cerebellar cortex, which your cut may have separated from the rest of the cerebellum. This is the **lingula of the cerebellum.**

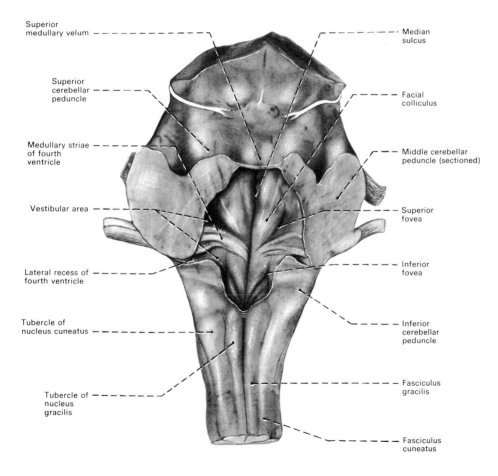

Fig. 6.10 The rhomboid fossa. BRAIN B. Posterior view of the brain stem after total removal of the cerebellum.

The floor of the fourth ventricle [Fig. 6.10]

Now examine the floor of the fourth ventricle, and note that on either side of a **median sulcus** is a faint sinuous groove, the **sulcus limitans,** which is partly obliterated at the level of the lateral recesses by transverse streaks known as the **medullary striae of the fourth ventricle.** Caudal to the medullary striae the sulcus limitans presents a shallow pit, the **inferior fovea,** from which two grooves diverge, one passing medially towards the central canal of the medulla, and the other, which is the sulcus limitans, continuing caudally, parallel with the median sulcus. Another shallow pit in the sulcus limitans, the **superior fovea,** lies rostral to the medullary striae and in a more lateral position than the inferior fovea.

Immediately subjacent to the floor of the fourth ventricle is a layer of grey matter which contains motor and sensory **nuclei of the cranial nerves** that are attached to the brain stem. The organization of this grey matter is fairly simple. In general, the motor nuclei, or **nuclei of origin,** lie medial, and the sensory nuclei, or **nuclei of termination,** lie lateral to the sulcus limitans. The area medial to the caudal part of the sulcus limitans overlies the nuclei of origin of the hypoglossal and vagus nerves. Medial to the superior fovea is a rounded elevation, the **facial colliculus,** which overlies the nucleus of the abducent nerve. The elevation is called the facial colliculus because motor fibres of the facial nerve partly encircle the nucleus of the abducent nerve as they pass from their nucleus of origin to their point of exit at the cerebellopontine angle [p. 6.6]. Lateral to the sulcus limitans, both rostral and caudal to the medullary striae, is the **vestibular area,** beneath which lie the (sensory) nuclei of the vestibular part of the vestibulocochlear nerve.

Sections of the brain stem

Although the disposition of the grey and white matter in the brain stem cannot be studied adequately without a micro-scope and stained preparations, with which you should be provided in a later part of your course, a few of the principal landmarks can be made out with the naked eye.

Make a series of transverse sections of the undivided brain stem (BRAIN B) at the following levels:

1. Through the lower half of the inferior colliculus of the midbrain.
2. Through the attachment of the trigeminal nerve to the pons.
3. Through the upper half of the olive in the medulla oblongata.

The cut surfaces of these sections should now be examined, beginning with the lowest.

The medulla oblongata [Fig. 6.11]

In the ventral part of the section through the medulla oblongata, you should have no difficulty in seeing the white matter of the **pyramids** [Fig. 6.11]. Within the **olive** you will see a sinuous U-shaped line of grey matter embedded in white matter. This is the **inferior olivary nucleus,** whose length is the same as that of the olive. The inferior olivary nucleus sends fibres to the cerebellum through the opposite **inferior cerebellar peduncle,** which you will see as white matter that caps the bulge dorsal to the olive. In the dorsal part of the section, immediately beneath the floor of the fourth ventricle, you should be able to see a lamina of grey matter. Between this and the inferior olivary nucleus is a region of fairly evenly-mixed grey and white matter called the **reticular formation.**

The pons [Fig. 6.12]

Examine the section of the pons. It is divided into a posterior third called the **dorsal part** of the pons and an anterior two-thirds called the **basilar part** of the pons [Fig. 6.12]. The basilar part comprises bundles of longitudinal and trans-

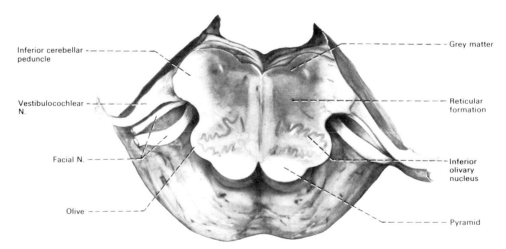

Fig. 6.11 **Transverse section through the upper half of the olive in the medulla oblongata.** BRAIN B. Semischematic. The section is viewed from below.

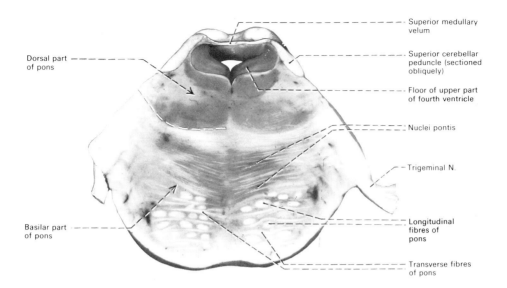

Fig. 6.12 Transverse section through the pons. Brain B. Semischematic. The curved broken white line indicates the boundary between the dorsal and basilar parts of the pons.

verse fibres interspersed with irregular patches of grey matter known as the **nuclei pontis.** The **transverse fibres of the pons** originate in these nuclei, cross the midline and pass into the **middle cerebellar peduncle** of the opposite side. In cross-section the bundles of **longitudinal fibres of the pons** may appear as round patches of white matter. Many of the fibres are corticospinal fibres which pass into the pyramid of the medulla oblongata.

The dorsal part of the pons is an upward continuation of the parts of the medulla oblongata which lie dorsal to the pyramids. Beneath the ventricular floor in this region is a layer of grey matter, and between this and the basilar part of the pons is an area of mixed grey and white matter, also called the **reticular formation.** The **superior cerebellar peduncles** are likely to be seen in this section of the brain stem, lying on either side of the lumen of the ventricle as they pass rostrally into the dorsal part of the upper segment of the pons.

The midbrain [Figs 6.13 and 6.14]

Identify the **cerebral aqueduct** in the section through the lower half of the midbrain. The aqueduct is surrounded by a zone of grey matter, the **central grey matter** [Fig. 6.13]. Dorsal to this is the roof, called the **tectum of the midbrain,** which bears the four **colliculi.** You will see that the inferior colliculi are formed mostly of grey matter. Ventral to the central grey matter are the two **cerebral peduncles,** each of which is divided into two parts by a very distinct layer of deeply pigmented neurons, called the **substantia nigra.** Anterior to the substantia nigra is the base of the peduncle, or **basis pedunculi** (crus cerebri), which is composed of white matter through which run the corticospinal nerve fibres that descend through the basilar part of the pons and into the pyramids of the medulla oblongata. Dorsal to the substantia

nigra is the **tegmentum,** which mostly consists of **reticular formation.** In the tegmental parts of the two peduncles you should be able to make out an oval area of white matter on each side of the midline. These are the **superior cerebellar peduncles,** which decussate at this level.

Look at the upper surface of the divided midbrain. The appearance of this section is similar to that through the inferior colliculi, but, in place of the superior cerebellar peduncles in the medial part of the tegmentum, you will find, on each side, a large circular mass of grey matter, the **red nucleus,** which has a pink colour in the fresh brain. The red nucleus extends from the upper part of the midbrain into the diencephalon, and is cigar-shaped in longitudinal section. Above the level at which they decussate, the fibres of the superior cerebellar peduncles ascend to the thalamus, passing through the region of the red nucleus, where some of the fibres end.

(If you are dissecting one brain, turn to the special instructions for the study of the cerebellum which start on page 6.32.)

The cerebellum

Examine the cerebellum, which you detached from the brain stem (Brain B), and note the three parts into which it is subdivided for descriptive purposes (the subdivision has no functional significance): an unpaired median part called the **vermis,** and two lateral masses, the **cerebellar hemispheres.** The vermis forms a rounded crest on the superior surface of the cerebellum, where it is hardly distinguishable from the two hemispheres [Fig. 6.15]. On the inferior surface the vermis lies in a deep midline groove, called the **vallecula of the cerebellum.**

As you have already seen, the cerebellar cortex is folded

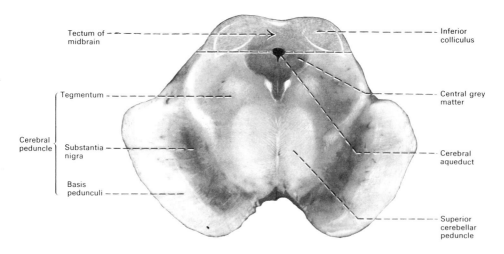

Fig. 6.13 Transverse section through the inferior colliculus of the midbrain. BRAIN B. Semischematic. The horizontal broken line, passing through the cerebral aqueduct, indicates the ventral boundary of the tectum.

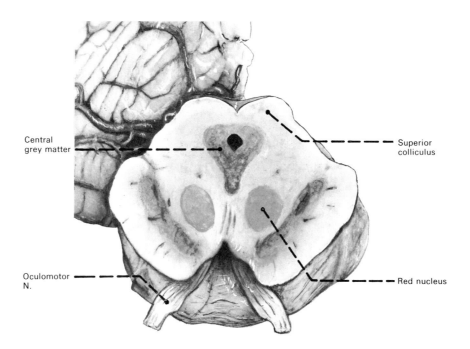

Fig. 6.14 Transverse section through the superior colliculus of the midbrain (viewed from above). The left half of the cerebellum has been removed; see 'one-brain' dissection on p. 6.30.

into long narrow convolutions, or **foliae,** separated by parallel **fissures.** Many of the fissures extend transversely across the vermis from one hemisphere to the other. The deeper fissures subdivide the vermis, and to each subdivision of the vermis there are attached corresponding parts of the hemispheres.

The anterior lobe

Examine the sagittal surface of the bisected brain stem (BRAIN A). The small part of the vermis resting on the superior medullary velum is the **lingula of the cerebellum** [Fig. 6.16]. The most posterior of the deep fissures that cut

the superior surface of the vermis is called the **primary fissure.** Trace this fissure into the adjoining hemisphere, removing arachnoid and blood vessels to do this; also identify the fissure on the unbisected cerebellum (BRAIN B) [Fig. 6.15]. The parts of the cerebellum anterior to this fissure form an anterior lobe of the cerebellum. Morphologically, the anterior lobe is an unpaired structure which has certain functions which are distinct from those of other parts of the cerebellum.

The flocculonodular lobe

Now identify on the bisected brain stem (BRAIN A) the three

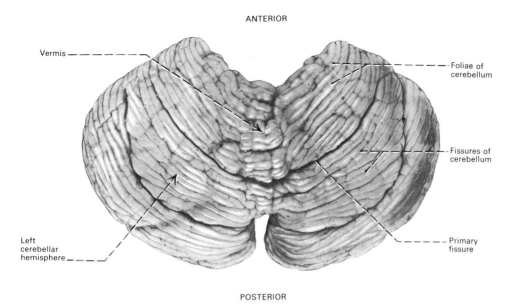

Fig. 6.15 The superior surface of the cerebellum. BRAIN B.

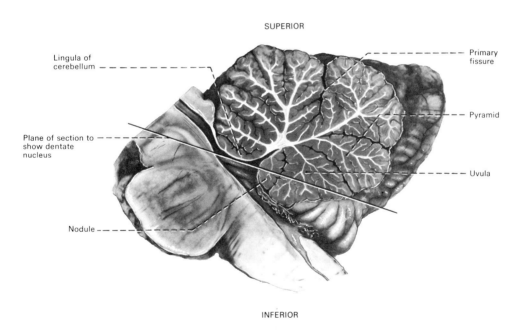

Fig. 6.16 Median section of brain stem and cerebellum. Right half of BRAIN A.

small lobules into which the inferior part of the vermis is divided. Anteriorly is the **nodule,** and immediately behind it the **uvula,** and then the **pyramid** [Fig. 6.16].

On the inferior surface of the cerebellum (BRAIN B), immediately inferior and lateral to the middle cerebellar peduncle, is a small tufted outgrowth, called the **flocculus** [Fig. 6.17]. This is the part of the hemisphere which corresponds to, and is connected with, the nodule. It lies close behind the facial and vestibulocochlear nerves. Identify the flocculus on your bisected specimen first (BRAIN A), and then on the detached cerebellum (BRAIN B). The flocculus

is connected to the nodule by a slender peduncle. The nodule and the paired flocculi form a functionally-distinct small part of the cerebellum, which is sometimes called the flocculonodular lobe. This lobe is concerned with the maintenance of balance. The cortex of this lobe receives nerve fibres from the vestibular part of the vestibulocochlear nerve and the vestibular nuclei in the brain stem.

The posterior lobe

Note that on either side of the uvula each hemisphere presents a low rounded projection, the **tonsil** of the

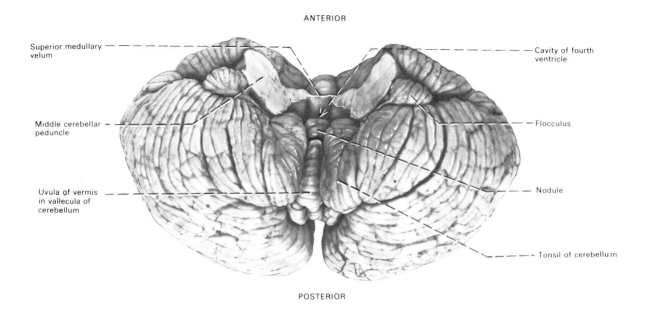

Fig. 6.17 **The inferior surface of the cerebellum.** Brain B.

cerebellum, the folds of which are disposed longitudinally [Fig. 6.17].

The parts of the cerebellum between the anterior lobe on the superior surface and the flocculonodular lobe on the in-

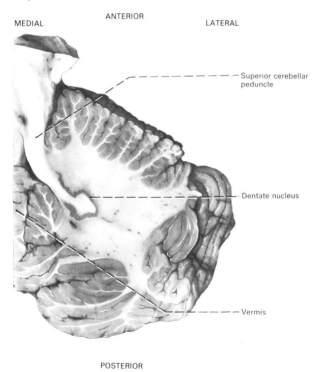

Fig. 6.18 **The right dentate nucleus.** Brain A. Superior view of the right half of the cerebellum, sectioned in the plane shown in Fig. 6.16.

ferior surface constitute a posterior lobe of the cerebellum. The uvula and pyramid belong to the posterior lobe but have functional affinities with the flocculonodular lobe, with which they are sometimes grouped. The rest of the posterior lobe forms the largest part of the human cerebellum. It is called the **neocerebellum,** because it is the youngest part of the cerebellum from the evolutionary point of view. The neocerebellum (like the pons to which it is connected) is relatively larger in man than in other animals.

The cerebellar nuclei

The information which passes to the cerebellum is carried by afferent fibres which enter through the inferior and superior cerebellar peduncles and go directly to the cortex of the anterior lobe, pyramid, uvula, and flocculonodular lobe. The neocerebellar cortex receives fibres from the nuclei pontis through the middle cerebellar peduncle.

The efferent fibres from the cerebellum do not arise in the cerebellar cortex, but from small masses of grey matter deep to the cortex called the **cerebellar nuclei.** The largest of these nuclei is the **dentate nucleus.** To see this nucleus, slice the cerebellum on the bisected brain stem (Brain A) in the plane shown in Fig. 6.16. The dentate nucleus resembles the inferior olivary nucleus of the medulla oblongata, and appears as a sinuous line of grey matter embedded in the white matter [Fig. 6.18]. The nerve fibres from this nucleus pass through the superior cerebellar peduncle to the red nucleus and thalamus of the opposite side of the brain.

Other deep nuclei of the cerebellum lie medial to the dentate nucleus and project their fibres to the pons and medulla oblongata.

The forebrain

The cerebral arteries [Figs 6.19 and 6.20]

The following dissection should be carried out on the bisected hemispheres (BRAIN A). (If you were provided with only one brain and have followed the instructions on pages 5.30 to 5.35 you will be able to pursue these instructions on the intact hemisphere still at your disposal.)

The anterior cerebral artery

Divide the anterior cerebral artery close to its origin, and follow it on to the medial surface of the hemisphere, separating the artery from the brain as you do so. The arachnoid and pia mater will be peeled off at the same time. Note that the branches of the anterior cerebral artery supply the medial surface of the hemisphere as far back as the splenium of the corpus callosum. Also note that they extend over the supero-medial border of the medial surface to supply a narrow strip of the supero-lateral surface of the hemisphere close to the longitudinal fissure.

The posterior cerebral artery

Now follow the posterior cerebral artery, removing more of the arachnoid and pia mater as you do so. Its branches pass laterally over the inferior surface of the posterior two-thirds of the hemisphere, and backwards over the medial surface of the occipital region, extending on to the supero-lateral surface around the occipital pole.

The middle cerebral artery

Lay the hemisphere down on its flat medial surface, and peel off the arachnoid and pia mater covering the whole of its supero-lateral surface. This will allow you to see more clearly the deep **lateral sulcus** of this surface, in which the middle cerebral artery lies. Follow the stem of the middle cerebral artery into the sulcus, separating the lips of the sulcus to facilitate the removal of the artery. Later you will see that there is a large area of buried cortex (the **insula**) in this fissure, which, together with most of the cortex on the supero-lateral surface of the hemisphere, is supplied by the middle cerebral artery.

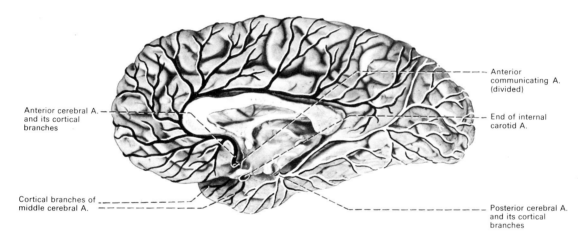

Anterior communicating A. (divided)

End of internal carotid A.

Anterior cerebral A. and its cortical branches

Cortical branches of middle cerebral A.

Posterior cerebral A. and its cortical branches

Fig. 6.19 Medial surface of the right cerebral hemisphere with the cerebral arteries superimposed.

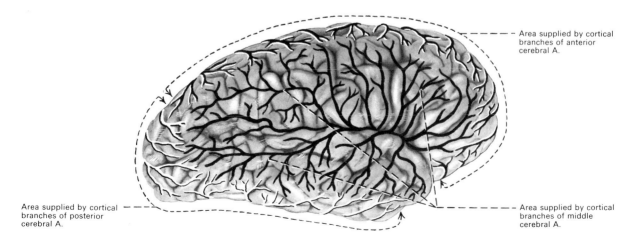

Area supplied by cortical branches of anterior cerebral A.

Area supplied by cortical branches of posterior cerebral A.

Area supplied by cortical branches of middle cerebral A.

Fig. 6.20 Supero-lateral surface of the right cerebral hemisphere with the cerebral arteries superimposed.

6.17

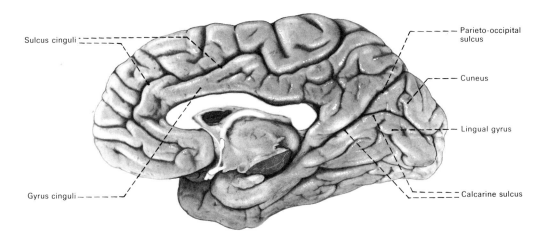

Parieto-occipital sulcus

Cuneus

Lingual gyrus

Calcarine sulcus

Sulcus cinguli

Gyrus cinguli

Fig. 6.21 Medial surface of the right cerebral hemisphere. BRAIN A.

The sulci and gyri of the cerebral hemispheres

The medial surface of the cerebrum [Fig. 6.21]

Turn the hemisphere on to its supero-lateral surface and carefully remove all the remaining arachnoid and pia mater from the medial surface of the hemisphere. The pattern of the convolutions, or cerebral gyri, and of the cerebral sulci between them, varies considerably from one brain to another, and only the more constant folds need be studied.

The principal sulcus of the medial surface starts below the genu of the corpus callosum and curves upwards and then backwards, more or less parallel to the convex border of the corpus callosum, and about 1 cm distant from it. This, the **sulcus cinguli** [Fig. 6.21], ends posteriorly by turning upwards to cross and fade into the supero-medial border of the hemisphere. Between the corpus callosum and the sulcus cinguli is the **gyrus cinguli.**

Below the splenium of the corpus callosum you should find the anterior end of a deep sulcus, the **calcarine sulcus,** which passes posteriorly towards the occipital pole. The calcarine sulcus is joined by another deep sulcus, the **parieto-occipital sulcus,** which ascends to the supero-medial border of the hemisphere almost at a right-angle to the calcarine sulcus. Separate the lips of the calcarine and parieto-occipital sulci and note their considerable depth. The cortex of the lips and walls of the calcarine sulcus has the specific function of receiving the visual information that is first transmitted along the optic nerves. It is therefore called the visual area of cortex [Fig. 6.25]. The triangular convolution which lies between the diverging calcarine and parieto-occipital sulci is called the **cuneus.** Ventral to the calcarine sulcus is another constant and well-defined convolution, the **lingual gyrus.** This gyrus extends on to the inferior surface of the hemisphere, where it is bounded laterally by the **collateral sulcus** [Fig. 6.22].

The inferior surface of the cerebrum [Fig. 6.22]

Turn the brain and examine the inferior surface of the hemisphere. Note the long collateral sulcus which starts near the occipital pole and runs forwards near the midline, towards the temporal pole. Anteriorly, the collateral sulcus forms the lateral boundary of a convolution called the **parahippocampal gyrus,** which lies against the lateral surface of the cerebral peduncle. Follow the parahippocampal gyrus forwards. At its anterior end this gyrus turns sharply round upon itself, forming a hook, called the **uncus.** The cortex of the uncus and the anterior end of the parahippocampal gyrus are concerned with the perception of olfactory sensations.

The supero-lateral surface of the cerebrum [Fig. 6.23]

Follow the sulcus cinguli upwards to the point where it notches the supero-medial border of the posterior part of the hemisphere. There is usually another sulcus which notches this border just anterior to the sulcus cinguli. Follow this second sulcus, and you will see that it passes antero-laterally across the supero-lateral surface of the hemisphere, towards the midpoint of the lateral sulcus. The sulcus you are following is the **central sulcus** [Fig. 6.23]. It is usually kinked, and it never quite joins the **lateral sulcus** below.

The central sulcus separates two parallel convolutions. The one anterior to the sulcus is called the **precentral gyrus,** and the one posterior, the **postcentral gyrus.**

The areas of the cortex [Figs 6.24 and 6.25]

The cortex of the postcentral gyrus is called the **somaesthetic area** of the cortex [Fig. 6.24]. It is concerned with the accurate perception of such sensations as touch and the position of joints. It is thus a projection area for information entering the central nervous system through all the spinal nerves

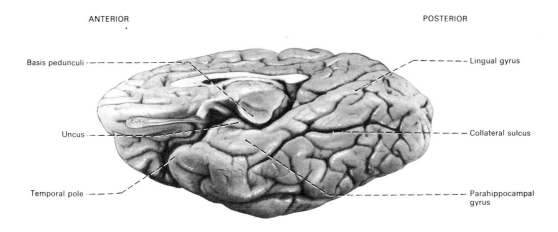

ANTERIOR   POSTERIOR

Basis pedunculi

Uncus

Temporal pole

Lingual gyrus

Collateral sulcus

Parahippocampal gyrus

Fig. 6.22 Inferior and medial surfaces of the right cerebral hemisphere. BRAIN A, viewed obliquely from below.

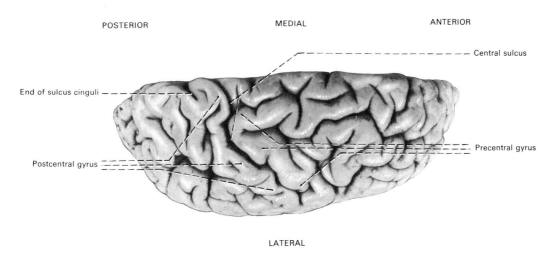

POSTERIOR   MEDIAL   ANTERIOR

End of sulcus cinguli

Postcentral gyrus

Central sulcus

Precentral gyrus

LATERAL

Fig. 6.23 Superior view of the right cerebral hemisphere. BRAIN A.

and also through the trigeminal, facial, glossopharyngeal, and vagus nerves. The **visual area,** or calcarine cortex, is concerned in a corresponding way with the information that is conveyed by the optic nerves, as is the **olfactory area,** or uncinate (uncus) cortex, with the impulses relayed by the olfactory nerves [Fig. 6.25].

The cortex of the precentral gyrus, and of an area extending a variable distance anterior to it, is concerned with motor function, and specifically with the neural mechanisms which control the movements of joints and the tone of muscles. This part of the cerebral cortex is referred to as the **motor area** [Fig. 6.24].

The only sensory area of the cortex which remains to be identified is the one concerned in the reception of auditory information, which enters the central nervous system through the cochlear part of the vestibulocochlear nerve. The **auditory area** of cortex lies in the floor and lower lip of the lateral sulcus, opposite the lower end of the postcentral gyrus, and is part of a convolution, the **superior temporal gyrus,** that lies below and parallel to the lateral sulcus.

This gyrus is bounded inferiorly by the **superior temporal sulcus** [Fig. 6.24].

The lobes of the cerebral hemispheres [Fig. 6.26]

Now that the principal sulci and gyri of the hemispheres have been identified, it is possible to define the four lobes into which each hemisphere is arbitrarily subdivided. The lobes are named after the bones of the skull to which they are principally related.

The **frontal lobe** is that part of the hemisphere that is superior to the lateral sulcus and anterior to the central sulcus [Figs 6.25 and 6.26]. You will see that the central sulcus lies so far posteriorly that part of the frontal lobe is related to the parietal bone.

The **occipital lobe** can be defined as the area between the parieto-occipital sulcus and the occipital pole. Between the parieto-occipital sulcus and the central sulcus lies the **parietal lobe.** The **temporal lobe** lies below the lateral sulcus, and has no distinct posterior boundary to separate it from the parietal and occipital lobes.

6.19

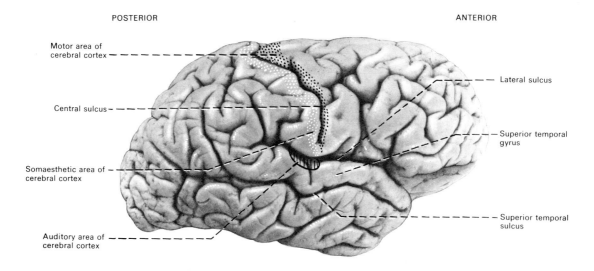

ANTERIOR

Motor area of
cerebral cortex

Central sulcus

Somaesthetic area of
cerebral cortex

Auditory area of
cerebral cortex

Lateral sulcus

Superior temporal
gyrus

Superior temporal
sulcus

Fig. 6.24 The motor and sensory areas of the right cerebral hemisphere. Supero-lateral surface of BRAIN A.

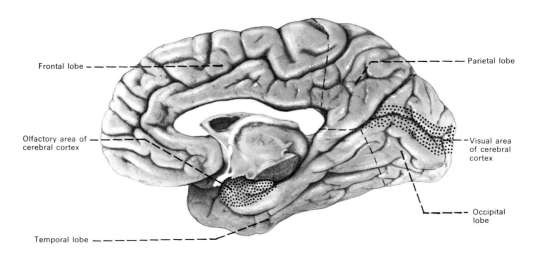

Frontal lobe

Olfactory area of
cerebral cortex

Temporal lobe

Parietal lobe

Visual area
of cerebral
cortex

Occipital
lobe

Fig. 6.25 Medial surface of the right cerebral hemisphere. BRAIN A. The broken white lines mark the boundaries between the lobes.

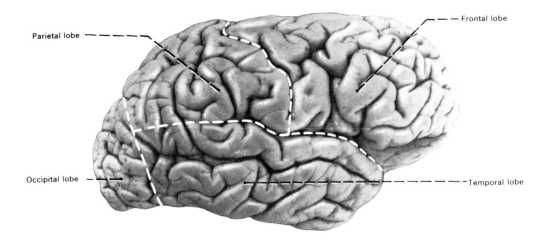

Parietal lobe

Occipital lobe

Frontal lobe

Temporal lobe

Fig. 6.26 The lobes of the right cerebral hemisphere. BRAIN A. The broken white lines mark the boundaries between the lobes.

6.20

The gyrus cinguli, the parahippocampal gyrus, and the uncus on the medial surface of the hemisphere are sometimes collectively referred to as the 'limbic lobe'.

The geniculate bodies [Fig. 6.27]

Identify the optic tract on one of the separated hemispheres (BRAIN A), and follow it posteriorly, displacing the parahippocampal gyrus laterally to do so. The optic tract passes round the upper end of the crus cerebri and ends in a slight elevation called the **lateral geniculate body** [Fig. 6.27]. Medial and a little posterior to the lateral geniculate body is a more prominent elevation, the **medial geniculate body,** which may have been cut when the brain stem was divided. Both geniculate bodies are on the under-surface of the thalamus, of which they are part. They consist of collections of neurons whose axons project on to the cerebral cortex. Those of the lateral geniculate body convey visual information to the visual area of cortex in the region of the calcarine sulcus; those of the medial geniculate body convey auditory information to the auditory area of cortex of the superior temporal gyrus.

Behind the geniculate bodies the posterior free margin of the thalamus presents a rounded projection, called the **pulvinar.**

Frontal sections of the cerebral hemisphere

Now make five serial frontal sections through one of the separated hemispheres (BRAIN A) [Fig. 6.28], starting anteriorly and placing the incisions so as to pass through:

1. The rostrum of the corpus callosum.
2. The posterior border of the anterior commissure.
3. The mamillary body.
4. The lateral geniculate body (approximately the upper opening of the cerebral aqueduct).
5. The middle of the splenium of the corpus callosum.

Examine the anterior of the two cut surfaces through the rostrum of the corpus callosum, i.e. the posterior surface of the frontal pole. You will see that the **corpus callosum** is continuous with the white matter of the cerebral hemisphere, which is surrounded by the grey matter of the cerebral cortex. The lateral ventricle extends forwards into a cul-de-sac called the **anterior horn of the lateral ventricle** [Fig. 6.29], which is bounded anteriorly by the genu of the corpus callosum. The **septum pellucidum** forms the medial wall of the ventricle. Below the sloping floor of the ventricle is a large mass of grey matter, called the **head of the caudate nucleus,** which is incompletely separated by a striated band of white matter from a smaller mass of grey matter lying lateral to it.

Now identify the head of the caudate nucleus in the section which passes through the anterior commissure [Fig. 6.30]. It is smaller here. The mass of grey matter below and lateral to it is the **lentiform nucleus,** which is now clearly

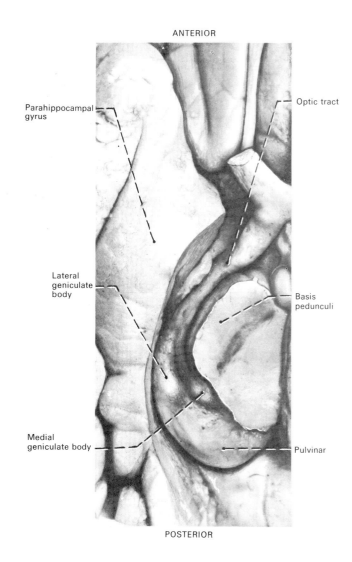

Fig. 6.27 **The right optic tract and the geniculate bodies.** Part of the parahippocampal gyrus and uncus have been excised.

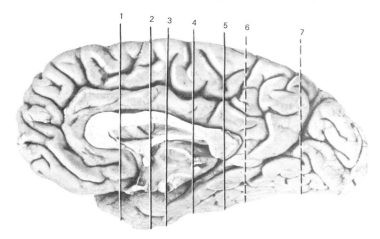

Fig. 6.28 **Medial surface of the right cerebral hemisphere showing positions of the frontal sections referred to in the text.** BRAIN A.

6.21

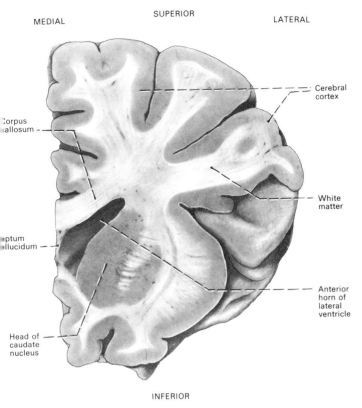

MEDIAL SUPERIOR LATERAL

Cerebral cortex

Corpus callosum

White matter

septum llucidum

Anterior horn of lateral ventricle

Head of caudate nucleus

INFERIOR

Fig. 6.29 Frontal section of the right cerebral hemisphere through the rostrum of the corpus callosum (looking anteriorly at Section 1 of Fig. 6.28). The temporal pole has been removed.

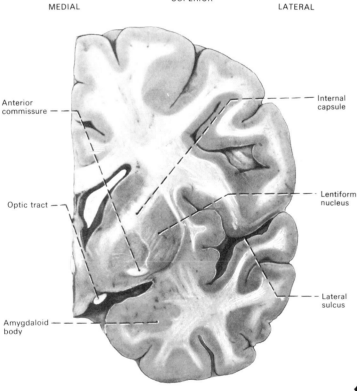

MEDIAL SUPERIOR LATERAL

Anterior commissure

Internal capsule

Optic tract

Lentiform nucleus

Lateral sulcus

Amygdaloid body

INFERIOR

separated from the caudate nucleus by a band of white matter, which is called the **internal capsule.** The narrower band of white matter running horizontally below the lentiform nucleus is the **anterior commissure,** some of whose fibres pass into the temporal lobe.

The caudate nucleus is smaller still in the section that passes through the mamillary bodies [Fig. 6.31]. Here the head of the nucleus, which lies in the lateral half of the floor

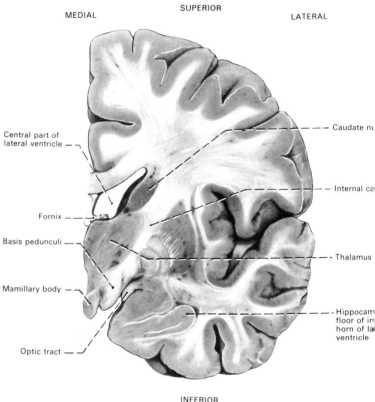

MEDIAL SUPERIOR LATERAL

Central part of lateral ventricle

Caudate nu

Fornix

Internal ca

Basis pedunculi

Thalamus

Mamillary body

Optic tract

Hippocam floor of in horn of la ventricle

INFERIOR

Fig. 6.31 Frontal section of the right cerebral hemisphere through the mamillary body (looking anteriorly at Section 3 of Fig. 6.28).

of the central part of the lateral ventricle, tapers off into the **tail of the caudate nucleus.** Medial to the tail the floor of the ventricle overlies the **thalamus,** which appears as a large mass of grey matter. The internal capsule now separates the lentiform nucleus, which in this plane of section appears triangular, from the lateral surface of the thalamus. The **fornix** forms the lower boundary of the septum pellucidum, but is separated from the thalamus by the **choroid fissure,** into which is invaginated the **choroid plexus of the lateral ventricle.**

Trace the thalamus, the tail of the caudate nucleus, and the fornix posteriorly through the next two sections [Figs 6.32 and 6.33]. You will reach the posterior extremity or

Fig. 6.30 Frontal section of the right cerebral hemisphere through the posterior border of the anterior commissure (looking anteriorly at Section 2 of Fig. 6.28).

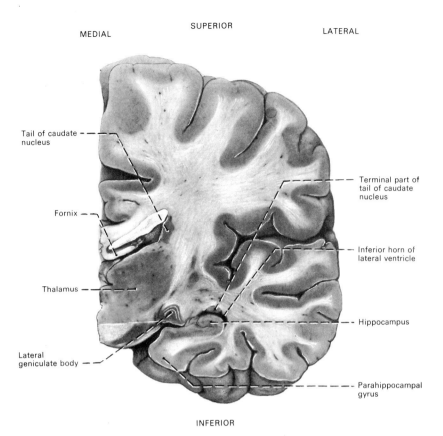

SUPERIOR

MEDIAL   LATERAL

Tail of caudate
nucleus

Fornix

Thalamus

Lateral
geniculate body

Terminal part of
tail of caudate
nucleus

Inferior horn of
lateral ventricle

Hippocampus

Parahippocampal
gyrus

INFERIOR

Fig. 6.32   Frontal section of the right cerebral hemisphere through the lateral geniculate body (looking anteriorly at Section 4 of Fig. 6.28).

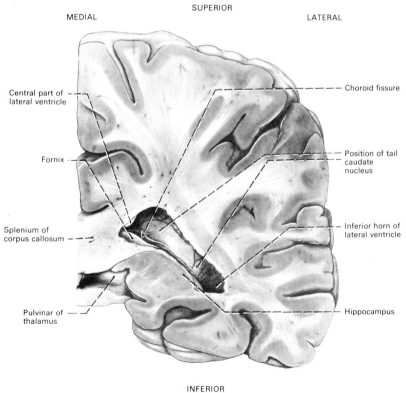

SUPERIOR

MEDIAL   LATERAL

Central part of
lateral ventricle

Fornix

Splenium of
corpus callosum

Pulvinar of
thalamus

Choroid fissure

Position of tail
caudate
nucleus

Inferior horn of
lateral ventricle

Hippocampus

INFERIOR

Fig. 6.33   Frontal section of the right cerebral hemisphere through the splenium of the corpus callosum (looking anteriorly at Section 5 of Fig. 6.28). The choroid plexus has been removed.

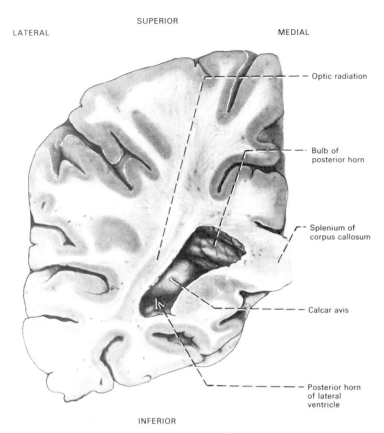

SUPERIOR

LATERAL   MEDIAL

— Optic radiation

— Bulb of
posterior horn

— Splenium of
corpus callosum

— Calcar avis

— Posterior horn
of lateral
ventricle

INFERIOR

Fig. 6.34 Frontal section of the right cerebral hemisphere through the splenium of the corpus callosum (looking posteriorly at Section 5 of Fig. 6.28).

pulvinar of the thalamus in the slice between the lateral geniculate body and the splenium of the corpus callosum. Open up the choroid fissure between the thalamus and fornix, and carefully remove the choroid plexus. Follow the fornix backwards. It and the ventricle loop round the back of the thalamus, and curve gently downwards and forwards, swinging laterally into the temporal lobe. This extension of the lateral ventricle is called the **inferior horn of the lateral ventricle.** Follow the inferior horn forwards through the slices of brain to its termination. Now follow the lower part of the fornix forwards, and you will see that it flattens out to become the upper surface of a rounded longitudinal elevation, known as the **hippocampus,** in the floor of the inferior horn.

In frontal section it can be seen that the hippocampus is directly related to the **parahippocampal gyrus,** which lies below and medial to it. The layers of grey and white matter in the hippocampus, which can be regarded as a strip of cortex that has invaginated the ventricle, give it a whorled appearance.

Trace the tail of the caudate nucleus round the thalamus. In section it appears as a very small area of grey matter in the roof of the inferior horn of the ventricle. The tail of the caudate nucleus continues forwards to end in a small mass

of grey matter, called the **amygdaloid body** [Fig. 6.30], which lies in the roof of the termination of the inferior horn, and which is continuous with the grey matter of the adjacent cortex. You may be able to see this nucleus in the frontal section that passes through the anterior commissure.

Look at the cut surface of the most posterior portion of the hemisphere. Here you will see the **posterior horn of the lateral ventricle** extending into the occipital lobe [Fig. 6.34]. The longitudinal elevation in the upper part of its medial wall is formed by bundles of fibres from the splenium of the corpus callosum. The elevation is called the **bulb of the posterior horn.** Below is a larger elongated elevation, the **calcar avis,** which is formed by the very deep **calcarine sulcus** invaginating the ventricle [Fig. 6.35]. Confirm this by making a frontal section of the hemisphere through the calcar avis [Section 6, Fig. 6.28].

Now make a further frontal section through the junction of the calcarine and parieto-occipital sulci [Section 7, Fig. 6.28]. Examine the cut surface of the cerebral cortex bordering the calcarine sulcus, and identify a line or stria of white matter which runs parallel with the surface, embedded in the grey matter. This stria reflects the structural specialization of the visual area of cortex which, consequently, is sometimes referred to as the **striate cortex** [Fig. 6.36].

The optic tract and the lateral geniculate body

Place the slices of the hemisphere together in their proper order, and again identify the optic tract, following the tract posteriorly. Now examine the section which passes through the lateral geniculate body, which you will see is composed of a small mass of interlaminated grey and white matter [Fig. 6.32]. The nerve fibres originating in the lateral geniculate body pass laterally through the white matter above the inferior horn of the lateral ventricle, before sweeping first posteriorly and then medially to the calcarine cortex. They form the optic radiation [Fig. 6.34], which you will soon see more clearly in a horizontal section of the hemisphere.

The insula [Fig. 6.37]

Place the slices of brain together again, and identify the lateral sulcus. You will see that the floor of this fissure is formed by a fairly extensive convex area of hidden cerebral cortex. This area of cortex is called the insula, and has its own sulci and gyri.

The basal nuclei [Figs 6.37 and 6.38]

The lentiform nucleus lies medial to the insula, separated from it by white matter in which you will see a line of grey matter. This grey matter forms the **claustrum.** Between the claustrum and the lentiform nucleus is the **external capsule** of white matter.

Examine the **lentiform nucleus** in the section which passes through the mamillary bodies, and note that it has a medial segment, the **globus pallidus,** which is paler than the lateral

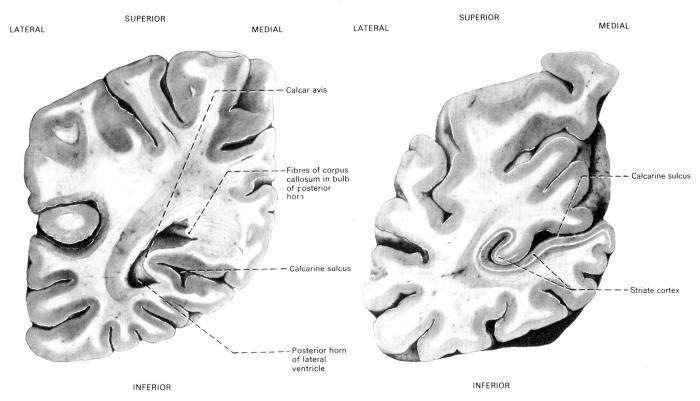

SUPERIOR

LATERAL   MEDIAL

— Calcar avis

— Fibres of corpus callosum in bulb of posterior horn

— Calcarine sulcus

- - Posterior horn of lateral ventricle

INFERIOR

Fig. 6.35 Frontal section of the right cerebral hemisphere through the calcar avis (looking posteriorly at Section 6 of Fig. 6.28).

SUPERIOR

LATERAL   MEDIAL

— Calcarine sulcus

- - Striate cortex

INFERIOR

Fig. 6.36 Frontal section of the right cerebral hemisphere through the junction of the calcarine and parieto-occipital sulci (looking posteriorly at Section 7 of Fig. 6.28).

segment, called the **putamen** [Fig. 6.37]. Look again at the more anterior slices of brain, noting that the putamen extends farther forwards than the globus pallidus. At its anterior extremity the putamen is continuous with the inferior part of the head of the **caudate nucleus.** Bands of grey matter also stretch across the internal capsule from the caudate nucleus to the putamen, giving a striated appearance to the capsule. This is especially well seen in the frontal section which passes through the anterior commissure. The mass formed by the caudate nucleus, the lentiform nucleus, and the white matter between them is consequently called the **corpus striatum.** The caudate and lentiform nuclei, the **amygdaloid body,** and the claustrum are also collectively termed the basal nuclei. They help to control muscular activity.

The blood supply of the corpus striatum is partly provided by the central branches of the anterior and middle cerebral arteries, which pierce the anterior perforated substance [see p. 6.4]. You will find that the anterior perforated substance underlies the lentiform nucleus.

The nerve fibres of the white matter

Now examine the slice of brain between the mamillary and lateral geniculate bodies, and note that the basis pedunculi is continuous with the internal capsule. Nerve fibres which pass from the cerebral cortex to the brain stem and spinal

medulla descend through the internal capsule, and converge on the basis pedunculi. Among them are fibres from the motor area which pass to the nuclei of origin of the cranial nerves in the brain stem (**corticonuclear tract**), and to the nuclei of origin of the spinal nerves in the spinal medulla (**corticospinal tracts**). The internal capsule also contains many fibres which arise in the thalamus and fan out to pass to all parts of the cerebral cortex, and fibres that pass in the reverse direction from the cerebral cortex to the thalamus and the basal nuclei. All these fibres connect the cerebral cortex with more caudal parts of the nervous system, and are collectively called **projection fibres.**

In addition to the projection tracts of the internal capsule and the transversely-running **commissural fibres** of the corpus callosum and anterior and posterior commissures, which link the cortex of the two hemispheres, there are also fibres which connect different parts of the cortex of the same hemisphere. These, collectively, are called **association fibres.** Some of them form longitudinal bundles of considerable size.

The horizontal section of the cerebral hemisphere

Divide the second isolated hemisphere (BRAIN A) horizontally, making your incision so that it passes through the upper part of the interventricular foramen. (If you were given only one brain, you may be supplied with an

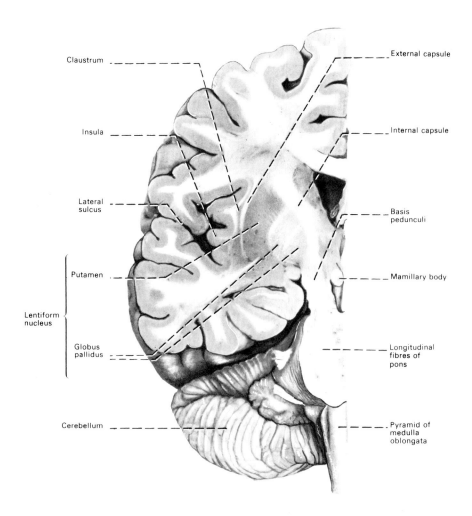

Fig. 6.37 Frontal section of the right half of a brain in the plane of the basis pedunculi (viewed from the front).

additional half-brain on which to make the horizontal cut referred to above. Failing this, examine Fig. 6.38.)

The internal capsule [Fig. 6.38]

Examine the anterior horn and the central part of the lateral ventricle. Confirm the presence of the posterior and inferior horns by passing a seeker into them. Identify the head and tail of the caudate nucleus, the thalamus, the lentiform nucleus, the claustrum, and the insula. You will see that the internal capsule is bent at the point where the head of the caudate nucleus comes into contact with the thalamus. This bend is called the **genu of the internal capsule** [Fig. 6.38]. Anterior to the genu, between the caudate and lentiform nuclei, is the **anterior limb of the internal capsule;** behind the genu, between the thalamus and the lentiform nucleus, is the **posterior limb of the internal capsule.** The **optic radiation** occupies the most posterior part of the posterior limb of the capsule, and may be seen as a faintly paler zone of white matter which sweeps backwards, lateral to the ventricle, before turning medially towards the calcarine sulcus.

Most of the fibres of the radiation pass below, or behind, the posterior horn of the ventricle.

Dissection of the internal capsule [Figs 6.39–6.41]

Turn now to BRAIN B (the one which was not bisected) and remove the arachnoid, pia mater, and blood vessels from the surfaces of both hemispheres. Expose the **insula** of one side by making a large circular incision with a scalpel in the supero-lateral surface of the hemisphere. The centre of your cut should fall about the midpoint of the lateral sulcus. You should remove as much of the frontal, parietal, and temporal lobes as is necessary to expose the insula completely [Fig. 6.39].

Use the handle of a scalpel to scrape away the gyri of the insula, working in an upward direction. Do not hesitate to remove gyri of the convex surface of the hemisphere at the periphery of the insula as you follow the planes of cleavage that your scalpel creates. The underlying white matter will peel off in thin ridged sheets. The ridging will be particularly apparent at the upper border of the insula, where you must scrape firmly towards the superficial cortex of the hemisphere. Firm deliberate strokes with the handle of your scalpel will make a better dissection than timid nibbles.

If you now refer to the frontal slices of the hemisphere, you will see that you have been stripping white matter (and claustrum) from the lateral surface of the **lentiform nucleus.** You will also see that the upper border of the insula coincides with the upper border of the lentiform nucleus, so that, in this region, you have been scraping away many fibres of the internal capsule. Return to the brain you are dissecting, and try to make out the anterior, superior, and posterior parts of the border of the lentiform nucleus. Beyond this border the projection fibres of the internal capsule fan out towards the frontal, parietal, and occipital lobes, and form what is called the **corona radiata** [Fig. 6.40]. These projection fibres intermingle with those of the corpus callosum. The **optic radiation** forms a well-defined band which can be found by scraping backwards from the lower border of the insula. Trace the optic radiation to the medial surface of the occipital lobe, removing the overlying gyri where necessary.

Now, starting in the frontal lobe in front of the anterior end of the lateral sulcus, and carrying the handle of your scalpel backwards across the lateral sulcus to the temporal lobe, scrape or peel off a layer of white matter. This will reveal bundles of association fibres connecting the different parts of the cortex with each other. Some of these fibres (the uncinate fasciculus) hook sharply round the anterior end of the lateral sulcus, while others pass posteriorly towards the occipital lobe.

Peel off what remains of the white matter covering the lentiform nucleus, and then scoop or scrape out the grey matter of the nucleus, this time scraping horizontally, at right-angles to the fibres of the internal capsule, whose lateral surface now comes into view [Fig. 6.41]. Complete the removal of the lentiform nucleus by digging down medial to the association fibres you have just revealed connecting the frontal and temporal lobes. As you reach the inferior boundary of the lentiform nucleus you will encounter the **anterior commissure** running postero-laterally to the temporal lobe. It forms a narrow but distinct bundle of fibres.

Make a transverse incision through the association fibres that connect the frontal and temporal lobes at the point where they cross the lateral sulcus, carrying the blade of your scalpel as far as the lateral border of the optic tract. Make a second incision in the frontal plane, passing through the temporal lobe about 2 cm behind the first cut, and extending to, but not including, the optic tract. Join the medial ends of the two incisions with a third incision which should follow the lateral border of the optic tract, and remove the part of the temporal lobe you have isolated. You can now see that the internal capsule is continuous with the **basis pedunculi** medial to the optic tract [Fig. 6.42].

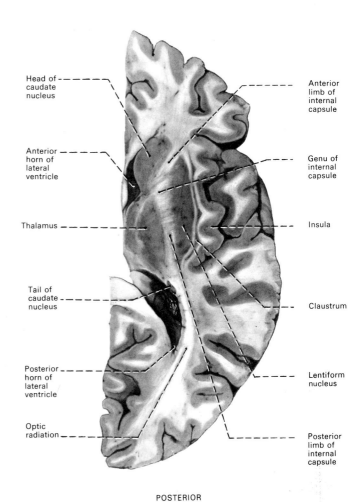

Head of caudate nucleus

Anterior horn of lateral ventricle

Thalamus

Tail of caudate nucleus

Posterior horn of lateral ventricle

Optic radiation

Anterior limb of internal capsule

Genu of internal capsule

Insula

Claustrum

Lentiform nucleus

Posterior limb of internal capsule

POSTERIOR

Fig. 6.38 Horizontal section of the right cerebral hemisphere through the upper part of the interventricular foramen. BRAIN A, viewed from above.

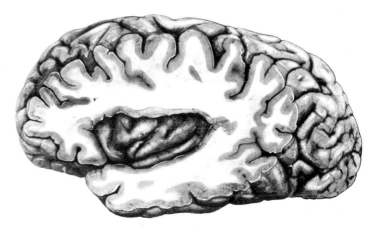

Fig. 6.39 Lateral view of the left cerebral hemisphere with the insula exposed. BRAIN B. Parts of the frontal, parietal, and temporal lobes have been excised.

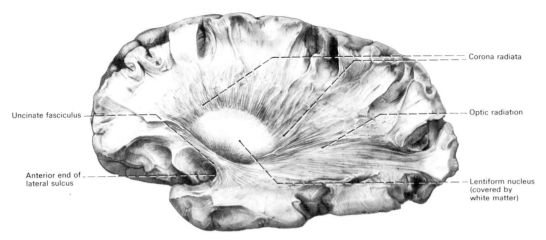

Fig. 6.40 The left lentiform nucleus and corona radiata. BRAIN B.

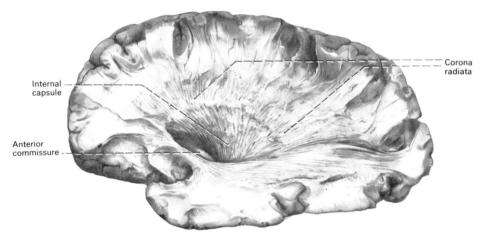

Fig. 6.41 Lateral view of the left internal capsule. BRAIN B. The lentiform nucleus has been removed from the dissection shown in Fig. 6.40.

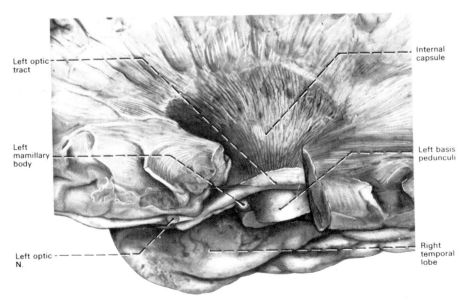

Fig. 6.42 Lateral view of the left internal capsule with optic tract and basis pedunculi exposed. BRAIN B. Part of the left temporal lobe has been excised.

6.28

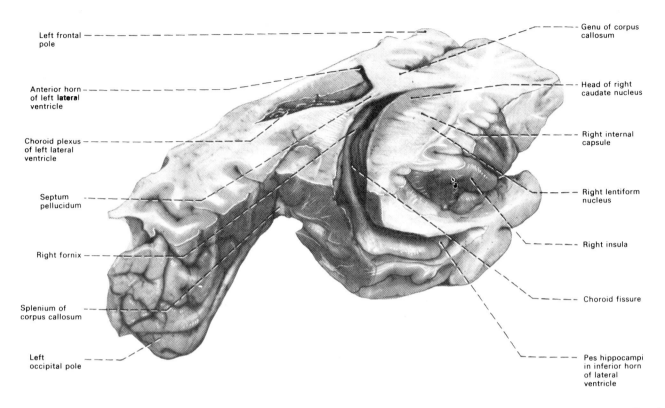

Left frontal pole

Anterior horn of left **lateral** ventricle

Choroid plexus of left lateral ventricle

Septum pellucidum

Right fornix

Splenium of corpus callosum

Left occipital pole

Genu of corpus callosum

Head of right caudate nucleus

Right internal capsule

Right lentiform nucleus

Right insula

Choroid fissure

Pes hippocampi in inferior horn of lateral ventricle

Fig. 6.43 Postero-lateral view of the right lateral ventricle. BRAIN B. The cerebral hemispheres have been sectioned horizontally. The right insula and the left internal capsule have been exposed, and the right occipital lobe and the lateral wall of the inferior horn of the right lateral ventricle have been removed.

Dissection of the lateral ventricle [Fig. 6.43]

Turn now to the hemisphere (BRAIN B) which you have not dissected so far, and expose the insula as you did on the opposite side. Then place the brain with the insula uppermost, and with a long-bladed knife, divide the brain horizontally 2 to 3 mm below the upper border of the insula, carrying your incision through both hemispheres. Remove the occipital lobe of the hemisphere facing you by making a frontal section flush with the posterior margin of the splenium of the corpus callosum, terminating your cut at the midline. Use scissors to remove the white matter between the two parts of the lateral ventricle that have been exposed by these incisions. Open up the inferior horn of the lateral ventricle by carefully removing its lateral wall with scissors [Fig. 6.43].

Identify the **choroid plexus of the lateral ventricle,** and then carefully tear it out. In so doing you will open up the **choroid fissure,** which will now appear as a curved slit in the medial wall of the ventricle, extending all the way from the interventricular foramen to the inferior horn of the lateral ventricle. Gently separate the roof and floor of the inferior horn, and you will see the rounded longitudinal elevation of the **hippocampus** in the medial part of the floor. Anteriorly it expands to form the **pes hippocampi** before it terminates abruptly at the tip of the inferior horn of the ventricle. Note how the **fornix** arises from the upper surface of the hippocampus and arches up and over the thalamus, coming to lie in the inferior border of the **septum pellucidum.**

Note that the anterior horns and central parts of the lateral ventricles lie close to each other, separated only by the thin septum pellucidum. Identify the **interventricular foramen** on each side. Posteriorly, the ventricles diverge as each wraps itself round the back of the thalamus, internal capsule, basal nuclei, and insula. This block of structures forms the 'core' of the hemisphere, and is clearly exposed by this dissection.

Section 6.2

The 'one-brain' dissection

Only those instructions that are specially required for the 'one-brain' dissection are given in this section. For the rest you will turn to the text for the 'two-brain' dissection as follows:

to p. 6.2 for the examination of the external anatomy of the undivided brain;
to p. 6.12 for sections of the brain stem;
to p. 6.8 for the third ventricle;
and to p. 6.17 to complete the study of the forebrain.

Begin by following the instructions for the 'two-brain' dissection from p. 6.2 until the end of the section on 'The corpus callosum and dorsal surface of the midbrain' on p. 6.6. With only one brain at your disposal your next step will be the dissection of the brain stem which you must now separate from the cerebral hemispheres.

The brain stem

Lay the brain down on its superior surface so that you are looking at its base. Your cut will be made between the mamillary bodies and the oculomotor nerves at right-angles to the long axis of the brain stem. Place the heel of the blade of your scalpel against the ventral surface of one of the two cerebral peduncles with the point of the blade directed laterally. Begin your cut by moving the point of the blade backwards, then across the midline through the dorsal part of the midbrain. Then cut forwards through the other peduncle and complete the separation of the cerebrum from the cerebellum and the brain stem.

Grey and white matter

Look at the cut surface of the midbrain [Fig. 6.14] and you will see that it is not uniform in colour. Some parts of the surface are almost pale. This is especially so near the ventral margin of the cerebral peduncle. In this area bundles of nerve fibres which form the **white matter** are running longitudinally down the brain stem.

Identify the lumen of a canal that pierces the midbrain. Around this is a darker area of **grey matter** which comprises aggregations of the cell bodies (perikarya) of neurons. In addition you will see ventrolateral to the lumen a band of black material on each side. This also is grey matter but it is uncharacteristic in that it contains many neurons which are unusual in that they contain pigment.

The ventricular system in the brain stem

The brain and spinal medulla develop in the embryo from a tubular structure called the **neural tube,** whose lumen is filled with **cerebrospinal fluid.** Except in rare pathological conditions, the lumen of the tube never becomes occluded in the brain. You have already identified a narrow part of this lumen in the cut surface of the midbrain at the rostral end of your specimen. This is the **cerebral aqueduct** [Fig. 6.13] which connects two larger cavities, the **third ventricle** in the midline of the forebrain and the **fourth ventricle** in the hindbrain.

Now look at the lower end of the specimen, gently separating the cerebellum from the medulla oblongata. In the midline you will find a wide opening into the lower end of the fourth ventricle. This is the **median aperture of the fourth ventricle.** Place one seeker in the aperture and pass another into the cerebral aqueduct from above. With a scalpel cut through the cerebellum (but not the midbrain) in the median plane on the line connecting the seekers. Cut carefully, gently separating the two halves of the cerebellum as you go, until you can see into the cavity of the fourth ventricle.

The next step is to remove one half of the cerebellum from the brain stem. On one side only, incise the middle cerebellar peduncle just posterior to the roots of the trigeminal, facial, and vestibulocochlear nerves, cutting in a postero-medial direction. The line of incision is shown (on both sides) in Fig. 6.9. Hold the brain stem so that the half of the cerebellum you are removing tends to fall away from it, and cut towards the midline, but no further. Detach the half of the cerebellum thus freed and set it aside for later study.

Through the large window that has been made you can see the whole of the fourth ventricle [Fig. 6.44]. Posteriorly the cerebellum forms an apex to the roof of the fourth ventricle. Rostral to this, the roof is formed by a thin sheet of white matter, the **superior medullary velum.** Now gently separate the medulla oblongata from the part of the cerebellum to which it is still attached, and you will see that the inferior part of the roof of the fourth ventricle is formed by delicate membrane which has possibly been torn. This membrane consists only of the lining epithelium of the ventricle, called **ependyma,** with pia mater on its external surface. This particular area of pia mater is rich in blood vessels and is called the **tela chorioidea of the fourth ventricle.** The median aperture of the fourth ventricle, which you identified before removing half of the cerebellum, is a midline perforation in this membrane. (The **inferior medullary velum** is a narrow and thin sheet of white matter which is interposed between the ependyma and pia mater at the upper lateral margin of the tela chorioidea.)

Cerebrospinal fluid is secreted in the fourth ventricle, and in all the other dilatations or ventricles of the brain, by vascular structures called choroid plexuses, which comprise tufts of vessels which invaginate the thin membranes formed where ependyma and pia mater come into apposition. The **choroid plexus of the fourth ventricle** is the long dark granular structure which you will find attached to the thin part of the roof of the ventricle.

The rhomboid fossa [Fig. 6.10]

Anteriorly (ventrally) the pons and medulla oblongata form a floor to the fourth ventricle. Identify the boundaries of the floor. Because of its shape the floor of the fourth ventricle is called the **rhomboid fossa.** There is a superior angle where the ventricle continues into the cerebral aqueduct, and an inferior angle where it joins a central canal in the lower part of the medulla oblongata. At the level of the junction between the medulla oblongata and the pons are two lateral angles, called the **lateral recesses of the fourth ventricle** [Figs 6.10 and 6.44]. Cerebrospinal fluid escapes from the ventricular system into the subarachnoid space through the median aperture of the fourth ventricle and also through **lateral apertures of the fourth ventricle,** one in each lateral recess. With a seeker confirm the presence of this aperture on the side to which the cerebellum is still attached.

Again gently separate the cerebellum and the medulla oblongata on the intact side and note that the thin roof of the caudal half of the ventricle extends laterally to meet a thick bundle of nervous tissue, which diverges from the median plane to enter the cerebellum higher up. This is the **inferior cerebellar peduncle** [Figs 6.10 and 6.44].

Now examine the posterior aspect of the medulla oblongata. Its lower part resembles the spinal medulla, but the **posterior median sulcus,** by which it is marked, soon splays open into the caudal part of the fourth ventricle.

Carefully nibble away the tightly-adherent pia mater off the posterior surface of the lower part of the medulla oblongata and try to make out on the infero-lateral boundaries of the ventricle two slight elevations on each side, formed by aggregations of nerve cells (nuclei). The medial elevation is the **tubercle of the nucleus gracilis,** and the lateral elevation, the **tubercle of the nucleus cuneatus.** These two nuclei are relay stations for the tracts of nerve fibres, the one the **fasciculus gracilis,** the other the **fasciculus cuneatus,** which ascend in the white matter of the posterior part of the spinal medulla. You can easily make out these tracts just caudal to the tubercles.

The nerve fibres arising in these nuclei cross over to the opposite side in the so-called **sensory decussation** and run up the brain stem to the forebrain.

The inferior cerebellar peduncle [Fig. 6.10]

Now examine the inferior cerebellar peduncle of the side on which the ventricle has been exposed. You will see that it lies between the upper part of the infero-lateral boundary

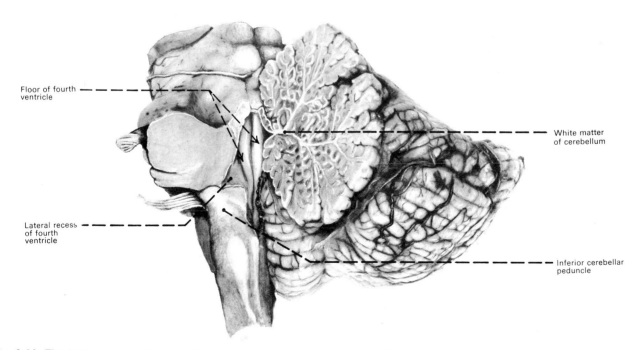

Floor of fourth
ventricle

White matter
of cerebellum

Lateral recess
of fourth
ventricle

Inferior cerebellar
peduncle

Fig. 6.44 The brain stem with the left half of the cerebellum removed. 'One-brain' dissection. Postero-lateral view from the left.

of the fourth ventricle and the groove from which the root-lets of the glossopharyngeal, vagus, and accessory nerves emerge behind the olive. The peduncle passes up from the medulla oblongata into the cerebellum, where it lies on the medial side of the much larger **middle cerebellar peduncle.**

Both peduncles have been divided at this point by the in-cision which removed half of the cerebellum.

The superior cerebellar peduncle [Fig. 6.10]

The supero-lateral boundary of the ventricle is mostly formed by the superior cerebellar peduncle. This is a flat bundle of fibres which passes forwards and upwards from the cerebellum to the midbrain. Like the inferior cerebellar peduncle, this peduncle will also have been divided obli-quely on one side of the brain stem.

Stretching between the well-defined medial borders of the superior cerebellar peduncles, and forming the roof of the ventricle in this region, is the thin **superior medullary velum.**

The floor of the fourth ventricle [Fig. 6.10]

Now examine the floor of the fourth ventricle, and note that on either side of a **median sulcus** is a faint sinuous groove, the **sulcus limitans,** which is partly obliterated at the level of the lateral recesses by transverse streaks known as the **medullary striae of the fourth ventricle.** Caudal to the medul-lary striae the sulcus limitans presents a shallow pit, the **in-ferior fovea,** from which two grooves diverge, one passing medially towards the central canal of the medulla, and the other, which is the sulcus limitans, continuing caudally, parallel with the median sulcus. Another shallow pit in the sulcus limitans, the **superior fovea,** lies rostral to the medul-lary striae and in a more lateral position than the inferior fovea.

Immediately subjacent to the floor of the fourth ventricle is a layer of grey matter which contains motor and sensory **nuclei of the cranial nerves** that are attached to the brain stem. The organisation of this grey matter is fairly simple. In general, the motor nuclei, or **nuclei of origin,** lie medial, and the sensory nuclei, or **nuclei of termination,** lie lateral to the sulcus limitans. The area medial to the caudal part of the sulcus limitans overlies the nuclei of origin of the hypoglossal and vagus nerves. Medial to the superior fovea is a rounded elevation, the **facial colliculus,** which overlies the nucleus of the abducent nerve. The elevation is called the facial colliculus because motor fibres of the facial nerve partly encircle the nucleus of the abducent nerve as they pass from their nucleus of origin to their point of exit at the cere-bellopontine angle [p. 6.6]. Lateral to the sulcus limitans, both rostral and caudal to the medullary striae, is the **ves-tibular area,** beneath which lie the (sensory) nuclei of the vestibular part of the vestibulocochlear nerve.

The ventral surface of the medulla oblongata [Fig. 6.4]

Now examine the ventral surface of the medulla oblongata.

You have already identified the anterior median fissure, the pyramids, and the olives of the medulla oblongata.

The pyramids are made up of longitudinal bundles of nerve fibres. Chief among these are the **corticospinal tracts** of motor nerve fibres, which arise from cells in the cerebral cortex and end by forming connections with neurons at all levels of the grey matter of the spinal medulla. Towards the lower end of the medulla oblongata the greater part of each corticospinal tract crosses over the midline to the opposite side.

Splay open the rostral end of the anterior median fissure by inserting the closed points of a pair of blunt forceps. Fol-low the fissure downwards, opening it up as you go. If the brain stem was cut off low enough when the brain was re-moved from the cadaver, you will see that the lower end of the anterior median fissure is interrupted by the decussa-tion of the two corticospinal tracts called the **pyramidal decussation** or **motor decussation.** It lies immediately caudal to the sensory decussation.

You will now complete your study of the brain stem by examining it in transverse sections. For this purpose turn to the instructions set out on pages 6.12 to 6.13 under the heading 'Sections of the Brain Stem'.

The cerebellum

In order to study the rhomboid fossa you divided the cere-bellum in two and detached one half from the brain stem. The half attached to the brain stem is now in three pieces. Fit the pieces together; then place the halves of the cerebel-lum together and study its unpaired median part. This is called the **vermis.** The vermis forms a rounded crest on the superior surface of the cerebellum where it is hardly dis-tinguishable from the two lateral masses on each side which constitute the **cerebellar hemispheres** [Fig. 6.15]. On the in-ferior surface the vermis lies in a deep median groove, called the **vallecula of the cerebellum.** Note on either side of the vallecula a low rounded projection, the folds of which are disposed longitudinally [Fig. 6.17]. This is the **tonsil** of the cerebellum.

Examine the cut surface of the half of the cerebellum which was removed from the brain stem. Note the small central core of white matter which branches towards the highly-folded surface from which, however, it is always separated by a thin rind or **cortex** of grey matter [Fig. 6.6], the **cerebellar cortex.** A corresponding arrangement of grey and white matter characterizes the cerebral hemispheres, the surface of which is not as finely folded as is that of the cere-bellum. In the cerebellum the long narrow ridges or con-volutions into which the cortex is folded are called **foliae,** separated by parallel **fissures.** Many of the fissures extend transversely across the vermis from one hemisphere to the other. The deeper fissures subdivide the corresponding parts of the hemispheres. Some of these subdivisions are identified in the alternative dissection using two brains [pp. 6.14 to 6.16].

You have made two transverse incisions through the other half of the cerebellum, the first at the level at which the trigeminal nerve is attached to the pons, and the second at the level of the upper half of the olive in the medulla oblongata. Examine both cut surfaces of the slice between these two planes of section and look for the grey matter of the **cerebellar nuclei** embedded in the white core of the cerebellum. Deeply-enfolded cortex should not be taken for the grey matter of these nuclei. If there is no evidence of buried grey matter on either surface of the slice, slit the latter into two thinner slices. The fresh section thus made will reveal the **denate nucleus** [Fig. 6.18] which resembles the inferior olivary nucleus of the medulla oblongata. Figure 6.18 depicts the dentate nucleus as it appears when the cerebellum is sectioned in the plane of the superior cerebellar peduncle (not in a plane transverse to the axis of the brain stem). Postero-medial to the dentate nucleus are other smaller cerebellar nuclei in the white matter that forms the roof of the fourth ventricle.

The cerebellar nuclei contain the cell bodies of the vast majority of the nerve fibres that carry impulses from the cerebellum. The fibres from the dentate nucleus pass through the superior cerebellar peduncle to the red nucleus and the thalamus of the opposite side of the brain.

The forebrain

Before it is divided into two, the forebrain should be dissected on one side only, preferably the left, which is shown in all the figures that illustrate this dissection. After bisection the cerebral arteries and the sulci and gyri of the cortex are examined on the remaining half, which is then divided into a series of frontal sections so that you can re-examine the deep grey matter.

The grey and white matter of the forebrain

As you will be carrying out the dissection of the forebrain without the benefit of a preliminary examination of sections of the hemisphere, you need to have some understanding of the general arrangement of its grey and white matter.

Each cerebral hemisphere develops from a sac-like dilatation, the **cerebral vesicle,** which extends laterally from the rostral end of the embryonic neural tube. The lumen of the vesicle becomes the ventricle of the hemisphere, called the **lateral ventricle,** and the walls of the vesicle thicken and fold as grey and white matter develop. Grey matter comes to lie just beneath the folded external surface of the hemisphere and forms the **cerebral cortex.** In addition grey matter collects close to the lumen of the ventricle, particularly its ventral floor, to form the **basal nuclei** or **basal ganglia.**

The midline part of the neural tube from which the two cerebral vesicles sprout becomes the **diencephalon.** This lies ventrally between the two cerebral hemispheres. Its cavity is the **third ventricle.** Collections of grey matter develop in the lateral walls of the third ventricle, the largest mass being the **thalamus.** The infundibulum and the mamillary bodies are parts of the diencephalon which you have already identified.

Many millions of nerve fibres connect these various areas of grey matter with each other and with the brain stem. They are collected together into a thick layer of white matter which lies between the superficial grey matter of the cortex and the deep grey matter of the basal and diencephalic nuclei.

Gently separate the frontal and temporal lobes of one side of the brain sufficiently to tear the arachnoid that veils the deep **lateral sulcus** which lies between them [Fig. 6.24]. Trace the fissure to its end. Using scissors and forceps peel back the arachnoid and pia mater and blood vessels from the surface of the hemisphere for about 8 cm on each side of the lateral sulcus, but do not pull vessels out of the fissure. In the depths of the sulcus there is an extensive area of buried cortex which is called the **insula** (i.e. island) on account of its relative isolation from the outer surface of the hemisphere [Fig. 6.39].

With the centre of your cut about the midpoint of the lateral sulcus make a circular incision with a scalpel in the surface of the hemisphere in order to expose the insula. Carve away as much of the frontal, parietal, and temporal lobes as is necessary to expose the insula completely in the floor of a shallow excavation with gently-sloping walls [Fig. 6.39]. If you feel unsure about how deep to go refer to Figures 6.37 and 6.38 which show the insula in horizontal and frontal (coronal) sections, and also keep your eyes on the undissected hemisphere.

Now carefully remove the blood vessels overlying the insula, dividing them with scissors where they arise from their stem vessels towards the lower and anterior end of the lateral sulcus.

Use the handle of a scalpel to scrape away the gyri of the insula, working in an upward direction. Do not hesitate to remove gyri of the convex surface of the hemisphere at the periphery of the insula as you follow the planes of cleavage that your scalpel creates. The underlying white matter will peel off in thin ridged sheets. The ridging will be particularly apparent at the upper border of the insula, where you must scrape firmly towards the surface of the hemisphere. Firm deliberate strokes with the handle of your scalpel will make a better dissection than timid nibbles.

Continue scraping until you expose a mass of grey matter with roughly the same size and shape as the insula. This is the **lentiform nucleus,** which is one of the basal nuclei. The white matter above its upper curved border radiates upwards, forwards, and backwards to all parts of the cerebral cortex, and is called the **corona radiata.** Scrape away until you can see the fan-shaped arrangement of these fibres.

They are continuous with a dense mass of fibres, called the **internal capsule,** which lies deep to the lentiform nucleus and so cannot yet be seen.

As you follow the radiating fibres towards the cortex you will tear across other tracts of fibres that are passing through them. You will encounter particular difficulty in following the fibres which radiate to the frontal and parietal lobes because of the presence of bundles of fibres which connect with the opposite hemisphere through the corpus callosum. Open the longitudinal fissure between the hemispheres and check the level at which the corpus callosum is attached to the medial surface of the hemisphere which you are dissecting. This will give you an idea of where you are likely to come across callosal fibres.

The fibres which radiate to the occipital lobe are much easier to trace. Scrape backwards from the lower border of

the lentiform nucleus and you will expose a well-defined band of fibres extending into the occipital lobe. This is the **optic radiation.** It carries visual impulses to the cortex on the medial surface of the occipital lobe [Fig. 6.40].

Now turn to the anterior end of the lateral sulcus, and with the handle of your scalpel scrape backwards across the lateral sulcus into the temporal lobe, peeling off a layer of white matter. By so doing you will reveal bundles of fibres connecting the frontal lobe with the temporal and occipital lobes. Some of these fibres (the uncinate fasciculus) hook sharply round the anterior end of the lateral sulcus, while others pass posteriorly towards the occipital lobe.

The superior half of the hemisphere you are dissecting is now to be removed. Place a long-bladed knife in a horizontal plane at the level of the upper border of the lentiform nucleus and cut into the hemisphere, carrying the incision

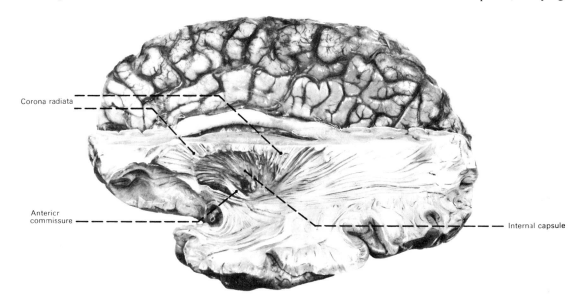

Fig. 6.45 Lateral view of the left internal capsule. 'One-brain' dissection similar to that shown in Fig. 6.41, followed by removal of the superior quadrant of brain after horizontal section of the hemisphere.

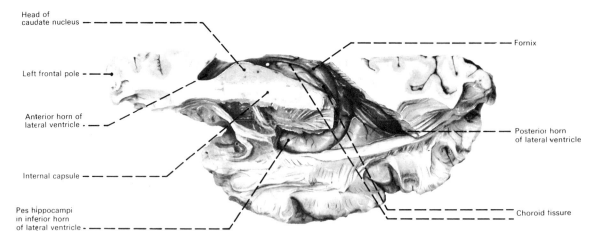

Fig. 6.46 Supero-lateral view of the left lateral ventricle. The right cerebral hemisphere has been removed. The left hemisphere has been sectioned horizontally, the interanl capsule has been exposed, and the lateral wall of the inferior horn of the lateral ventricle has been removed.

through the hemisphere as far as the midline. Then place the knife between the two hemispheres and cut down through the corpus callosum to meet your horizontal incision. Remove the quadrant of brain that you have severed [Fig. 6.45]. The incision will have opened up a cavity in the hemisphere. This is the **lateral ventricle.** On the horizontal cut surface lateral to the ventricle and medial to the corona radiata is a mass of grey matter. This is the **caudate nucleus,** which is another one of the basal nuclei. Medial to the caudate nucleus in the floor of the exposed part of the ventricle is the convex upper surface of the **thalamus.**

Next scoop out the grey matter of the lentiform nucleus, scraping horizontally from its posterior end at right-angles to the fibres of the corona radiata, whose downward extension into the internal capsule now comes into view [Fig. 6.45]. Complete the exposure of the lateral surface of the internal capsule by digging down and removing the lentiform nucleus medial to the fibres, which you have already revealed, that connect the frontal and temporal lobes. As you reach the inferior boundary of the lentiform nucleus you will see a narrow but distinct bundle of fibres running postero-laterally to the temporal lobe. This is the **anterior commissure** [Fig. 6.45]. In front of it you will see a group of small vessels, the **thalamostriate arteries.**

Follow the anterior commissure towards the midline, carefully removing the grey matter by which it is surrounded. As you trace the anterior commissure to the midline it is possible that you will break into a space between the two hemispheres immediately posterior to the commissure. This space, which is bounded anteriorly by the commissure, is the third ventricle.

The ventricles of the forebrain

If you look into the part of the lateral ventricle which was opened by the horizontal section through the hemisphere and direct your gaze forwards and medially, you may be able to identify the anterior commissure where it crosses the midline. You may also be able to see into the anterior end of the third ventricle, through the **interventricular foramen** which connects it with the lateral ventricle.

Turn the brain over so that you are looking at its ventral surface. Place the blade of a long knife in the midline, being sure that the sharp edge lies in the middle of the optic chiasma, between the two mamillary bodies and in line with the cerebral aqueduct behind. Now cut deeply to meet the incision you have already made in the corpus callosum. Your specimen will now be in two halves. Set the hemisphere which has been dissected on one side. On the medial surface of the intact hemisphere examine the lateral wall of the **third ventricle** as you follow the description given on pages 6.8 to 6.9.

The lateral ventricle [Fig. 6.46]

Now return to the hemisphere which you have been dissecting and with a probe or your little finger explore in a posterior direction the cavity of the lateral ventricle. You will find that the cavity diverges from the median plane. The full extent of the ventricle cannot be seen without removing some of its walls. During your dissection of the corona radiata and internal capsule on this hemisphere you will have reduced the lateral wall of the ventricle to a sheet of white matter only a few millimetres thick. To expose completely the cavity of the ventricle you should now remove this wall piece by piece using scissors and a scalpel to cut out sections of the wall about 7 mm wide and 10 mm long. Start posteriorly and proceed backwards and downwards towards the occipital pole and then forwards into the remains of the temporal lobe. You should now be able to identify the extensions of the ventricle:

into the frontal lobe—the **anterior horn,** which is separated from its fellow only by the septum pellucidum;

into the occipital lobe—the **posterior horn;**

into the temporal lobe—the **inferior horn,** which diverges from the midline most.

Identify the choroid plexus of the lateral ventricle, and then carefully tear it out. In so doing you will open up the **choroid fissure,** which is a curved slit in the medial wall of the ventricle, extending all the way from the interventricular foramen to the inferior horn of the lateral ventricle. In the upper or central part of the ventricle the choroid fissure separates the **fornix** from the upper surface of the thalamus which forms a floor to the ventricle here. Follow the fornix backwards and trace it round the back of the thalamus into the inferior horn of the ventricle. You will see that it merges with a rounded longitudinal elevation in the floor of the inferior horn. This elevation is called the **hippocampus.** Anteriorly the hippocampus expands to form the **pes hippocampi** [Fig. 6.46] before it terminates abruptly at the tip of the inferior horn of the ventricle.

Note that the anterior horn and central parts of the lateral ventricles lie close to each other, separated only by the thin septum pellucidum. Posteriorly, the ventricle diverges from the midline as it wraps itself round the back of thalamus, internal capsule, basal nuclei, and insula. From this block of structures, which form the 'core' of the hemisphere, you have removed by dissection the insula and the lentiform nucleus.

For the remainder of your dissection of the forebrain the instructions you will follow are the same as those laid out on pages 6.17 to 6.25 for the 'two-brain' dissection.

Appendix

The lymphatic system

The lymphatic system is made up of a network of channels through which flows a fluid called **lymph.** The peripheral part of the network consists of a mesh of minute capillaries, lying close to the blood capillaries, and in intimate relation with the interstitial fluid spaces. The lymphatic capillaries unite to form increasingly larger vessels all of which ultimately feed into collecting ducts which open, either singly or jointly, into the venous system near the beginning of the two brachiocephalic veins. The larger lymphatic vessels are interrupted by (or pass through) small filtering organs, called **lymph nodes.** These are irregular ovoid bodies, of varying size, which are situated in certain specific regions along the vessels. Until it passes through a lymph node the fluid in a lymph vessel is known as peripheral lymph.

All but the largest **lymphatic vessels** are so thin-walled as to be indiscernible and undissectable in the cadaver, unless they have been specially injected. Yet from a clinical point of view they are important. They exist in all vascular tissues except the brain, the spinal medulla, the bone-marrow, and possibly skeletal muscle and the parenchyma of the spleen. In most parts of the body the lymphatic vessels are arranged in a superficial set, whose collecting vessels penetrate the deep fascia to feed into a deep set. The **thoracic duct** [p. 3.45] and the **right lymphatic duct** are the two main collecting ducts of the whole lymphatic system. Lymph nodes and the thoracic duct are the only parts of the lymphatic system which you are certain to see in the course of your dissection.

The lymph nodes are masses of **lymphoid tissue** which consists of aggregations of **lymphocytes** in a framework of specialized fibrous tissue. Lymphoid tissue also occurs, in different form, in the **tonsils** [p. 5.78], and in the wall of the intestines [p. 4.51]. The **thymus** consists essentially of lobes of lymphoid tissue, while the **spleen** also consists largely of lymphoid tissue.

The lymph

The cells which make up the tissues of the body are always bathed in fluid which exudes from the blood capillaries. This interstitial fluid contains salts and sugars which are readily absorbed by the blood capillaries after they have played their part in the nutrition of the tissues. It also contains a little protein which has escaped from the blood capillaries, but which cannot be directly reabsorbed into them. The protein-containing fluid passes, instead, into the lymphatic capillaries as **peripheral lymph.** When it reaches, and then passes through, the lymph nodes, it receives an addition of white blood cells, mainly lymphocytes, and an occasional red blood cell. The **central lymph** which is formed in this way is colourless, but lymph from the intestines is usually opalescent or even milky because of the fat it contains.

Lymphoid tissue

Lymphoid tissue is the source of the lymphocytes found in the blood. It is also concerned in a number of reactions whereby the body protects itself from invasion by bacteria and viruses. Exactly how lymphoid tissue exercises its effects in this role is not completely understood, any more than is the function of the lymphocytes themselves. What is certain is that lymphoid tissue acts as a filter to the passage of particulate matter, such as bacteria and cancer cells. For this reason the disposition of the lymph nodes is of considerable importance to the surgeon. In the case of infection, or cancer, the surgeon always examines the lymph nodes draining the area involved. When he removes a cancerous growth he tries to take away any lymph nodes in which cancer cells have been trapped, and from which they could spread. Painful swelling of lymph nodes, for example in the axilla, may correspondingly draw attention to some minute focus of infection, say in a finger, which has spread to the axillary nodes by the lymphatic vessels of the arm.

Lymph nodes [Fig. A.1]

The region on each lymph node where the blood vessels enter and leave is called the **hilum.** Here an **efferent lymphatic vessel** emerges to pass either into wider collecting lymphatic channels, or to another lymph node in the same or another chain, so as to allow further filtration of the lymph. In the latter case efferent vessels from more than one node usually converge as **afferent vessels** on another node, the afferent lymph vessels piercing the capsule to enter a diffuse **sub-capsular sinus** from which the lymph percolates through the tissue of the node, from which it is collected, yet again, in a single efferent channel which leaves at the hilum. Most lymph nodes are found near large veins or arteries, as in the axilla, and they are also numerous on the lymph vessels in the mesenteries of the stomach and intestines. Some are superficial to the deep fascia, but most of the lymph nodes of the body lie more deeply.

The disposition of the main groups of lymph nodes, which are usually greyish in colour, is fairly constant, but their

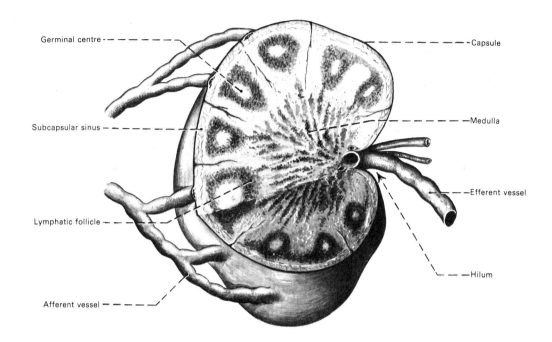

Germinal centre

Capsule

Subcapsular sinus

Medulla

Efferent vessel

Lymphatic follicle

Hilum

Afferent vessel

Fig. A.1 A schematic section of a lymph node.

number and size vary considerably from person to person. They also vary in prominence with age, a general process of lymphoid atrophy setting in after puberty. The thymus, for example, is all but completely involuted in the aged cadaver [see p. 3.17]. Some groups of lymph nodes, for example those of the inguinal region [p. 2.21], are again always larger than others (e.g. those of the popliteal region [p. A. 5]). Those of the lungs are invariably darker in colour than those of other parts of the body [see p. 3.16], because of the trapped particles of dust, including carbon, carried to them from the alveoli of the lungs along the pulmonary lymphatics. This is especially marked in coal-miners, and to a lesser degree, in city dwellers.

The following description of the lymphatic system focuses predominantly on the regional disposition of the main groups of lymph nodes. It must be understood that these are either linked by lymphatic vessels with other groups of nodes distal or proximal to them (the term proximal referring to groups less distant from the main collecting ducts), or that their efferent channels lead without further filtration barriers to the two main terminal collecting ducts of the body.

The main collecting ducts

The lymph from the lower limbs, the pelvis, and the lower parts of the abdominal wall is collected into a pair of **lumbar trunks** [Fig. A.2]. One or more **intestinal trunks** drain lymph from the field of the portal circulation. The lumbar and in-

testinal trunks open into the lower end of the **thoracic duct,** which is the largest of the collecting ducts. The lower end of the thoracic duct is sometimes dilated to form the **cisterna chyli** [p. 4.75]. The thoracic duct ascends from the abdomen, passes through the thorax [p. 3.45, Fig. 3.46], and ends on the left side of the root of the neck by opening into the left brachiocephalic vein at the angle formed by the union of the internal jugular and subclavian veins [p. 5.94, Fig. 5.93].

Lymph from all parts of the upper limb, and the lymph which flows in the superficial lymphatics of the trunk above the umbilicus drains into a **subclavian trunk** on each side [Figs A.2 and A.4]. A **jugular trunk** collects lymph from each half of the head and neck. The lymph from the lungs, mediastinum, and most of the thoracic wall is collected into a **bronchomediastinal trunk** on each side of the trachea [Figs A.2 and A.8]. The left jugular and subclavian trunks join the thoracic duct close to its termination. The left broncho-mediastinal trunk usually opens into the left brachio-cephalic vein close to, but separately from, the thoracic duct. On the right side, the jugular, subclavian, and broncho-mediastinal trunks may open into the great veins separately, but they often coalesce in the neck to form the very short **right lymphatic duct** which opens into the right brachio-cephalic vein in the angle between the right subclavian and internal jugular veins [Fig. A.2].

This description of the main collecting ducts should make it clear that all the lymph, except that from the right half of the body above the level of the umbilicus, reaches the venous system by way of the thoracic duct [Fig. A.3].

The upper limb

The skin and subcutaneous tissues of the fingers and palm are richly supplied with lymphatics, which coalesce with the collecting channels from the superficial lymphatic plexuses of the rest of the hand and forearm, to form main collecting channels which run up the medial and lateral borders of the limb, in relation to the basilic and cephalic veins respectively. A small group of superficial lymph nodes, called the **cubital lymph nodes** [Fig. A.4], is situated near the basilic vein, just above the medial epicondyle, and another small group of **deltopectoral nodes** lies between the upper parts of the deltoid and pectoralis major muscles. A small group of **infraclavicular nodes** lies on the clavipectoral fascia, close to the termination of the cephalic vein [pp. 1.13 and 1.14].

The axillary lymph nodes [Figs A.4 and A.5]

The main nodes of the upper limb with which you should concern yourself are the axillary lymph nodes. These receive not only the superficial lymphatics of the upper limb but also the deep lymph vessels which have accompanied the radial, ulnar, interosseous, and brachial vessels. The axillary lymph nodes also receive lymph from the breast and the superficial tissues of the trunk above the level of the umbilicus. Their main practical significance relates to the surgical treatment of cancer of the breast, whose lymphatic drainage is dealt with separately on page A.5.

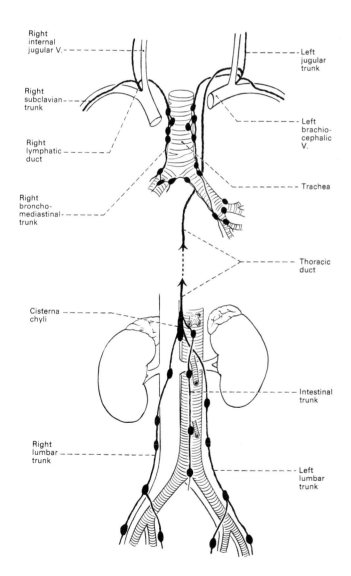

Fig. A.2 Schema of the main lymphatic collecting ducts.

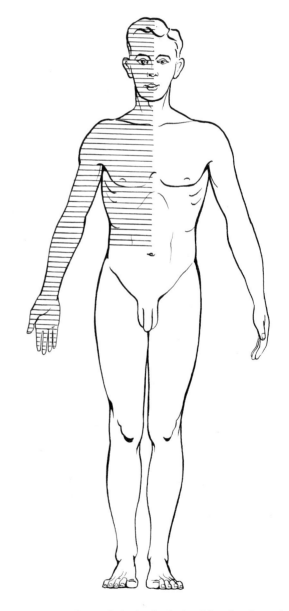

Fig. A.3 The regions of the body drained by the thoracic and right lymphatic ducts. Lymph from the shaded area enters the right lymphatic duct; all that from the unshaded area of the body eventually reaches the thoracic duct.

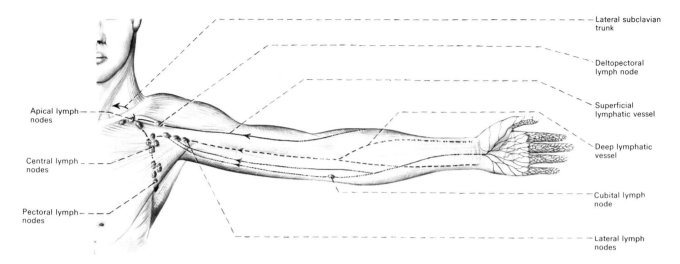

Fig. A.4 Schema of the lymphatic drainage of the left upper limb.

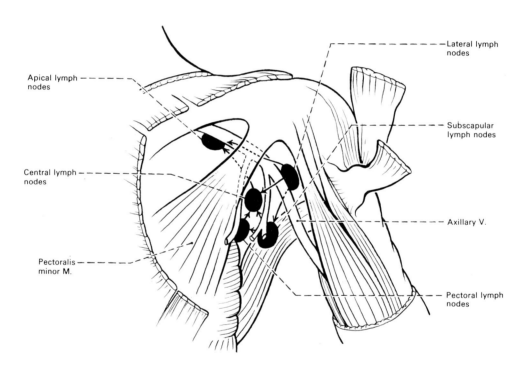

Fig. A.5 Schema of the left axillary lymph nodes.

The axillary lymph nodes, like most other lymph nodes in the body, usually appear as irregularly ovoid grey structures matted into the fascia or connective tissue in which they are embedded, and through which their afferent and efferent channels flow. They are all close to the axillary vein or its tributaries, but five groups are usually distinguished, without any more than an arbitrary anatomical significance. The most superior, near the apex of the axilla, are called the **apical nodes** [Fig. A.4]; they lie above the pectoralis minor muscle and deep to the clavipectoral fascia [p. 1.13]. Through them passes the lymph which has filtered

from the other axillary lymph nodes, and also lymph which flows directly from the breast. Their efferent vessel is the **subclavian trunk,** which drains in a variable way either into the thoracic duct or right lymphatic duct, or into the big veins at the base of the neck, or through the lower of the deep cervical lymph nodes.

The four other groups of axillary nodes lie below (i.e. distal to) the pectoralis minor muscle [Fig. A.5]. The group called the **lateral nodes** lies most distally behind and on the medial side of the axillary vein. These nodes receive lymph from the upper limb. Another group, called the **pectoral**

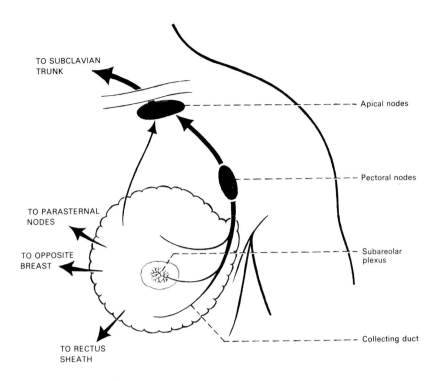

Fig. A.6 Schema of the lymphatic drainage of the left breast.

nodes, lies along the lateral (lower) border of the pectoralis minor muscle, and is of particular importance in the drainage of the breast. **Subscapular nodes** lie more posteriorly along the lateral border of the subscapularis muscle, and a group of **central nodes** lies in the fascia which forms the floor or base of the axilla. There are numerous lymphatic connections between the lateral, pectoral, subscapular, and central nodes, and their lymph finally drains through the apical nodes.

The number of nodes in each group is very variable (from one to about fifteen), the lateral and central groups being the largest. As already stated, the main efferent channel from the apical group of glands is called the subclavian trunk; it may consist of either a single channel or of two or three lymphatic vessels.

The breast [Fig. A.6]

Lymph from the breast drains into a superficial lymphatic plexus deep to the areola, called the **subareolar plexus,** and into a deep lymphatic plexus on the pectoralis major muscle. From both plexuses collecting trunks pass laterally around the lateral border of the pectoralis major muscle to the pectoral group of axillary nodes. Other channels pierce the pectoral muscles to reach the apical axillary nodes, either directly or through the infraclavicular nodes, and also the parasternal lymph nodes, which are associated with the internal thoracic artery inside the thorax [see p. A.6]. There are also connections with the lymphatic plexuses of the opposite breast, and with deep lymphatics of the abdominal wall in the region of the xiphoid process of the sternum and the upper part of the rectus sheath.

The lower limb

The superficial lymphatic vessels of most of the lower limb, including the gluteal region, the anterior abdominal wall (below the level of the umbilicus), the perineum, and the external genitalia, follow the course of the main veins and end as afferent channels to a large series of **superficial inguinal nodes** [p. 2.21, Fig. A.7]. These are arranged in an upper (proximal) row which lies below and parallel to the inguinal ligament, and a lower (distal) set which lies along the terminal part of the great saphenous vein. The superficial inguinal nodes also receive some lymph which drains from the body of the uterus along the round ligament [p. 4.85], and also lymph from the lower ends of the vagina and anal canal.

The efferents from the superficial inguinal nodes pass through the cribriform fascia and the femoral canal and end in the **external iliac nodes** [Figs A.7 and A.9], which lie around the vessels of the same name.

The deep lymphatic vessels of the leg accompany the tibial and peroneal vessels and end in the **popliteal nodes** [Fig. A.7]. This group consists of a small number of lymph nodes which lie around the popliteal vessels, deep to the deep fascia of the popliteal fossa. The popliteal nodes also receive a few superficial lymphatic vessels, which accompany the small saphenous vein on the posterior aspect of the leg. Their efferents, with the deep lymphatic vessels of the thigh, accompany the blood vessels upwards, and end in the **deep inguinal nodes** [Fig. A.7]. These vary in number from one to three, and may be found beneath the fascia lata on the medial side of the femoral vein, in the femoral canal, or near the femoral ring. Some of the lymph from the glans penis (clitoris) also drains through them. The efferents of the deep inguinal nodes pass behind the inguinal ligament and become afferents to the external iliac nodes.

The thorax

The thoracic wall

Lymph from the superficial parts of the thoracic wall passes to the axillary nodes. That from deeper parts of the left

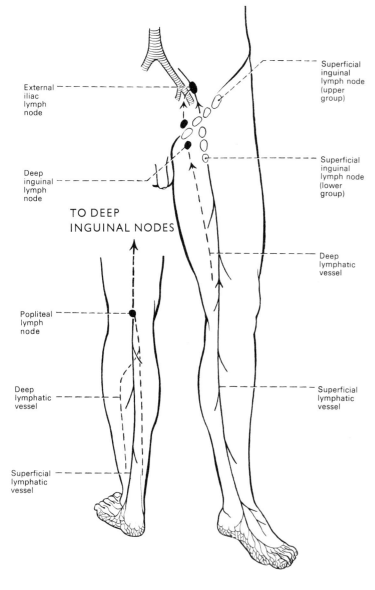

Fig. A.7 Schema of the lymphatic drainage of the left lower limb. Superficial lymph nodes are drawn in outline; deep lymph nodes are shown black.

side of the thorax mostly reaches the thoracic duct or cisterna chyli [p. A.2], while that from the right side drains into the right bronchomediastinal trunk. There are several groups of parietal lymph nodes on the course of the deeper lymphatics of the chest wall. Small **intercostal nodes** are found near the heads of the ribs, and **parasternal nodes** are found on the course of the internal thoracic vessels. There are also **diaphragmatic nodes** on the thoracic surface of the diaphragm.

The lungs [Fig. A.8]

Most of the lymph from the right lung and the inferior lobe of the left drains into the right lymphatic duct [p. A.2], while that from the superior lobe of the left lung drains largely into the thoracic duct. The pulmonary lymphatic vessels are associated with numerous black lymph nodes within the lung, in the root of the lung, on the main bronchi, and on the bifurcation of the trachea. These nodes form part of a continuous lymphatic pathway which is subdivided into the following four groups of lymph nodes [Fig. A.8]: **pulmonary nodes,** within the lungs; **bronchopulmonary nodes,** in the hila of the lungs; **tracheobronchial nodes,** around the principal bronchi, and in the bifurcation of the trachea; and **paratracheal nodes,** along the trachea, extending up into the neck. The **bronchomediastinal trunk** usually emerges on each side from the paratracheal nodes [see p. A.2]. There are numerous lymphatic vessels which connect together the tracheobronchial and paratracheal nodes of each side.

The mediastinum

Apart from the lymph nodes associated with the lungs, there

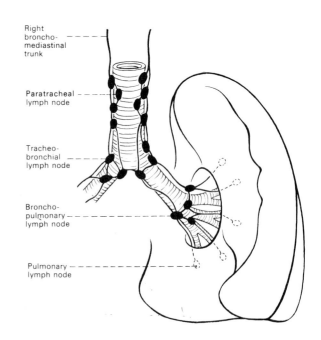

Fig. A.8 Schema of the lymphatic drainage of the left lung.

are other groups of nodes to which lymph from the mediastinal structures drains. There are **anterior mediastinal nodes,** which lie in the superior mediastinum, in front of the brachiocephalic veins, and **posterior mediastinal nodes,** lying behind the pericardium, in close relation to the oesophagus and the descending aorta.

Lymph from the right side of the heart and pericardium drains largely into the anterior mediastinal nodes, while that from the left side drains to the tracheobronchial nodes.

The final path of the lymph from the thoracic viscera to the thoracic duct and the bronchomediastinal trunks is very variable.

The abdomen

The abdominal wall

As already noted [p. A.5], the superficial vessels of the abdominal wall below the level of the umbilicus drain to the superficial inguinal nodes; those above this level pass to the axillary nodes. The deep lymphatics of the abdominal wall follow the blood vessels, to enter lymph nodes within the abdominal and thoracic cavities.

The abdominal and pelvic viscera

The lymphatic vessels of the abdominal viscera are associated with their corresponding blood vessels, and a variable and plentiful number of lymph nodes are almost always to be found along their paths. The various groups of nodes derive their names from the blood vessels (e.g. inferior mesenteric, left gastric, hepatic nodes), and only occasionally from their positions (e.g. the pyloric nodes of the stomach). The only groups of lymph nodes which need special mention in this Appendix are the external iliac, internal iliac, and common iliac nodes, and the lumbar (lateral aortic) and pre-aortic nodes [Fig. A.9].

The **external iliac nodes** lie around the external iliac vessels and receive their main afferents from the lymph nodes of the lower limb. Their efferents pass to the **common iliac nodes,** which also receive those of the **internal iliac nodes.** The latter nodes lie around the corresponding vessels, and drain most of the pelvic viscera.

The common iliac lymph nodes, which again are associated with the corresponding blood vessels, drain to the **lumbar lymph nodes.** The latter constitute a large number of nodes which lie at the sides of the abdominal aorta and

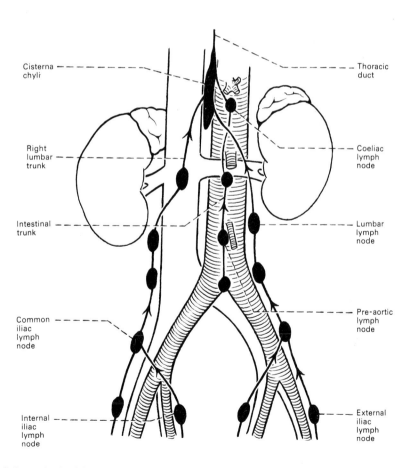

Fig. A.9 Schema of the principal lymphatic collecting ducts and lymph nodes of the posterior abdominal wall.

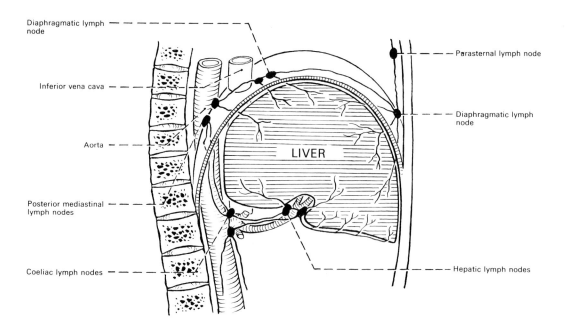

Diaphragmatic lymph node

Inferior vena cava

Aorta

Posterior mediastinal lymph nodes

Coeliac lymph nodes

LIVER

Parasternal lymph node

Diaphragmatic lymph node

Hepatic lymph nodes

Fig. A.10 Schema of the lymphatic drainage of the liver.

inferior vena cava. Into them pass, either directly or indirectly, the lymph from the lower limbs, the urogenital organs and the walls of the pelvis and lower part of the abdomen. The efferents of the lumbar nodes form the **lumbar trunks,** which join the lower end of the thoracic duct, sometimes forming the **cisterna chyli** [see p. 4.75].

A number of nodes lie along the front of the aorta, especially in relation to the coeliac, superior mesenteric and inferior mesenteric arteries. These are collectively known as the **pre-aortic nodes** [Fig. A.9]. They receive lymph from the stomach, intestines, pancreas, spleen, and parts of the liver, and their efferents unite to form the **intestinal trunk** which passes to the cisterna chyli.

The lymphatic drainage of some of the abdominal organs is discussed separately below.

The stomach

The lymph from the lymphatic plexuses which drain the walls of the stomach passes through nodes lying on the greater and lesser curvatures, close to the blood vessels which supply the stomach and after which they are named. Other specially-named nodes lie around the pylorus **(pyloric nodes)** and along the borders of the pancreas **(pancreatic nodes).** Nearly all the lymph from the stomach eventually reaches the **coeliac nodes,** which constitute the upper end of the pre-aortic group.

The liver [Fig. A.10]

The main lymphatic vessels from the liver pass via the **hepatic nodes,** lying in the porta hepatis, and accompany the hepatic artery to the coeliac nodes. Some lymph reaches the

thorax either by passing from the subperitoneal plexus to the lower parasternal nodes, or by accompanying the inferior vena cava to the posterior mediastinal lymphatic nodes [Fig. A.10]. Some of this lymph may pass through diaphragmatic nodes.

The pelvic organs

The lymphatic vessels that drain the pelvic organs connect freely with each other and accompany the arteries from which these organs receive their blood supply. Efferents from the majority of the pelvic organs pass to the **internal, external,** and **common iliac nodes** [Fig. A.9]. Efferents from the ovary, testis, and uterine tube (which are supplied by arteries arising directly from the aorta) and the upper part of the uterus, pass to the **lumbar nodes.**

Efferents from the lower part of the vagina, the scrotum, the penis (except some from the glans [see p. A.6]), and the lower part of the anal canal pass to the **superficial inguinal nodes.** So, too, do a few lymphatics from the body of the uterus, which pass down the inguinal canal with the round ligament. Other efferents from the uterus, vagina, bladder, seminal vesicles, the lower part of the rectum, and the upper part of the anal canal pass to the external and internal iliac nodes, while those from the upper part of the rectum and from the colon pass to the **inferior mesenteric nodes** of the pre-aortic group.

The head and neck

All the lymph vessels of the head and neck drain directly or indirectly either into the **deep lateral cervical nodes** which

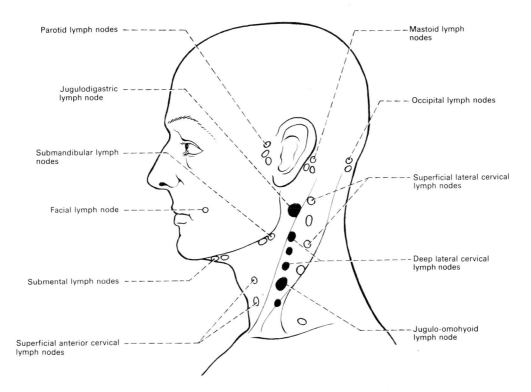

Parotid lymph nodes

Jugulodigastric lymph node

Submandibular lymph nodes

Facial lymph node

Submental lymph nodes

Superficial anterior cervical lymph nodes

Mastoid lymph nodes

Occipital lymph nodes

Superficial lateral cervical lymph nodes

Deep lateral cervical lymph nodes

Jugulo-omohyoid lymph node

Fig. A.11 Schema of the lymphatic drainage of the head and neck. Superficial lymph nodes are drawn in outline; deep lymph nodes are shown in black.

lie close to the internal jugular vein [Fig. A. 11] or into the **deep anterior cervical nodes** which lie close to the larynx and trachea. The **retropharyngeal nodes** behind the nasal part of the pharynx are the uppermost of the deep lateral cervical nodes. Belonging to the same group is the **jugulodigastric node** which lies high up behind the angle of the mandible at the point where the posterior belly of the digastric muscle is crossed by the anterior border of the sternocleidomastoid muscle. Much lower down in the chain is the **jugulo-omohyoid node,** situated near the intermediate tendon of the omohyoid muscle.

The efferents from the deep cervical nodes form the **jugular trunk,** which drains into the thoracic duct on the left side and the right lymphatic duct on the right side.

Lymph from the superficial tissues of the head drains into a 'collar' of superficial lymph nodes whose positions are indicated by their names. Thus there are **occipital, mastoid, parotid, facial, submental,** and **submandibular nodes** [Fig.

A.11]. Lymph from superficial structures of the neck drains into **superficial lateral** and **superficial anterior cervical nodes** associated with the external and anterior jugular veins respectively. Efferent lymph vessels from all these nodes pass to the deep cervical group of lymph nodes.

Lymph from deeper structures drains directly into the deep cervical group, as well as indirectly through deeper groups of distal nodes. The lymph vessels of the palatine tonsil, and of the posterior one-third and median parts of the tongue, pass directly to the jugulodigastric node. On the other hand, vessels from the tip and frenulum of the tongue pass to the submental nodes, while those from the margins of the tongue pass to the submandibular nodes. A few lymph vessels from the tip of the tongue pass directly to the jugulo-omohyoid node. Lymph from structures near the midline may drain to nodes on both sides of the neck. This should be remembered especially with respect to the lymphatic drainage of the tongue.

Index

This index lists the English terms used in the book and their Latin (4th edition *Nomina Anatomica*) equivalents. Each entry is given in both terms, before the reference to pages and figures. The index thus serves as an English-Latin, Latin-English dictionary for those anatomical terms used in the text.

Where the English term is identical with the NA term the latter is not indexed separately (e.g. Abdomen). There are English terms which do not have an equivalent Latin term in the 4th edition NA. A few Latin terms from earlier editons of the NA have been retained. Occasionally officially recognized NA alternatives have been added in brackets where they help to explain usage (e.g. Stomach, *ventriculus (gaster)*).

The alphabetical order in which the English and NA terms are indexed is set by their first, and, where necessary, second and third words, e.g.

Angulus mandibulae, angle of mandible
Angulus oculi lateralis, lateral angle of eye
Angulus oculi medialis, medial angle of eye
Anterior arch of atlas, *arcus anterior atlantis*
Anterior belly of digastric M., *venter anterior m. digastrici*
Anterior cerebral A., *a. cerebri anterior*

Exceptions to this ordering are:

1. English terms beginning with 'right' and 'left', when the second and subsequent words have been used to determine the sequence, e.g.
    Common carotid A., *a. carotis communis*
        left
        right
    Lymphatic duct, right, *ductus lymphaticus dexter*

2. Plurals. These are ordered according to the spelling of the corresponding singular form, e.g.
    Articulatio cubiti, elbow joint
    Articulationes fibrosae, fibrous joints
    Articulatio genus, knee joint

3. English terms which start with the same word as their NA equivalents but are otherwise different. Such terms are grouped in alphabetical order immediately following the NA terms, e.g.
    Foramen sphenopalatinum, sphenopalatine foramen
    Foramen spinosum, *foramen spinosum*
    Foramen v. cavae, foramen for vena cava
    Foramen zygomatico-orbitale, zygomatico-orbital foramen
    Foramen caecum of tongue, *foramen caecum linguae*
    Foramen for vena cava, *foramen v. cavae*
    Foramen ovale of base of skull, *foramen ovale basis cranii*

Such terms as mandible, *oculus*, eye, vena cava, and tongue which appear in these sample lists are, of course, indexed separately.

Roman type is used for English terms and page references, the more important being shown in bold roman figures. *Italic type* is used for NA terms and figure references. The latter are also enclosed by square brackets. In both English and NA terms, artery, vein, nerve, and muscle are contracted to A., V., N., and M. *Ligamentum* is contracted to *lig*.

1

3

Superficial part of cardiac plexus, 3.44

Superficial part of external anal sphincter, *pars superficialis m. sphincteris ani externi*, [*5.6b*]

Superficial part of masseter M., *pars superficialis m. masseteris*, 5.46, [*5.42, 5.46*]

Superficial perineal space, *spatium perinei superficiale*, 4.11, 4.14, [*4.7, 4.11*]

Superficial peroneal N., *n. peroneus superficialis*, 2.49, 2.57, [*2.56a and b, 2.59, 2.62, 2.64*]

Superficial temporal A., *a. temporalis superficialis*, 5.36, 5.47, 5.68, [*5.41, 5.44, 5.64*]

Superficial temporal Vs, *vv. temporales superficiales*, 5.47, [*5.43*]

Superficial transverse perineal M., *m. transversus perinei superficialis*, 4.11, 4.12, [*4.7, 4.11*]

Superior alveolar Ns, *nn. alveolares superiores*, 5.57

Superior angle of scapula, *angulus superior scapulae*, 1.3

Superior aperture of thorax, *apertura thoracis superior*, 3.7

Superior articular facet of lateral mass of atlas, *fovea articularis superior massae lateralis atlantis*, [*5.2a*]

Superior articular process of sacrum, *processus articularis superior oss. sacri*, [*2.7a and b*]

Superior articular process of vertebra, *processus articularis superior vertebrae*, 3.3, [*3.2–3, 3.4a*]

Superior belly of omohyoid M., *venter superior m. omohyoidei*, 5.19, [*5.20*]

Superior border of scapula, *margo superior scapulae*, 1.3, [*1.2b*]

Superior branch of oculomotor N., *ramus superior n. oculomotorii*, 5.104, [*5.104*]

Superior cerebellar A., *a. cerebelli superior*, 6.3, [*6.3*]

Superior cerebellar peduncle, *pedunculus cerebellaris superior*, **6.11**, 6.13, 6.16, [*6.10, 6.12–13, 6.18*]

Superior cervical ganglion, *ganglion cervicale superius*, 5.95, [*5.94*]

Superior colliculus, *colliculus superior*, 6.6, 6.13, [*6.5, 6.14*]

Superior constrictor M. of pharynx, *m. constrictor pharyngis superior*, 5.72, **5.79**, 5.82, 5.88, [*5.78, 5.80, 5.84*]

Superior costal facet of thoracic vertebra, *fovea costalis superior vertebrae thoracicae*, [*3.2b*]

Superior costotransverse ligament, *lig. costotransversarium superius*, 3.50, [*3.49*]

Superior dental arch, *arcus dentalis superior*, 5.38

Superior epigastric A., *a. epigastrica superior*, 3.10, 4.20, 4.30, 4.32, [*3.11, 4.28*]

Superior extensor retinaculum, *retinaculum mm. extensorum superius*, 2.50, [*2.57*]

Superior fascia of pelvic diaphragm, *fascia diaphragmatis pelvis superior*, 4.8, 4.88

Superior fascia of urogenital diaphragm, *fascia diaphragmatis urogenitalis superior*, 4.12

Superior fornix of conjunctiva, *fornix conjunctivae superior*, 5.101

Superior fovea of rhomboid fossa, *fovea superior fossae rhomboideae*, 6.12, [*6.10*]

Superior gluteal A., *a. glutea superior*, 2.10, 2.11, 4.87, [*2.11, 4.78, 4.81, 4.91*]

Superior gluteal N., *n. gluteus superior*, 2.11, [*2.11, 2.14–15, 4.91*]

Superior gluteal Vs, *vv. gluteae superiores*, 2.10, 2.11

Superior horn of thyroid cartilage, *cornu superius cartilaginis thyroideae*, 5.85, [*5.82*]

Superior hypogastric plexus, *plexus hypogastricus superior*, 4.75, **4.76, 4.101**, [*4.64–5*]

Superior intercostal V.,
  left, *v. intercostalis superior sinistra*, 3.17, 3.19, [*3.19, 3.21*]
  right, *v. intercostalis superior dextra*, 3.20, [*3.18*]

Superior laryngeal N., *n. laryngeus superior*, 5.69, **5.86**, [*5.68, 5.78, 5.84*]

Superior lateral cutaneous N. of arm, *n. cutaneus brachii lateralis superior*, 1.29

Superior lobe bronchus,
  left, *bronchus lobaris superior sinister*, 3.42
  right, *bronchus lobaris superior dexter*, 3.15, 3.42, [*3.18, 3.43a*]

Superior lobe of left lung, *lobus superior pulmonis sinistri*, 3.39, [*3.16a, b and c, 3.17, 3.42b*]

Superior lobe of right lung, *lobus superior pulmonis dextri*, 3.39, [*3.16a, b and d, 3.17, 3.42a*]

Superior mediastinum, *mediastinum superius*, 3.17, 3.43, [*3.20–2*]

Superior medullary velum, *velum medullare craniale (superius)*, 6.8, 6.11, [*6.6, 6.10, 6.12, 6.17*]

Superior mesenteric A., *a. mesenterica superior*, 4.41, **4.49**, 4.58, 4.61, 4.65, 4.72, [*4.45–7, 4.54, 4.56, 4.58, 4.66*]

Superior mesenteric plexus, *plexus mesentericus superior*, 4.75

Superior mesenteric V., *v. mesenterica superior*, 4.41, 4.61, 4.64, 4.74, [*4.46, 4.58, 4.60, 4.68*]

Superior nasal concha, *concha nasalis superior*, 5.113, [*5.116–17*]

Superior nasal meatus, *meatus nasi superior*, 5.113, [*5.116*]

Superior nuchal line, *linea nuchae superior*, 5.3, [*5.1*]

Superior oblique M., *m. obliquus superior*, **5.103**, 5.107, [*5.100, 5.103–4*]

Superior ophthalmic V., *v. ophthalmica superior*, **5.106**, 5.110

Superior orbital fissure, *fissura orbitalis superior*, 5.30, 5.97, [*5.30, 5.95*]

Superior pancreaticoduodenal A., *a. pancreaticoduodenalis superior*, 4.47, 4.61, 4.72, [*4.46*]

Superior parathyroid gland, *glandula parathyroidea superior*, 5.93

Superior part of duodenum, *pars superior duodeni*, 4.49, 4.62, [*4.38, 4.46*]

Superior peroneal retinaculum, *retinaculum mm. peroneorum superius*, 2.51, 2.59, [*2.57a*]

Superior petrosal sinus, *sinus petrosus superior*, **5.109**, 5.110, [*5.108, 5.110, 5.113*]

Superior pubic ligament, *lig. pubicum superius*, 4.88

Superior pulmonary V.,
  left, *v. pulmonalis superior sinistra*, 3.16, 3.42, [*3.19, 3.36, 3.43b*]
  right, *v. pulmonalis superior dextra*, 3.15, [*3.18, 3.43a*]

Superior ramus of pubis, *ramus superior oss. pubis*, 2.3, 2.40, 4.3, [*2.2, 2.45, 4.2b*]

Superior rectal A., *a. rectalis superior*, 4.59, 4.83, 4.97, 4.99, [*4.54, 4.77, 4.88*]

Superior rectal V., *v. rectalis superior*, 4.97, 4.99, [*4.68*]

Superior rectus M., *m. rectus superior*, **5.103**, 5.107, [*5.101–3*]

Superior root of ansa cervicalis, *radix superior ansae cervicalis*, 5.19, 5.63, [*5.20, 5.65*]

Superior sagittal sinus, *sinus sagittalis superior*, **5.30**, 5.34, [*5.27, 5.108*]

Superior suprarenal A., *a. suprarenalis superior*, 4.71, 4.77, [*4.69*]

Superior surface of cerebellum, *facies superior cerebelli*, [*6.5, 6.15*]

Superior temporal gyrus, *gyrus temporalis superior*, 6.19, [*6.24*]

Superior temporal line, *linea temporalis superior*, 5.38, [*5.34, 5.45*]

Superior temporal sulcus, *sulcus temporalis superior*, 6.19, [*6.24*]

Superior thyroid A., *a. thyroidea superior*, 5.63, [*5.22, 5.42, 5.52, 5.63–4, 5.92*]

Superior thyroid V., *v. thyroidea superior*, 5.63, 5.93

Superior transverse scapular ligament, *lig. transversum scapulae superius*, 1.23, [*1.24, 1.42, 1.44*]

Superior trunk of brachial plexus, *truncus superior plexus brachialis*, 1.15, [*1.15*]

Superior ulnar collateral A., *a. collateralis ulnaris superior*, 1.33

Superior vena cava, *v. cava superior*, **3.18**, 3.26, 3.31, [*3.18, 3.21, 3.28–9, 3.33*]

Superior vesical As, *aa. vesicales superiores*, 4.86, 4.89, [*4.77–8, 4.81*]

Superior wall of orbit, *paries superior orbitae*, 5.97

Supero-lateral surface of cerebrum, *facies superolateralis cerebri*, 6.18, [*6.24*]

Supinator crest, *crista m. supinatoris*, 1.47

Supinator M., *m. supinator*, **1.47**, 1.62, [*1.41, 1.53, 1.57, 1.78*]

Supraclavicular Ns, *nn. supraclaviculares*, **1.11**, 5.13, [*5.12*]

Supraglenoid tubercle, *tuberculum supraglenoidale*, [*1.2c*]

Suprahyoid Ms, *mm. suprahyoidei*, 5.21, [*5.22*]

Suprameatal triangle, *foveola suprameatica*, 5.135

Supraorbital foramen *or* notch, *foramen sive incisura supraorbitalis*, 5.97, [*5.95*]

Supraorbital margin, *margo supraorbitalis*, 5.97

Supraorbital N., *n. supraorbitalis*, 5.100, 5.101, [*5.98, 5.100*]

Suprapatellar bursa, *bursa suprapatellaris*, 2.69, [*2.81a*]

Suprarenal gland, *glandula suprarenalis (adrenalis)*, 4.77, [*4.59–60, 4.65, 4.69*]

Suprarenal impression of liver, *impressio suprarenalis hepatis*, 4.55

Suprarenal plexus, *plexus suprarenalis*, 4.75

Suprarenal V.,
  left, *v. suprarenalis sinistra*, 4.77, [*4.67, 4.69*]
  right, *v. suprarenalis dextra*, 4.74, 4.77, [*4.67*]

Suprascapular A., *a. suprascapularis*, 1.23, **5.14**, 5.92, [*1.24, 5.13, 5.91*]

Suprascapular N., *n. suprascapularis*, 1.23, 1.31, [*1.24, 1.44*]

Supraspinatus M., *m. supraspinatus*, 1.30, [*1.24, 1.36, 1.43–4, 1.46*]

Supraspinous fossa, *fossa supraspinata*, 1.3, 1.30, [*1.2a*]

Supraspinous ligament, *lig. supraspinale*, 1.7, **5.125**, [*5.125*]

Supratrochlear N., *n. supratrochlearis*, 5.101, [*5.98, 5.100*]

Supravaginal portion of cervix of uterus, *portio supravaginalis cervicis uteri*, 4.95

Sura, calf, 2.57, 2.59, [*2.67–8*]

Sural N., *n. suralis*, 2.34, 2.49, 2.57, [*2.56b and c, 2.59, 2.62*]

Surface, *facies*, 0.10

Surgical neck of humerus, *collum chirurgicum humeri*, 1.4, [*1.4b*]